Apply and review t̲ ̲ ̲ ̲ ̲nt you've covered in ̲ ̲ ̲ ̲ ̲

D0116135

The workbook for **Radiographic Image Analysis, 3rd Edition** helps you get more from your text with extra practice and images to further develop your imaging and evaluation skills. This workbook enables you to:

- **Review evaluation criteria** by studying additional images not provided in the textbook.

- **Practice and apply material covered in the text** with study questions, in-depth image analyses, and additional practice images.

- **Explore study questions on positioning** to ensure you know how to capture the best image every time.

- **See a list of necessary features** so you know what needs to consistently appear in your radiographic images.

- **Analyze what makes images unacceptable** and be confident that your images are always useful and relevant.

Use your workbook to see better results!

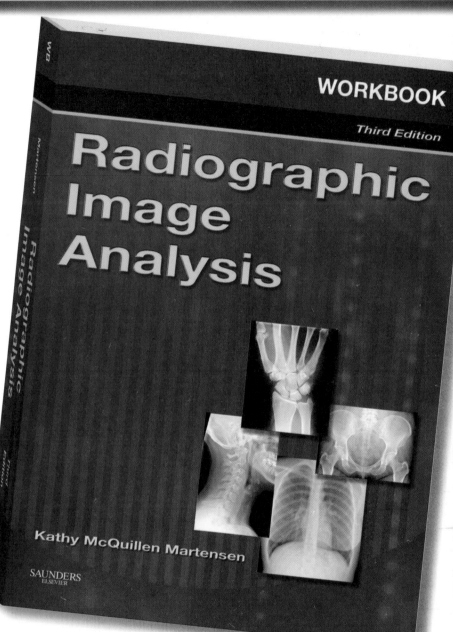

WORKBOOK

Third Edition

Radiographic Image Analysis

Kathy McQuillen Martensen

SAUNDERS
ELSEVIER

ISBN: 978-1-4377-0337-5

Get the resources you need now!

- **Visit your local bookstore**
- **Order online at www.elsevierhealth.com**
- **Call toll-free 1-800-545-2522**

SL100020 TR/KB

Radiographic Image Analysis

Third Edition

Kathy McQuillen Martensen, MA, RT(R)
Director, Radiologic Technology Education
University of Iowa Hospitals and Clinics
Iowa City, Iowa

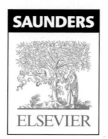

SAUNDERS

ELSEVIER

SAUNDERS
ELSEVIER

3251 Riverport Lane
St. Louis, Missouri 63043

RADIOGRAPHIC IMAGE ANALYSIS, THIRD EDITION   ISBN: 978-1-4377-0336-8
Copyright © 2011, 2006, 1996 by Saunders, an imprint of Elsevier Inc. All rights reserved.

No part of this publication may be reproduced or transmitted in any form or by any means, electronic or mechanical, including photocopying, recording, or any information storage and retrieval system, without permission in writing from the publisher. Details on how to seek permission, further information about the Publisher's permissions policies and our arrangements with organizations such as the Copyright Clearance Center and the Copyright Licensing Agency can be found at our website: www.elsevier.com/permissions.

This book and the individual contributions contained in it are protected under copyright by the Publisher (other than as may be noted herein).

Notice

Knowledge and best practice in this field are constantly changing. As new research and experience broaden our understanding, changes in research methods, professional practices, or medical treatment may become necessary.

Practitioners and researchers must always rely on their own experience and knowledge in evaluating and using any information, methods, compounds, or experiments described herein. In using such information or methods they should be mindful of their own safety and the safety of others, including parties for whom they have a professional responsibility.

With respect to any drug or pharmaceutical products identified, readers are advised to check the most current information provided (i) on procedures featured or (ii) by the manufacturer of each product to be administered, to verify the recommended dose or formula, the method and duration of administration, and contraindications. It is the responsibility of practitioners, relying on their own experience and knowledge of their patients, to make diagnoses, to determine dosages and the best treatment for each individual patient, and to take all appropriate safety precautions.

To the fullest extent of the law, neither the Publisher nor the authors, contributors, or editors, assume any liability for any injury and/or damage to persons or property as a matter of products liability, negligence or otherwise, or from any use or operation of any methods, products, instructions, or ideas contained in the material herein.

Library of Congress Cataloging-in-Publication Data
McQuillen-Martensen, Kathy.
    Radiographic image analysis / Kathy McQuillen Martensen. — 3rd ed.
        p. ; cm.
    Includes bibliographical references and index.
    ISBN 978-1-4377-0336-8 (hardcover : alk. paper) 1. Radiography, Medical. I. Title.
    [DNLM: 1. Technology, Radiologic. 2. Radiography—methods.   WN 160 M479r 2011]
    RC78.M3265 2011
    616.07′572—dc22
                                                                              2009046752

Vice President and Publisher: Andrew Allen
Publisher: Jeanne Olson
Associate Developmental Editor: Luke Held
Publishing Services Manager: Patricia Tannian
Project Manager: Claire Kramer
Designer: Paula Catalano

Working together to grow
libraries in developing countries

www.elsevier.com | www.bookaid.org | www.sabre.org

ELSEVIER   BOOK AID International   Sabre Foundation

Printed in the United States of America

9 8 7 6 5 4 3 2 1

To my husband, Van,
and to our family,
Nicole, Zachary, Adam, Phil, and Haley

Dennis Bowman, RT(R)
Clinical Instructor/Staff Radiographer
Community Hospital of the Monterey
    Peninsula
Monterey, California

**Donna J. Crum, MS, RT(R)(CT),
    ARRT**
Associate Professor and Program
    Director—Radiography
St. Catharine College
Catharine, Kentucky

Kendall DeLacerda, MSRS, RT(R)
Assistant Professor
Northwestern State University
Shreveport, Louisiana

**Merryl N. Fulmer, BS, RT(R)(M)
    (MR)(QM)(CT)**
Clinical Trials Trainer, Diagnostic
    Imaging Specialist
American College of Radiology
Philadelphia, Pennsylvania

Stephanie A. Harris, BS, RT(R)(M)(CT)
Imaging Educator
University of Iowa Hospitals
    and Clinics
Iowa City, Iowa

Angela Lambert, ARRT, AFAA
Assistant Professor
Bluefield State College
Bluefield, West Virginia

Staci Marie Maier, BS, RT(R)
Radiology Program
Holy Cross Hospital School of
    Radiologic Technology
Silver Spring, Maryland

Starla L. Mason, MS, RT(R)(QM)
Program Director
Radiography Department
Laramie County Community College
Cheyenne, Wyoming

Robert E. McClung, MS, RT(R)
Term Assistant Professor
University of Alaska Anchorage
Anchorage, Alaska

Kristi G. Moore, MS, RT(R)(CT)
Program Instructor
University of Mississippi Medical Center
    School of Health Related Professions
    Radiologic Sciences Program
Jackson, Mississippi

Marcia Moore, BS, RT(R)(CT)
Instructor
St. Luke's College
Sioux City, Iowa

Debra J. Poelhuis, MS, RT(R)(M)
Radiography Program Director
Montgomery County Community
    College
Pottstown, Pennsylvania

Kenneth A. Roszel, MS, RT(R)
Program Director
Geisinger Medical Center
Danville, Pennsylvania

Jayme S. Rothberg, MS, RT(R)(M)
Associate Professor
Radiography Program Coordinator
Pasco-Hernando Community College
New Port Richey, Florida

**Erica Koch Wight, MEd, RT(R)(M)
    (QM)**
Program Director, Medical Imaging
    Sciences
University of Alaska
Anchorage, Alaska

Paula B. Young, BS, RT(R)(M)
Clinical Coordinator, Radiologic
    Technology Program
University of Mississippi Medical
    Center
Jackson, Mississippi

After 10 years of experience as a radiologic technologist, I accepted a position as an educator and was given the task to instruct the radiographic procedures course. My first thoughts were that instructing a procedures course would not be too difficult because I had been producing radiographic images for over 10 years. Once into the course, though, I realized that there was uncertainty about what constituted the "correct way" to position for the different procedures, and that added a level of confusion I had not anticipated. There were three imaging procedure textbooks in the library that showed small variations in how the procedures should be performed. About 60 technologists in the Radiology Department, where the students completed their clinical experience, also had their own slight variations. Then there were my own "tricks of the trade." The most common question from the students at the time was, "Which way is the correct way?" as they were preparing for a test or wondering why a technologist had changed their positioning to something different from what they had been taught. This uncertainty as to how to answer this question lead me on a path of discovery, taking me to radiology textbooks, the cadaver lab, and the film archives as I researched the material that eventually became the information that you will find in this textbook. As I researched each procedure, I found that the focus of my procedures course was changing from discussions about how to position the patient to discussions about how each positioning step correlates with the resulting image and how the anatomic relationships on that image should appear for optimal diagnosis. This deeper understanding empowers the students because they now are able to visualize the anatomic relationship differences that occur on the image if positioning steps are accomplished differently. They are also better able to problem-solve when imaging the nonroutine patient.

This textbook has been designed to provide educators, students, and radiographers with the information needed to analyze radiographic images for exposure and positioning accuracy, to adjust the technical equipment or mispositioning to produce an optimal image when a less than optimal one has been obtained, to prepare for the certification examination by the ARRT, and to develop a high degree of problem-solving ability. This textbook also serves as a practical image analysis reference for working technologists.

Although new information is included in the third edition, the content and organization of the textbook have not been significantly changed. Chapters 1 and 2 lay the foundations for evaluating all images, outlining the technical and screen-film and digital imaging concepts that are to be considered when studying the procedures that are presented in the subsequent chapters. Chapters 3 through 12 detail the analysis criteria for the most commonly performed radiographic procedures. For each procedure, this textbook provides an accurately positioned image with labeled anatomy, many examples of poorly positioned images, photographs of models demonstrating accurate and inaccurate patient positioning, and an image analysis criteria list. For each criterion listed, a discussion is provided that correlates the analysis criteria with the corresponding patient or central ray set-up procedure that defines how the resulting image will appear if the correct patient or central ray set-up procedure is followed and explains radiographic principles as they relate to the criterion. Following this are a discussion and supporting poorly positioned images that focus on how the image will look if the patient is positioned incorrectly. The images for each procedure that demonstrate poor patient and central ray positioning are grouped together, and next to each of these images is a synopsis discussing the mispositioning and how the patient or central ray should be repositioned to obtain an optimal image. Grouping the poorly positioned images together at the end of each procedure instead of next to the referring text is irregular and requires the first-time reader to flip a couple of pages to see the image, but I have used this arrangement to help the student and the practicing technologist see all the images together so that they can be used easily as a reference and to compare subtle differences.

I designed the textbook to guide the reader in a systematic order through the body structures. After the first two chapters have been studied, it is not necessary to follow the textbook as it is written. One can freely skip from chapter to chapter or procedure to procedure and fully comprehend the material.

NEW TO THIS EDITION

The third edition has grown by including descriptions of digital imaging and through elaboration of some previous content to accommodate an improved understanding. In the third edition the reader will notice the following:

- Chapter 1 has been expanded to include additional technical and exposure-related criteria. Subsequent chapters reference the concepts addressed in Chapter 1 and no longer repeat the information. A section on imaging the obese patient has been added, and the nonroutine/trauma and pediatric imaging guidelines have been expanded.

- Chapter 2 is a new chapter. This chapter defines the guidelines to follow when producing and evaluting images obtained with a digital imaging system.
- A quick reference image analysis criteria table has been added for each procedure presented to streamline the analysis. Tables that contain condensed versions of frequently mentioned information have also been added for quick reference.
- Chapter objectives and a key word list have been added at the start of each chapter, and a glossary has been added at the end of the textbook.
- Images with improved detail resolution and updated positioning and skeletal bone photographs have been replaced or added as needed to better clarify concepts.
- An increased number of nonroutine/trauma and pediatric images have been included throughout the textbook.

ANCILLARIES

Ancillary materials are provided online on Elsevier's Evolve website. Evolve is an interactive learning environment designed to work in coordination with *Radiographic Image Analysis*. Instructors may use Evolve to provide an Internet-based course component that reinforces and expands on the concepts delivered in class. Evolve may be used to publish the class syllabus, outlines, and lecture notes; set up "virtual office hours" and e-mail communication; share important dates and information through the online class calendar; and encourage student participation through chat rooms and discussion boards. Evolve allows instructors to post examinations and manage their grade books online. For more information, visit http://evolve.elsevier.com/Martensen/imageanalysis/ or contact an Elsevier sales representative.

Instructor Resources

Instructor resources accompany the textbook and are available on Evolve. The resources include:

- Instructor's Manual, which includes chapter outlines, learning activities, and laboratory activities
- Test Bank, which includes over 600 questions in the ExamView format.
- Textbook Electronic Image Collection, which includes all the images from the textbook.

- Workbook Electronic Image Collection, which includes all the images from the workbook.
- Instructor Electronic Image Collection, which includes 330 images that are not included in the textbook or workbook and that can be used for testing purposes.

Student Resources

The *Workbook for Radiographic Image Analysis*, third edition, is available for separate purchase and provides the learner with ample opportunities to practice and apply the information presented in the textbook. The workbook includes images beyond those in the textbook for analysis, so the student can further hone imaging and evaluation skills. Students also have access to the Evolve website, including a set of links to relevant imaging websites.

ACKNOWLEDGMENTS

I am pleased to acknowledge and recognize my friend and colleague Stephanie Harris, BS, RT(R)(CT)(M), for the help she provided in locating needed images, reviewing the textbook, and providing support in areas too numerous to list. Stephanie is a dedicated educator with whom I am honored to work.

I would also like to thank the following individuals who have helped with this edition.

My newest model, Sawyer Kirby, who will be too small to remember that he did not like having his photograph taken.

The University of Iowa Hospitals and Clinics' Radiologic Technology Classes of 1988 to 2009, who have been my best teachers because they have challenged me with their questions and insights.

Luke Held, Jeanne Olson, and the entire Elsevier Saunders team for their support, assistance, and expertise in planning and developing this project.

The professional colleagues, book reviewers, educators, and technologists who have evaluated the book, sent me compliments and suggestions, and questioned concepts in the first and second editions. Please continue to do so.

—Kathy

CONTENTS

Image Analysis Guidelines

OBJECTIVES

After completion of this chapter, you should be able to:

- State the characteristics of an optimal projection.
- Properly display projections of all body structures.
- State the demographic requirements for projections and explain why this information is needed.
- Discuss how to mark projections accurately and explain the procedure to be followed if a projection has been mismarked or the marker is only faintly seen.
- Discuss why good collimation practices are necessary, and list the guidelines to follow to ensure good collimation.
- Describe how positioning of anatomic structures in reference to the x-ray beam and image receptor affects how they are visualized on the image.
- State how similarly appearing structures can be identified on images.
- Determine the amount of patient or central ray adjustment required when poorly positioned projection are obtained.
- Explain the procedural factors that affect the recorded detail sharpness of an image and how they are identified on the resulting image.

- Describe the radiation protection practices that are followed to limit patient dose and discuss how to identify whether adequate shielding was used.
- Discuss the factors that affect radiographic density and contrast and state how they should be adjusted, and to what degree, when an image is produced that demonstrates poor density or contrast.
- List and describe the different artifact categories and discuss how they can be prevented.
- State the procedures to follow after an examination has been completed.
- Discuss the difference between an optimal and acceptable projection.
- List the guidelines for obtaining mobile and trauma projections and state how technical factors should be adjusted to adapt for different mobile and trauma-related conditions.
- Describe the differences to consider when performing procedures and evaluating images of pediatric and obese patients.

KEY TERMS

additive disease
air-gap technique
ALARA
anode heel effect
anterior
artifact
automatic exposure control
backup timer
body habitus
caudal
cephalic
compensating filter
contrast
decubitus
density
destructive disease

differential absorption
distal
distortion
dose equivalent limits
elongation
entrance skin exposure (ESE)
flexion
foreshortening
grid
grid cutoff
image receptor
inferior
inverse square law
involuntary motion
ionization chamber
lateral

law of isometry
medial
midcoronal plane
midsaggital plane
minimum response time
nonstochastic effects
object–image receptor distance (OID)
optimum kilovoltage peak (kVp)
posterior
profile
project
proximal
radiolucent
radiopaque
recorded detail
resolution

scatter radiation
source–image receptor distance (SID)
source-object distance (SOD)

source-skin distance (SSD)
square law
stochastic effects

subject contrast
superior
voluntary motion

WHY IMAGE ANALYSIS?

Radiographic images are such that slight differences in quality do not necessarily rule out the diagnostic value of the image. Radiologists can ordinarily make satisfactory adjustment by reason of their experience and knowledge, although passing less than optimal images may compromise the diagnosis and treatment and result in additional imaging at a higher expense and radiation dose to the patient. Historically, the purpose of image analysis has been to teach technologists how to evaluate an image for passability. The problem with this approach is that it fails to consider the large impact of small variations in positioning and technical factors on what can be demonstrated on an image.

Why should a technologist care about creating optimal images and studying all the small, seemingly insignificant aspects of image analysis? The most important answer to this question lies in why most technologists join the profession—to help people. From the patient's point of view, it provides the reviewer with images that contain optimal diagnostic value, prevents the anxiety that occurs when additional images or studies need to be performed, and prevents the radiation dosage that might be caused by additional imaging. From a societal point of view, it helps prevent additional increases in health care costs that could result because of the need for additional, more expensive imaging procedures and because of the malpractice cases that might result from a poor or missed diagnosis. From a technologist's point of view, it would be the preventable financial burden and stress that arise from legal actions, a means of protecting professional interest as more diagnostic procedures are being replaced with other modalities, and the personal satisfaction gained when our patients, employer, and ourselves benefit from and are recognized for our expertise.

Consider how accuracy in positioning and technical factors affect the diagnostic value of the image. It is estimated that in the United States, 68 million chest imaging procedures are performed each year to evaluate the lungs, heart, and thoracic viscera as well as disease processes such as pneumonia, heart failure, pleurisy, and lung cancer.[2] The reviewer must consider all the normal variations that exist in areas such as the mediastinum, hila, diaphragm, and lungs. Should they also have to consider how the appearance of these structures are different with preventable positioning and technical errors? It takes only 2 or 3 degrees of rotation to affect the appearance of the lungs, causing differences in density along the lateral borders of the chest image (Figure 1-1). Similarly, certain conditions such as mediastinal widening or cardiac size

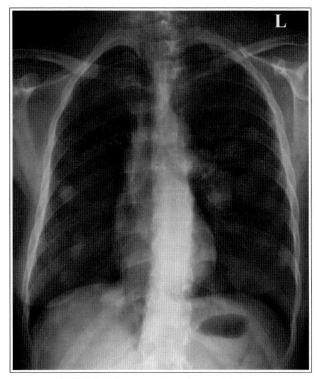

FIGURE 1-1 Rotated PA chest projection.

cannot be evaluated properly on a rotated posteroanterior (PA) chest projection. The normal heart shadow on such an image will occupy slightly less than 50% of the transverse dimension of the thorax (Figure 1-2). This is evaluated by measuring the largest transverse diameter of the heart on the PA or AP projection and relating that to the largest transverse measurement of the internal dimension of the chest. When the PA chest projection is rotated, bringing a different heart plane into profile, this diagnosis becomes compromised.

According to an article written by Elizabeth Church[3] in the *Radiologic Technology* Journal, a 1999 report from the Institute of Medicine, up to 98,000 Americans die each year from medical errors and remedial care for adverse medical events costs as much as $30 billion annually in the United States.[1] The radiology field employs the professionals who are sued most frequently, not because they have the deepest pockets or are the least competent, but because radiologists and radiologic technologists have contact with the vast majority of patients for imaging services. Radiologic technologists are the second in line in regard to imaging responsibilities and competency and should be aware that they may also be named in lawsuits. The article states that radiology-related malpractice cases fall into the

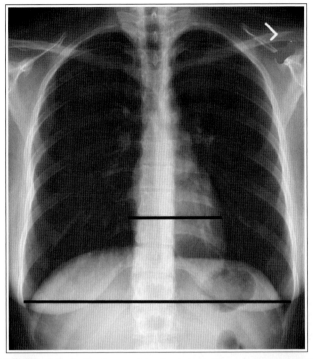

FIGURE 1-2 Evaluating a PA chest projection for mediastinal widening.

following categories: 42%, radiographic misdiagnosis; 22%, failure to order imaging studies; 16%, radiographic procedure complications; 8%, radiation oncology complications; and 5% of patients injured during transportation. Historically, there has been a tendency to place legal responsibility on the highest authority possible and, in the case of a radiographer, actions would typically result in lawsuits against his or her employer or against the physician with whom he or she works. In recent years, however, the rule of personal responsibility has been increasingly applied. This means that everyone is liable for their own negligent conduct. Although radiographers are seldom named specifically in malpractice lawsuits, the rule of personal responsibility has resulted in some unfavorable judgments against radiographers as individuals.

When such judgments are brought forward, the claimant must prove to the court's satisfaction that four conditions are met:

1. The person being sued had a duty to provide reasonable care to the patient.
2. The patient sustained some loss or injury.
3. The person being sued is the responsible party for the loss.
4. The loss is attributable to negligence or improper practice.

The American Society of Radiologic Technologists (ASRT) has developed a code of ethics for the radiography profession and the Canadian Association of Medical Radiation Technologists (CAMRT) has adopted a similar

code of ethics. These codes define the ethical responsibilities and the appropriate conduct toward others to which the imaging professional should adhere. It is these codes that are used by lawyers in medical malpractice and negligence claims to determine the accepted level of care and to show whether the professional conducted himself or herself in an ethical manner. To avoid a malpractice suit, professionals must remain vigilant. There is a natural human tendency to let down one's guard or ignore red flags when there have been no recent mistakes. It was also suggested that professionals carefully observe the system that they use and consider their responsibilities carefully, taking a leadership role.[3]

The number of computed tomography (CT) examinations has increased about 600% from the mid-1980s to the mid-1990s and has continued to rapidly grow each year since then. Whereas CT represents only about 5% of all x-ray imaging procedures, it is responsible for 40% to 67% of all medical radiation. Although this increase may be justified considering the diagnostic information that can be gained through such procedures, the effect of the quality of diagnostic images on the increased use of alternative imaging modalities must be considered. A 2008 article in the *American Journal of Roentgenology* written by R.D. Welling and colleagues[5] summarizes a study in which the researchers defined the number and type of wrist fractures diagnosed using diagnostic radiography compared with the use of multidetector computed tomography (MDCT). They examined the records of 60 patients who underwent radiographic and MDCT examinations of the wrist. Two musculoskeletal radiologists and one emergency radiologist reviewed the MDCT results and categorized each of the bones in the wrist as normal or fractured. The study revealed that radiography missed 30% of wrist fractures visible on MDCT. Of the patients demonstrating wrist bone fractures in the distal carpal row, only 33% of the trapezium, 0% of the trapezoidal and capitate, and 60% of the hamate fractures were diagnosed on radiographs. Small variations in wrist positioning can have a large effect on how well the carpal bones are visualized.

If instead of being evaluated for passability, images are evaluated for optimalism, could more consistent and improved diagnoses be made from diagnostic images? For example, Figures 1-3 and 1-4 demonstrate three lateral and PA wrist projections, all of which were determined to be passable and sent to the radiologist for review. Note how the trapezium is visualized only on the first lateral wrist projection but is not demonstrated on the other two, and observe how the carpometacarpal (CMC) joints and distal carpal bones are well visualized on the first PA wrist projection but are not seen on the other two images. The first lateral wrist projection was obtained with the patient's thumb depressed until the first metacarpal was aligned with the second metacarpal (MC), whereas the other lateral wrist projections were

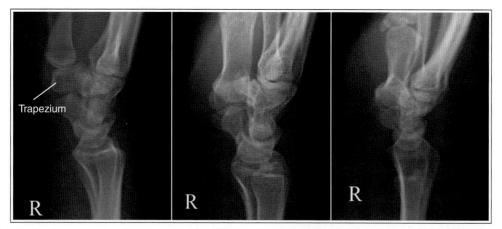

FIGURE 1-3 Lateral wrist projections demonstrating the difference in trapezium visualization with thumb depression and elevation.

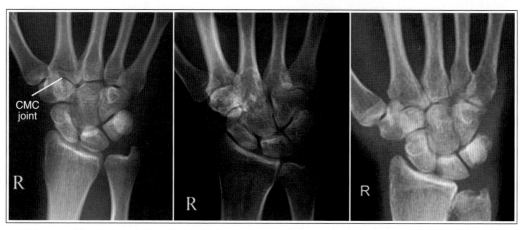

FIGURE 1-4 PA wrist projections demonstrating the difference in carpometacarpal (CMC) joint visualization with variations in metacarpal alignment with the image receptor.

obtained with the first metacarpal elevated. The first PA wrist image was obtained with the metacarpals aligned at a 10- to 15-degree angle with the image receptor (IR), the second PA wrist image was taken with the metacarpals aligned at an angle greater than 15 degrees, and the third image was taken with the metacarpals aligned at an angle less than 10 degrees. If the radiologist cannot arrive at a conclusive diagnosis from the images that the technologist provides, he or she must recommend other imaging procedures or follow-up images.

TERMINOLOGY

Many terms are used in radiography to describe the path of the x-ray beam, the patient's position, the precise location of an anatomic structure, the position of one anatomic structure in relation to another, and the way a certain structure will change its position as the patient moves in a predetermined direction. Familiarity with radiography terminology will help you understand statements made throughout this text and to converse competently with other medical professionals. At the beginning of each chapter, there is a list of key terms that should be reviewed prior to reading the chapter. The glossary at the end of the textbook provides definitions of these terms.

CHARACTERISTICS OF THE OPTIMAL IMAGE

The skills needed to obtain optimal images of all body structures are taught in radiographic procedures, image analysis, and radiographic exposure (imaging) courses.

An optimal image of each projection demonstrates all the most desired features, which should include the following:

- Demographic information (e.g., patient and facility name, time, date)
- Correct markers in the appropriate position without superimposing anatomy of interest
- Desired anatomic structures in accurate alignment with each other
- Maximum geometric integrity
- Appropriate radiation protection
- Best possible density, contrast, and gray scale, with minimal noise
- No preventable artifacts

Unfortunately, because of a patient's condition, equipment malfunction, or technologist error, such perfection is not obtained for every image that is produced. A less than optimal image should be thoroughly evaluated to determine the reason for error so that the problem can be corrected before the examination is repeated. An image that is not optimal but is still passable according to a facility's standards should be carefully studied to determine whether skills can be improved before the next similar examination; continuous improvement is sought. An image should never have to be taken a third time because the error was not accurately identified and the proper adjustment made from the first image.

This book cannot begin to identify the standards of acceptability in all the different imaging facilities. What might be an acceptable standard in one facility may not be acceptable in another. As you study the images in this book, you may find that many of them are acceptable in your facility, even though they do not meet optimal standards. The goal of this text is not to dictate to your facility what should be acceptable and unacceptable images. It is to help you focus on improving your image analysis, positioning, and exposure skills and to provide guidelines on how the image may be improved when a less than optimal image results.

DISPLAYING IMAGES

Before an image is evaluated for accuracy, it is displayed on a digital display monitor or made available in the form of a hard-copy radiograph and displayed on a view box. Box 1-1 lists the guidelines to follow when displaying images.

IMAGE ANALYSIS FORM

Once an image is correctly displayed, it should be evaluated for positioning and technical accuracy. This should follow a systematic approach so that all aspects of the analytic process are considered, reducing the chance of missing important details and providing a structured pattern for the evaluator to use in a stressful situation. The image analysis form shown in Figure 1-9 is designed to be used when evaluating images to ensure that all aspects of the image are evaluated. Under each item in the image analysis form, there is a list of questions to explore while evaluating an image. The following discussions explore each of these question areas in depth. The answers to all the questions, taken together, will determine whether the image is optimal, acceptable, or needs repeating. The discussions presented in this chapter will focus primarily on

---

BOX 1-1	Image Displaying Guidelines

- Display torso, vertebral, cranial, shoulder, and hip images as if the patient were standing in an upright position.
- **AP, PA, and AP-PA oblique projections** of the torso, vertebrae, and cranium should be displayed as if the viewer and the patient are facing one another. The right side of the patient's image is on the viewer's left, and the left side of the patient's image is on the viewer's right. Whenever AP or AP oblique projections are taken, the R (right) or L (left) marker appears correct when the image is accurately displayed, as long as the marker was placed on the IR face-up before the image was taken (Figure 1-5). When PA or PA oblique projections are taken, the R or L marker appears reversed if placed face-up when the image is accurately displayed (Figure 1-6).
- The marker placed on **lateral projections** of the torso, vertebrae, and cranium represents the side of the patient positioned closer to the IR. If the patient is positioned with the left side against the imaging table for a lateral lumbar vertebrae projection, a left marker should be placed on the IR (Figure 1-7). In general, accurately displayed lateral projections demonstrate a correct marker as long as the marker was placed on the IR face-up before the image was taken. One exception to this guideline may be when left lateral chest projections are displayed; often, reviewers prefer the left lateral

projection to be displayed as if taken in the right lateral projection.
- **AP/PA (lateral decubitus) chest and abdominal projections** are generally displayed so that the side of the patient that was positioned upward when the image was taken is upward on the displayed image.
- **Inferosuperior (axial) shoulder and axiolateral hip projections** are displayed so the patient's anterior surface is up and posterior surface is down.
- **Extremity projections** are displayed as if the viewer's eyes were going through the image in the same manner the central ray went through the extremity when the image was taken. For example, a right PA hand projection is displayed with the thumb positioned toward the viewer's left side and a right lateral hand projection is displayed so the palmar side of the hand is positioned toward the viewer's left side (Figure 1-8).
- Display finger, wrist, and forearm images as if the patient were hanging from his or her fingertips.
- Display elbow and humerus images as if they were hanging from the patient's shoulder.
- Display toe and AP and AP oblique foot projections as if the patient were hanging from his or her toes.
- Display lateral foot, ankle, lower leg, knee, and femur projections as if they were hanging from the patient's hip.

AP, Anteroposterior; *IR*, image receptor; *L*, left; *PA*, posteroanterior; *R*, right.

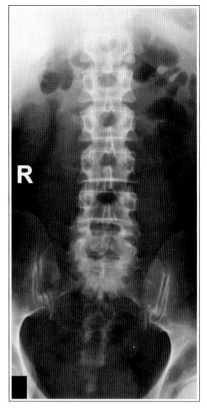

FIGURE 1-5 Accurately displayed and marked AP lumbar vertebrae projection.

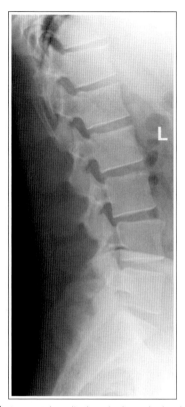

FIGURE 1-7 Accurately displayed lateral lumbar vertebrae projection.

screen-film imaging systems, and those unique to digital radiography will be presented in Chapter 2.

Demographic Requirements

Patient and Facility Identification. The correct patient's name and age or birth date, and the facility's name, should be permanently photoflashed onto the identification (ID)

plate or displayed on the digital display monitor. This information should be typed and legible. Evaluate all the images within a routine series to ensure that these have been correctly imprinted or displayed on the image. Never assume that an image has been correctly photoflashed or assigned to the correct patient. Always double-check. Flash cards can be easily switched or forgotten.

If the wrong information has been photoflashed onto the ID plate when using a screen-film system, a corrected information sticker should be placed over the

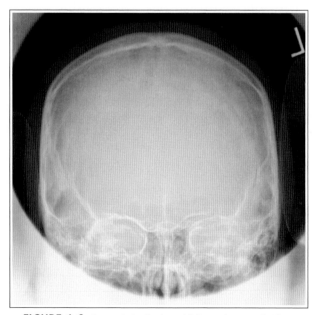

FIGURE 1-6 Accurately displayed PA cranium projection.

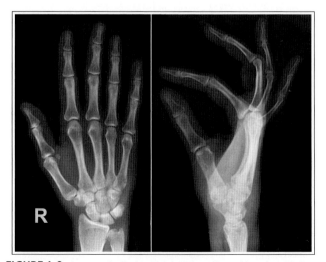

FIGURE 1-8 Accurately displayed right PA and lateral hand projections.

IMAGE ANALYSIS FORM

_____ Demographic requirements are visualized on the image.
- Are the patient's name and age or birth date visible and is it accurate?
- Is the facility's name visible?
- Are the examination time and date visible and accurate?
- Is the ID plate positioned so it does not obscure anatomy of interest?

_____ Correct marker (e.g., R/L, arrow) is visualized on image and demonstrates accurate placement.
- Is the marker visualized within the collimated field and is it positioned as far away from the center as possible?
- Have specialty markers been added and correctly placed if applicable?
- Is the marker clearly seen without distortion and is it positioned so it does not superimpose anatomy of interest?
- Does the R or L marker correspond to the correct side of the patient?
- If more than one image is on IR, have both images been marked if they are different sides of the patient?

_____ Required anatomy is present and correctly placed in image.
- Are all of the required anatomical structures visible on the image?
- Was the IR positioned CW or LW correctly to accommodate required anatomy and/or patient's body habitus?
- Was the smallest possible IR used?
- Were as many projections as possible placed on the same IR without collimation field overlap and were the parts all aligned in the same direction?
- Is a collimated border present on all four sides of the image when applicable?
- Is collimation within ½ inch (1.25 cm) of the patient's skinline on all extremity, chest, and abdominal images?
- Is collimation to the specific anatomy desired on images involving structures within the torso?

_____ Relationships between the anatomical structures are accurate for the projection demonstrated.
- Are the anatomical structures accurately displayed on the image for the projection demonstrated, as indicated in the procedural analysis sections of book or defined by your imaging facility?
- Are the anatomical structures of interest in the center of the image?
- Does the image demonstrate the least possible amount of size distortion?
- Does the image demonstrate undesirable shape distortion?
- Are the joints of interest open or fracture lines well demonstrated?
- If the image is less than optimum, how should the patient's positioning or the central ray alignment be adjusted and by how much before the image is repeated or another similar projection is obtained?

_____ Image demonstrates maximum recorded detail sharpness.
- Was a small focal spot used when indicated?
- Was the appropriate SID used?
- Was the part positioned as close to the IR as possible?
- Was the correct screen-film IR system used for the body part being imaged?
- Does evidence suggest poor screen-film contact?
- Does the image demonstrate signs of undesirable patient motion or unhalted respiration?
- Are there signs of a double-exposure?
- CR: Was the smallest possible IR used?

_____ Radiation protection is present on image when indicated, and good radiation protection practices were used during procedure.
- Was the exam explained to the patient and were clear, concise instructions given during the procedure?
- Were immobilization devices used to prevent patient motion when needed?
- Was the minimal source-skin distance of at least 12 inches (30 cm) maintained for mobile radiography?
- Was a compensating filter used when applicable?
- Was a grid used when indicated and was the grid ratio used the lowest possible for the kVp range employed?
- S/F: Was the fastest screen-film IR speed used without compromising recorded detail?
- Was the possibility of pregnancy determined of all females of childbearing age?
- Is gonadal shielding evident and accurately positioned when the gonads are within the primary beam and shielding is therefore indicated?
- Were radiation protection measures used for patients whose radiosensitive cells were positioned within 2 inches (5 cm) of the primary beam?
- Was the field size tightly collimated?
- Were exposure factors (kVp, mA, and time) set to minimize patient exposure?
- If the AEC was used, was the backup time set to prevent overexposure to the patient?
- Are there anatomical artifacts demonstrated on the image?
- Were personnel or family who remained in the room during the exposure given protective attire, positioned as far from the radiation source as possible, and present only when absolutely necessary and for the shortest possible time?

FIGURE 1-9 Image analysis form.   *(Continued)*

_____ Radiographic density is adequate to visualize bony and soft tissue structures of interest.
- Is the radiographic density too light or too dark to visualize the soft tissue structures of interest? What adjustment should be made if density is inadequate?
- Does the image have adequate penetration to demonstrate the cortical outlines of the structures of interest? How much adjustment in kVp should be made if penetration is inadequate?
- If the AEC was used, was the mA station set to prevent exposure times less than the minimum response time?
- If the AEC was used, was the backup time set at 150 – 200% of the expected manual exposure time for the exam?
- If the AEC was used, was the activated ionization chamber(s) completely covered by the anatomy?
- If the AEC was used, is there any radiopaque hardware or prosthetic devices positioned in the activated chamber(s)?
- If the AEC was used, is the AEC calibrated for the screen-film IR system that was used?
- If the AEC was used, was the density control on 0?
- Was the correct SID used for the exposure set?
- Was the OID kept to a minimum and if not was the mAs adjusted for the reduction in scatter radiation when applicable?
- Was the appropriate technique used for the grid chosen?
- Are there grid line artifacts demonstrated?
- S/F: Was the appropriate technique used for the screen-film IR system chosen?
- Does the image demonstrate quantum noise?
- If collimation was significantly reduced, was the mAs adjusted for the reduction in scatter radiation when applicable?
- Has a compensating filter been used when indicated and has homogeneous density been realized across the structure?
- If a 17-inch IR was used, was the thinnest end of a long bone or vertebral column positioned at the anode end of the tube?

_____ Radiographic contrast is adequate to demonstrate the subject contrast of structure imaged.
- Is subject contrast sufficient to record each tissue composition on the image and if not, how should the kVp be adjusted?
- Is the scale of contrast appropriate for procedure and if not, how should kVp be adjusted?
- Has image fog been kept to a minimum?
- Was the appropriate grid ratio used?
- Was the exposure field size kept to a minimum?

_____ Image histogram was accurately produced. (Digital Radiography Only)
- CR: Is the exposure indicator within the acceptable parameters?
- Was the correct body part and projection chosen from the workstation menu?
- Was the central ray centered to the VOI?
- Was collimation as close to VOI as possible, leaving minimum background in the exposure field?
- Was scatter controlled with lead sheets, grids, tight collimation, etc.?
- CR: If collimating smaller than the IR, was the VOI in the center of the IP and are all four collimation borders seen?
- Was at least 30% of the IP covered?
- CR: If multiple projections are on one IP, is collimation parallel and equidistant from the edges of the IP and are they separated by at least 1 inch (2.5 cm)?
- CR: Was the IP left in the imaging room while other exposures were made and was the IP read shortly after exposure?
- CR: Was the IP erased if the IR was not used within a few days?

_____ No preventable artifacts are present on the image.
- Are any artifacts visible on the image?
- What is the location of any present artifact with respect to a palpable anatomical structure?
- Does the image have to be repeated because of the artifact?

_____ Ordered procedure and the indication for the exam have been fulfilled.
- Has the routine series for the body structure ordered been completed as determined by your facility?
- Do the images in the routine series fulfill the indication for the examination, or must additional images be taken?

_____ Requisition and other post-procedure requirements have been completed, and the repeat/reject analysis information has been provided as indicated by your facility.

Image is: _____ optimal   _____ acceptable, but not optimal
              _____unacceptable

If image is acceptable, but not optimal or unacceptable, describe what measures should be taken to produce an optimal image.

FIGURE 1-9 cont'd Image analysis form.

incorrect patient information before the images are sent to be interpreted.

Time and Date. The examination time and date must be accurate to distinguish the images in a timed series and to match images with their accompanying requisition and report.

Identification Plate Placement Guidelines. Box 1-2 provides guidelines to help prevent the ID plate from superimposing the anatomy of interest when using screen-film radiography. In digital radiography, the ID plate placement is not as sensitive as it is for a screen-film radiograph because after the image is displayed,

BOX 1-2	Identification (ID) Plate Placement Guidelines

- When the IR is positioned LW, the ID plate is placed in the upper right or lower left corner.
- When the IR is positioned CW, the ID plate is placed in the lower right or upper left corner.
- Place the ID plate outside the collimated field whenever possible.
- Position the ID plate away from the direction in which the central ray is angled.
- Position the ID plate next to the narrowest anatomic structure.

CW, Crosswise; *IR,* image receptor; *LW,* lengthwise.

the blocker location can be moved to a location away from the anatomy of interest.

Marking Images

Lead markers are used to identify the patient's right and left sides, indicate variations in the standard procedure, or show the amount of time that has elapsed in timed procedures, such as small bowel studies. The markers are constructed of lead so as to be radiopaque. Whenever a marker is placed on the image receptor (IR) within the collimated light field, radiation will be unable to penetrate it, resulting in an unexposed white area on the image where the marker was located. Each image must include the correct marker. Mismarking an image can have many serious implications, including treatment of the incorrect anatomic structure. The marker must also be included on the image for it to be considered a legal document in a court of law. After an image has been produced, evaluate it to determine whether the correct marker has been placed properly on the image. Box 1-3 lists guidelines to follow when marking and evaluating marker accuracy on images.

Using the Collimator Guide for Marker Placement. When collimating less than the size of the IR used, it can be difficult to determine exactly where to place the marker on the IR so that it will remain within the collimated field and not obscure anatomic areas of interest. The best way of accomplishing this is first to collimate the desired amount and then use the collimator guide (Figure 1-20) to determine how far from the IR's midline to place the marker. Although different models of x-ray equipment have different collimator

BOX 1-3	Marker Placement Guidelines

- Position marker in the exposure field (area within collimated light field) as far away from the center as possible.
- Avoid placing marker beneath the anatomy of interest or lead shielding, or over the ID plate.
- Place markers on the IR and not on the imaging table or patient. This placement avoids marker distortion and magnification, prevents scatter radiation from undercutting the marker, and ensures that the marker will not be projected off the IR (Figure 1-10).
- For **AP and PA projections** of the torso, vertebrae, and cranium, place the R or L marker laterally on the side being marked. The patient's vertebral column is the dividing plane for the right and left sides. If marking the right side, position the R marker to the right of the vertebral column; if marking the left side, position the L marker to the left of the vertebral column (see Figure 1-5).
- For **lateral projections** of the torso, vertebrae, and cranium, the marker placed on the IR indicates the side of the patient positioned closer to the IR. If the patient's left side is positioned closer to the IR for a lateral lumbar vertebrae projection, place an L marker on the IR (Figure 1-11). Whether the marker is placed anteriorly or posteriorly to the lumbar vertebrae does not affect the accuracy of the image's marking, although the images of markers placed posteriorly are often overexposed (Figure 1-12).
- For **AP/PA (lateral decubitus) projections** of the torso, vertebrae, and cranium, the marker placed on the IR identifies the side of the patient positioned closer to the IR and is placed on the correct side of the patient (Figure 1-13). As with the AP-PA projections, the vertebral column is the plane used to divide the right and left sides of the body.
- For **decubitus projections** of the torso, place the R or L marker laterally on the correct side. If marking the right side, position

the R marker to the right of the vertebral column; if marking the left side, position the L marker to the left of the vertebral column. The marker will be better visualized and less likely to obscure the anatomy of interest if the side of the patient that is positioned up, away from the cart or imaging table on which the patient is lying, is the side marked. Along with the right or left marker, use an arrow marker pointing up toward the ceiling or lead lettering to indicate which side of the patient is positioned away from the cart or imaging table (Figure 1-14).

- For **extremity projections**, mark the side of the patient being imaged. When multiple projections are placed on the same IR, it is necessary to mark only one of the projections placed on the IR as long as they are all images of the same anatomic structure (Figure 1-15). If positions of a right anatomic structure and its corresponding left are placed on the same IR, mark both images with the correct R or L marker (Figure 1-16).
- For **AP and AP oblique shoulder and hip projections**, the marker placed on the IR should indicate the side of the patient being imaged (Figure 1-17). It is best to place the marker laterally to prevent it from obscuring medial anatomic structures and to eliminate possible confusion about which side of the patient is being imaged. Figure 1-18 demonstrates an AP hip projection with the marker placed medially. Because the marker is placed at the patient's midsagittal plane, the reviewer might conclude that the technologist was marking the right hip.
- For **cross-table lateral projections**, position the marker anteriorly to prevent it from obscuring structures situated along the posterior edge of the IR. The marker used should indicate the right or left side of the patient when the extremities, shoulder, or hip is imaged (Figure 1-19) and the side of the patient positioned closer to the IR when the torso, vertebrae, or cranium is imaged (see Figure 1-11).

AP, Anteroposterior; *IR,* image receptor; *L,* left; *PA,* posteroanterior; *R,* right.

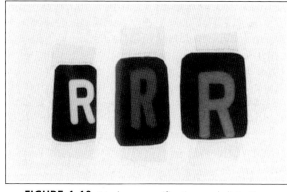

FIGURE 1-10 Marker magnification and distortion.

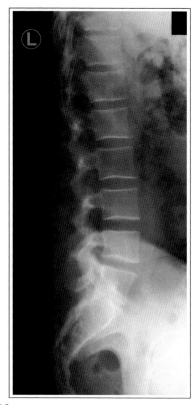

FIGURE 1-12 Poor marker placement in lateral lumbar vertebrae projection.

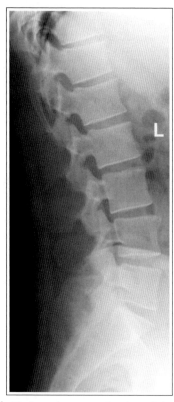

FIGURE 1-11 Marker placement for lateral lumbar vertebrae projection.

guides, the information displayed by all is similar. Each guide explains the IR coverage for the source–image receptor distance (SID) and amount of longitudinal and transverse collimation being used. If a 14- × 17-inch (35- × 43-cm) IR is placed in the Bucky tray at a set SID, and the collimator guide indicates that the operator has collimated to an 8- × 17-inch (20- × 43-cm) field size, the marker should be placed 3.5 to 4 inches (10 cm) from the IR's longitudinal midline to be included in the collimated field (Figure 1-21). If the field was also longitudinally collimated, the marker would also have to be positioned within this dimension. In the preceding example, if the collimator guide indicates that the longitudinal field is collimated to a 15-inch

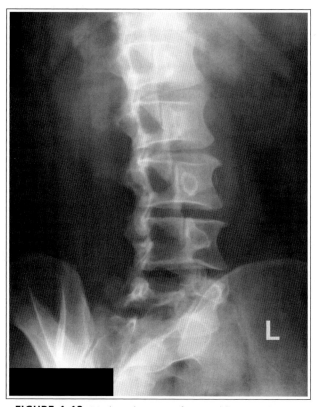

FIGURE 1-13 Marker placement for AP oblique projection.

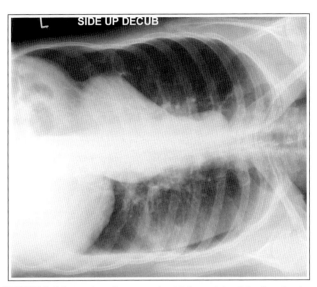

FIGURE 1-14 Marker placement for AP (lateral decubitus) projection.

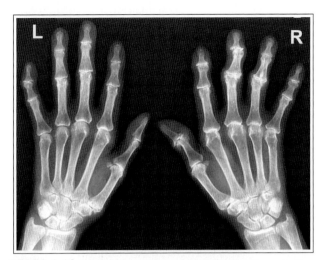

FIGURE 1-16 Marker placement for bilateral extremity projections.

(38-cm) field size, the marker would have to be placed 7.5 inches (19 cm) from the IR's transverse midline (see Figure 1-21).

Determining Mismarking Using the Identification Plate. If both sides of the body are demonstrated on the same radiograph, as with an anteroposterior (AP) projection of the pelvis or abdomen, evaluate it to ensure that an R marker is placed to the right of the vertebral column or an L marker is placed to the left of the vertebral column. When the screen-film system is used, this can be accomplished by using the patient ID plate because it is permanently built into the cassette and is always in the same place. Begin by displaying the image on the view box in the same manner that the IR was placed in the Bucky diaphragm. (For posteroanterior [PA] projections, display the image as if the patient's back were facing you. This is not the proper way to display such an image but is a method for determining

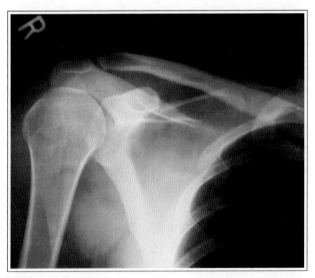

FIGURE 1-17 Marker placement for an AP projection of shoulder.

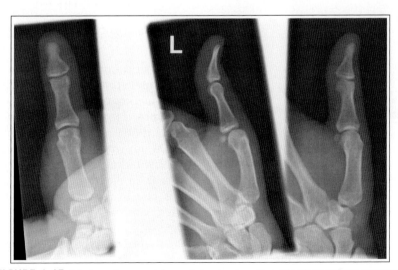

FIGURE 1-15 Marker placement for unilateral extremity projections on one receptor.

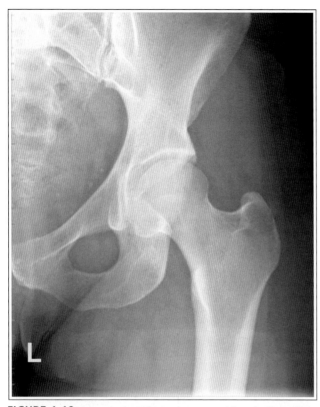

FIGURE 1-18 Poor marker placement on an AP projection of hip.

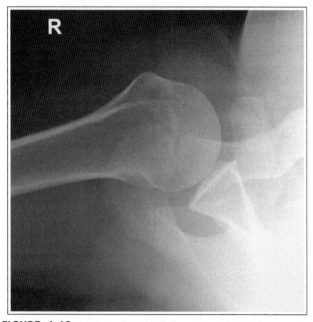

FIGURE 1-19 Marker placement for cross-table (inferosuperior axial) lateral shoulder projection.

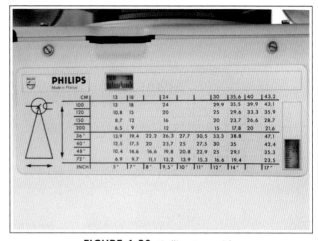

FIGURE 1-20 Collimator guide.

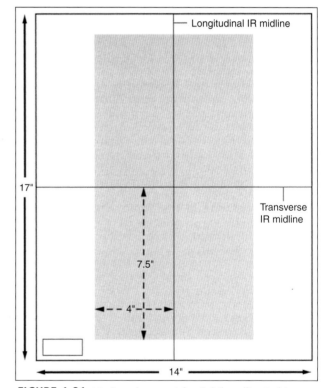

FIGURE 1-21 Marker placement for tightly collimated image.

marker accuracy.) The ID plate is in the lower left corner or the upper right corner on a lengthwise image and in the upper right or lower left corner on a crosswise image. Then, position yourself as the patient was positioned with respect to the IR. If the patient was in an AP projection, turn your back to the image; if the patient was in a PA projection, face the image.

The marker on the image should correspond to your right or left side—an R marker on your right side or an L marker on your left side.

When a marker on an image is only faintly visible, circle it and rewrite the information it displays next to it. Do not write the information over it (Figure 1-22).

Mismarked Images. If the R or L marker does not appear on the image or the image has been mismarked, it is best to repeat the image. Do not guess or rely on what you may believe to be a sure sign. The heart shadow, which is normally located on the left side of the thorax, may be shifted toward the right because of a disease process or because the patient has situs inversus (total or partial reversal of the body organs).

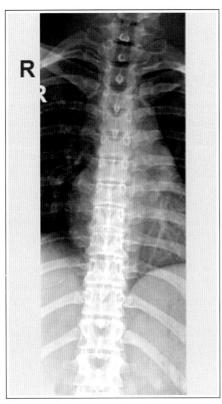

FIGURE 1-22 Partially visible marker.

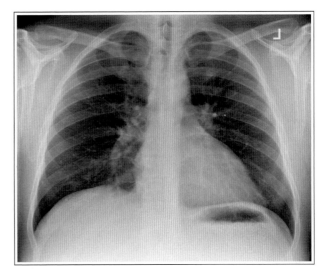

FIGURE 1-23 PA chest projection of hypersthenic patient.

Anatomic Structure Requirements and Placement

Each image requires that the area of interest be included, as well as a certain amount of the surrounding anatomic structures. For example, because radiating wrist pain may be a result of a distal forearm fracture, all wrist positions require that one fourth of the distal forearm be included with the wrist examination. A lateral ankle projection should include 1 inch (2.5 cm) of the fifth metatarsal base to rule out a Jones fracture.

Size Selection and Placement of Image Receptor. The IR used for a procedure should be just large enough to include the region being examined. Deciding whether to place the long axis of the IR crosswise (CW), lengthwise (LW), or diagonally in respect to the long axis of the part being examined is a simple matter of positioning it so that all the required anatomy can easily be demonstrated on the IR size chosen. This is mostly dictated by the body habitus, part length, and IR system used. As a general rule, the long axis of the part is aligned with the long axis of the IR.

Body Habitus. There are four types of body habitus to consider when positioning a patient for a PA-AP chest or AP abdomen projection—hypersthenic, sthenic, hyposthenic, and asthenic. The hypersthenic patient has a wide, short thorax and a broad peritoneal cavity, with a high diaphragm (Figure 1-23). This body habitus requires the IR to be placed CW for PA-AP chest projections to include the entire lung field and requires two CW

IRs to be used for an AP abdomen projection to demonstrate the entire peritoneal cavity. The asthenic patient has a long, narrow thoracic cavity and narrow peritoneal cavity, with a lower diaphragm (Figure 1-24). The sthenic and hyposthenic types of body habitus have thoracic and peritoneal cavities, with lengths and widths that are between those of the hypersthenic and asthenic body habitus (Figures 1-25 and 1-26). The sthenic, hyposthenic, and asthenic types of body habitus require the IR to be placed LW for the PA-AP chest and AP abdomen

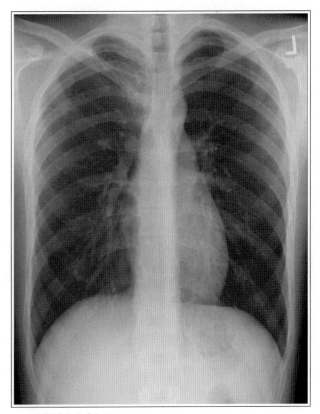

FIGURE 1-24 PA chest projection of asthenic patient.

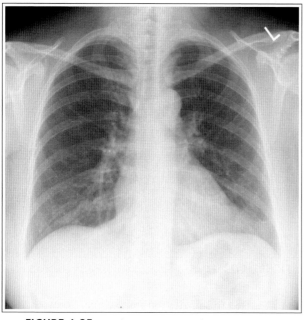

FIGURE 1-25 PA chest projection of sthenic patient.

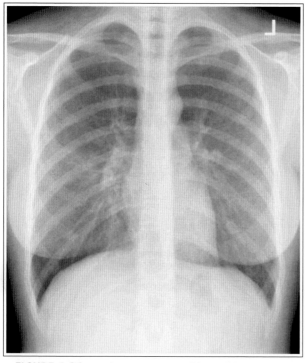

FIGURE 1-26 PA chest projection of hyposthenic patient.

projections to include the entire lung field and peritoneal cavity, respectively.

Long Bones. When imaging long bones, such as the forearm, humerus, lower leg, or femur, which require one or both joints to be included on the image, choose an IR that is long enough to allow 1 to 2 inches (2.5 to 5 cm) of the IR to extend beyond each joint space. This is needed to prevent the off-centered joint(s) from being projected off the IR because they will move in

the direction in which the diverged x-ray beams that are used to record them on the image are moving (Figure 1-27).

Images of the humerus and lower leg may be placed diagonally on the IR to have enough length that both joints can be included on a single image when a screen-film IR system is used (Figure 1-28). This is not advisable when using a cassette-based computed radiography (CR) system because an exposure field that is not parallel with the edges of the imaging plate may result in poor exposure field recognition and histogram analysis errors. For CR systems, when the structure is too long for the part to fit on one cassette, two separate images should be obtained, with each including a joint and portion of the midshaft and with overlapping of at least 2 inches (5 cm) between the images.

Multiple Projections on Same Image Receptor. How the IR is placed (LW or CW) often dictates how many images can be placed on the IR. For example, a 10- × 12-inch (24- × 30-cm) IR placed CW can accommodate three images of the wrist, but the same-sized IR placed LW has space available for only two images. When an extremity is imaged and more than one projection of the structure is exposed on the same IR, the images should be evenly spaced on the IR and similar anatomic structures should be located at the same end of the IR. For example, when the AP and lateral projections of the forearm are placed on the same 14- × 17-inch (35- × 43-cm) IR, the AP is positioned on half of the IR and the lateral on the other, with a defined collimated border around each, and the elbows in the two images are to be demonstrated at the same end of the IR (Figure 1-29). Failure to keep this alignment makes displaying and viewing of the image difficult (Figure 1-30).

Collimation. Proper collimation is accomplished when the beam of radiation is narrow enough to include only the areas of interests. Good collimation practices result in the following: (1) decrease the radiation dosage by limiting the amount of patient tissue exposed; (2) improve the visibility of recorded details by reducing the amount of scatter radiation that reaches the IR; and (3) reduces histogram analysis errors when using digital radiography. As a general rule, each image should demonstrate a small collimated border around the entire image of interest. The only time that this rule does not apply is when the entire IR must be used to prevent clipping of needed anatomy, as in chest and abdominal imaging. This collimated border not only demonstrates good collimation practices but also can be used to determine the exact location of central ray placement. Make an imaginary X on the image by diagonally connecting the corners of the collimated border (Figure 1-31). The center of the X indicates the central ray placement for the image.

Accurate placement of the central ray and alignment of the long axis of the part with the collimator's longitudinal light line are two positioning practices that will aid

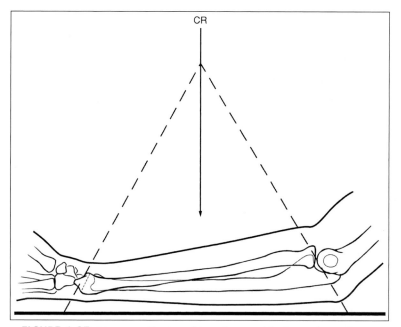

FIGURE 1-27 Proper positioning of long bones with diverged x-ray beam.

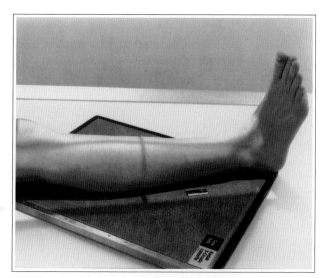

FIGURE 1-28 Diagonally positioning long bones on the IR to include both joints.

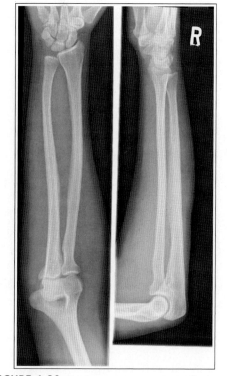

FIGURE 1-29 Proper receptor-anatomy alignment.

in obtaining tight collimation. When collimating, do not allow the collimator's light field to mislead you into believing that you have collimated more tightly than what has actually been done. When the collimator's central ray indicator is positioned on the patient's torso and the collimator is set to a predetermined width and length, the light field demonstrated on the patient's torso does not represent the true width and length of the field set on the collimator. This is because x-rays (and the collimator light, if the patient was not in the way) continue to diverge as they move through the torso to the IR, increasing the field size as they do so (Figure 1-32).

The thicker the part being imaged, the smaller the collimator's light field that appears on the patient's skin surface. On a very thick patient, it is often difficult to collimate the needed amount when the light field appears so small but, on these patients, tight collimation demonstrates the largest improvement in the visibility of the recorded details.

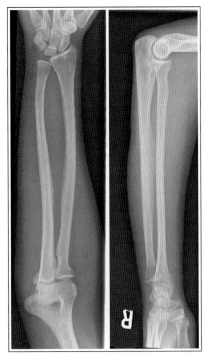

FIGURE 1-30 Poor receptor-anatomy alignment.

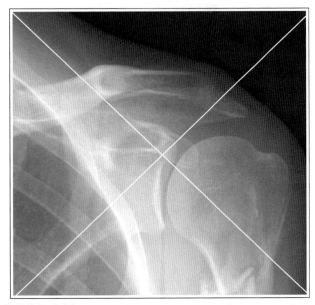

FIGURE 1-31 Using collimated borders to locate central ray placement.

Learn to use the collimator guide (see Figure 1-20) to determine the actual IR coverage. For example, when an AP lumbar vertebral projection is taken, the transversely collimated field should be reduced to an 8-inch (20-cm) field size. Because greater soft tissue thickness has nothing to do with an increase in the size of the skeletal structure, the transverse field should still be reduced when a thick patient part is being imaged. Accurately center the patient by using the centering light field and then set the transverse collimation length to 8 inches

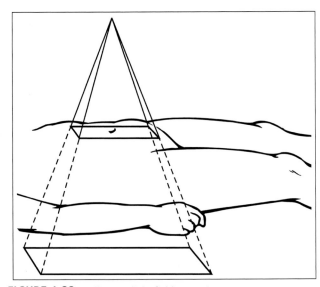

FIGURE 1-32 Collimator light field versus image receptor coverage.

by using the collimator guide. Be confident that the IR coverage will be sufficient, even though the light field appears small.

Box 1-4 lists guidelines to follow when collimating and evaluating collimation accuracy on images.

Rotating Collimator Head. On some x-ray equipment, the collimator head can be rotated without rotating the entire tube column. This capability allows the technologist to increase collimation on anatomic structures such as the clavicle, which is not aligned directly with the longitudinal or transverse axis of the light field. Rotating just the collimator head does not affect the alignment of the beam with the grid; this alignment is affected only when the tube column is rotated and is demonstrated on the image by visualization of grid lines artifacts and grid cutoff. Rotation of the collimator head should be avoided when using cassette-based digital radiography because it may affect the exposure field recognition process.

Overcollimation. Evaluate all images to determine whether the required anatomic structures have been included. Poor centering or overcollimation can result in the clipping of required anatomy (Figure 1-36).

BOX 1-4 | **Collimation Guidelines**

- For **extremity projections**, collimate to within 0.5 inch (1.25 cm) of the skin line of the thickest area of interest. (Figure 1-33).
- For **chest and abdomen projections**, collimate to within 0.5 inch (1.25 cm) of the patient's skin line (Figure 1-34).
- When collimating **structures within the torso**, bring the collimated borders as close to the structures of interest as possible. Use palpable anatomic structures around the area of interest to determine how close the borders are to the structure of interest (In Figure 1-35, the collimation field was closed to the palpable symphysis pubis and ASISs to frame the sacrum).

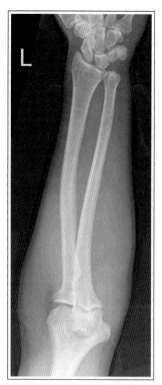

FIGURE 1-33 Proper "to skin line" collimation on an AP forearm projection.

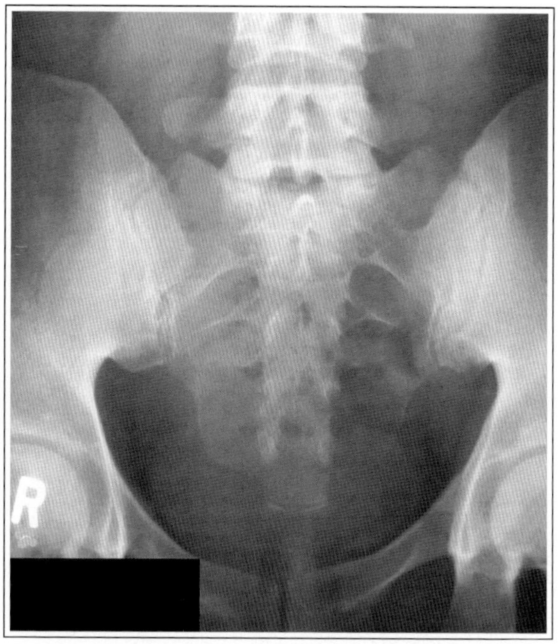

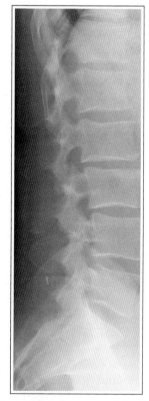

FIGURE 1-35 Proper collimation on an AP sacral projection.

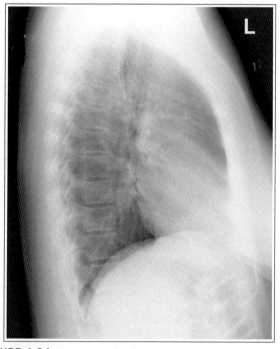

FIGURE 1-34 Proper "to skin line" collimation on a lateral chest projection.

FIGURE 1-36 Poor collimation on a lateral lumbar vertebral projection.

Clipping of required anatomy can also result from overcollimation on a structure that is not placed in direct contact with the IR, such as for a lateral third or fourth finger or lateral hand projection. Clipping occurs because the divergence of the x-ray beam has not been taken into consideration during collimation. To prevent clipping, view the shadow of the object projected onto the IR by the collimator light (Figure 1-37). It will be magnified. This magnification is similar to the magnification that the x-ray beam undergoes when the image is created. Allow the collimated field to remain open enough to include the shadow of the

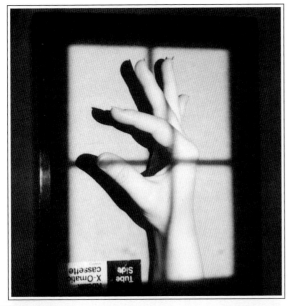

FIGURE 1-37 Viewing an object's shadow to determine proper collimation.

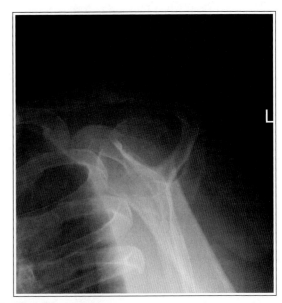

FIGURE 1-38 Properly positioned tangential (supraspinatus outlet) shoulder projection.

object, ensuring that the object will be shown in its entirety on the image.

Anatomic Relationships

Evaluate each image for proper anatomic alignment, as defined in the procedural analysis sections of this text. Each projection should demonstrate specific bony relationships that will best facilitate diagnosis. For example, an AP ankle projection demonstrates an open talotibial joint space (medial mortise), whereas the AP oblique projection demonstrates an open talofibular joint space (lateral mortise), and the lateral projection demonstrates the talar domes and soft tissue fat pads.

Positioning Routines and Understanding the Reason for the Procedure. Most positioning routines require AP-PA and lateral projections to be taken to demonstrate superimposed anatomic structures, localize lesions or foreign bodies, and determine alignment of fractures. When joints are of interest, oblique projections are also added to this routine to visualize obscured areas better. In addition to these, special projections may be requested for more precise demonstration of specific anatomic structures and pathologic conditions.

To appreciate the importance of the anatomic relationships on an image, one must understand the clinical reason for what the procedure is to demonstrate for the reviewer. This is particularly important when obtaining special projections that are not commonly performed and require specific and accurate anatomic alignment to be useful. For example, an optimally positioned tangential (supraspinatus outlet) shoulder projection (Figure 1-38) should demonstrate the supraspinatus outlet (opening formed between acromion and humeral head)

and the posterior aspects of the acromion and acromioclavicular (AC) joint in profile. The technologist produces these anatomic relationships when the patient's midcoronal plane is positioned vertically and can be ensured that the proper positioning was obtained when the superior scapular angle is positioned at the level of the coracoid tip on the image. From this optimal image, the radiologist can evaluate the supraspinatus outlet for narrowing caused by variations in the shape (spur) or slope of the acromion or AC joint, which has been found to be the primary cause of shoulder impingements and rotator cuff tears. If instead of being vertical, the patient's upper midcoronal plane was tilted toward the IR, the resulting image would demonstrate the superior scapular angle positioned above the coracoid tip, preventing clear visualization of the acromion and AC joint deformities, because their posterior surfaces would no longer be in profile and would narrow or close the supraspinatus outlet (Figure 1-39). Because the reviewer would be unable to diagnose outlet narrowing that results from variations in the shape or slope of the acromion or AC joint, this image would not be of diagnostic value.

Correlating the Anatomic Relationships and Positioning Criteria. For each projection in the procedural analysis sections of this book, there is a list of analytic criteria to use when evaluating the anatomic relationships that should be seen on an optimal image of that projection, an explanation that correlates it with the specific positioning procedure, and a description of related positioning errors. This information is needed to reposition the patient properly if a poorly positioned image is obtained because only the aspect of the positioning procedure that was inaccurate should be

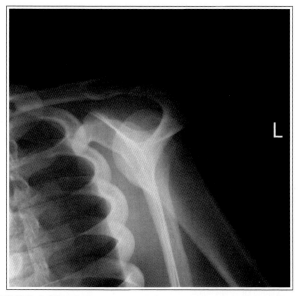

FIGURE 1-39 Poorly positioned tangential (supraspinatus outlet) shoulder projection.

changed when repeating the image. For example, a PA chest projection that is demonstrated without foreshortening visualizes the manubrium superimposed by the fourth thoracic vertebra, with approximately 1 inch (2.5 cm) of the apical lung field visible above the clavicles. This analysis criterion is demonstrated on the image when the patient's midcoronal plane is positioned vertically. If a PA chest projection demonstrates all the required analysis criteria, with the exception of the manubrium and fourth thoracic vertebral alignment, the technologist who understands the correlation between the analysis criteria and positioning procedure would know to adjust only the positioning of the patient's midcoronal plane before repeating the image.

Identifying Anatomic Structures. An optimal image should appear as much like the real object as possible, but because of unavoidable distortion that results from the shape, thickness, and position of the object and beam, part, and IR alignment, this is not always feasible, resulting in some anatomic structures appearing different than the real object. Using skeletal bones positioned in the same manner as the projection will greatly aid in identification of the anatomic structures on an image. Closely compare the visualization of the anatomic structures on the skeletal scapular bone photograph and x-ray image shown in Figure 1-40. Note that the superior scapular angle and lateral borders of this surface on the skeletal image are well demonstrated, obscuring the coracoid, but on the x-ray image the superior scapular angle is seen as a thin cortical line, its lateral borders are not demonstrated, and the coracoid can be clearly visualized. Also, note that the superior surface of the spine is visualized on the skeletal bone image between the lateral and medial scapular spine borders, but is not seen on the x-ray image.

When identifying anatomic structures, one must consider how anatomy may appear different from the real object. The following concepts, when understood and applied to how the procedure was obtained, can help with identification of the anatomic structures on the image.

Off-Centering. X-rays used to create an image are emitted from the x-ray tube's focal spot in the form of a fan-shaped beam. The central ray is the center of this beam; it is used to center the anatomic structure and IR. It is here that the x-ray beam has the least divergence and the image of an anatomic structure demonstrates the least amount of distortion. As one moves away from the center of the beam, the x-rays used to record the image diverge and expose the IR at an angle (Figure 1-41). The farther one moves away from the

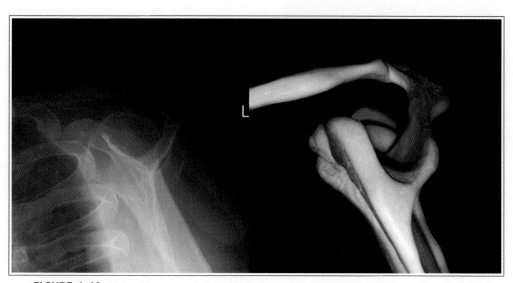

FIGURE 1-40 Skeletal bones and shoulder in the tangential (supraspinatus outlet) projection.

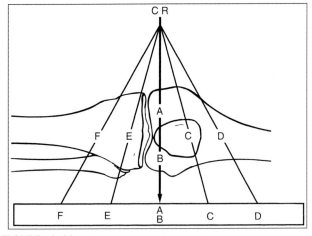

FIGURE 1-41 Effect of central ray placement on anatomic alignment.

central ray, the larger is the angle of divergence. Whether straight or angled beams are used to record the anatomic structures, and how those beams traverse the structures, will determine where and how they are visualized on the image.

Compare the relationship of the symphysis pubis and coccyx, and how differently the sacrum is visualized on accurately positioned AP abdominal and pelvic projections (Figure 1-42). Both images are taken with a perpendicular central ray, but the central ray is centered to the midpoint of the abdomen at the level of the iliac crest for the abdominal image and is centered at the midpoint of the sacrum for the pelvic image. The symphysis pubis and coccyx on both images were recorded using diverged beams, but because the central ray is centered more

superiorly and beams with greater angle of divergence were used to record the symphysis pubis and coccyx on the abdomen image, the symphysis pubis is moved more inferiorly to the coccyx on this image when compared with its alignment with the coccyx on the pelvic image. Also, compare sacral visualization on these two images. Because of the more inferior centering used in the pelvic image, the x-rays recording the sacrum are angled cephalically into the curve of the sacrum and those recording the sacrum for the abdominal image are angled caudally, against the sacral curve. This results in decreased sacral foreshortening on the pelvic image and increased sacral foreshortening on the abdominal image. The off-centered diverged beams will affect structures in the same manner that an angled central ray will (see preceding section for discussion of angled central ray). According to an experiment on beam divergence that is indicated in Q.B. Carroll's *Practical Radiographic Imaging* textbook, at a 40-inch SID, the divergence of x-rays is 2.5 degrees for every inch (1 degree/cm) off-centered in any direction from the central ray; at a 72-inch SID, beam divergence is off-centered about 1.5 inches (3.75 cm).

Angled Central Ray. When an angled central ray or diverged beam is used to record an object, the object will move in the direction in which the beams are traveling. The more the central ray is angled, the more the object will move. Also, note that objects positioned on the same plane but at different distances from the IR, which would have been superimposed if a perpendicular central ray were used, will be moved different amounts. Figure 1-43 demonstrates this concept. Point A is farther away from the IR than point C. Even though point A is horizontally aligned with point C, an angled

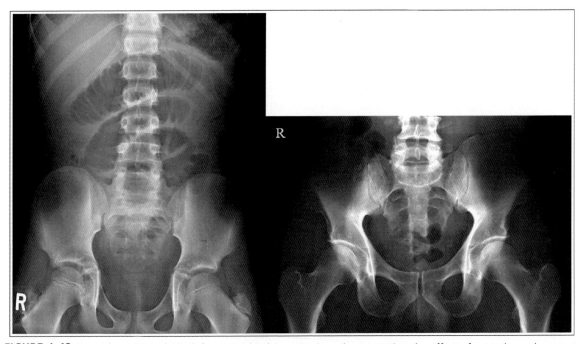

FIGURE 1-42 Properly positioned AP abdomen and pelvis projections demonstrating the effect of central ray placement.

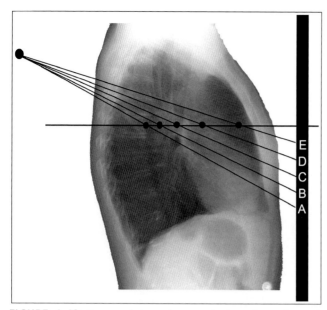

FIGURE 1-43 On angulation, the part farthest from the IR is projected the most.

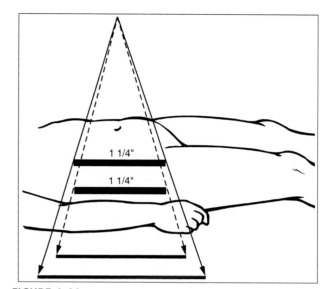

FIGURE 1-44 The part farthest from the IR will be magnified the most.

central ray used to record these two images would project point A farther inferiorly than point C. If these two structures were closer together (points A and B on Figure 1-43), the amount of separation on the image would be less. If these two structures were farther apart (points A and E on Figure 1-43), the separation on the image would be greater.

Magnification. Magnification, or size distortion, is present on an image when all axes of a structure demonstrate an equal percentage of increase in size over the real object. Because of three factors—no image is taken with the part situated directly on the IR, no anatomic structure imaged is flat, and not all structures are imaged with a perpendicular beam—all images demonstrate some type of size distortion. The amount of magnification mostly depends on how far each structure is from the IR at a set source–image receptor distance (SID). The farther away the part is situated, the more magnified the structure will be (Figure 1-44). Magnification also results when the same structure, situated at the same object–image receptor distance (OID), is imaged at a different SID. Size distortion should be kept to a minimum by using the shortest possible OID and the longest feasible SID.

Differences in magnification can be noticed between one side of a structure when compared with the opposite side if they are at significantly different OIDs. This can be seen on an accurately positioned lateral chest image, which demonstrates about 0.5 inch (1 cm) of space between the right and left posterior ribs, even though both sides of the thorax are of equal size. Because the right lung field and ribs are positioned at a greater OID than the left lung field and ribs on a left lateral projection, the right lung field and ribs are more magnified (Figure 1-45).

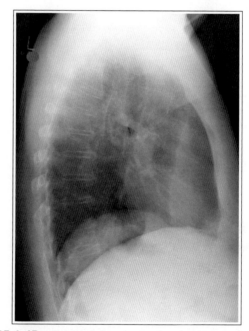

FIGURE 1-45 Left lateral chest image showing increased magnification of right lung field.

Elongation. This is the most common shape distortion and occurs when one of the structure's axes appears disproportionately longer on the image than the opposite axis (Figure 1-46). The least amount of elongation occurs when the central ray, part, and IR set up is ideal as demonstrated in Figure 1-47, *A,* and is most noticeable in the following situations:

• The central ray is perpendicular to the part and the IR is parallel with the part (Figure 1-47, *B*), but the part is not centered to the central ray (off-centered). The greater the off-centering, the greater the elongation.

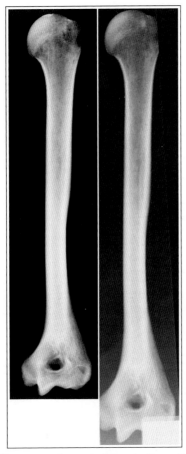

FIGURE 1-46 Humerus bones in AP projection without and with elongation.

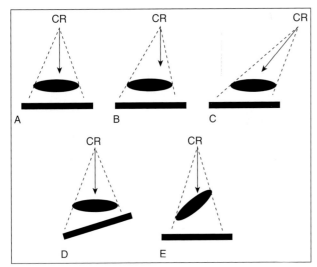

FIGURE 1-47 A-E, Causes of image distortion. See text for details.

- The central ray is angled and is not aligned perpendicular to the part, but the IR and the part are parallel with each other (Figure 1-47, *C*). The greater the central ray angulation, the greater the elongation.
- The central ray and part are aligned perpendicular to each other, but the IR is not aligned parallel with the part (Figure 1-47, *D*). The greater the angle of the IR, the greater the elongation.

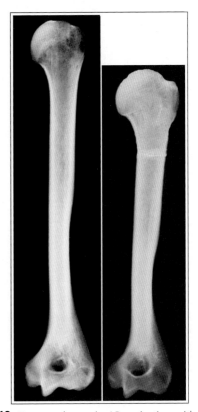

FIGURE 1-48 Humerus bones in AP projection without and with foreshortening.

Foreshortening. This is another form of shape distortion and is demonstrated when one of the structure's axes appears disproportionately shorter on the image than the opposite axis (Figure 1-48). Foreshortening occurs when the central ray and IR are perpendicular to each other, but the part is inclined (see Figure 1-47, *E*). The greater the incline, the greater will be the foreshortening.

Distinguishing Between Structures of Similar Shape and Size. The most difficult structures to identify are those that are identical in shape and size, such as the femoral condyles or talar domes. For these structures, three methods may be used to distinguish the structures from one another.

1. Use the structures that surround the area of interest. For example, if a poorly positioned lateral ankle image demonstrates inaccurate anterior alignment of the talar domes and a closed tibiotalar joint space, one cannot view the joint space to determine which talar dome is the more anterior, but the relationship of the tibia and fibula can easily be used to deduce this information.
2. Use bony projections such as tubercles to identify a similar structure. For example, the medial femoral condyle can be distinguished from the lateral condyle on a lateral knee image by locating the adductor tubercle situated on the medial condyle (Figure 1-49).
3. Identify the more magnified of the two structures. The anatomic structure situated farthest from the IR is magnified the most (see Figure 1-44).

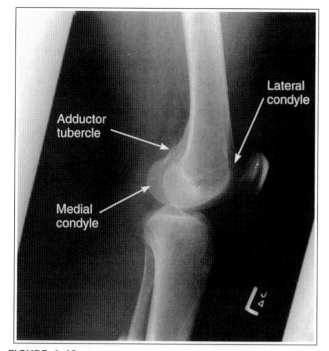

FIGURE 1-49 Poorly positioned lateral knee projection with the medial condyle posterior.

Determining the Degree of Patient Obliquity. To align the anatomic structures correctly, it is necessary to demonstrate precise patient positioning and central ray alignment. How accurately the patient is placed in a true AP-PA, lateral, or oblique projection, whether the structure is properly flexed or extended, and how accurately the central ray is directed and centered in relation to the structure determines how properly the anatomy is aligned. Because few technologists carry protractors, there must be

a method for determining whether the patient is in a true AP-PA or lateral projection, or specific degree of obliquity. For every projection described, an imaginary line (e.g., for the midsagittal or midcoronal plane, a line connecting the humeral or femoral epicondyles) is given that can be used to align the patient with the IR or imaging table. When the patient is in an AP-PA projection, the reference line should be aligned parallel (0-degree angle) with the IR (Figure 1-50, *A*) and, when the patient is in a lateral projection, the reference line should be aligned perpendicular (90-degree angle) to the IR (see Figure 1-50, *B*). For a 45-degree AP-PA oblique projection, place the reference line halfway between the AP-PA projection and the lateral position (see Figure 1-50, *C*). For a 68-degree AP-PA oblique projection, place the reference line halfway between the 45- and 90-degree angles (see Figure 1-50, *D*). For a 23-degree AP-PA oblique projection, place the reference line halfway between the 0- and 45-degree angles (see Figure 1-50, *E*). Even though these five angles are not the only angles used when a patient is positioned for images, they are easy to locate and can be used to estimate almost any other angle. For example, if a 60-degree AP-PA oblique projection is required, rotate the patient until the reference line is positioned at an angle slightly less than the 68-degree mark. I have used the torso to demonstrate this obliquity principle, but it can also be used for extremities. When an AP-PA oblique projection is required, always use the reference line to determine the amount of obliquity. Do not assume that a sponge will give you the correct angle. A 45-degree sponge may actually turn the patient more than 45 degrees if it is placed too far under the patient or if the patient's posterior or anterior soft tissue is thick.

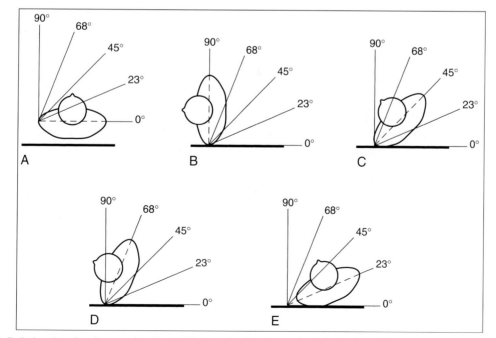

FIGURE 1-50 A-E, Estimating the degree of patient obliquity, viewing the patient's body from the top of the patient's head. See text for details.

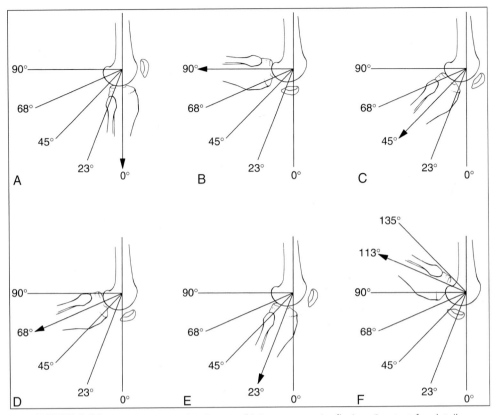

FIGURE 1-51 A-F, Estimating the degree of joint or extremity flexion. See text for details.

Determining the Degree of Extremity Flexion. For many examinations, a precise degree of structure flexion or extension is required to adequately demonstrate the desired information. Technologists need to estimate the degree to which an extremity is flexed or extended when positioning the patient and when evaluating images. When an extremity is in full extension, the degree of flexion is 0 (Figure 1-51, *A*), and when the two adjoining bones are aligned perpendicular to each other, the degree of flexion is 90 degrees (see Figure 1-51, *B*). As described in the preceding discussion, the angle found halfway between full extension and 90 degrees is 45 degrees (see Figure 1-51, *C*). The angle found halfway between the 45- and 90-degree angles is 68 degrees (see Figure 1-51, *D*), and the angle found halfway between full extension and a 45-degree angle is 23 degrees (see Figure 1-51, *E*). Because most flexible extremities flex beyond 90 degrees, the 113- and 135-degree angles (see Figure 1-51, *F*) should also be known.

Demonstrating Joint Spaces and Fracture Lines. For an open joint space or fracture line to be demonstrated, the central ray or diverged rays recording the area must be aligned parallel with the joint or fracture line of interest (Figures 1-52 and 1-53). Failure to accomplish this alignment will result in closed joint or poor fracture visualization because the surrounding structures are projected into the space or over the fracture line (Figures 1-54 and 1-55).

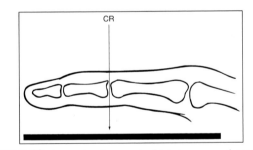

FIGURE 1-52 Accurate alignment of joint space and central ray.

STEPS FOR REPOSITIONING THE PATIENT FOR REPEAT IMAGES

1. Identify the two structures that are mispositioned (e.g., the medial and lateral femoral condyles for a lateral knee projection or the petrous ridges and supraorbital rims for an AP axial (Caldwell method) cranial projection.
2. Determine the number of inches or centimeters that the two mispositioned structures are "off." For example, the anterior surfaces of the medial and lateral femoral condyles should be superimposed on an accurately positioned lateral knee projection, but a 0.5-inch (1.25-cm) gap is present between them on the produced image (see Figure 1-49). Or, consider

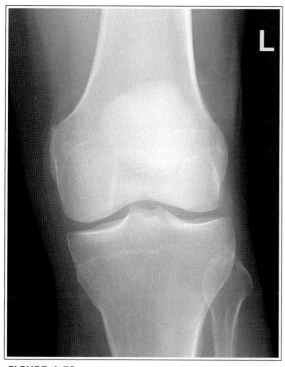

FIGURE 1-53 AP knee projection with open knee joint.

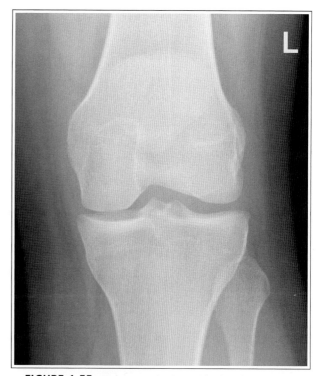

FIGURE 1-55 AP knee projection with closed knee joint.

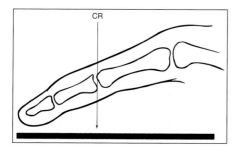

FIGURE 1-54 Poor alignment of joint space and central ray.

how the supraorbital margins should be demonstrated 1 inch (2.5 cm) superior to the petrous ridges on an accurately positioned AP axial cranial projection, but they are superimposed on the produced image (Figure 1-56).

3. Determine if the two structures will move toward or away from each other when the main structure is adjusted. For example, when the medial femoral condyle is moved anteriorly, the lateral condyle moves in the opposite direction (posteriorly). Also, when the patient's chin is elevated away from the chest, the supraorbital margins move superiorly, whereas the petrous ridges, being located at the central pivoting point in the cranium, do not move.

4. Begin the repositioning process by first positioning the patient as he or she was positioned for the poorly positioned image. From this position, move the patient as needed for proper positioning.

5. If the structures move in opposite directions from each other when the patient is repositioned, adjust the patient half the distance that the structures are off. For example, if the anterior surface of the lateral femoral condyle is situated 0.5 inch (1.25 cm) anterior to the anterior surface of the medial femoral condyle on a poorly positioned lateral knee projection (see Figure 1-49), the medial condyle should be rotated anteriorly 0.25 inch (0.6 cm).

6. If only one structure moves when the patient is repositioned, adjust the patient so that the structure that moves is adjusted the full amount. For example, if the petrous ridges should be located 1 inch (2.5 cm) inferior to the supraorbital margins on an accurately positioned AP axial cranial projection but they are superimposed (see Figure 1-56), then adjust the patient's chin 1 inch (2.5 cm) away from the chest, moving the supraorbital margins superiorly and 1 inch (2.5 cm) above the petrous ridges.

STEPS FOR REPOSITIONING THE CENTRAL RAY FOR REPEAT IMAGES

1. Identify the two structures that are mispositioned—for example, the medial and lateral femoral condyles for a lateral knee projection.

2. Determine which of the identified structures is positioned farthest from the IR. This is the structure that will move the most when the central ray angle is adjusted. For example, the medial femoral condyle is positioned farthest from the IR for a lateral knee projection.

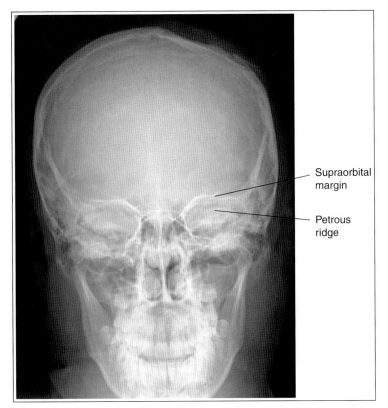

FIGURE 1-56 AP axial (Caldwell method) cranial projection showing poor positioning.

3. Determine the direction in which the structure situated farthest from the IR must move to be positioned accurately with respect to the other structure. For example, in Figure 1-49, the medial femoral condyle must be moved anteriorly toward the lateral condyle to obtain accurate positioning.

4. Determine the number of inches or centimeters that the two mispositioned structures are off on the image. For example, the anterior surfaces of the medial and lateral femoral condyles should be superimposed on an accurately positioned lateral knee projection, but a 0.5-inch (1.25-cm) gap is present between them on the produced image (see Figure 1-49).

5. Estimate how much the structure situated farthest from the image will move per 5 degrees of angle adjustment placed on the central ray. How much the central ray angulation will project two structures away from each other depends on the difference in the physical distance of the structures from each other, as measured on the skeletal bone, and the IR.

Box 1-5 lists guidelines that can be used to determine the degree of central ray adjustment required when dealing with different anatomic structures. For example, the physical space between the femoral condyles of the knee, as measured on a skeletal bone, is approximately 2 inches (5 cm). Using the central ray adjustment guidelines in Box 1-5, we find that structures that are 2 inches apart will require a 5-degree central ray angle adjustment to move the part situated farthest from the IR 0.25 inch (0.6 cm) more than the structure situated closer to the IR.

6. Place the needed angulation on the central ray, as determined by steps 4 and 5 above, and direct the central ray in the direction indicated in step 3 above. For example, if a lateral knee image demonstrates a separation between the medial and lateral femoral condyle of 0.5 inch (1.25 cm), then the central ray would need to be adjusted 10 degrees and directed toward the part farthest from the IR that needs to be moved to superimpose the condyles on the image. To obtain an optimal lateral knee projection for Figure 1-49 using the central ray only to improve positioning, it should be angled 10 degrees and directed anteriorly. This will move the medial condyle 0.5 inch (1.25 cm) anteriorly.

Figure 1-56 demonstrates a poorly positioned AP axial projection (Caldwell method). To obtain an optimal AP axial projection using the central ray, the technologist will do the following:

- Identify that the petrous ridges and supraorbital margins are superimposed on the image in Figure 1-56 and the supraorbital margins should be 1 inch (2.5 cm) superior to the petrous ridges on an optimal projection.
- Determine that the supraorbital margins are the farthest from the IR and that they will need to be moved 1 inch (2.5 cm) superiorly to obtain optimal alignment with the petrous ridges.

BOX 1-5	Central Ray Adjustment Guidelines for Structures Situated at the Central Ray*

- If the identified physical structures (actual bone, not as seen on radiographic image) are separated by 0.5-1.25 inches, a 5-degree central ray (CR) angle adjustment will move the structure situated farthest from the IR by about 0.125 inch (0.3 cm).
- If the identified physical structures are separated by 1.5-2.25 inches, a 5-degree CR angle adjustment will move the structure situated farthest from the IR about 0.25 inch (0.6 cm).
- If the identified physical structures are separated by 2.5-3.25 inches, a 5-degree CR angle adjustment will move the structure situated farthest from the IR about 0.5 inch (1.25 cm).
- If the identified physical structures are separated by 3.5–4.5 inches, a 5-degree CR angle adjustment will move the structure situated farthest from the IR about 0.75 inch (1.9 cm).

*Structures situated away from the CR will also be affected by divergence of the x-ray beam and the amount of the source-image receptor distance used, and may require less adjustment than indicated earlier. *IR*, image receptor.

- Measure the physical distance between the petrous ridges and supraorbital margins on a skeletal structure, which will be found to be about 3 inches (7.5 cm), and then use the chart in Box 1-5 to determine the degree of angulation adjustment that is needed to move the supraorbital margins 1 inch (2.5 cm) superiorly.
- Adjust the central ray angulation by 10 degrees cephalically before repeating the image.

Recorded Detail

Recorded detail refers to the sharpness of the lines of the image. If the lines are recorded as sharp, the image demonstrates good recorded detail. Poor recorded detail is visualized as a blurry edge around the lines. The factors that influence how well the recorded details are resolved include the focal spot size, SID, OID, speed of the image receptor system, contact between the film and intensifying screen, motion, and double exposure.

Focal Spot Size. A detail that is smaller than the focal spot used to produce the image will not be visible. This is why a small focal spot is recommended when fine detail demonstration is important, such as images of the extremities. Compare the trabecular patterns on the ankle images in Figures 1-57 and 1-58. Figure 1-57 was taken using a large focal spot and Figure 1-58 was taken using a small focal spot. Note how the use of a small focal spot increases the visibility of the bony trabeculae.

Using a small focal spot may not be feasible when imaging structures that require a high milliampere-seconds (mAs) setting because milliamperage (mA) settings of 300 mA or below can only be used when the small focal spot is chosen and the need for a long exposure time to obtain the density required may result in patient motion. Weigh the expected exposure time and the possibility of motion against the advantages gained by choosing a small

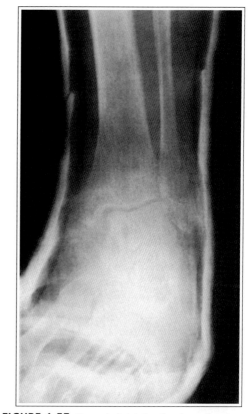

FIGURE 1-57 Recorded detail using large focal spot.

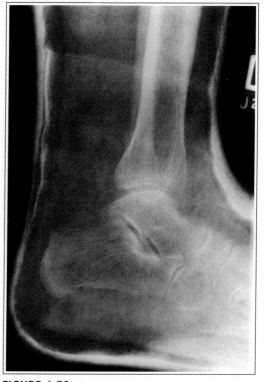

FIGURE 1-58 Recorded detail using small focal spot.

focal spot. If the patient's thickness measurement is large or the patient's ability to hold still is not reliable, a large focal spot and high milliamperage is the better choice.

Distances. By using the shortest possible OID and the longest feasible SID, size distortion can be kept to a minimum. This is especially important, because size distortion reduces an object's recognizability and blurs the recorded details.

In nonroutine clinical situations, the technologist may be unable to get the part as close to the IR as possible. For example, if a patient lying flat on the imaging table were unable to straighten his or her knee and had to keep it bent, the knee would be up off the table and have an increased OID. The technologist can compensate for this by increasing the SID above the standard used. It is often not feasible to increase the SID the needed amount to offset the magnification completely because the ratio between the OID and SID must remain the same for equal magnification to result. For example, an image taken at a 1-inch OID and 40-inch SID would demonstrate the same magnification as one taken at a 4-inch OID and 160-inch SID because both have a 1:40 ratio. When the SID is increased to offset magnification, it is also necessary to increase the mAs using the square law to maintain density.

Image Receptor Systems. Image receptors are chosen for their ability to demonstrate fine recorded details or for their speed. For maximum recorded detail sharpness, choose a single-emulsion film with a low-speed single-screen IR. This single-emulsion system (referred to as a slow detail system) eliminates the unsharpness caused by the parallax and crossover effects seen when a thick or large crystal screen emulsion is used to increase speed. Figure 1-59 demonstrates a hand image exposed using a slow detail screen and a fast screen system. Compare the trabecular patterns on these hand images. As a general rule, the higher the relative speed of the intensifying screen used, the lower will be the sharpness of detail demonstrated. Use a low-speed system for most extremity examinations. This system is for tabletop work only and should not be used when a grid is used or when a thick body part is being imaged. A medium-speed system should be used when the detail capability provides little benefit. For example, hands and feet can have hairline fractures that may be visualized only on a detail screen; because a fracture of the femoral bone is very obvious, however, we do not need to see small details to identify it. Use a high-speed system for examinations such as those performed for scoliosis, in which the bony cortical outlines are all that need to be demonstrated for measurements to be taken. Such a system should not be used when information about the structure itself is desired.

Poor Screen-Film Contact. This results when a screen-film system is used and a foreign object is wedged between the IR and the screen or the cassette is damaged or warped. Radiographically, poor screen-film contact is demonstrated by a blurred image only in the area in which the screen and film are not making direct contact. Figure 1-60 demonstrates a PA oblique hand projection. Note how the hand image is sharp everywhere, except at the fourth and fifth digits. Because it would be impossible for these two fingers to move without also causing the rest of the hand to move, it can be concluded that this blurring is a result not of patient motion but of poor screen-film contact. The screen should be thoroughly

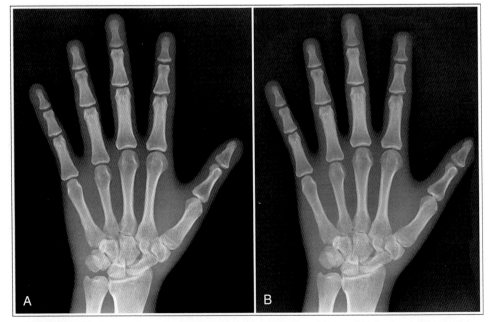

FIGURE 1-59 Comparing recorded detail between low-speed (**A**) and high-speed (**B**) screens.

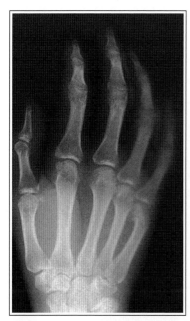

FIGURE 1-60 Poor screen-film contact.

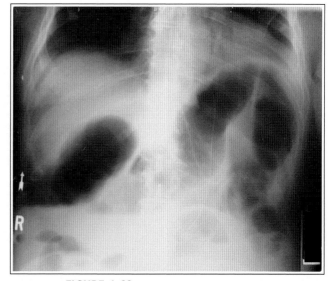

FIGURE 1-62 Involuntary patient motion.

cleaned and tested on a phantom. If the test radiograph does not demonstrate improved screen-film contact, the cassette should be replaced.

Motion. The term *motion unsharpness* refers to lack of detail sharpness in an image that is most often caused by patient movement during the exposure. This movement can be voluntary or involuntary. Voluntary motion refers to the patient's breathing or otherwise moving during the exposure. It can be controlled by explaining to the patient the importance of holding still, making the patient as comfortable as possible on the imaging table, using the shortest possible exposure time, and using positioning devices. Voluntary motion can be identified on an image by blurred bony cortical outlines (Figure 1-61). Involuntary motion is movement that the patient cannot control. Its effects will appear the same as those of voluntary motion in most situations, with the exception of within the abdomen. In the abdomen, peristaltic activity of the stomach and small or large intestine can be

identified on an image by sharp bony cortices and blurry gastric and intestinal gases (Figure 1-62). The only means of decreasing the blur caused by involuntary motion is to use the shortest possible exposure time, which in some cases is not good enough. At times, normal voluntary motions such as breathing or shaking can become involuntary motions. For example, an unconscious patient is unable to control breathing and a patient with severe trauma may be unable to control shivering.

Double-Exposed Image. A double-exposed image may also appear blurry and can easily be mistaken for an image affected by patient motion (Figure 1-63). When evaluating a blurry image, look at the cortical outlines of bony structures that are lying longitudinally and transversely. Is there only one cortical outline representing each bony structure, or are there two? Is one outline lying slightly above or to the side of the other? If one outline is demonstrated, the patient moved during the exposure, but if two are demonstrated, the image was exposed twice, and the patient was in a slightly different position for the second exposure.

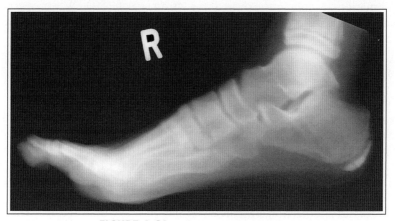

FIGURE 1-61 Voluntary patient motion.

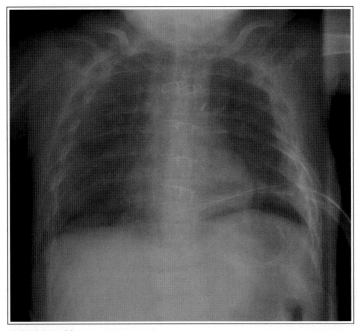

FIGURE 1-63 Double-exposed screen-film pediatric AP chest projection.

Radiation Protection

Diagnostic imaging professionals have a responsibility to adhere to effective radiation protection practices for the following reasons: (1) to prevent the occurrence of radiation-induced nonstochastic effects by adhering to dose-equivalent limits that are below the threshold dose-equivalent levels and (2) to limit the risk of stochastic effects to a reasonable level compared with non-radiation risks and in relation to society's needs, benefits gained, and economic factors.[3]

More than adults, children are susceptible to low levels of radiation because they possess many rapidly dividing cells and have a longer life expectancy. In rapidly dividing cells, the repair of mutations is less efficient than in resting cells. When radiation causes DNA mutations in a rapidly dividing cell, the cell cannot repair the damaged DNA sufficiently and continue to divide; therefore, the DNA remains in disrepair. The risk of cancer from radiologic examinations accumulates over a lifetime, and because children have a longer life expectancy, they have more time to manifest radiation-related cancers. This is particularly concerning because many childhood diseases require follow-up imaging into adulthood.

Continually evaluating one's radiation protection practices is necessary because radiation protection guidelines for diagnostic radiology assume a linear, nonthreshold, dose-risk relationship. Therefore any radiation dose, whether small or large, is expected to produce a response. Even when radiation protection efforts are not demonstrated on the image, good patient care standards dictate their use. Following are radiation protection practices that should be evaluated to provide images that can be obtained by following the ALARA (as low as reasonably achievable) philosophy.

Effective Communication. Taking the time to explain the procedure to the patient and giving clear, concise instructions during the procedure will help the patient understand the importance of holding still and maintaining the proper position, reducing the need for repeat radiographic exposures and additional radiation dose.

Immobilization Devices. If the patient moves during a procedure, the resulting image will be blurred. Such images have little or no diagnostic value and need to be repeated with additional exposure to the patient. Using appropriate immobilization devices can eliminate or minimize patient motion, which is especially important when imaging children, who may have a limited ability to understand and cooperate.

Source-Skin Distance. Mobile radiography units do not have the SID lock that department equipment is required to have to prevent exposures from being taken at an unsafe SID. When operating mobile radiography units, the technologist must maintain a source-skin distance (SSD) of at least 12 inches (30 cm) to prevent an unacceptable entrance skin dose. The entrance skin dose represents the absorbed dose to the most superficial layers of skin. As the distance between the source of radiation and the person increases, radiation exposure decreases. The amount of exposure decrease can be calculated using the inverse square law.

Compensating Filters. Compensating filters are constructed of aluminum or lead-acrylic and are used to create more homogeneous density across objects that vary in thickness. The filter absorbs x-ray photons before they reach the IR. The thicker part of the filter absorbs more photons than the thinner part. When a compensating filter is used, a technique is set that will adequately expose the thickest part being examined. If the filter has been accurately positioned, it will absorb the excessive radiation directed toward the thinnest structures, resulting in uniform image density throughout the image. Compensating filters that are positioned between the focal spot and the patient will reduce radiation dose to structures positioned beneath the filter.

Grids. Grids are used to improve radiographic contrast by eliminating some of the scatter radiation before it exposes the IR and should be used when imaging anatomic parts that are 4 inches (10 cm) or larger and using tube potentials above a 60-kilovoltage peak (kVp). When a grid is added, the mAs must be increased to compensate for the density loss that occurs as scatter is reduced. This increase will cause a direct increase in patient dose. To keep patient exposure as low as possible, grids should be used only when appropriate and the grid ratio should be kept to the lowest possible value that will provide sufficient contrast improvement as based on the kVp range used (see later, Table 1-1).

Screen-Film Image Receptor Speed. Relative screen speed is a major factor in reducing the radiation dose to the patient. By changing to a faster screen that requires less radiation to produce the image, the technologist can significantly reduce the patient's radiation dose. Unfortunately the reduction in dose gained from switching to a higher speed screen must be weighed against the sharpness of detail loss that occurs.

Possible Pregnancy. When imaging a female of childbearing age, it is essential that the technologist question the patient regarding the possibility of pregnancy. In some departments this is required of all females older than 11 years. Teenage girls may not admit to being pregnant until they reach the radiology department. If there is hesitancy rather than denial, additional questioning should occur, with follow-up questions such as, "Are you sexually active? If so, are you taking precautions?" If the patient is to have a procedure that requires significant pelvic exposure and there is some doubt as to her pregnancy status, it is recommended that a pregnancy test be performed.

Avoiding unnecessary radiation exposure or limiting it during the embryonic stage of development is essential because it is in this stage that the embryonic cells are dividing and differentiating and they are extremely radiosensitive and easily damaged by ionizing radiation.

Gonadal Shielding. Proper gonadal shielding practices have been proven to reduce radiation exposure of the female and male gonads. Gonadal shielding is recommended in the following situations:

- When the gonads are within 2 inches (5 cm) of the primary x-ray beam
- If the patient is of reproductive age
- If the gonadal shield does not cover information of interest

Professional technologists must always strive to improve skills and develop better ways to ensure good patient care while obtaining optimal images. All images should be evaluated for the accuracy of gonadal shielding.

Gonadal Shielding in the AP Projection for Female Patients. Shielding the gonads of the female patient for an AP projection of the pelvis, hip, or lumbar vertebrae requires more precise positioning of the shield to prevent the obscuring of pertinent information. The first step in understanding how to shield a woman properly is to know which organs should be shielded and their location. These are the ovaries, uterine (fallopian) tubes, and uterus. The uterus is found at the patient's midline, superior to the bladder. It is approximately 3 inches (7.5 cm) in length; its inferior aspect begins at the level of the symphysis pubis and it extends anterosuperiorly. The uterine tubes are bilateral, beginning at the superolateral angles of the uterus and extending to the lateral sides of the pelvis. Tucked between the lateral side of the pelvis and the uterus and inferior to the uterine tubes are the ovaries. The exact level at which the uterus, uterine tubes, and ovaries are found varies from patient to patient. Figures 1-64 and 1-65 show images from two different hysterosalpingograms. Note the variation in the location of the uterus, uterine tubes, and ovaries in these two patients. Because the location of these organs within the inlet pelvis cannot be determined with certainty, the entire inlet pelvis should be shielded to ensure that all the reproductive organs' have been protected.

To shield the female gonads properly, use a flat contact shield made from at least 1 mm of lead and cut to the shape of the inlet pelvis (Figure 1-66). Oddly shaped and male (triangular) shields do not effectively protect the female patient (Figure 1-67). The dimensions of the

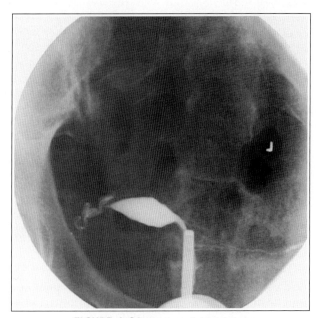

FIGURE 1-64 Hysterosalpingogram.

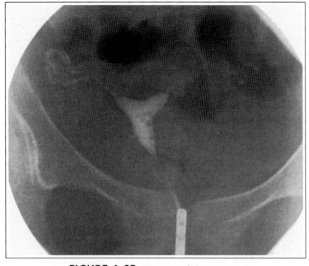

FIGURE 1-65 Hysterosalpingogram.

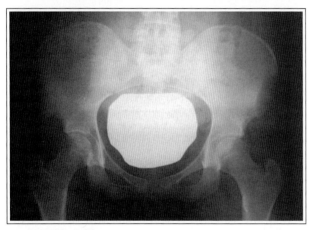

FIGURE 1-66 Proper gonadal shielding in the female.

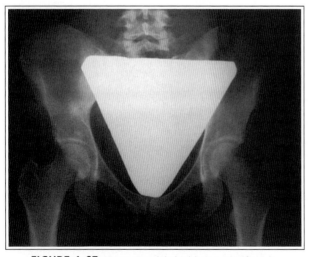

FIGURE 1-67 Poor gonadal shielding in the female.

shield used should be varied according to the amount of magnification that the shield will demonstrate, which is determined by the OID and SID and by the size of the patient's pelvis, which increases from infancy to

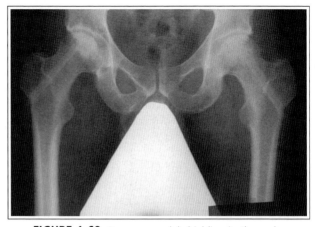

FIGURE 1-68 Proper gonadal shielding in the male.

adulthood. Each department should have different-sized contact or shadow shields for variations in female pelvic sizes for infants, toddlers, adolescents, and young adults.

To position the shield on the patient, place the narrower end of the shield just superior to the symphysis pubis and allow the wider end of the shield to lie superiorly over the reproductive organs. Side-to-side centering can be evaluated by placing an index finger just medial to each anterior superior iliac spine (ASIS). The sides of the shield should be placed at equal distances from the index fingers. When imaging children, do not palpate the pubic symphysis because they are taught that no one should touch their "private parts." Instead use the greater trochanters to position the shield because they are at the level of the superior border of the pubic symphysis. It may be wise to tape the shield to the patient. Patient motion such as breathing may cause the shield to shift to one side, inferiorly, or superiorly.

Gonadal Shielding in the AP Projection for Male Patients. The reproductive organs that are to be shielded on the male are the testes, which are found within the scrotal pouch. The testes are located along the midsagittal plane inferior to the symphysis pubis. Shielding the testes of a male patient for an AP projection of the pelvis or hip requires more specific placement of the lead shield to avoid obscuring areas of interest. For these examinations, a flat contact shield made from vinyl and 1 mm of lead should be cut out in the shape of a right triangle (one angle should be 90 degrees). Round the 90-degree corner on this triangle. Place the shield on the adult patient with the rounded corner beginning approximately 1 to 1.5 inches (2.5 to 4 cm) inferior to the palpable superior symphysis pubis. When accurately positioned, the shield frames the inferior outlines of the symphysis pubis and inferior ramus and extends inferiorly until the entire scrotum is covered (Figure 1-68). Each department should have different-sized male contact shields for the variations in male pelvic sizes for infants, youths, adolescents, and young adults.

Gonadal Shielding in the Lateral Projection for Male and Female Patients. When male and female patients are imaged in the lateral projection, use gonadal shielding whenever (1) the gonads are within the primary radiation field and (2) shielding will not cover pertinent information. In the lateral projection, male and female patients can be similarly shielded with a large flat contact shield or the straight edge of a lead apron. Begin by palpating the patient's coccyx and elevated ASIS. Next, draw an imaginary line connecting the coccyx with a point 1 inch posterior to the ASIS, and position the longitudinal edge of a large flat contact shield or half-lead apron anteriorly against this imaginary line (Figure 1-69). This shielding method can be safely used on patients being imaged for lateral vertebral, sacral, or coccygeal projections without fear of obscuring areas of interest (Figure 1-70).

Shielding of Radiosensitive Cells Not Within Primary Beam. Shielding of radiosensitive cells should be done whenever they lie within 2 inches (5 cm) of the primary beam. Radiosensitive cells are the eyes, thyroid, breasts, and gonads. To protect these areas, place a flat contact shield constructed of vinyl and 1 mm of lead or the straight edge of a lead apron over the area to be protected. Because the atomic number of lead is so high, radiation used in the diagnostic range will be readily absorbed in the shield.

Collimation. Tight collimation reduces the radiation exposure of anatomic structures that are not required on the image. For example, its use on chest images will reduce exposure of the patient's thyroid; on a cervical vertebral image, it will reduce exposure of the eyes; on a thoracic vertebrae image, it will reduce exposure of the breasts; and, on a hip image, it will reduce exposure of the gonads.

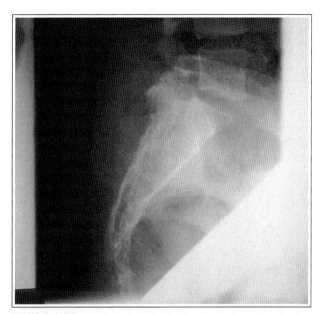

FIGURE 1-70 Proper gonadal shielding in the lateral projection.

Exposure Factors to Minimize Patient Exposure. Selection of appropriate technical exposure factors for a procedure should focus on producing an image of diagnostic quality with minimal patient dose. This is accomplished by selecting the highest practical kilovoltage and the lowest mAs that will produce an image with sufficient information. Also, when the patient has difficulty holding still or halting respiration, the shortest possible exposure time should be used by selecting a high-milliampere station.

Automatic Exposure Control Backup Timer. The backup timer is a safety device that prevents overexposure to the patient when the automatic exposure control (AEC) is not properly functioning or the control panel is not set correctly. When using the AEC, set the AEC backup time at 150% to 200% of the expected manual exposure time. Once the backup time is reached, the exposure will automatically terminate.

Anatomic Artifacts. These are anatomic structures of the patient or x-ray personnel that are demonstrated on the image but should not be there (Figure 1-71). Note in the figure how the patient's other hand was used to help maintain the position. This is not an acceptable practice. Many sponges and other positioning tools are available to aid in positioning and immobilizing the patient. Whenever the hands of the patient, x-ray personnel, or others must be within the radiation field, they must be properly attired with lead gloves.

Personnel and Family Members in Room During Exposure. Appropriate immobilization devices should be used and all personnel and family members should leave the room before the x-ray exposure is made. If the patient cannot be effectively immobilized or left alone in the room during the exposure, lead protection attire such as aprons, thyroid shields, glasses, and gloves should be worn by the personnel during any x-ray exposure. Anyone

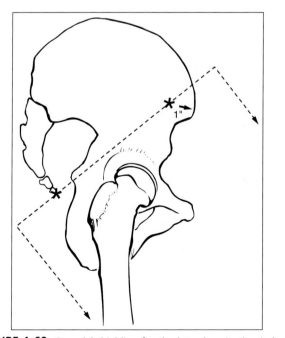

FIGURE 1-69 Gonadal shielding for the lateral projection in both male and female.

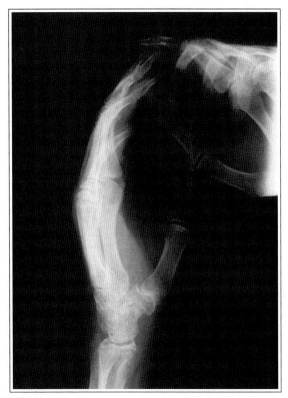

FIGURE 1-71 Anatomic artifact—poor radiation protection.

remaining in the room should also stand out of the path of the radiation source and as far from it as possible.

Radiographic Density

Radiographic density is a visibility of detail factor that describes the amount of overall blackness seen on the image and is directly related to the quantity of radiation that reaches the IR. The technologist evaluates each image for sufficient density by determining whether the bony and soft tissue structures of interest are visualized. If the anatomic structures of interest are not adequately seen, the technologist must determine which factors contributed to the density error. Before making any changes and repeating an examination because the image is too dark or light, evaluate all factors that affect radiographic density:

- Did you read the technique chart correctly and set the mAs and kVp as stated on the technique chart?
- Was the patient measured correctly?
- Was the patient properly positioned in respect to the activated ionization chamber(s)?
- Was the SID set correctly?
- Was the OID at a minimum?
- Was a grid used, if required, and was it positioned correctly with the central ray?
- Did you use the correct receptor system, and was the correct IR placed in that system?
- Did you use maximum collimation?
- Was a compensating filter used when applicable?
- Did you position the part to use the anode heel effect to your advantage?

Only if all of these factors are considered can one be ensured that the correct adjustment was made prior to repeating the image.

The following discussion will present the factors that cause excessive and insufficient radiographic density. Tables 1-1 and 1-2 can be used when evaluating the causes of poor radiographic density on images and determining how to improve the image.

Milliampere-Seconds. Density is directly related to the quantity of radiation that reaches the IR and mAs is the controlling factor for quantity. With adequate penetration, an increase in mAs will cause an increase in radiographic density and a decrease in mAs will cause a decrease in radiographic density. If an image is exposed using excessive mAs, it demonstrates density that is so dark that some or all of the bony and soft tissue structures of interest are not well visualized. A dark image produced using excessive mAs can be distinguished from one that was produced using very high kVp by evaluating the contrast on the image.

An overexposed image obtained using excessive mAs will demonstrate acceptable contrast as long as the kVp is optimal. Even though the overall image will be dark, the cortical outlines of the bone should remain high in contrast. Figure 1-72 demonstrates an accurately exposed and overexposed AP pelvic projection.

An underexposed image obtained using insufficient mAs will demonstrate density that is so light that some or all of the anatomic structures cannot be evaluated. Evaluating the visualization of the bony trabecular patterns is valuable when determining acceptability of such an image because usually on light images, unless underexposure is extreme, the demonstration of the soft tissue structures is better. Because underexposed and underpenetrated images demonstrate low density, it is necessary to learn to identify each technical error. One way to distinguish whether an image has been underexposed rather than underpenetrated is to study the bony cortical outlines of the structures of interest. On an image that has been underexposed, the cortical outlines are visible, even though their density is light, whereas an underpenetrated image will not demonstrate areas of the cortical outlines that were not penetrated. Figure 1-73 shows accurately exposed and underexposed AP pelvic projections.

When image density is inadequate, mAs is the controlling factor of choice. How much adjustment in mAs should be made to obtain an optimal image is directly proportional to the amount of increase or decrease in density that is needed. Typically, three adjustments are made when making density changes:

- A 30% change in mAs adjusts the image density just enough for the eyes to be able to visualize that a change has been made. This amount of adjustment should never be used when an image needs to be repeated because the density is too light or dark. However, it is an ideal adjustment to make when the image demonstrates acceptable but not

TABLE 1-1	Excessive Radiographic Density
Technical Factor	**Causes and Adjustments**
mAs	**mAs too high** • If borderline too dark, decrease mAs by 50% (divide mAs by 2 and subtract from original) • If very dark, decrease mAs 3 to 4 times (divide by 3 or 4 and subtract from original)
kVp	**kVp too high** • If borderline too dark, decrease the original kVp used by 15%. Be careful not to stray too far from optimal kVp so insufficient penetration does not result. • If image is 3 to 4 times too dark, do a combination kVp and mAs change by reducing the kVp by 15% and making the remainder of the density adjustment using mAs.
AEC	**Wrong Bucky was activated and the backup timer shut the exposure off.** • Activate correct Bucky **Exposure time needed was less than the minimum response time.** • Reduce mA station until time needed for exposure is above minimum response time. **Density control was left on + setting from the previous patient.** • Reduce the density control setting. **Ionization chamber(s) chosen was beneath a structure that has a higher atomic number or is denser or thicker than tissue of interest.** • Select ionization chamber(s) centered beneath anatomical structure(s) of greatest interest. **A radiopaque artifact or appliances is included within or over the anatomy of interest.** • Do not use AEC. Manual set technique controls. **A faster screen speed was used when the AEC was calibrated for a slower screen speed.** • Use the screen-film IR system the AEC's thyristor is calibrated for.
SID	**SID was decreased without an equivalent decrease in mAs** • Use the density maintenance formula to adjust mAs when SID is changed: $$\frac{\text{Old mAs}}{\text{New mAs}} = \frac{\text{old SID}^2}{\text{new SID}^2}$$
Grid	**Used a grid technique without a grid or used a high grid ratio technique with a lower grid ratio** • Use the grid conversion factor (GCF) to determine the mAs adjustment needed for grid variations: *Nongrid to grid*: New GCF × old mAs = new mAs with new grid ratio *Grid to grid*: New GCF × old mAs = new mAs with new grid ratio old GCF <table><tr><th>Grid Ratio</th><th>GCF at 70 kVp</th><th>GCF at 90 kVp</th><th>GCF at 120 kVp</th></tr><tr><td>6:1</td><td>2</td><td>2.5</td><td>3</td></tr><tr><td>8:1</td><td>3</td><td>3.5</td><td>4</td></tr><tr><td>12:1</td><td>3.5</td><td>4</td><td>5</td></tr><tr><td>16:1</td><td>4</td><td>5</td><td>6</td></tr></table>
Screens	**Used mAs for a slow speed screen system with a fast speed screen system** • Use the correct slow speed screen system or adjust mAs for the fast speed screen system. To determine adjustment needed, use the mAs conversion factor formula for screens. $$\frac{\text{Old mAs}}{\text{New mAs}} \times \frac{\text{new relative screen speed}}{\text{old relative screen speed}}$$ Rare earth receptor speeds: extremity, 80; medium, 300; regular, 400; high, 800.
Anode heel effect	**Thicker end of long body part (forearm, lower leg, etc.) was positioned at anode end of tube and thinnest at end positioned at cathode end, resulting in underexposure of thick body part end and overexposure of thinnest body part end.** • Position the thicker end of the long body part at the cathode end of the tube and the thinnest at the anode end of the tube.

AEC, Automatic exposure control; *kVp*, kilovoltage peak; *mAs*, milliampere-seconds; *SID*, source–image receptor distance.

optimal density and needs to be repeated because of a factor other than density, such as an artifact, patient motion, or mispositioning. To calculate a 30% change, multiply the original mAs value by 0.30; then, add the result to the original mAs value to increase density or subtract the result from the original mAs value to decrease density.

• An image that is borderline too light requires a 100% increase in mAs (see Figure 1-73) and an image that is borderline too dark requires a 50% decrease in mAs (see Figure 1-72). To calculate a 100% increase in density, multiply the original mAs by 2 and add the result to the original mAs. If the original mAs were 20, the new mAs would

TABLE 1-2	Insufficient Radiographic Density

Technical Factor	Causes and Adjustments
mAs	**mAs too low** • If borderline light, increase mAs by 100% (multiply mAs by 2 and add to original) • If very light, increase mAs 3 to 4 times (multiply by 3 or 4 and add to original)
kVp	**kVp too low** • Increase kVp by 15% (multiply kVp by 0.15 and add to original) to change penetration enough to double the density.
AEC	**Backup time was shorter than the needed exposure time.** • Set backup timer at 150% – 200% of the expected manual exposure time. **Density control was left on the minus setting from the previous patient.** • Increase density control setting. **Ionization chamber(s) chosen was beneath a structure having a lower atomic number or was less dense or thinner than tissue of interest.** • Select ionization chamber(s) centered beneath anatomical structure(s) of greatest interest. **Inadequate collimation caused excessive scatter radiation to reach the ionization chamber(s) and prematurely shut off exposure.** • Increase collimation. **A small anatomic part was imaged and the activated ionization chamber was not fully covered by anatomy of interest.** • Do not use AEC. Manual set technique controls **AEC was used on a peripheral anatomic part and the activated ionization chamber was not fully covered by the anatomy of interest.** • Do not use AEC. Manual set technique controls **A slower screen speed was used when the AEC was calibrated for a faster screen speed.** • Use the screen-film IR system the AEC's thyristor is calibrated for.
SID and OID	**Increased SID without an equivalent increase in mAs** • Use the density maintenance formula to adjust mAs for the SID change: $$\frac{\text{Old mAs}}{\text{New mAs}} = \frac{\text{old SID}^2}{\text{new SID}^2}$$ **Increased OID without an increase in mAs (Only if procedure would produce a significant amount of scatter radiation that will not reach IR when OID is increase)** • Increase the mAs 10% for every centimeter of OID increase.
Grid	**Used a nongrid technique but left the grid in or used a low ratio grid technique with a high ratio grid** • Repeat exposure with correct grid ratio. • Use the grid conversion factor (GCF) to determine the mAs adjustment needed for grid variations: *Nongrid to grid*: New GCF × old mAs = new mAs with new grid ratio *Grid to grid*: New GCF × old mAs = new mAs with new grid ratio old GCF

Grid Ratio	GCF at 70 kVp	GCF at 90 kVp	GCF at 120 kVp
6:1	2	2.5	3
8:1	3	3.5	4
12:1	3.5	4	5
16:1	4	5	6

Technical Factor	Causes and Adjustments
	Grid is off-level or the central ray (CR) is angled toward grid's lead strips, demonstrating grid cutoff on the side that CR is angled toward if parallel grid was used and across the entire image if focused grid was used. • Level the grid, bringing it perpendicular to the CR. **SID is outside grid's focusing range, demonstrating grid cut-off on each side of the image.** • Increase or decrease SID to bring distance in the grid's focusing range. **Focused grid inverted, demonstrating grid cut-off on each side of the image.** • Flip grid around. **Focused grid off-center, demonstrating grid cut-off across entire image; image will not be in the center of the IR but will be to one side.** • Center the CR to the center of the grid.
Screens	**Used mAs for a fast speed screen system with a slow speed screen system** • Use the correct fast speed screen system or adjust mAs for the slow speed screen system. To determine adjustment needed, use the mAs conversion factor formula for screens. $$\frac{\text{Old mAs}}{\text{New mAs}} \times \frac{\text{new relative screen speed}}{\text{old relative screen speed}}$$ Rare earth receptor speeds: extremity, 80; medium, 300; regular, 400; high, 800.
Collimation	**A large decrease in field size was made without an increase in mAs (Only if procedure would produce a significant amount of scatter radiation that will not reach IR when OID is increase)** • 14- × 17-inch IR size to a 10- × 12-inch IR size: increase mAs by 35%. • 14- × 17-inch IR size to an 8- × 10-inch IR size: increase mAs by 50%.

AEC, Automatic exposure control; *mAs*, milliampere-seconds; *IR*, image receptor; *OID*, object–image receptor distance; *SID*, source–image receptor distance.

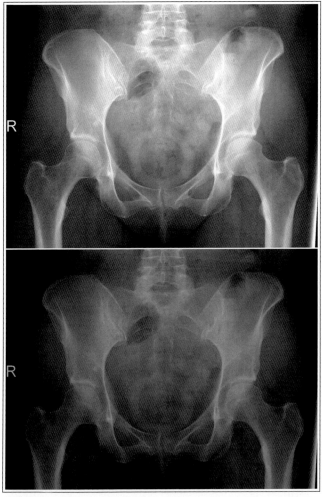

FIGURE 1-72 Accurately exposed *(top)* and overexposed, by 100% *(bottom)*, AP pelvic projections.

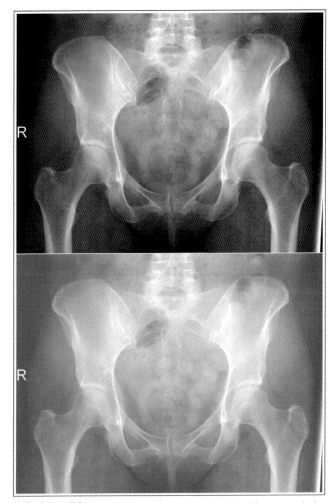

FIGURE 1-73 Accurately exposed *(top)* and underexposed, by 100% *(bottom)*, AP pelvic projections.

be 40. To calculate a 50% decrease in density, divide the original mAs by 2 and subtract the result from the original mAs, so that if the original mAs were 20, the new mAs would be 10.

• An image that is so light or dark that you immediately know absolutely that it needs to be repeated requires a 3 or 4 times increase in mAs if it is too light (Figure 1-74) and a 3 or 4 times decrease in mAs if it is too dark (Figure 1-75). To calculate a 3 or 4 times increase in density, multiply the original mAs by 3 or 4, respectively, and add the results to the original mAs. To calculate a 3 or 4 times decrease in density, multiply the original mAs by 3 or 4 times, respectively, and subtract the result from the original mAs.

Kilovoltage. The penetrating ability of the primary x-ray beam is controlled by the kilovoltage peak that is used. Radiographic density is affected by a change in kVp because it alters the quality of photons, which changes the ratio of penetrated to absorbed photons. The higher the kVp, the greater is the number of photons that penetrate the patient and reach the IR, resulting in greater image density; the lower the kVp, the greater is the number of photons absorbed in the patient, decreasing the numbers reaching the IR and image density. Because no amount of mAs will ever compensate for insufficient kVp, an optimum kVp level based on the tissue's composition and thickness is required for each body part. Optimum kVp is defined as the kVp that will provide adequate body part penetration and sufficient gray scale.

An image that has been adequately penetrated demonstrates the cortical outlines of the thinnest and thickest bony structures of interest. If these structures have not been penetrated (not enough kVp used), the image demonstrates too little density but, in comparison with an underexposed image, the cortical outlines of the thickest parts of the structure are not visible. Compare the bottom images in Figures 1-76 and 1-73. Note that if a transparency were laid over the images and an outline of the bony structures drawn on the transparency, with lines made only where the cortical outlines of the bone were clearly visible, many of the hip structures around the acetabulum would not be drawn. If the cortical outlines of the structure of interest can be seen even though the image density is light, it can be concluded

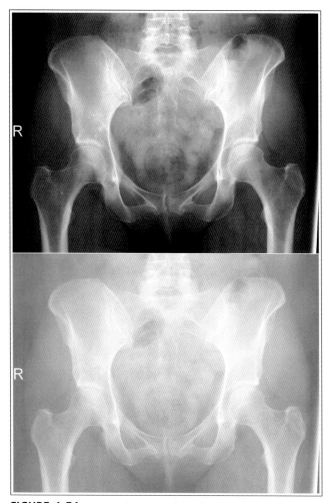

FIGURE 1-74 Accurately exposed *(top)* and underexposed, by 3 to 4 times *(bottom)*, AP pelvic projections.

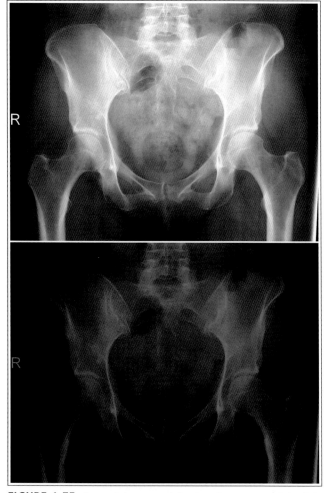

FIGURE 1-75 Accurately exposed *(top)* and overexposed, by 3 to 4 times *(bottom)*, AP pelvic projections.

that the mAs needs adjusting; if the cortical outlines of the structure cannot be seen and the image density is light, a kVp adjustment is required.

An underpenetrated image may also demonstrate inadequate density. The amount of density adjustment needed must also be considered when deciding how much kVp adjustment is to be made:

- If an image has to be repeated because it was underpenetrated and the density (see earlier, density discussion, for the explanation) was 100% too light, increase the kVp by at least 15%. (If 50 kVp was the level used on the original image, the new kVp level is calculated by multiplying 50 by 0.15 and adding the result [7.5] to the original 50 kVp; the new kVp value would be 57.5.) The mAs should remain the same as that used on the original image, because a 15% kVp change will also increase density by 100% (see Figure 1-76).
- If an image is underpenetrated and light enough to require a 3 or 4 times density adjustment, a

combination kVp and mAs change is indicated. Figure 1-77 demonstrates an underpenetrated AP pelvic projection. How much of the adjustment should be with kVp in this situation depends on your departmental standard for contrast; it can be determined by using the optimal kVp level for the structure being imaged as a guideline. As a general rule, the kVp should be kept relatively close to the optimal level. First, calculate a 15% increase in the kVp. Is this new kVp reasonably close to the optimal level for the structure being imaged? If so, you know that there will be a significant penetration change, and any additional density adjustment could be made with mAs without negatively affecting image contrast. Increasing the kVp too far above optimum results in an increase in scatter radiation being directed toward the IR and a decrease in image contrast.

Patient Condition.   Additive and destructive patient conditions that result in change to the normal bony

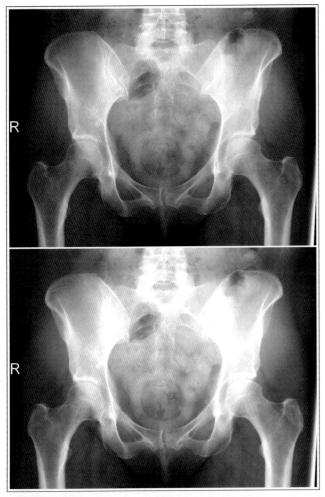

FIGURE 1-76 Accurately penetrated *(top)* and underpenetrated (100% density difference; *bottom*) AP pelvic projections.

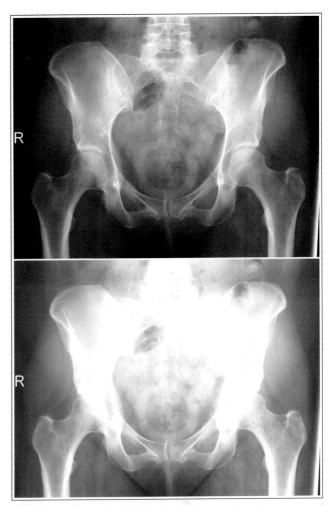

FIGURE 1-77 Accurately penetrated *(top)* and underpenetrated (3 to 4 times density; *bottom*) AP pelvic projections.

structures, soft tissues, or air or fluid content of the patient may require technical changes as compensation before exposing the patient. Additive diseases cause tissues to increase in mass density or thickness, resulting in them being more radiopaque, whereas destructive diseases cause tissues to break down, resulting in them being more radiolucent. Table 1-3 lists common additive and destructive diseases that may require technique adjustments and provides a starting point for adjusting technical factors for the condition.

Automatic Exposure Control. The AEC allows the mAs to be automatically determined by controlling the exposure time, but it is the technologist's responsibility to set an optimum kVp and optimal mA manually. Optimum mA refers to using a high enough mA at a given focal spot size to minimize motion, but not so high that the exposure times are shorter than the AEC's minimum response time. The minimum response time is the time that it takes for the circuit to detect and react to the radiation received; this is determined by the AEC manufacturer.

Guidelines for Using Automatic Exposure Control and Evaluating Images Produced

- Set optimum kVp for body part being imaged to obtain appropriate part penetration and contrast scale. kVp must be set to assure accurate part penetration and the desired contrast.

See earlier discussions of kVp, penetration, and contrast scale to determine the appropriate adjustment in kVp to be made when penetration and contrast scale are inadequate. If less than optimum kVp is used for the anatomy of interest, this anatomy will be underpenetrated and underexposed, although the radiographic density of any anatomic structures that were penetrated may be adequate as long as the backup time is long enough to accommodate the increased exposure time needed to compensate. An underexposed light image will result if the kVp is so low that inadequate penetration occurred in all anatomic structures beneath the activated chamber(s). No amount of mAs will compensate for inadequate penetration.

TABLE 1-3	**Adjusting Technical Factors for Patient Conditions**		
Additive Diseases		**Destructive Diseases**	
Condition	Amount to Increase	Condition	Amount to Decrease
Acromegaly	8%-10% kVp	Aseptic necrosis	8% kVp
Ascites	50% mAs	Blastomycosis	8% kVp
Cardiomegaly	50% mAs	Bowel obstruction	8% kVp
Fibrous carcinomas	50% mAs	Emphysema	8% kVp
Hydrocephalus	50%-75% mAs	Ewing's tumor	8% kVp
Hydropneumothorax	50% mAs	Exostosis	8% kVp
Osteoarthritis	8% kVp	Gout	8% kVp
Osteochondroma	8% kVp	Hodgkin's disease	8% kVp
Osteopetrosis	8% kVp	Hyperparathyroidism	8% kVp
Paget's disease	8% kVp	Osteolytic cancer	8% kVp
Pleural effusion	35% mAs	Osteomalacia	8% kVp
Pneumonia	50% mAs	Osteoporosis	8% kVp
Pulmonary edema	50% mAs	Pneumothorax	8% kVp
Pulmonary tuberculosis	50% mAs	Rheumatoid arthritis	8% kVp

From Carroll QB. *Practical radiographic imaging*, ed 8, Springfield, Ill, 2007, Charles C Thomas.
kVp, Kilovoltage peak; *mAs*, milliampere-seconds.

- Set mA at the highest station for the focal spot size needed, but not so high that the exposure time required for proper radiographic density is less than the minimum response time.

Exposures taken with an exposure time that is less than the minimum response time will result in overexposed, dark images. This is because the AEC circuit does not have enough time to detect and react to the radiation received to shut the exposure off in the time needed to produce the ideal image. The mA station should be decreased until exposure times are sufficient to produce the desired density.

- Set backup time at 150% to 200% of the expected manual exposure time. As a general guideline, use 0.2 seconds for all chest and proximal extremities, 1 second for abdominal and skull projections, and 2 – 4 seconds for very large torso projections.

The backup timer is the maximum time that the x-ray exposure will be allowed to continue. Once the backup time is met the exposure will automatically terminate. If the set backup time is too short the exposure will prematurely stop before adequate exposure has reached the ionization chamber(s), resulting in an underexposed, light image. If the set backup time is too long and the AEC is not functioning properly or the control panel is not correctly set, the exposure will continue much longer than needed to produce adequate density, resulting in an overexposed, dark image and excessive radiation dose to the patient.

- Select and activate the ionization chamber(s) that will be centered beneath the anatomic structures of greatest interest.

Recommendations for ionization chamber selection can be found at the beginning of each procedural analysis chapter of the book. Failure to properly activate the correct ionization chamber(s) and center the anatomic structures of greatest interest beneath them will result in images that are over- or underexposed. An overexposed image results when the ionization chamber chosen is located beneath a structure that has a higher atomic number or is thicker or denser than the structure of interest. For example, when an AP abdomen projection is taken, the outside ionization chambers should be chosen and situated within the soft tissue, away from the lumbar vertebrae, to yield the desired abdominal soft tissue density. If the chamber situated under the lumbar vertebrae is used instead, the capacitor (device that stores energy) requires a longer exposure time to reach its maximum filling level and terminate the exposure. This occurs because of the high atomic number of bone and the higher number of photons that bone absorbs compared with soft tissue. The result will be an image with adequate bone density but overexposed soft tissue (Figure 1-78).

An underexposed image results, however, when the ionization chamber chosen is located beneath a structure that has a lower atomic number or is thinner or less dense than the structure of interest. When an AP lumbar vertebral projection is taken, the center ionization chamber is chosen and centered directly beneath the lumbar vertebrae. If one or both of the outside chambers are used or the center ionization chamber is off center, the image is underexposed, because soft tissue, which has a lower atomic number than bone, is above the activated chamber (Figure 1-79).

- Do not use AEC on peripheral or very small anatomy where the activated chamber(s) is not completely covered by the anatomy, resulting in a portion of the chamber(s) being exposed with a part of the x-ray beam that does not go through the patient.

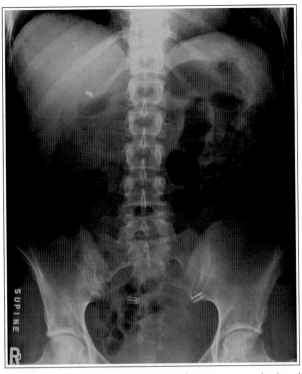

FIGURE 1-78 AP abdomen projection that was exposed using the center AEC chamber.

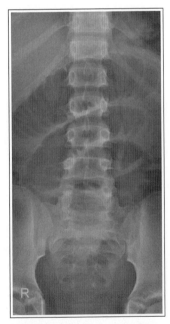

FIGURE 1-79 AP lumbar vertebrae projection exposed using the two outside AEC chambers.

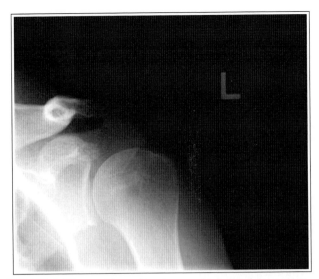

FIGURE 1-80 AP oblique (Grashey method) shoulder projection that was exposed with the center AEC chamber positioned too peripherally.

- Tightly collimate to the area of interest to reduce scatter radiation from the table or body that may cause the AEC to shut off prematurely.

For example, an AP thoracic vertebrae projection that has inadequate side-to-side collimation will demonstrate too much scatter through the lungs, hitting the AEC before the vertebrae can be adequately exposed.

- Do not use the AEC when the structures of interest are in close proximity to thicker structures and both will be situated above the activated ionization chamber.

For example, it is best not to use the AEC on an AP atlas and axis (open-mouthed) projection of the dens. With this examination, the upper incisors, occipital cranial base, and mandible add thickness to the areas superior and inferior to the dens and atlantoaxial joint. This added thickness causes the area of interest to be overexposed, because more time is needed for the capacitor to reach its maximum level as photons are absorbed in the thicker areas (Figure 1-81).

- Never use the AEC when any type of radiopaque hardware or prosthetic device will be positioned above the activated chamber(s). For these situations, use a manual technique.
- Make certain that no external radiopaque artifacts such as lead sheets or sandbags are positioned over the activated chamber(s).

Radiopaque materials, such as metal, lead sheets, or sandbags, have a much higher atomic number than that of the bony and soft tissue structures of the body. When a radiopaque material is situated within the activated chamber(s), the AEC will attempt to expose the radiopaque structure adequately, resulting in the anatomic structures being overexposed and a dark image (Figure 1-82).

Each activated ionization chamber measures the average amount of radiation striking the area it covers. The part of the chamber not covered with tissue will collect radiation so quickly that it will charge the capacitor to its maximum level, terminating the exposure before proper density has been reached, resulting in an underexposed light image (Figure 1-80).

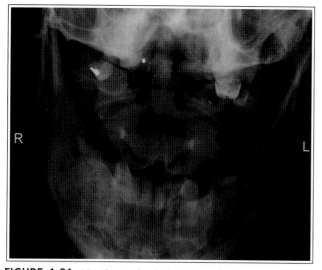

FIGURE 1-81 AP atlas and axis (open-mouthed) projection that was exposed using the center AEC chamber.

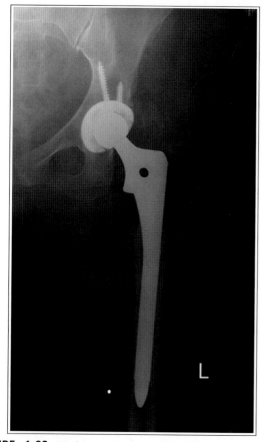

FIGURE 1-82 AP hip projection with radiopaque prosthesis exposed using the center AEC chamber.

• Use only the screen-film IR combination that the AEC's thyristor (device used to set the maximum capacitor charge) is calibrated to accommodate.

If a higher speed screen-film IR system is used with an AEC that is calibrated for a lower screen-film system, an

overexposed dark image will result; if a lower speed screen-film IR system is used with an AEC that is calibrated for a higher screen-film system, an underexposed light image will result. The AEC will not adjust for changes in receptor system speeds without the thyristor being recalibrated for the system.

• Density controls can temporarily be used when AEC equipment is out of calibration and to fine tune radiographic density when the anatomic structure of interest and activated chamber(s) are only slightly misaligned.

The density controls change the preset thyratron sensitivity so that the exposure time will be increased or decreased, adjusting radiographic density by the density control setting amount. Typical density control settings change the exposure level by increments of 25%, with the +1 and +2 buttons increasing the exposure and the −1 and −2 buttons decreasing the exposure. The 1 buttons will result in a 25% density change and the 2 buttons in a 50% density change. Some facilities have the AEC density controls set to obtain a 100% density increase and a 50% density decrease.

Correcting Poor Automatic Exposure Control Images. Tables 1-1 and 1-2 list reasons why an AEC image may have inadequate density. When an unacceptable AEC image is produced, the technologist needs to consider each potential cause to determine the correct adjustment to make before repeating the image. Many imaging units include an mAs readout display, on which the amount of mAs used for the image is shown after the exposure. In situations in which it is not advisable to repeat an unacceptable image using the AEC, the technologist can revert to a manual technique by using this readout to adjust the mAs to the value needed.

Source–Image Receptor Distance. Increasing the SID will decrease radiographic density. Decreasing the SID will increase density by the inverse square law, because the area through which the x-rays are distributed is spread out or condensed, respectively, with distance changes. It takes only a 20% change in SID for a visible density change to occur. When the technologist uses a manual technique and varies the SID from the standard, the mAs should be adjusted by using the direct square law ([new mAs]/[old mAs] = [new distance squared]/[old distance squared]), preventing an over- or underexposed image. Failure to make this adjustment may require the image to be repeated. If this occurs, leave the SID at the same setting and adjust the mAs the needed amount (see Tables 1-1 and 1-2).

Object–Image Receptor Distance. Although it is standard to maintain the lowest possible OID, there are situations in which increasing the OID is unavoidable. Increasing the OID may result in a noticeable density loss because of the reduction in the amount of scatter radiation detected by the IR when a portion of the scattered x-rays generated in the patient are scattered away from the IR. The amount of density loss will depend on the degree of OID increase and the amount of scatter that would typically reach the IR for such a procedure, which is determined by the kVp selected, field size, and patient thickness. As tube potentials are raised above 60 kVp, scatter radiation is directed in a more increasingly forward direction, so the image will demonstrate significant density loss as the OID is increased and the scatter is diverged away from the IR. With tube potentials below 60 kVp, there is a decrease in the number of scatter photons that are scattered in a forward direction, so an increase in OID will not result in a significant enough change in the amount of scatter reaching the IR or image density to be noticeable. A larger field size and body part thickness will affect the amount of scatter produced, with more production resulting in increased reduction of scatter reaching the IR as the OID increases. When the OID is increased, causing significant scatter radiation to be diverted from the IR, the mAs should be increased by about 10% for every centimeter of OID to compensate for the loss in density that such a change will cause.

Grids. When a grid is added or the technologist changes from one grid ratio to another, radiographic density will be inadequate unless the mAs is adjusted (see Table 1-2) to compensate for the resulting change in scatter radiation cleanup. When changing to a higher grid ratio, an increase in mAs is needed or insufficient radiographic density will result; when changing to a lower grid ratio, a decrease in mAs is needed or excessive radiographic density will be demonstrated.

Inadequate radiographic density will also be seen when the grid and central ray are misaligned, causing a decrease in the number of transmitted photons that reach the IR. The density decrease caused by grid cutoff can be distinguished from other density problems by the appearance of grid lines (small white lines) on the image where the cutoff is demonstrated. (See later, "Equipment-Related Artifacts," for examples of grid cutoff.)

Air-Gap Technique. An alternative to using a grid is to use the air-gap technique. To use the air-gap technique, move the IR 10 to 15 cm from the patient. The long OID will cause scatter radiation that would typically expose the IR at a short OID to scatter away from the IR. Because much of the scatter radiation is not being directed toward the IR, density is decreased and contrast is enhanced. When the air-gap technique is used, increase the mAs by about 10% for every centimeter of air gap. It is usually equivalent to using an 8:1 grid.

Screen-Film Receptor System Speed. Intensifying screens convert x-ray energy into light energy through fluorescence. The more light that is emitted for a given x-ray exposure, the greater is the relative speed value of the intensifying screen. Rare earth receptor systems are the most commonly used today and are defined with the descriptive names of extremity, medium speed,

regular speed, and high speed, with relative speeds of 80, 300, 400 and 800, respectively. When changing from one intensifying screen speed to another, a new mAs must be calculated because each relative speed value produces a different density or the image will be too dark or too light. Each screen has a conversion factor that is calculated by forming a fraction with 100 in the numerator and the relative speed value of the screen in the denominator. Then divide the numerator by the denominator; the decimal produced is the conversion factor (e.g., a rare earth screen at a relative speed value of 400 would have a conversion factor of 100/400 = 0.25). Tables 1-1 and 1-2 list the rare earth receptors conversion factors and the formula for calculating the new mAs when changing from one screen speed to another.

Collimation. An increase or decrease in the area exposed on the patient, as determined by collimation, changes the amount of scatter radiation produced and hence the amount of scatter reaching the IR and the overall radiographic density. The amount of density change will depend on the field size and the amount of scatter that would typically reach the IR for such a procedure, which is determined by the kVp selected and patient thickness (see earlier). The mAs needs to be changed to compensate for density changes when the collimation field size is changed and the part produces significant scatter radiation. If the field size is changed from a size that will cover a 14- × 17-inch IR to a size that will cover a 10- × 12-inch IR, the mAs should be increased by about 35%. If the change is to an 8- × 10-inch IR, the mAs should be increased by about 50%. Failure to make a mAs adjustment may result in an image with inadequate density.

Compensating Filter. With some examinations, when an exposure is set that will adequately demonstrate one structure of interest, other structures of interest are overexposed. This occurs because of the differences in thickness among the structures being imaged. AP projections of the shoulder, feet, and thoracic vertebrae are three examples that demonstrate this problem. To offset this thickness difference and obtain homogeneous density, place a compensating filter over or under the thinnest structures (Figure 1-83). A compensating filter absorbs x-ray photons before they reach the IR. The thicker part of the filter absorbs more photons than the thinner part. Set a technique that will adequately expose the thickest part being examined. If the filter has been accurately positioned, it will absorb the excessive radiation directed toward the thinnest structures, resulting in uniform image density throughout the image. Figures 1-84 and 1-85 show AP foot projections. The image in Figure 1-84 was taken without using a compensating filter, whereas the image in Figure 1-85 was taken with a compensating filter positioned over the distal metatarsals and phalangeal regions. Note the increased visibility of anatomic structures covered by the compensating filter.

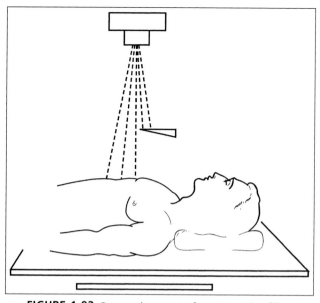

FIGURE 1-83 Proper placement of compensating filter.

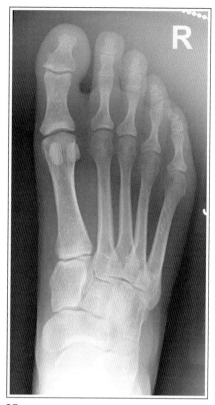

FIGURE 1-85 AP foot projection taken with compensating filter placed over toes.

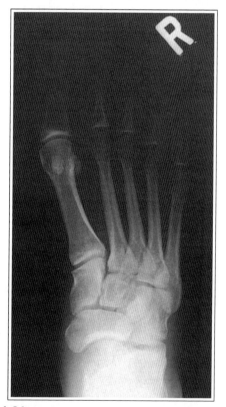

FIGURE 1-84 AP foot projection taken without compensating filter placed over toes.

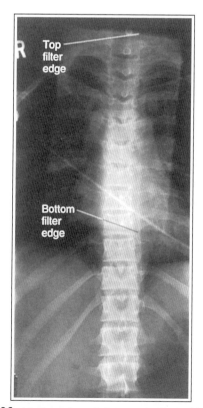

FIGURE 1-86 AP thoracic vertebrae projection with poor compensating filter placement.

If the compensating filter is inaccurately positioned, there will be a density variation defining where the filter was and was not placed over the structures (Figure 1-86). Having too much of the filter positioned over or under a structure that does not need it will result in too many of the photons being absorbed and too little radiographic density in the area.

Anode Heel Effect. Another exposure factor that should be considered when positioning long bones and the vertebral column, when a long 17-inch (43-cm) field length is used to accommodate the structure, is the anode heel effect. When this field length is used, a noticeable density variation occurs across the entire field size that is significant enough between the ends of the field that when they are compared, it can be seen. This density variation is a result of the greater photon absorption that occurs at the thicker "heel" portion of the anode compared with the thinner "toe" portion when a long field is used. Consequently, radiographic density at the anode end of the tube is lower because fewer photons emerge from that end of the tube than at the cathode end.

Using this knowledge to our advantage can help produce images of long bones and vertebral column that demonstrate uniform density at both ends. Position the thinner side of the structure at the anode end of the tube and the thicker side of the structure at the cathode end. Set an exposure (mAs) that will adequately demonstrate the midpoint of the structure (where the central ray is centered). Because the anode will absorb some of the photons aimed at the anode end of the IR and the thinnest structure, but not as many of the photons aimed at the cathode end and the thickest structure, a more uniform density across that part will be demonstrated (Figure 1-87). Table 1-4 provides guidelines for

TABLE 1-4	Guidelines for Positioning to Incorporate the Anode Heel Effect	
Projection(s)	**Placement of Anode**	**Placement of Cathode**
AP and lateral forearm	Wrist	Elbow
AP and lateral humerus	Elbow	Shoulder
AP and lateral lower leg	Ankle	Knee
AP and lateral femur	Knee	Hip
AP thoracic vertebrae	Cephalic	Caudal
AP lumbar vertebrae	Cephalic	Caudal

AP, Anteroposterior.

positioning structures to take advantage of the anode heel effect. Because the density variation between the ends of the IR is only approximately 30%, the anode heel effect will not adequately adjust for large thickness differences but will help improve images of the structures listed in Table 1-4.

Most imaging rooms are designed so that the patient's head is positioned on the technologist's left side (when facing the imaging table), placing the anode end of the x-ray tube at the head end of the patient. The placement of the anode end of the tube may vary in reference to the patient as the tube is moved into the horizontal position. To identify the anode and cathode ends of the x-ray tube, locate the + and − symbols attached to the tube housing where the electrical supply enters. The + symbol is used to identify the anode end of the tube and the − symbol indicates the cathode end (Figure 1-88).

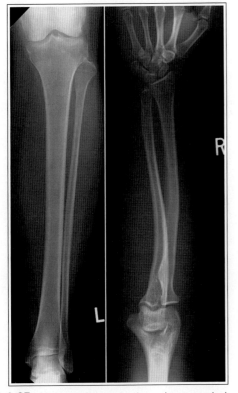

FIGURE 1-87 AP lower leg projection where anode heel effect was used properly (knee positioned at cathode end) and AP forearm projection where the anode heel effect was not used properly (wrist positioned at cathode end).

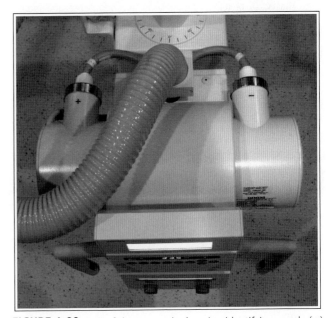

FIGURE 1-88 Top of the x-ray tube housing identifying anode (+) and cathode (−) ends of the x-ray tube.

Radiographic Contrast

Radiographic contrast is a visibility of detail factor that describes the difference between adjacent densities on an image. For an anatomic structure to be visualized on an image as a separate and distinct entity, it must exhibit a contrasting shade of black, white, or gray compared with the structures surrounding it. Images that display just a few gray shades and appear mostly black and white are considered to have a short contrast scale and images with many shades of gray and fewer blacks and whites are considered to have a long contrast scale.

Subject contrast plays a significant role in the production of radiographic contrast and is the contrast caused by the atomic density, atomic number, and thickness composition differences of the patient's body parts and how differently each tissue composition will absorb x-ray photons (differential absorption). Box 1-6 describes the different appearances of tissues on images.

Controlling Factor (Kilovoltage). The kVp is the factor that determines the energy of the x-ray photons produced and consequently the differential absorption that occurs in the patient's tissue as the photons traverse the body. High kVp produces high-energy photons that penetrate through body tissues, decreasing differential absorption and producing low-contrast (long-scale) images (Figure 1-94). Low kVp produces low-energy photons that are easily absorbed in the patient's tissues, increasing differential absorption and producing high-contrast (short-scale) images (Figure 1-95).

BOX 1-6	Subject Contrast Appearances on Images

- Patients who are in good physical shape, with strong muscles, low fat content, and dense bones, usually display the highest subject contrast (Figure 1-89).
- Patients whose bodies have deteriorated because of disease or age and obese patients will ordinarily display less subject contrast because their muscles have lost strength and have become the consistency of fat. On an image of this patient, subject contrast will be low because the densities representing fat and muscle will be more alike (Figure 1-90).
- Images of bony structures that have lost minerals and are less dense because of disease appear gray on images rather than white, blending in more with the surrounding structures and demonstrating reduced subject contrast (Figure 1-91).
- Patients who have retained fluid because of disease or injury display decreased subject contrast because the fluid surrounds the body tissues and causes their tissue densities to become more alike (Figure 1-92).
- The bones of infants and children are less dense and more porous than adult bones, resulting in less image contrast being demonstrated between the bone and soft tissue in children's images than on adults' images (Figure 1-93).

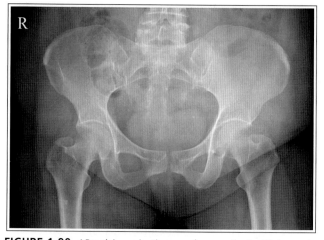

FIGURE 1-90 AP pelvic projection on obese patient with low subject contrast.

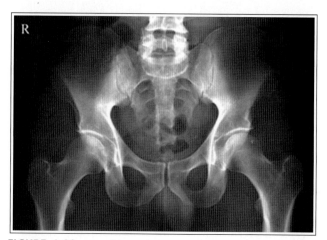

FIGURE 1-89 AP pelvic projection on patient with high subject contrast.

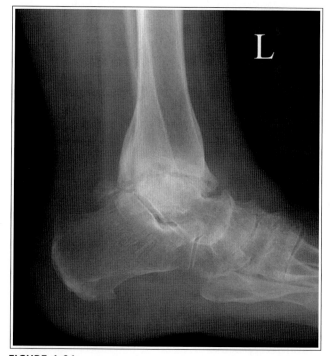

FIGURE 1-91 Lateral ankle projection demonstrating low subject contrast caused by a destructive disease.

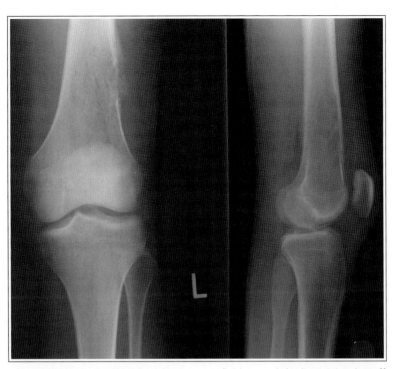

FIGURE 1-92 AP and lateral knee projections that demonstrate fluid around the knee joint that affects subject contrast.

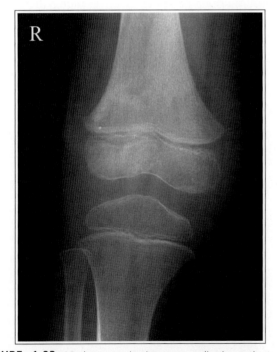

FIGURE 1-93 AP knee projection on pediatric patient that demonstrates low subject contrast.

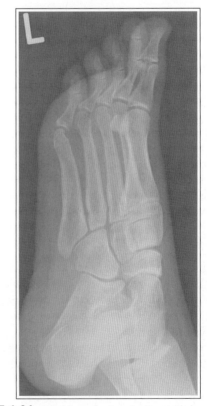

FIGURE 1-94 AP oblique foot projection with low contrast.

To obtain the desired level of radiographic contrast and gray scale, the technologist must evaluate the composition of the body part to be imaged and select a kVp level that will produce the appropriate differential absorption. Recommendations for the optimal kVp level to use for each body part can be found at the beginning of each procedural analysis chapter in this book. Optimal kVp is the kVp that will provide adequate body part penetration and sufficient image contrast.

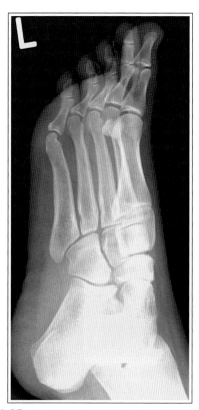

FIGURE 1-95 AP oblique foot projection with high contrast.

Adjusting Contrast With kVp Using the 15% Rule. Even when optimum kVp levels are used, there are different situations and patient conditions that occur in which this kVp level does not provide the best penetration or contrast. In these cases the kVp must be adjusted from the routinely used optimal level (see Table 1-3). In situations in which the density on the image is adequate but the contrast level is not sufficient to visualize all the anatomic structures adequately, the contrast level can be adjusted by varying the kVp and the density can be maintained by counteracting the kVp adjustment with a comparable mAs adjustment.

- If higher contrast is desired, decrease the original kVp used by 15% and increase the mAs value used by 100%. For example, if the original settings were 80 kVp at 10 mAs, the new settings would be 68 kVp at 20 mAs.
- If lower contrast is desired, increase the original kVp used by 15% and decrease the mAs value used by 50%. For example, if the original technique was 80 kVp at 10 mAs, the new technique would be 92 kVp at 5 mAs.

In both these situations the image density has remained the same as in the original image, because the density adjustment made with kVp is offset by an equal mAs adjustment. The amount of kVp adjustment depends on how dramatic a contrast change is desired. As a general rule, you should stay relatively close to the optimal kVp

level for the structure being imaged to prevent insufficient penetration or excessive image fogging.

Scatter Radiation. Radiographic contrast is also affected by the amount of scatter radiation that reaches the IR, which is determined by the kVp, field size, and patient thickness. Scatter radiation degrades the radiographic contrast by putting a blanket of density, also referred to as fog, over the image. The once individual and distinct gray shades of the image become blended with each other when fog is added to an image, resulting in a very gray low-contrast image. As the amount of scatter radiation reaching the IR increases, the greater is the decrease in radiographic contrast and decrease in detail visibility. Technologists can control the amount of scatter that reaches the IR and improve radiographic contrast by reducing the amount of tissue irradiated, decreasing the field size, and using a grid. The higher the grid ratio, the greater will be the scatter cleanup and the higher the radiographic contrast.

Flat contact shields made of lead can also be used to control the amount of scatter radiation that reaches the IR by eliminating scatter produced in the table from being scattered toward the area of interest. When the anatomic structures being examined demonstrate an excessive amount of scatter fogging along the outside of the collimated borders (e.g., the lateral lumbar vertebrae), place a large, flat contact shield or the straight edge of a lead apron along the appropriate border. This greatly improves the visibility of the recorded details. Compare the lateral lumbar vertebral projections in Figure 1-96 and Figure 1-97. Figure 1-96 was

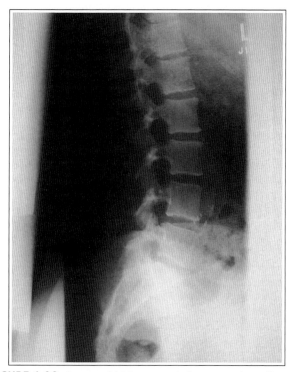

FIGURE 1-96 Contact shield was used along posterior collimated border.

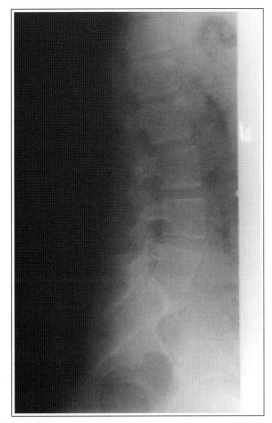

FIGURE 1-97 Contact shield was not used along posterior collimated border.

taken with a lead contact shield placed against the posterior edge of the collimator's light field, but a contact shield was not used for Figure 1-97. Note the improvement in visualization of the lumbar spinous processes using a contact shield.

Artifacts

An artifact is any undesirable structure or substance recorded on an image. They may be grouped into several categories: (1) anatomic structures that obscure the area of interest or have no purpose for being there and can be removed from the image; (2) externally removable objects, such as patient or hospital possessions; (3) internal objects, such as prostheses or monitoring lines; and (4) appearances that result from improper use of equipment.

Before an image is taken, it may be wise to have the patient change into a hospital gown and to ask whether any patient belongings are in or around the area being imaged. Patients are often nervous and may forget to remove articles of clothing or, for sentimental reasons they may not remove jewelry, so you should recheck the area of interest, even after the patient has changed into a gown. Once the patient is positioned and the IR is ready to be exposed, take a last look to make sure that all hospital possessions that can be moved out of the imaging field have been moved. Check that those items

that must remain in the field, such as heart monitoring leads, have been shifted so that they will superimpose the least amount of information.

It would be impossible to delineate in this book all the possible artifacts that can appear on an image, but it is important for technologists to familiarize themselves with as many artifacts as possible. It might be wise for your department to keep a folder of images that had to be repeated because of artifacts. These can be studied occasionally to help keep all technologists updated on the possibilities for facility-related artifacts.

Most possession-related artifacts are demonstrated on the image as lighter densities than the anatomic structures that surround them. Artifacts that are related to poor film or phosphor plate handling, such as film creases, static, and light leaks, most often exhibit greater density. The following discussion concerns different categories of image artifacts and common examples of each.

Anatomic Artifacts. An anatomic artifact is any anatomic structure that is within the image that could have been removed. These include those that are superimposed over an area of interest, as well as those that are not superimposed over an area of interest but are still located within the collimated field and could easily have been excluded. A common anatomic artifact is the patient's own hand or arm. Figure 1-98 shows an AP abdomen projection obtained in the supine position in which the patient's hands are superimposed over the upper abdominal region. More than likely the patient was not positioned in this manner when the technologist left the room. After the

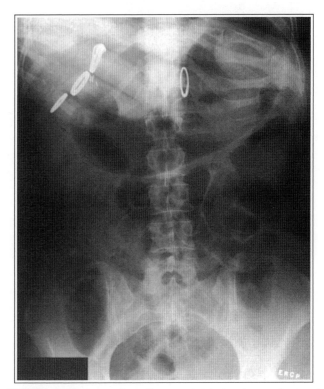

FIGURE 1-98 Anatomic artifact—patient's hands superimposed on AP abdomen projection.

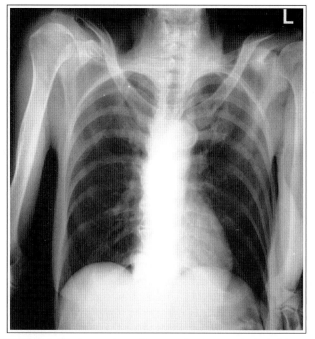

FIGURE 1-99 Anatomic artifact—patient's arms included in AP chest projection.

technologist positioned the patient and before the exposure was taken, however, the patient found a more comfortable position. This example stresses the importance of explaining examinations to patients so that they understand how important it is for them to remain in the position in which the technologist placed them. This also shows the importance of rechecking each patient's position before the exposure is taken if much time has elapsed between positioning the patient and exposing the image. It is also not uncommon for a patient who is experiencing hip or lower back pain from lying on the imaging table to place a hand beneath an affected hip. This will result in superimposition of the hip and hand on the image. Remember, the patient does not know that repositioning because of discomfort is not acceptable. Figure 1-99 shows an AP chest projection produced with a mobile x-ray machine, which was taken with the patient's arms positioned tightly against the sides. Because humeri are not evaluated on a chest image, there is no reason for them to be included, and they could easily have been shifted out of the imaging field.

Double-Exposure Artifacts. A double-exposed image occurs when two exposures are taken on the same IR without processing having been done between them. The images exposed on the IR can be totally different and easy to identify, such as AP and lateral lumbar vertebrae projections (Figure 1-100), or they may be the same image, with almost identical overlap. Double-exposures of images of the same procedure typically appear blurry and can easily be mistaken for patient motion (Figure 1-101). When evaluating a blurry image,

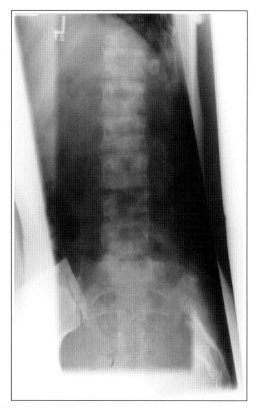

FIGURE 1-100 Screen-film double-exposure (AP and lateral vertebral projections).

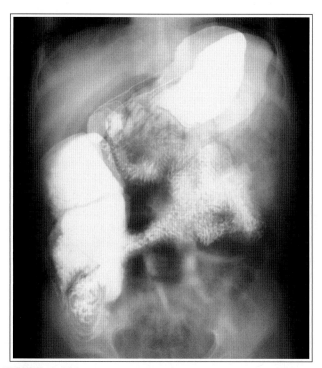

FIGURE 1-101 Screen-film double-exposure (two AP abdomen projections with barium in stomach and intestines).

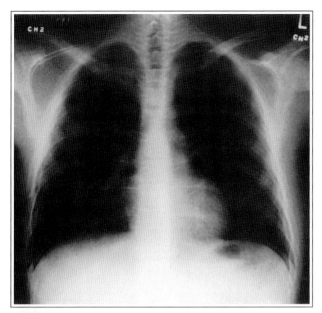

FIGURE 1-102 Screen-film double exposure (two PA chest projections).

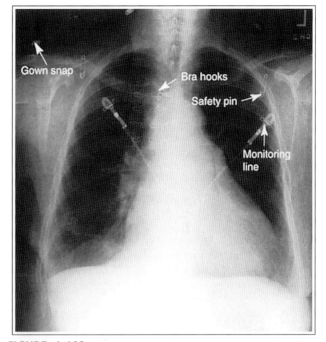

FIGURE 1-103 AP chest projection showing external artifacts from patient clothing and hospital monitoring equipment.

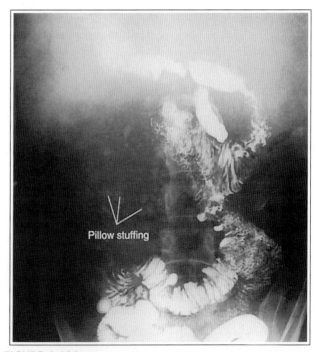

FIGURE 1-104 AP abdomen projection showing an external artifact from a pillow.

look at the cortical outlines of bony structures that are lying longitudinally and transversely:

- Is there only one cortical outline to represent each bony structure, or are there two?
- Is one outline lying slightly above or to the side of the other?

If one outline is demonstrated, the patient moved during the exposure, but if two are demonstrated, the image was exposed twice and the patient was in a slightly different position for the second exposure. Another indication of a double-exposed image in conventional radiography is its density (Figure 1-102). When the screen-film system is used, a double-exposed image will result in high image density because the film was exposed to radiation twice.

External Artifacts. An external artifact is found outside the patient's body, such as a patient's possession that remained in a pocket or a hospital possession (e.g., needle cap, ice bag) that was lying on top of or beneath the patient. Common external artifacts include earrings, rings, necklaces, bra hooks, dental structures, hairpins, heart monitoring lines, and gown snaps (Figure 1-103). Two external artifacts that are not as common but that do occasionally appear are caused by pillows (Figure 1-104) and by the imprinted designs on shirts and pants (Figure 1-105). Most of these artifacts can easily be avoided with proper patient preparation and positioning. Being aware of as many objects as possible that can create artifacts on the image is the best way of preventing them.

Internal Artifacts. Internal artifacts are found within the patient. They cannot be removed and must be accepted. Examples of commonly seen internal artifacts

are the prosthesis (Figures 1-105 and 1-106), pacemaker (Figure 3-16), central venous catheter (Figures 3-12 and 3-13), pleural drainage tube (Figures 1-107 and 3-11), and endotracheal tube (Figure 3-9).

If an artifact that is normally not found within the body is identified on an image, it is the technologist's duty to discretely search and interview the patient or to consult the ordering physician to determine whether

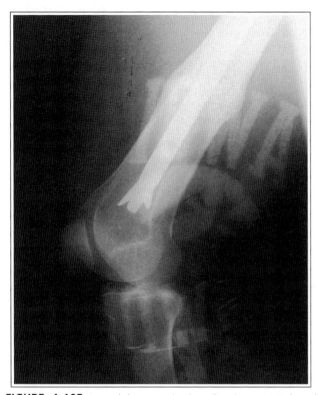

FIGURE 1-105 Lateral knee projection showing external and internal artifacts caused by imprint of patient clothing and leg prosthesis.

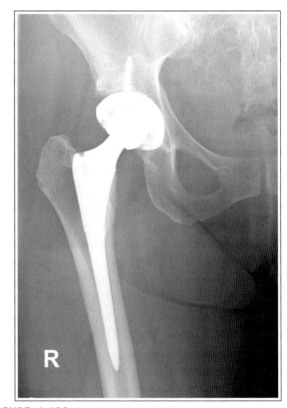

FIGURE 1-106 AP hip projection showing an internal artifact caused by prosthesis.

the artifact can be located outside the patient's body. If it is not found, it may have been introduced into the patient through one of the body orifices. Your search and interview discoveries should be recorded on the patient's requisition. Figure 1-108 shows a pelvic image of a patient who had swallowed several batteries.

Equipment-Related Artifacts. Equipment-related artifacts are caused by improper use of the imaging equipment.

Grid Alignment Artifacts. Grid alignment artifacts are grid lines that result from the use of stationary grids and the improper use of all grid types. They occur because the grid's lead strips absorb primary radiation

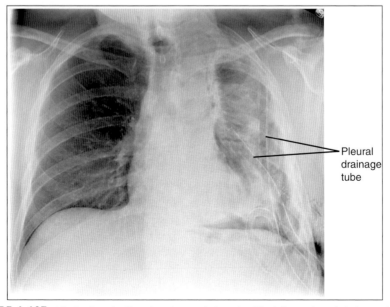

Pleural drainage tube

FIGURE 1-107 AP chest projection showing an internal artifact (two pleural drainage tubes).

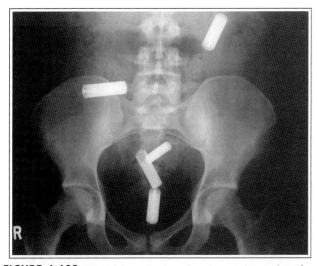

FIGURE 1-108 AP pelvis projection showing an internal artifact (five swallowed batteries).

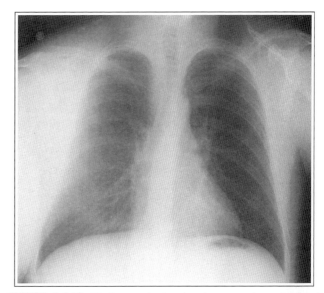

FIGURE 1-110 AP chest projection showing an equipment-related artifact. Parallel grid was tilted or the central ray was angled toward the grid's lead strips.

and are visible as small white lines on the image. Grid line artifacts caused by improper grid alignment are more noticeable with higher ratio grids and can be avoided by choosing a moving grid whenever possible and by properly aligning the central ray and grid.

Causes of grid cut-off include the following:

- If a parallel grid was tilted (off level) or the central ray was angled toward the grid's lead strips, the image demonstrates grid lines on the side toward which the central ray was angled (Figures 1-109, *A*, and 1-110).
- If a parallel or focused grid was off focus (taken at an SID outside focusing range), the image demonstrates grid lines on each side of the image (Figure 1-111; see Figure 1-109, *B*).

- If a focused grid was tilted (off level) or the central ray was angled toward the grid's lead strips, the image demonstrates grid lines across the entire image (Figure 1-112; see Figure 1-109, *C*).
- If a focused grid was upside down, the image demonstrates grid lines on each side of the image (Figure 1-113; see Figure 1-109, *D*).
- If a focused grid was off center (central ray not centered on the center of the grid), the image demonstrates grid lines across the entire image (Figure 1-114; see Figure 1-109, *E*). If the image was

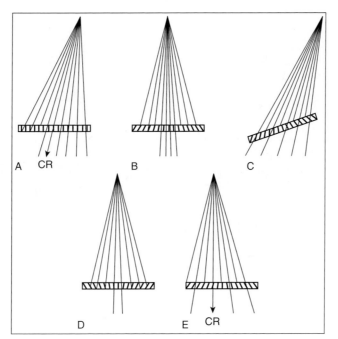

FIGURE 1-109 Causes of grid cutoff. **A,** Central ray angled against grid's lead lines. **B,** Off focus. **C,** Off level. **D,** Inverted. **E,** Off center.

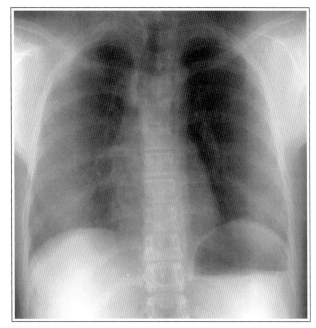

FIGURE 1-111 AP chest projection showing an equipment-related artifact. Off-focused grid cutoff.

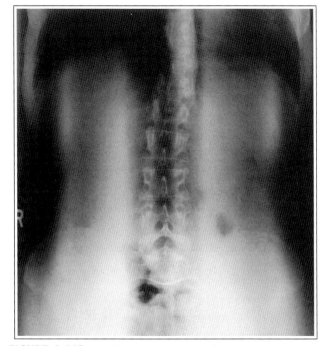

FIGURE 1-113 AP abdomen projection showing an equipment-related artifact. Focused grid was inverted.

taken with the table Bucky, the image will not be in the center of the IR but will be demonstrated to one side.

When conventional screen-film radiography is used, an image taken with a grid alignment artifact demonstrates a loss in density where the grid lines are shown.

The degree of density loss will be greater on the side toward which the central ray is angled and will increase with increased severity of misalignment. Density loss will also be greater when higher grid ratios are used.

Film Handling and Processing Artifacts. Improper film handling and processing can cause artifacts such as

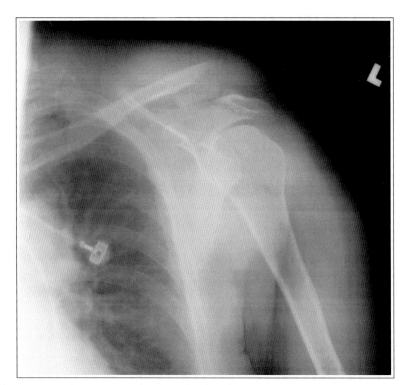

FIGURE 1-112 AP shoulder projection showing an equipment-related artifact. Focused grid was tilted or the central ray was angled toward the grid's lead strips.

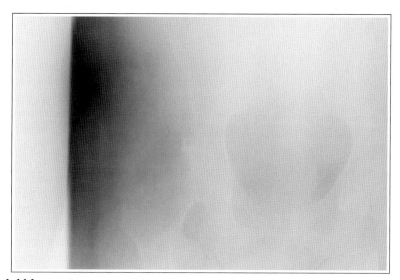

FIGURE 1-114 AP pelvis projection showing an equipment-related artifact. Off-centered grid cutoff.

film creases, static (Figure 1-115), fog, stains, scratches (Figure 1-116), and hesitation marks (Figure 1-117). They can be avoided by following a good quality control program for the darkroom, film storage, and processor.

Locating and Repeating for Artifacts. Whenever an external or unidentifiable internal artifact is demonstrated on an image, discretely examine and interview the patient to determine the artifact's location. To pinpoint where to look for the artifact, study the image to locate a palpable anatomic structure situated close to the artifact. This is the area where the search should begin.

If an artifact that can be eliminated obscures any portion of the area of interest, the image needs to be repeated. A gown snap superimposed on an area of the lungs on a chest image can easily obscure a small lesion. A ring can easily obscure a hairline finger fracture.

If the artifact is located outside the field of interest, the image does not need to be repeated, although the patient should be discretely examined and interviewed to determine whether the artifact is located externally or internally.

Postprocedure Requirements

One of the last steps to take before deciding whether an image is acceptable is to make sure that you have taken all the images that are recommended by your facility for the body part being imaged. For example, many facilities require that AP and lateral projections are taken whenever images of the knee are requested. This series of images provides the reviewer with the needed information to accurately evaluate the patient's knee.

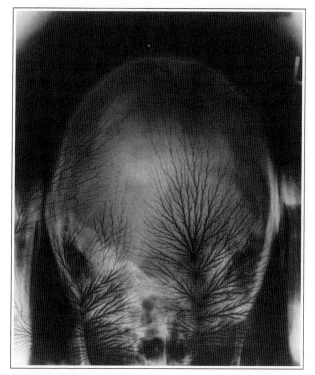

FIGURE 1-115 AP axial (Towne method) cranium projection showing a film-handling artifact—static.

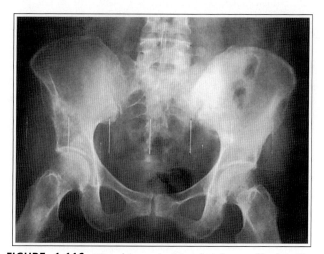

FIGURE 1-116 AP pelvis projection showing a film-handling artifact—scratches.

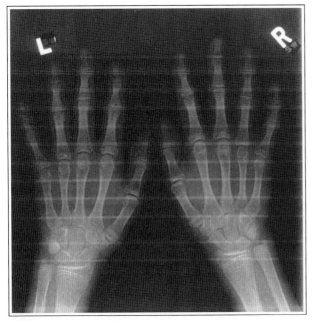

FIGURE 1-117 PA hand projection showing film-handling artifact—hesitation marks.

Not only should the entire series be taken, but you should also determine whether the indication for the examination has been fulfilled. If an elbow examination is ordered and the indication for the examination was to evaluate or rule out a radial head fracture, an additional external AP oblique or axiolateral (Coyle method) projection of the elbow may be needed to rule out this fracture definitively. Consult with the reviewer before allowing the patient to leave the imaging department.

Completing the Requisition Form. These are the sections of the requisition form that should be completed by the technologist: (1) the number and sizes of films that were used during conventional screen-film radiography; (2) the number of images obtained during digital imaging; (3) the mAs, kVp, and distance used; (4) the room number where the images were taken; (5) the technologist's name; (6) the date and time of the procedure; and (7) any additional patient history obtained from the patient-technologist interview (Figure 1-118).

Recording the number and sizes of films or images obtained on the requisition form tells the reviewer how many images are to be evaluated. The name(s) of the technologist(s) involved in the examination is valuable information if a question arises about the image or patient or if the patient is found to have a contagious disease and measures need to be taken to protect the technologist(s). Recording the same date and time of the procedure on the requisition form as are shown on the image, as well as double-checking that the name of the patient is correct, provides a means of verifying that the requisition form goes with a certain set of images.

The patient's history should be completed by the ordering physician before the requisition form arrives in the imaging facility; any information that the technologist has learned from interviewing and observing the patient that might assist the reviewer in the diagnosis should be added, however. This area of the form may also be used to note any situation necessitating departure from the routine examination procedure. For example, if a hand image was taken with the patient's ring still on the finger because the ring could not be removed, the technologist should record this fact in the patient history or notes section of the requisition form so that the reviewer understands why the ring appears on the image.

Repeat-Reject Analysis. The facility's repeat or reject analysis card, an example of which is shown in Figure 1-119, should be filled out to indicate any positioning or technical errors that occurred during the procedure. This information provides your facility with a means of distinguishing areas in which patient service can be improved through in-service personnel training or equipment repair.

Defining Image Acceptability. When an image meets all the necessary requirements, it is considered an optimal image and it should not be repeated. When an image is not optimal but may be acceptable, the question arises as to whether it is poor enough to repeat or whether the information needed can be obtained without exposing the patient to further radiation. Factors that should be considered when making this decision include the following:

- Your facility's standards
- The age and condition of the patient
- The conditions under which the patient was imaged
- Whether obvious pathology is evident
- Whether the indications for the examination have been fulfilled

Each facility has its own standards that will determine whether an image should be repeated. If standards are low, improving imaging skills can raise them, thereby increasing the accuracy of diagnosis. The age and condition of the patient, as well as the conditions under which the patient was imaged, are most important in the decision to repeat an image. Sometimes a less than optimal image must be accepted because repeating the image is impossible, as in a surgery case; at other times, the patient cannot or will not cooperate. Whenever an examination is accepted that does not meet optimal standards, record on the requisition form any information about the patient's condition or situation that resulted in acceptance of this examination. A less than optimal image may also be passed when the indication for the examination is clearly fulfilled by the images obtained. For example, a lower leg examination is taken without the required knee joint when the patient history states that the patient has had a distal fibular fracture and the indication for the examination is to evaluate the healing of the distal fibular fracture. In this case, it is obvious that the patient's knee is not being evaluated. As long as the distal fibula is included in its entirety on the original image, the image should not be repeated.

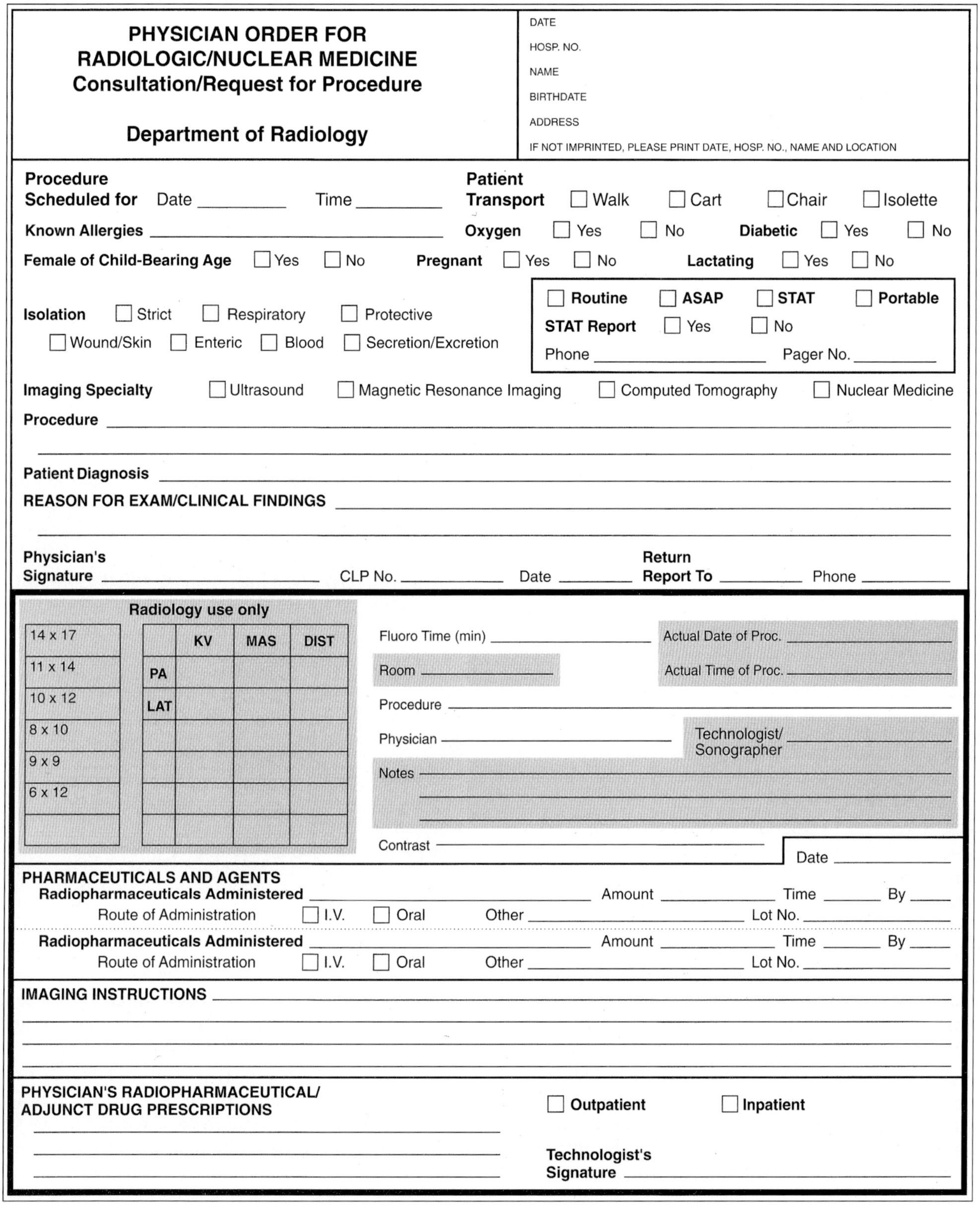

**PHYSICIAN ORDER FOR
RADIOLOGIC/NUCLEAR MEDICINE
Consultation/Request for Procedure**

Department of Radiology

DATE

HOSP. NO.

NAME

BIRTHDATE

ADDRESS

IF NOT IMPRINTED, PLEASE PRINT DATE, HOSP. NO., NAME AND LOCATION

**Procedure
Scheduled for**   Date _____   Time _____

Known Allergies _____

Female of Child-Bearing Age   ☐ Yes   ☐ No

**Patient
Transport**   ☐ Walk   ☐ Cart   ☐ Chair   ☐ Isolette

Oxygen   ☐ Yes   ☐ No   **Diabetic**   ☐ Yes   ☐ No

Pregnant   ☐ Yes   ☐ No   **Lactating**   ☐ Yes   ☐ No

Isolation   ☐ Strict   ☐ Respiratory   ☐ Protective
☐ Wound/Skin   ☐ Enteric   ☐ Blood   ☐ Secretion/Excretion

☐ **Routine**   ☐ **ASAP**   ☐ **STAT**   ☐ **Portable**
STAT Report   ☐ Yes   ☐ No
Phone _____   Pager No. _____

Imaging Specialty   ☐ Ultrasound   ☐ Magnetic Resonance Imaging   ☐ Computed Tomography   ☐ Nuclear Medicine

Procedure _____
_____

Patient Diagnosis _____

REASON FOR EXAM/CLINICAL FINDINGS _____

**Physician's
Signature** _____   CLP No. _____   Date _____   **Return
Report To** _____   Phone _____

Radiology use only

14 x 17		KV	MAS	DIST
11 x 14	PA			
10 x 12	LAT			
8 x 10				
9 x 9				
6 x 12				

Fluoro Time (min) _____

Room _____

Procedure _____

Physician _____

Notes _____

Actual Date of Proc. _____

Actual Time of Proc. _____

Technologist/
Sonographer _____

Contrast _____   Date _____

PHARMACEUTICALS AND AGENTS
  Radiopharmaceuticals Administered _____   Amount _____   Time _____ By ____
    Route of Administration   ☐ I.V.   ☐ Oral   Other _____   Lot No. _____
  Radiopharmaceuticals Administered _____   Amount _____   Time _____ By ____
    Route of Administration   ☐ I.V.   ☐ Oral   Other _____   Lot No. _____

IMAGING INSTRUCTIONS _____
_____
_____
_____

**PHYSICIAN'S RADIOPHARMACEUTICAL/
ADJUNCT DRUG PRESCRIPTIONS**

☐ **Outpatient**   ☐ **Inpatient**

_____

_____

**Technologist's
Signature** _____

FIGURE 1-118 The requisition form. The areas to be filled out by the technologist are shaded. *(Courtesy of the University of Iowa Hospital and Clinics, Iowa City, Iowa.)*

It is important that all unacceptable images and those less than optimal images that have been accepted are studied carefully to determine whether the situation(s) that caused them could be eliminated on future examinations. When an image is repeated, the overall radiation dose to the patient increases and the cost of patient care rises because reimaging requires more technologist time, supplies, and equipment use.

# OF EXAM FILMS	OVE	UNE	POS	PRO	ART	FOG	MOT	EQF	OTH
04 X 05	[ ]	[ ]	[ ]	[ ]	[ ]	[ ]	[ ]	[ ]	[ ]
06 X 12	[ ]	[ ]	[ ]	[ ]	[ ]	[ ]	[ ]	[ ]	[ ]
08 X 10	[ ]	[ ]	[ ]	[ ]	[ ]	[ ]	[ ]	[ ]	[ ]
09 X 09	[ ]	[ ]	[ ]	[ ]	[ ]	[ ]	[ ]	[ ]	[ ]
10 X 12	[ ]	[ ]	[ ]	[ ]	[ ]	[ ]	[ ]	[ ]	[ ]
11 X 14	[ ]	[ ]	[ ]	[ ]	[ ]	[ ]	[ ]	[ ]	[ ]
14 X 14	[ ]	[ ]	[ ]	[ ]	[ ]	[ ]	[ ]	[ ]	[ ]
14 X 17	[ ]	[ ]	[ ]	[ ]	[ ]	[ ]	[ ]	[ ]	[ ]
14 X 36	[ ]	[ ]	[ ]	[ ]	[ ]	[ ]	[ ]	[ ]	[ ]
14 X 51	[ ]	[ ]	[ ]	[ ]	[ ]	[ ]	[ ]	[ ]	[ ]
OTHER	[ ]	[ ]	[ ]	[ ]	[ ]	[ ]	[ ]	[ ]	[ ]

FIGURE 1-119 Example of a repeat or reject analysis card. ART, Artifact; EQF, equipment failure; FOG, film fog; MOT, patient motion; OTH, other; OVE, overexposure; POS, error in patient positioning; UNE, underexposure. *(Courtesy of the University of Iowa Hospital and Clinics, Iowa City, Iowa.)*

SPECIAL IMAGING SITUATIONS

Mobile and Trauma Imaging

The goal of mobile and trauma imaging is the same as that of routine imaging—to demonstrate accurate relationships among the anatomic structures for the projection imaged, without causing further patient injury and with minimal discomfort. The following are general guidelines for obtaining this goal.

1. Based on the requisition or request form, determine the projections that will be needed and the order in which they will be completed. First, obtain the projections that will provide information about the most life-threatening condition (cross-table lateral cervical vertebrae projection if a cervical fracture is questioned or when obtaining an AP chest projection for a patient having difficulty breathing). Speed is of the essence in many mobile and trauma situations, because the patient can be quite ill. Having a thought-out plan of action before starting allows the technologist to work in an organized and speedy manner. As a general rule, after the initial projections associated with life-threatening conditions have been exposed and checked by the radiologist or physician, the remaining projections are exposed in an order that will require the least amount of central ray adjustment. All AP projections are exposed, and then the central ray is moved horizontally for the lateral projections.

   It is important that projections be obtained that are at 90-degree angles from each other (AP-PA and lateral) when fractures and foreign bodies are suspected to determine the degree of bone displacement (Figure 1-120) and depth location.

2. Gather and organize the supplies (e.g., IRs, IR holders, positioning aides, disposable gloves, radiation protection supplies) that will be needed, and determine the

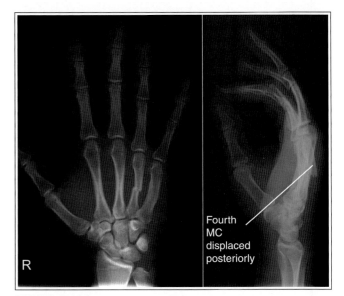

FIGURE 1-120 PA and lateral hand projections showing posterior displacement of the fourth metacarpal *(MC)* caused by a fracture.

starting technical factors (kVp, mAs, AEC) for the needed images. Cover the positioning aids and IRs to protect them from contamination.

3. Determine the degree of patient mobility, alertness, and ability to follow requests. Can the patient be placed in a seated position or be rotated to one side? Can the arm or leg fully extend or flex? When the patient is asked to breathe deeply, can he or she follow the request? Can the patient control movement?

4. Assess the site of interest for physical signs of injury (swelling, bruising, deformity, pain). Understanding the degree of injury will help the technologist prevent further injury during the positioning process.

5. Determine whether positioning devices (e.g., slings, backboards, and casts) and artifacts (e.g., heart leads, clothing, jewelry) may be removed and, if not, whether they will obscure the area of interest

on the ordered projections. If positioning devices or artifacts will obscure the area, consult with the radiologist or ordering physician about possible alternatives (e.g., taking a slight oblique instead of a true projection).

6. Set an optimal kVp and mAs or AEC for the anatomic structure and projection being imaged. Technical adjustments may also be needed as a result of the increase in absorption that may occur because of the positioning device or artifact. Either increase (+) or decrease (–) the kVp or mAs from the routine amount for the patient thickness measurement, as indicated in Table 1-5.

7. Obtain the requested images. The technologist should use the routine positioning guidelines such as for patient positioning, central ray centering, IR size, and collimation when obtaining mobile and trauma projections. For patients who are unable to follow the routine positioning requirements, adaptations to this setup can be made. Never force the patient into a position. Instead, adjust the central ray and IR. As long as the central ray, part, and IR form the same alignments, identical projections will result. The word *part* with regard to alignment refers to the specific plane, imaginary line, or anatomic structure used to position the patient with the central ray and IR in routine positioning.

GUIDELINES FOR ALIGNING CENTRAL RAY, PART, AND IMAGE RECEPTOR

• Whenever possible, set up the routinely used central ray, part, and IR alignments for the projection imaged.

Lateral Projections. Routine lateral foot projections require that the foot's lateral surface be aligned parallel to the IR and the central ray be aligned perpendicular to the part and the IR. In this situation the lateral foot

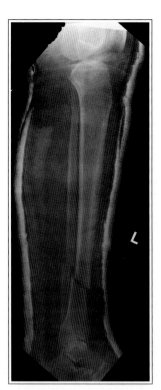

FIGURE 1-121 Lateral lower leg projection with fiberglass cast.

surface is the part, because this is what is used to position the foot in relation to the central ray and IR. If the lateral foot projection is taken on the imaging table, the patient will externally rotate his or her leg until the lateral foot surface is parallel to the IR, and the central ray will be aligned perpendicular to the IR and part (Figure 1-123).

If the lateral foot projection is taken in a standing position, the IR will be positioned vertically and the central ray horizontally. Even though the setup appears different, the central ray, part, and IR alignments are the same as in the previous setup. The lateral foot surface is positioned parallel to the IR, and the central ray is perpendicular to the IR and lateral foot surface. Often,

TABLE 1-5	Technical Adjustments for Trauma Patients		
Immobilization Device or Patient Condition		**kVp Adjustment**	**mAs Adjustment**
Small to medium plaster cast		+5–7 kVp	+50%- 60%
Large plaster cast		+8–10 kVp	+100%
Fiberglass cast (Figure 1-121)		No adjustment	No adjustment
Inflated air splint		No adjustment	No adjustment
Wood backboard (Figure 1-122)		+5 kVp	+25%- 30%
Ascites (accumulation of fluid in abdomen or swelled joint) (Figure 1-92)			+50%- 75%
Pleural effusion (fluid in pleural cavity)			+35%
Pneumothorax (air or gas in pleural cavity)		-8% kVp	
Postmortem imaging of head, thorax, and abdomen (because of pooling of blood and fluid)			+35%-50%
Soft tissue injury (used for foreign objects, such as slivers of wood, glass, or metal, embedded in the soft tissue and to demonstrate the upper airway)		-15% - 20% kVp	

kVp, Kilovoltage peak.

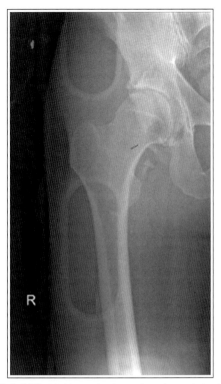

FIGURE 1-122 AP hip projection taken through backboard.

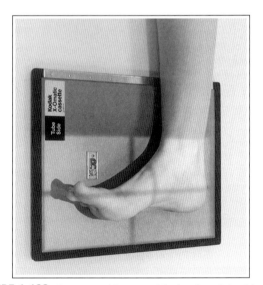

FIGURE 1-123 Accurate tabletop positioning for a lateral (mediolateral) foot projection.

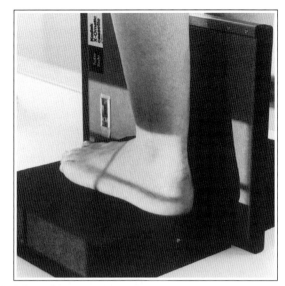

FIGURE 1-124 Accurate standing positioning for a lateral (lateromedial) foot projection.

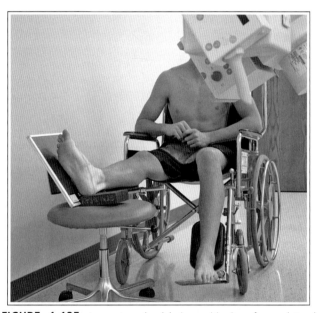

FIGURE 1-125 Accurate wheelchair positioning for a lateral (mediolateral) foot projection.

when a cross-table image is created, the projection taken is opposite. For a routine tabletop lateral foot projection, a mediolateral projection is performed, whereas a lateromedial projection is used for cross-table images. To obtain identical images for both pathways, the technologist must maintain the same central ray, part, and IR alignment. This means that the lateral surface of the foot must still be positioned parallel to the IR for a lateromedial projection, even if this surface is not placed directly adjacent to the IR. For a lateral foot projection,

this will require the medial aspect of the heel to be positioned slightly away from the IR (Figure 1-124).

If a patient arrives in the radiology department in a wheelchair and is unable to move to the imaging table for the lateral foot projection easily, the projection can be obtained with the patient remaining in the wheelchair. First, align the lateral foot surface with the IR and then align the central ray perpendicular to the IR and lateral foot surface. Again, because the relationships among the central ray, IR, and part are the same as in the two previous setups, the resulting image will be identical (Figure 1-125).

Oblique Projections. For trauma oblique images, begin by aligning the central ray with the plane, line, or anatomic structure that is used for an AP projection of the part being imaged. Next, adjust the central ray in the direction needed to set up the correct alignment between the central ray and structure. Because the degree of angulation in which patients are rotated for oblique projections is always referenced from the AP-PA projection, the amount of angle adjustment would be the same as the required degree of obliquity. For a routine internal AP oblique elbow projection, the central ray is aligned at a 45-degree angle with an imaginary line connecting the humeral epicondyles (the medial epicondyle is placed farther from the tube than the lateral). To obtain the same image in a patient who is unable to rotate his or her arm, the technologist first positions the central ray perpendicular to the line connecting the epicondyles and then adjusts the angle 45 degrees medially, positioning the medial epicondyle farther from the x-ray tube than the lateral epicondyle. The IR would then be angled so that it is perpendicular to the central ray (Figure 1-126).

- To obtain open joint spaces, clearly see fracture lines, or obtain specific anatomic relationships, the alignment of the central ray with the part must be accurate. This is more important than the alignment of the central ray or part with the IR.

When an open joint space or a particular anatomic relationship is required, it is the central ray alignment with the part that accomplishes the required results. Although IR alignment with the central ray and part is important to prevent distortion, it does not have an effect on the anatomic relationships that are demonstrated. After the central ray and part are accurately aligned, the IR should be positioned as close to perpendicular to the central ray as possible. If the central ray is not positioned perpendicular to the IR, the resulting image will demonstrate elongation in the direction toward which the central ray was angled, but the anatomic alignment of the structures should be demonstrated as required for the projection. The more acute the central ray and IR angle, the greater will be the elongation. In this situation, the IR will need to be offset from side to side or cephalocaudally in the direction toward which the central ray is angled more than what would occur if the IR were positioned perpendicular to the CR. Because of this offset, careful attention should be given to centering the central ray to the center of the IR.

- When imaging long bones the IR should be positioned as close to parallel with it as possible. If the bone and IR are not parallel, the law of isometry should be used to minimize shape distortion.

The law of isometry indicates that the central ray should be set at half of the angle formed between the object and IR to minimize shape distortion. If the patient's knee cannot be fully extended for an AP femur projection, causing the femur to be at a 30-degree angle with the IR, the central ray should be angled 15 degrees. The direction of the angle should be such that it brings the central ray closer to perpendicular with the IR (Figure 1-127).

- When imaging long bones that require both joints to be included on the same image, but the joints cannot be positioned in the true projection simultaneously because of a fracture, the joint closest to the fracture should be positioned in the true projection (Figure 1-128).

8. Use the smallest possible OID and increase the SID to compensate if a longer than routine OID is needed.

9. Use a grid if the patient part thickness is over 4 inches (10 cm) and over 60 kVp is used. When positioning latitude is narrow because of the patient's condition or when the mobile unit is used, choose a linear low-ratio grid to allow for the greatest positioning error latitude. Evaluate the alignment of the central ray and grid:

   - Is the central ray aligned accurately with the center of the grid?
   - If a central ray angle is used, is it angled with the grid lines?
   - Is the grid level?
   - Is the SID within the grid's focusing range?
   - Is the correct side of the grid facing the central ray?

10. Use good radiation protection practices. Ask female patients if there is any chance they could be pregnant. Never assume that other staff members have asked. Use gonadal shielding whenever possible, collimate tightly, and provide those assisting with patient holding during the exposure with aprons and lead gloves. Images of the extremity should

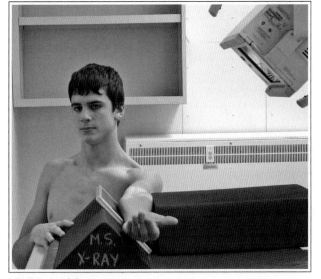

FIGURE 1-126 Accurate trauma positioning for an internal AP oblique elbow projection.

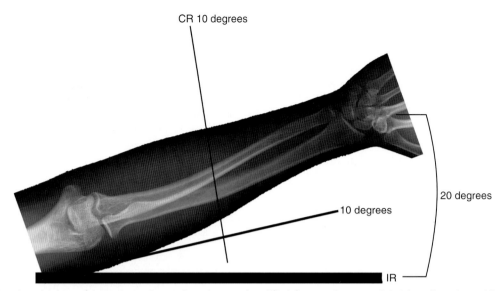

FIGURE 1-127 Using the law of isometry to image long bones. *(Modified from Holt MH. Minimizing distortion with geometry,* Radiol Technol *78:436–436, 2007.)*

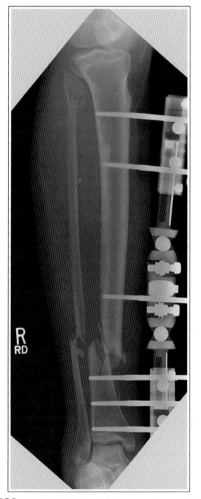

FIGURE 1-128 Trauma AP lower leg projection with joint closest to fracture demonstrating accurate positioning.

not be taken by placing the IR and part on the patient's torso unless it is the only means of obtaining accurate positioning. If this is the case, always place a lead apron between the IR and torso. Not all the radiation directed toward the IR is absorbed; high-energy beams will exit through the back of the IR, exposing structures beneath.

11. Never leave a confused patient or a trauma patient unattended in the imaging room.

12. Process the images and evaluate them for positioning and technical accuracy. Determine whether repeat images are needed and how much adjustment will be required. When the trauma is severe, all the evaluating criteria listed in the procedural sections of this textbook may not be evident. This is one of the reasons why I have often described more than one anatomic relationship to indicate accurate positioning in the evaluating criteria. For example, on the lateral ankle image in Figure 1-129, the tibial-fibular relationship cannot be used to determine accuracy of the positioning, but the domes of the talus are well visualized and indicate that the ankle was well positioned.

13. Repeat any necessary images.

14. Return the patient to the emergency room or, if the images were taken with the mobile unit, replace the bed, monitoring devices, and personal items to the positions they occupied when you entered the room or to positions that make the patient most comfortable.

15. Disinfect all equipment, IRs, and positioning devices used during the procedures.

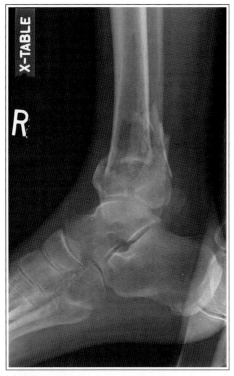

FIGURE 1-129 Trauma lateral ankle projection.

Pediatric Imaging

The images of pediatric patients are very different from those of adults and from each other during the various stages of bone growth and development (Figure 1-130). Bones throughout the body enlarge through the deposits of bone at cartilaginous growth regions, and long bones lengthen by the addition of bone material at the epiphyseal plate. Cartilaginous spaces and epiphyseal plates exist throughout the skeletal structure. They appear as dark spaces and lines on images and may look similar to an irregular fracture or joint space to those unfamiliar with pediatric imaging. The appearances of these spaces and lines are reduced as the child develops, until early adulthood, when they are replaced by bone and no longer are visible on the image. Round bones, such as the carpal and tarsal bones, are rarely formed at birth and therefore are not demonstrated on images of neonatal and very young pediatric patients. Because of this continual state of development, some anatomic relationships described in the imaging analysis sections may not be useful for determining accurate positioning for the pediatric patient. It is beyond our scope here to explain all the differences that could be demonstrated at different growth stages for each projection included in this text. When evaluating pediatric images for proper anatomic alignment, use only the analysis criteria that describe bony structures that are developed enough to use. For example, the section on PA wrist projection analysis describes the alignment of the carpal bones and metacarpals to determine accurate positioning. The carpal bone alignment cannot be used to evaluate young pediatric wrists, because all the carpal bones are not formed, but the metacarpals can be used to determine the accuracy.

Technical Considerations. Pediatric imaging requires lower technical values (kVp and mAs) when compared with those for adults. Box 1-7 lists guidelines to follow when selecting technical values for pediatrics patients.

Clothing Artifacts. Because lower kVp is used in pediatrics, clothing artifacts may be problematic in neonates and smaller children (Figure 1-131). The kVp used may not be high enough to burn out creases or folds, particularly in unlaundered material or flame-resistant clothing. It is best to image children without upper clothing or with a tee shirt when modesty is an issue. Skinfolds of neonates may also cause artifacts when they overlie the chest.

Obese Patients

According to the U.S. Centers for Disease Control and Prevention (CDC), approximately 64% of Americans are overweight. This has a direct impact on the health care system and imaging departments because these individuals have an increased incidence of diabetes, heart disease, and certain types of cancer and there is increasing popularity of bariatric surgery to help manage this

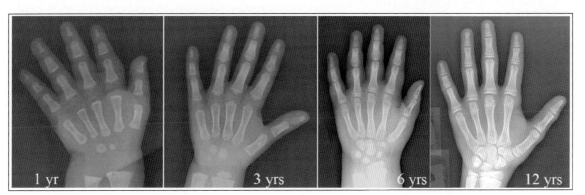

FIGURE 1-130 Pediatric PA hand and wrist projections at different ages of skeletal development.

| BOX 1-7 | **Guidelines for Setting Technical Values for Pediatric Patients** |

- Decrease the kVp value used for adults by at least 15% for skull imaging on patients younger than 6 years.
- A minimum of 50 kVp is needed to penetrate the premature infant's chest, 55 kVp for infants, and 60 kVp for toddlers and preschool children (ages 1 to 6 years)
- Decrease the mAs value used for adults by 50% for ages 0 to 5 years.
- Decrease the mAs value used for adults by 25% for ages 6 through 12.

From Fauber TL. *Radiographic imaging and exposure*, ed 3, St Louis, 2009, Mosby Elsevier.

kVp, Kilovoltage peak; *mAs*, milliampere-seconds.

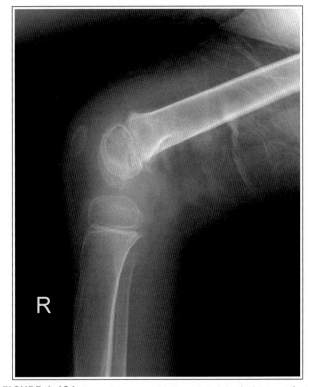

FIGURE 1-131 Lateral knee projection showing clothing artifacts around the distal femur on pediatric patient.

condition. The challenges facing technologists as they image obese patients include transporting and accommodating larger patients on the current equipment, and difficulties in acquiring quality images.[4] The following are considerations for imaging this population.

1. Obese patients often feel unwelcome in medical settings, where they encounter negative attitudes, discriminatory behavior, and a challenging physical environment. The emotional needs of these patients must be considered when they are imaged. Avoid making remarks about their size, being mindful of terms used such as "big" when referring to special equipment needs or requests for "lots of help" when transferring the patient.

2. Patient weight and body diameter are factors that should be evaluated before transporting the patient to the department or performing the examination. Use this information to determine whether the patient's weight exceeds any of the equipment weight limits, including waiting room chairs or support structures, or his or her diameter exceeds the wheelchair or cart dimensions.

3. Avoid injury to the patient and personnel by making certain that enough people are available to assist if the patient requires moving before or during the procedure. Use moving devices, such as table sliders and lifts, whenever possible.

4. Determine how the positioning procedure (IR size, CW-LW position of IR) will need to be adjusted from the routine to accommodate the increased structure size. For example, to include the entire abdomen on a morbidly obese patient may require a separate IR for each of the four abdominal quadrants, instead of one for the top and bottom.

5. Obese patients have inherently low subject contrast because their muscles have lost strength and have become the consistency of fat, so technical values must be set to enhance subject contrast while producing the lowest possible patient dose to produce an image with sufficient image contrast.

Technical Considerations. Thicker patients attenuate more of the primary x-ray photons than thin patients, requiring the technologist to increase mAs and/or kVp to compensate for the density loss that would result if a change were not made. Thicker patients also demonstrate a higher scatter–to–primary photon ratio (SPR) reaching the IR, causing a loss in image contrast. For example, a typical abdominal image taken on a patient measuring 20 cm will demonstrate a SPR of 3:1, meaning that 75% of the photons striking the IR are scattered photons that carry little or no useful information. For larger patients, the ratio in the abdomen can approach 5:1 or 6:1 (83% to 86%).

When determining how to adjust the technique for a thicker patient, the technologist must consider the effect that the change will have on patient dose and image contrast. As long as the kVp is set to allow penetration through the part, increasing the mAs will generate enough x-rays to provide more photons. As a general rule, for every 4 cm of added tissue thickness, the mAs should be doubled to maintain density. This technique adjustment will have a significant increase on patient dose because the increase in dose is directly proportional to the mAs increase. It will also demonstrate lower image contrast because the SPR will increase with increased thickness.

Another technique adjustment option is to increase the kVp. This will increase the penetration ability of the photons, resulting in more of them reaching the IR. As a general rule, for every centimeter of added tissue thickness, the kVp should be adjusted by 2 kV. With this option, the patient dosage will increase, but not directly, as with mAs, so the amount of dosage increase is significantly less. Image contrast will be also lowered, because an increase in kVp decreases subject contrast and causes scatter radiation to be directed at a forward angle toward the IR, which is difficult for the grid to remove.

For best results when adjusting technique for a thick patient, the kVp should be set as high as possible (to reduce radiation dose), but should not exceed a kVp value that will provide sufficient subject contrast. After the kVp value maximum has been attained, additional adjustments should be made with mAs.

Scatter Radiation Control. One of the biggest obstacles when imaging the obese patient is controlling scatter radiation enough to provide an image that has sufficient image contrast. This is accomplished by using very aggressive, tight collimation, using a high-ratio grid, or using an air-gap technique.

1. Tight collimation is often difficult when imaging obese patients because the collimator's light field demonstrated on the patient does not represent the true width and length of the field set on the collimator. The thicker the part being imaged, the smaller the collimator's light field that appears on the patient's skin surface. On a very thick patient, it is difficult to collimate the needed amount when the light field appears so small but, on these patients, tight collimation demonstrates the largest improvement in the visibility of recorded details. Learn to use the collimator guide (see Figure 1-20) to determine the actual IR coverage.

2. Many projections, such as the inferosuperior (axial) shoulder projection, which do not require a grid on the typical patient, will need to be performed using a grid. Measure all structures and use a grid when the part thickness is more than 10 cm.

Focal Spot Size. When using a small focal spot, the milliamperage is typically limited to 300 mA or less. Using such a small focal spot may not be feasible when imaging an obese patient because it would require a long exposure time to achieve the needed radiographic density and motion may result.

Automatic Exposure Control. Select a high mA to avoid long exposure times and the potential motion it causes. Also, adjust the backup timer to 150% to 200% of the expected manual exposure time.

1. When possible, remove overlapping soft tissue from the area being imaged to decrease the thickness of the tissue being penetrated. Figure 1-132 demonstrates an AP pelvis projection in which the soft tissue overlapping the hips could have been pulled superiorly and held with tape or by the patient, decreasing the soft tissue over the hips and allowing them to be demonstrated more effectively. Overlapping breast and arm tissue can also be held away from the shoulder during inferosuperior (axial) shoulder projections to decrease thickness and improve detail visibility.

2. Use palpable bony structures to position the patient and to collimate whenever possible. Remember, the skeletal structure does not increase in size with an increase in the soft tissue surrounding it. Figure 1-133 shows a bone scan on an obese patient that clearly illustrates this point. Using palpable bony

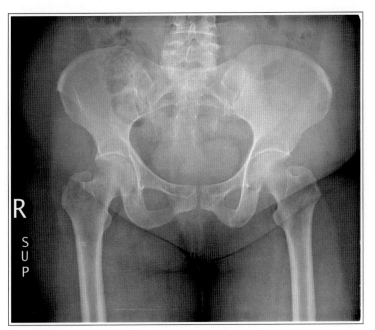

FIGURE 1-132 AP pelvis projection showing overlapping soft tissue, preventing uniform density of hip joints and proximal femurs.

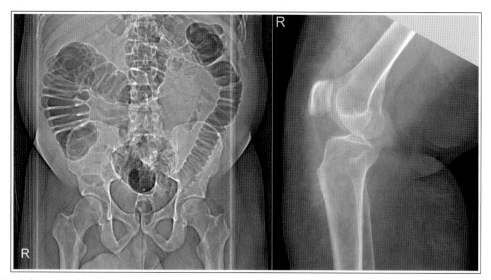

FIGURE 1-133 AP abdomen and lateral knee projections on an obese patient to show placement of skeletal structure within surrounding soft tissue.

structures to determine where structures are located whenever possible will help you to position accurately and collimate more specifically to the structures of interest.

When the soft tissue thickness prevents palpation of bony structures, use signs such as depressions or dimples in the soft tissue that suggest where the bony structures are located. Observe closely how the patient is positioned for each image so if a repeat is needed, you can adjust the amount needed from the original positioning.

REFERENCES

1. Church EJ: Legal trends in imaging, *Radiol Technol* 76:31–45, 2004.
2. Hobbs DL: Chest radiography for radiologic technologists, *Radiol Technol* 78:494–516, 2007.
3. Statkiewicz Sherer MA, Visconti PJ, Ritenour ER: *Radiation protection in medical radiography*, ed 5, St. Louis, 2006, Mosby Elsevier.
4. Upport RN, Sahani DV, Hahn PF, et al: Impact of obesity on medical imaging and image-guided intervention, *AJR Am J Roentgenol* 188:433–440, 2007.
5. Welling RD, Jacobson JA, Jamadar DA, et al: MDCT and radiography of wrist fractures: Radiographic sensitivity and fracture patterns, *AJR Am J Roentgenol* 190:10–16, 2008.

BIBLIOGRAPHY

Bushberg JT, Seibert JA, Leidholdt EM, Boone JM: *The essential physics of medical imaging*, ed 2, Philadelphia, 2002, Lippincott Williams & Wilkins.
Bushong SC: *Radiologic science for technologists*, ed 9, St. Louis, 2008, Mosby Elsevier.
Holt MH: Minimizing distortion with geometry, *Radiol Technol* May/June 78(5), 2007.

Digital Radiography

OBJECTIVES

After completion of this chapter, you should be able to do the following:

- Explain the difference between screen-film radiography and digital imaging.
- Describe the processing steps completed in computed radiography (CR) and direct-indirect digital radiography (DR).
- State why the exposure field recognition process is completed in CR and is not needed in DR.
- Identify the areas of an image histogram and list the guidelines to follow to produce an optimal histogram.
- Explain the relationship between the image histogram and the chosen lookup table in the automatic rescaling process.
- List the CR exposure indicator parameters and discuss what they are and when they are useful to improve image quality.

- State how the CR exposure indicators and the DR dose area product differ.
- Compare the factors that affect spatial resolution between CR and DR systems.
- Discuss how radiation dose is reduced using digital radiography.
- State the causes of overexposure and underexposure in digital radiography and the effect that each has on image quality.
- Discuss the causes of a histogram analysis error.
- Describe the factors that affect contrast resolution in digital radiography.
- List the different artifacts found in digital radiography and discuss how they can be prevented, when applicable.

KEY TERMS

algorithm
automatic rescaling
brightness
contrast resolution
detector element (DEL)
digitization
dose-area product (DAP)
dynamic range
exposure field recognition
exposure indicator

field of view (FOV)
histogram
histogram analysis error
image acquisition
imaging plate (IP)
lookup table (LUT)
matrix
moiré grid artifact
phantom image
pixel

quantization
quantum noise
raw data
shuttering
spatial frequency
spatial resolution
thin-film transistor (TFT)
volume of interest (VOI)
windowing

DIGITAL RADIOGRAPHY

Two types of digital imaging systems are used in radiography to acquire and process the radiographic image, the cassette-based system known as computed radiography (CR) and the cassetteless image detector system known as direct or indirect digital radiography (DR). The systems are unique in the methods that they use to acquire and process the image before sending it to the computer to be analyzed and manipulated. Understanding the acquisition

and processing steps of each system will help the technologist to prevent errors that cause poor processing of the image and understand the results seen on the image and exposure indicators when it is less than optimal.

The selection of milliampere-seconds (mAs), kilovoltage peak, (kVp), and distance for digital radiography are based on the same principles used in conventional screen-film radiography that were discussed in the previous chapter. The mAs is chosen for the number of photons needed to produce an image without quantum noise and the kVp is chosen for the desired subject contrast. It is recommended that when digital imaging is used, the kVp levels be increased by 15% above that used for screen-film radiography to optimize detector efficiency and reduce radiation exposure to the patient. For the most efficient detection and capture of radiation, the kVp is best set at the phosphor's K-edge. For example, the K-edge of the phosphor used in CR imaging plates (IPs) ranges from 30 to 50 keV, placing the optimal kVp range for the greatest detector efficiency at 60 to 110 kVp. The same optimal kVp range is used with DR systems. This increase in kVp can be accomplished without significant changes in scatter radiation production and narrowing of the angle of scatter divergence with the image receptor (IR).

Computed Radiography

Image (Data) Acquisition. CR is most like conventional radiography in that it uses a cassette that can be placed in the Bucky or on the tabletop. During the image acquisition process the radiographic exposure results in the IP storing trapped electrons in the plate's photostimulable phosphor. The amount of energy trapped in each area of the IP reflects the subject contrast of the body part imaged.

Image Sampling. Once the IP has been exposed, the examination or body part is selected from the menu choices on the CR workstation and the plate is placed in or sent to the reader unit. Selecting the correct examination or body part ensures that the correct lookup table (LUT) is applied when the image is rescaled. In the reader unit an infrared laser beam is scanned back and forth across the plate, releasing the stored energy in the form of visible light. The amount of light produced as each area of the plate is scanned is equivalent to the amount of energy that was stored in the plate during the acquisition process. The light is collected and converted to an electrical signal by the photomultiplier tube (PMT) and then sent to the analog-to-digital converter (ADC) to be digitized.

Digitization (Quantization). During digitization, the analog image is divided into a matrix and each pixel (cell) in the matrix is assigned a digital number (brightness value) that represents the amount of light that was emitted from that surface of the IP. Pixels that received greater radiation exposure are assigned values that represent less brightness, whereas the pixels receiving less exposure are assigned values that represent more brightness. All the brightness values together make up what is referred to as the raw or image data.

Exposure Field Recognition. In cassette-based digital systems the entire IP is scanned and brightness values are assigned for every area of the plate. The image data are then evaluated by the computer to distinguish the brightness values that represent the anatomic structures of interest (also referred to as the volume of interest) from the brightness values that are outside the exposure field. This process is called exposure field recognition; it is important to ensure that the histogram generated from the image data is shaped correctly and that the volume of interest (VOI) is accurately identified before automatic rescaling of the data occurs.

Histogram. After the image data from the exposure field has been discerned, a histogram graph is generated that has the pixel values on the x-axis and the number of pixels with that brightness value on the y-axis (Figure 2-1). The peaks and valleys of the graph represent the subject contrast of the structure imaged; the VOI is identified, with S1 representing the minimum useful signal and S2 representing the maximum useful signal. Because the subject contrast of a particular anatomic structure (e.g., chest, abdomen, shoulder) is fairly consistent from exposure to exposure, the shape of each structure's histogram should be fairly consistent as well. Metallic objects or contrast agents are recorded on the left in the graph, followed by bone, soft tissues near the center, fat, and finally gaseous or air densities on the right. The tail or high spiked portion on the far right of some histograms represents the background brightness value that is in the exposure field. This background value will be the darkest image data value because this area is exposed to primary radiation that does not go through any part of the patient, such as with extremity and chest images that have been collimated close to the skin line (Figure 2-2) but not within it. This spike is not visible on images in which the entire cassette is covered with anatomy, such as abdominal images or on

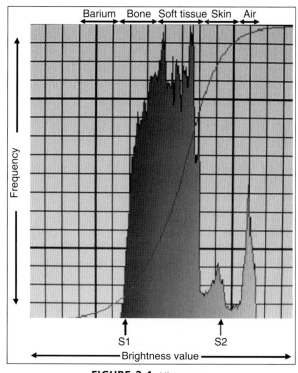

FIGURE 2-1 Histogram.

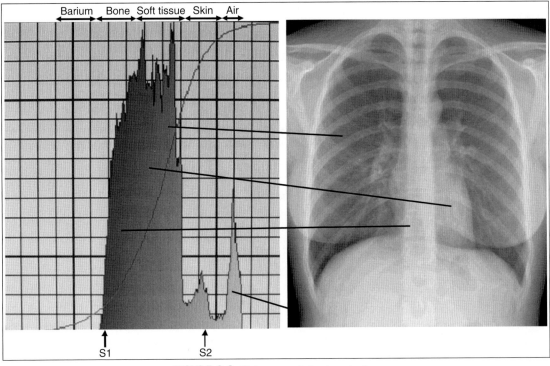

FIGURE 2-2 Histogram of chest projection.

images where the collimation field is within the skin line, such as for an AP lumbar vertebral image.

Poor histogram formation and subsequent histogram analysis errors will occur with poor positioning, collimation, or alignment of the part on the IR, with unusual pathologic conditions, with artifacts, by including anatomy that is not typically present or removing anatomy that is typically present, and with excessive scatter fogging. Box 2-1 lists guidelines for obtaining optimal image histograms.

BOX 2-1   Guidelines for Producing Optimal Image Histograms

- Set the correct technique factors for the projection.
- Choose the correct body part and projection from the workstation menu.
- Center the central ray to the center of the VOI.
- Collimate as closely as possible to the VOI, leaving minimum background in the exposure field.
- Control the amount of scatter reaching the IR (grids, collimation, lead sheets).
- If collimating smaller than the IR, center the image and show all four collimation borders.
- Use the smallest possible IR, covering at least 30% of the IR.
- When placing multiple projections on one IP, all collimation must be parallel and equidistant from the edges of the IP, make images at a distinct distance from each other.
- Do not leave the IP in the imaging room while other exposures are being made and read the IP shortly after the exposure.
- Erase the image plate if the IR has not been used within a few days.

IP, Imaging plate; *IR,* image receptor; *VOI,* volume of interest.

Automatic Rescaling. Included in the computer software is a lookup table (LUT), or "ideal" histogram for every part imaged. In the final phase of processing, automatic rescaling of the image occurs. In this phase, the computer compares the image histogram with the selected LUT and applies algorithms to the actual data as needed to align the image histogram with the LUT. For example, if the image histogram was positioned farther to the right than the LUT, representing an image where the brightness values are darker than they should be, the algorithm applied to the data would move the values toward the left, aligning them with the values in the LUT. The image that is then displayed on the display monitor is the rescaled image. Overexposures of 120% and underexposures as low as 60% from the ideal exposure can be rescaled without losing image quality.

For best rescaling results, the technologist must obtain images that produce histograms that clearly distinguish the VOI from other values and whose shape is similar to that of the LUT chosen. Including brightness values on the histogram that are other than those that are in the VOI will result in a misshapen histogram, which does not accurately represent the anatomic structure imaged and will not match the associated lookup table. If the image histogram and selected LUT do not have a similar shape, the computer software will be unable to align them, resulting in a histogram analysis error that produces a poor-quality image and provides an erroneous exposure indicator value.

Exposure Indicators. Exposure indicators are readings that express the amount of light given off by the IP and that denote the amount of exposure to the

TABLE 2-1	Computed Radiography Exposure Indicator Parameters					
System	Exposure Indicator	Acceptable Parameters	Ideal Exposure	Insufficient Exposure	Excessive Exposure	Change by Factor of 2
Kodak	Exposure index (EI)	1700–2300	2000	Below 1700	Above 2300	300
Fuji	Sensitivity (S) number	100–400	200	Above 400	Below 100	100
Phillips	Sensitivity (S) number	55–220	110	Above 220	Below 55	55
Agfa	Log median value (LgM)	2.2–2.8	2.5	Below 2.5	Above 2.8	0.3

patient and IP. It is not a measure of dose to the patient, but an indication of what the patient has received. After the histogram has been developed, the exposure indicator reading is read by the computer at the midpoint of the defined VOI (halfway between S1 and S2). The exposure indicator expression varies from one manufacturer to another and the technologist should be aware of those in their facility. Table 2-1 lists different manufacturers' exposure indicators and ranges for acceptable exposure for CR systems currently on the market.

Direct and Indirect Digital Radiography

Image Acquisition. Direct and indirect digital radiography use a cassetteless imaging capture system that is hard-wired to the image processing system. Thin-film transistor (TFT) detector arrays made up of many small detector elements (DELs) are located in the image receptor. During an exposure, the TFT receives the remnant radiation and converts it to electrical signals of varying intensity. These electrical signals are sent to the computer for processing and manipulation. Only the DELs in the TFT that have received radiation, which is determined when the technologist collimates, send electric signals and are included in the image. This eliminates the need for the exposure field recognition process that is completed in CR and the many histogram errors that poor recognition can cause.

Image Processing. Before the image is taken, the examination or body part must be accurately selected from the menu choices on the DR workstation panel to ensure that the correct LUT is applied when the image is rescaled. After the exposure is complete, the electrical signals are sent to the ADC to be digitized.

During digitization, each pixel's analog image is assigned a brightness value that represents the amount of radiation that reached the IP. As with CR, all the brightness values together make up the image data. After the brightness values have been recorded, a histogram graph is generated from the image data and then the computer applies algorithms to the actual data to align the image histogram with the selected LUT.

Producing a histogram that clearly distinguishes the VOI from the other values and whose shape is similar to that of the LUT chosen is as important in DR as it is in CR imaging. Poor histogram formation and subsequent histogram analysis errors will occur in DR in the following circumstances:

- With poor positioning and collimation
- With unusual pathologic conditions
- With artifacts
- By including anatomy that is not typically present or removing anatomy that is typically present
- With excessive scatter fogging

Box 2-1 lists guidelines for obtaining optimal image histograms. Although poor histogram formation and histogram analysis errors may result in CR when the image is not properly positioned in the center of the IR and collimation borders are not all shown or are not aligned accurately, this is not the case for DR, because only the pixels receiving exposure will send signals to the computer for processing.

Dose-Area Product. The dose-area product (DAP) is used in DR systems to monitor the radiation output and dose to the patient per volume of tissue irradiated. This measurement is obtained by a radiolucent measuring device positioned near the x-ray source below the collimator and in front of the patient. The DAP can be used to monitor the radiation intensity when overexposed and underexposed images are obtained, although it cannot be used to adjust exposure in the same way that the exposure indicators may be used in CR systems. The CR exposure indicators measure the exposure that reaches the IR after going through the patient, whereas DAP is a measure of the exposure before going through the patient.

Displaying Images

Image Receptor and Patient Orientation. Some CR system cassettes have orientation labels that indicate to the user which end of the cassette is the "top" and which side is the "right" or "left" side. These orientation indicators align the image orientation with the computer algorithm of a patient in the anatomic position (anteroposterior [AP] projection). The top indicator should be placed under the portion of the anatomy that should be up when the image is displayed and, for images of the torso, the right side of the patient should be placed over the right side indicator. The IP is read from left to right, starting at the top, and the image is displayed in the same manner as the IP is read. Thus, if the examination is taken in a position other than just described, the examination chosen (posteroanterior [PA] or AP chest) on the workstation must indicate this variation before the image is read for it to be displayed accurately.

The image receptor in the DR system also has top and side orientation indicators that should be followed when positioning the patient for accurate displaying of the image. Because the image is automatically displayed, the technologist must chose the correct examination from the workstation before exposing the image for it to be displayed accurately.

An examination taken without aligning the patient, IR, and workstation examination choice will be inverted top to bottom or rotated left to right relative to anatomic position. If this were to occur, the image can be flipped and rotated to the desired position.

Shuttering. The brightness of the areas outside the exposure field can be blackened by a postexposure manipulation called shuttering or black surround, which adds a black background around the exposure field. This is for image aesthetics only, providing a perceived enhancement of image contrast. As a rule, the technologist should only shutter to the exposed areas, matching the collimation borders, even though it is possible to shutter into the exposed areas. Because it is possible to shutter into the exposed areas, some facilities do not allow shuttering because of the possibility that the radiologist will not see information that has been included on the original image. Shuttering does not replace good collimation practices and should not be used to present a perceived radiation dose savings to the patient.

Display Stations. The resolution ability of the image may be different, depending on where the image is displayed in the department. Display station resolution refers to the maximum number of pixels that the screen can demonstrate. To display images at full resolution, the display monitor must be able to display the same number of pixels as those at which the digital system acquired the image. If the digital system matrix size is smaller than the display station's matrix size, the values of surrounding pixels will be averaged to display the whole image. The technologist's workstation display monitors typically do not demonstrate quality resolution as high as that of the radiologist's display monitor.

IMAGE ANALYSIS FORM

The image analysis form shown in Figure 1-9 is designed to work with screen-film and digital radiography images to ensure that all aspects of the image are evaluated. Under each item in the image analysis form, there is a list of questions to explore while evaluating an image. The following sections are extensions of those presented in Chapter 1 on screen-film radiography, with digital radiography being the focus in this chapter.

Demographic Requirements

Each CR cassette has a barcode label that is used to match the image data with the patient's identification barcode and examination request. For each examination, the cassette and patient barcodes must be scanned, connecting them with each other and the examination menu. With the DR system, the examination and patient are matched when the patient's information is pulled up on the workstation before the examination is obtained. It is important to select the correct patient and order number prior to beginning the examination.

Before selecting the patient and examination, compare the patient name and order number to be certain that they match. It may also be necessary to change the examination type (PA and lateral wrist may be shown, when a PA, lateral, and oblique wrist was ordered). If necessary, change the examination type prior to beginning the examination so that the correct view options are available. After the examination, double-check the order number again prior to sending to the picture archiving and communication system (PACS).

Once an image is sent to the archiving system, it is immediately available to whoever has access. Improperly connecting the patient and image will make it difficult to retrieve. If the image is associated with the wrong patient, the image may be seen or evaluated by a physician before the misassociation is noticed, resulting in an inaccurate diagnosis and unnecessary or inaccurate treatment of the wrong patient.

If incorrect patient information is assigned to an image, the technologist can reattribute the examination to the correct patient as long as the image has not been sent to the archiving system. If the images are sent to the PACS with the incorrect patient assigned to the examination, the PACS coordinator must be immediately notified to correct the error before the images are viewed.

Marking Images

Digital imaging systems allow the technologist to add annotations (e.g., R or L side, text words) after the exposure. For example, if the original R or L side marker was partially positioned outside the collimation field during the exposure, an annotated marker may be added to the image (Figure 2-3). When adding annotations, the original marker should not be covered up.

Even though marker annotations can be added after processing the image, using markers during the positioning process remains an important practice. Because images may be flipped and rotated in any manner and one can mark at any point on the image, markers added after processing may be less reliable. Once added, the image is not considered a legal document that will hold up in court.

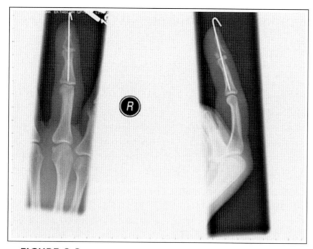

FIGURE 2-3 Adding marker with computed radiography.

Recorded Detail

The sharpness of the structural lines on an image is controlled in digital radiography in the same way that it is controlled in screen-film radiography—by using a small focal spot, the longest possible source–image receptor distance (SID), the shortest possible object–image receptor distance (OID), and halting motion.

Spatial Resolution. The quality of spatial resolution of a digital imaging system is mostly defined by the matrix size and the size of the pixels within the matrix. Spatial resolution refers to the ability of an imaging system to distinguish small adjacent details from each other in an image. The closer the details are to each other, with the image still showing them as separate objects, the better is the spatial resolution. At the point at which the objects are so close together that they appear as one, spatial resolution is lost. The term *spatial frequency* is used to describe spatial resolution and refers to how frequently the number of details changes in a set amount of space. This change is not expressed as the size of the object, but in terms of the largest number of line pairs per millimeter (lp/mm) that can be seen when a resolution line pair test tool is imaged using the system. As the spatial frequency number becomes larger, the ability to resolve smaller objects increases.

At its best, screen-film radiography is limited to approximately 10 lp/mm (100 relative speed system). This means that within 1 mm of distance, the system can visualize up to 10 details and the spaces between them, as long as the subject contrast is different between the detail and adjacent space. Resolution ability in screen-film radiography is superior to digital radiography, because a detail can be recorded in all areas in the film's phosphor, whereas in digital radiography, the IR is divided into specific squares or rectangles of area known as pixels. Each pixel can only visualize one gray shade, distinguishing only one detail, and two pixels are needed to make up a line pair. If the frequency of change in the image from detail to detail is closer together than

the width or height of the pixel, the details will not be resolved.

In the CR system, the pixel size is determined by the image field size relative to the image matrix size. The image matrix refers to the layout of pixels (cells) in rows and columns and is determined by the system's manufacturer. A larger matrix size will provide a higher number of pixels. The size of the pixels in the matrix is determined by the field of view (FOV). Because the entire IP is scanned during CR processing, the FOV is the entire plate for CR systems, and because different plate sizes are used, the size of the IP chosen influences the size of the actual pixels and the resulting spatial resolution. For example, a CR system using a matrix size of 1024 × 1024 will divide the image into 1,048,576 pixels. Spreading this matrix over a 14- × 17-inch FOV (image receptor) will result in larger pixel sizes than spreading the matrix over an 8- × 10-inch FOV (Figure 2-4). Because the 8- × 10-inch IR will contain pixels of smaller size, it will provide superior spatial resolution.

CR systems currently have resolution capabilities between 2.55 and 5 lp/mm, with the 14- × 17-inch FOV providing about 3 lp/mm and the 8- × 10-inch FOV providing about 5 lp/mm. Choosing the smallest possible IR is important when imaging structures for which small details, such as trabeculae, are needed to make an optimal diagnosis (Figure 2-5).

The spatial resolution capability of a CR system is also affected by the size of the laser spot used, and the divergence spreading of the laser light and photostimulated light during the scanning and collecting processes.

In DR systems there is an array of detectors linked together to form a matrix, in which the individual detector elements form the pixels of the matrix and their size determines the limiting spatial resolution of the system. The DELs contain the electronic components (e.g., conductor, capacitor, TFT) that store the detected energy

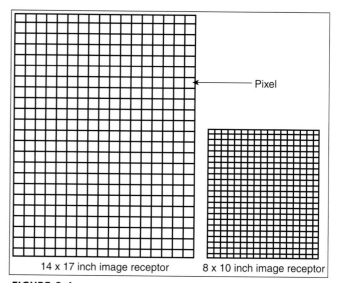

14 x 17 inch image receptor   8 x 10 inch image receptor

FIGURE 2-4 Image matrix and pixel sizes with different IR sizes.

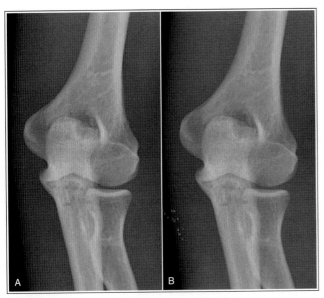

FIGURE 2-5 Comparing spatial resolution between large and small IR sizes using computed radiography. **A**, 8- ×10-inch IR. **B**, 14- ×17-inch IR.

BOX 2-2	**Reducing Dose With Digital Radiography**

- Exposure should not be repeated in digital radiography because of overexposure, brightness, or contrast concerns.
- Digital radiography systems cannot compensate for excessive noise caused by quantum noise.
- Watch dose or technique creep. As technologists try to avoid quantum noise, they use more exposure than necessary at a cost of increased dose to the patient.

From Bushong SC. *Radiologic science for technologists*, ed 9, St. Louis, 2008, Mosby Elsevier.

and link the detector to the computer. These components take up a fixed amount of the detectors' surfaces, limiting the amount of surface that is used to collect x-ray forming information. As the DELs become smaller, the spatial resolution capability increases, but the energy-collecting efficiency decreases. The ratio of energy-sensitive surface to the entire surface of each DEL is termed the *fill factor*. A high fill factor is desired, because energy that is not detected does not contribute to the image and an increase in radiation exposure may be required to make up the fill factor difference to prevent obtaining an image with quantum noise. Hence, this indicates a tradeoff between spatial and contrast resolution and between spatial resolution and radiation dose.

The spatial resolution capability of a DR system is affected by the size of the DELs and the spacing between them. It is not affected by a change in FOV (collimating smaller than the full detector array), because collimation only determines the DELs that will be used in the examination and does not physically change them. Current DR systems have spatial resolution capabilities of approximately 3.7 lp/mm.

Radiation Protection

Radiation protection procedures used in conventional screen-film radiography should be followed with digital systems as well. Digital radiography can reduce exposure to the overall population because repeats for overexposed and poor contrast images are not needed; the image can be adjusted to improve these through autoscaling and windowing. It is necessary for the technologist to avoid dose or technique creep, which results when technique values are elevated more than necessary

because of fear of producing images with quantum noise. Box 2-2 provides guidelines for reducing patient dose with digital radiography.

Relative Speed of Computed Radiography. Most CR systems are operated at a 200 speed in comparison to the most commonly used rare earth, 400-speed screen-film systems. This requires a doubling of the mAs to obtain equal density on an image. To reduce the radiation dose to the patient that this increase in exposure would cause, it is recommended that the kVp be increased by 15% instead of doubling the mAs.

Radiographic Brightness

In digital radiography, the term *brightness* is used to describe the degree of luminance seen on the display monitor. It refers to the degree of lightness (white) or lack of lightness (black) of the pixels in the image. This differs from the term *density* that is used in conventional radiography, which describes the degree of blackness of an area or structure on the radiograph.

Because of the automatic rescaling process that occurs when using digital radiography, adequate image brightness will usually result, even if a procedure is followed that would normally result in inadequate density in screen-film radiography. Low contrast is the indicator for high exposure values and quantum noise is the indicator for low exposure values in digital radiography. The CR exposure indicator values may also be used to indicate high and low exposure values as long as there is no suspected histogram analysis error.

Overexposure and Underexposure. The accuracy of technical factors used and positioning procedures followed greatly influence the resulting pixel brightness values, the shape and location of the VOI on the image histogram, and the amount of automatic rescaling that needs to be done to display an optimal image. Tables 2-2 and 2-3 list the causes of overexposure and underexposure when using digital systems and the effects that they have on image quality.

Adjusting for Underexposure and Overexposure Using the Exposure Indicator Number. The amount of automatic rescaling that takes place before the image is displayed can be estimated through the exposure

TABLE 2-2	Causes of Overexposure	
Parameter(s) Affected	**Causes**	**Effect on Image Quality**
mAs, kVp	• Used too much mAs and/or kVp was too high	• Brightness is acceptable • CR exposure indicator indicates excessive exposure* • Low contrast becomes increasingly grayer with increased exposure
AEC	• Wrong Bucky activated and backup time shuts AEC off • Density control left on plus (+) setting • Ionization chamber(s) chosen was beneath a structure having higher atomic number or is denser or thicker than tissue of interest • Radiopaque artifact in anatomy of interest	• Brightness is acceptable • CR exposure indicator indicates excessive exposure* • Low contrast becomes increasingly grayer with increased exposure
Distance	• Decrease in SID without a decrease in mAs	• Brightness is acceptable • CR exposure indicator indicates excessive exposure* • Low contrast becomes increasingly grayer with decreased SID
Grids	• Used technique for grid but forgot to add grid • Used mAs for a high grid ratio with a low grid ratio	• Brightness is acceptable • CR exposure indicator indicates excessive exposure* • Low contrast becomes decreasingly grayer with increasing grid ratio

*Useful only if no histogram analysis error is suspected.
AEC, Automatic exposure control; *CR*, computed radiography; *SID*, source–image receptor distance.

TABLE 2-3	Causes of Underexposure	
Parameter(s) Affected	**Causes**	**Effect on Image Quality**
mAs, kVp	• Did not use enough mAs and/or kVp was too low • If no histogram analysis error is indicated, determine the amount of change needed to bring the exposure indicator within acceptable parameters	• Brightness is acceptable • CR exposure indicator indicates insufficient exposure* • Quantum noise becomes more noticeable with decreasing exposure
AEC	• Backup timer was shorter than the needed exposure time • Density control left on minus (−) setting • Ionization chamber(s) chosen was beneath a structure having lower atomic number or is less dense or thinner than anatomy of interest • Small anatomic structure was imaged and activated ionization chamber was not fully covered by anatomy	• Brightness is acceptable • CR exposure indicator indicates insufficient exposure* • Quantum noise
Distance	• Increase in SID without an increase in mAs	• Brightness is acceptable • CR exposure indicator indicates insufficient exposure* • Quantum noise becomes more noticeable with increased distances
Grids	• Used technique for nongrid but left the grid in • Used mAs for a lower grid ratio with higher ratio grid • Grid off-level or central ray angled toward grid lines (Figure 2-23) • SID outside focusing range for grid used • Focused grid inverted (Figure 2-24) • Focused grid off-center	• Brightness is acceptable as long as grid cutoff is seen across the entire image • CR exposure indicator indicates insufficient exposure* • Quantum noise where grid cutoff is seen becomes more noticeable with increased grid ratio and degree of grid misalignment • Low contrast where grid cutoff is seen
Anode heel	• Thicker end of long body part positioned at anode end of tube and thinnest end of body part positioned at cathode end of tube	• Brightness is acceptable • Quantum noise at thicker end of body part

*Useful only if no histogram analysis error is suspected.
AEC, Automatic exposure control; *CR*, computed radiography; *SID*, source–image receptor distance.

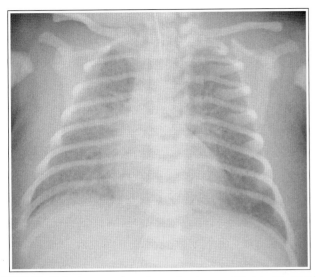

FIGURE 2-6 Computed radiography image (Kodak EI 1600) demonstrating quantum noise caused by underexposure.

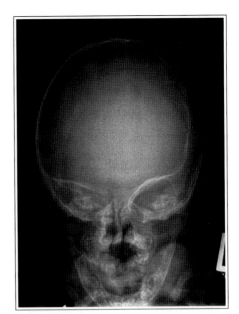

FIGURE 2-7 Computed radiography image (Kodak EI 1600) demonstrating quantum noise caused by underexposure.

indicator number as long as a histogram analysis error has not occurred. The more that this value is outside the ideal range for the system used, the more rescaling that occurred that resulted in the image presented. Images produced at exposure indicator numbers that specify lower than ideal exposure values may necessitate repeating the procedure because of the mottled image appearance (Figure 2-6). Quantum noise is a blotchy appearance on the image that results when an insufficient number of photons reach the IP, causing the random fluctuation of the photons striking the IP to be noticed. An increase in exposure factors (kVp and/or mAs) is needed to reduce the effects of quantum noise. Exposure indicator numbers that specify higher than ideal exposure values typically do not require repeating because of image quality unless they are so high above the ideal that the image demonstrates an excessive gray-scale, although the reason for this high value should be investigated, as excessive patient dosage was rendered to produce them. Exposures that are too high above the ideal to be rescaled adequately will require repeating due to excessive gray-scale. A decrease in mAs and/or kVp is needed. The farther the exposure indicator value is from the acceptable parameters and the ideal exposure, the greater will be the quantum noise demonstrated for underexposures (compare Figure 2-6 and Figure 2-7) and the grayness for overexposure.

Figure 2-8 shows a PA chest projection obtained using a Kodak system that demonstrates acceptable brightness resulting from automatic rescaling and quantum noise, with an exposure index (EI) of 1660. The image demonstrates tight collimation with only minimal abdominal structures included, the chest is centered to the center of the IP with all four collimated borders shown close to the skin line, contrast is high with little

scatter fogging, and no artifacts are present. These are all indications that good positioning procedures were followed, the image histogram was accurately shaped, and the VOI was accurately identified. Therefore the exposure indicator may be used to determine the amount of exposure adjustment required to produce an image without quantum noise. The acceptable EI range for images using the Kodak CR system is readings between 1700 and 2300, with an ideal exposure reading of 2000 (see Table 2-1). The 1660 reading obtained for the chest image in Figure 2-8 is below the 1700 parameter, indicating that the exposure was insufficient.

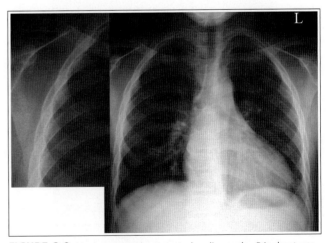

FIGURE 2-8 Underexposed computed radiography PA chest projection demonstrating acceptable brightness, proper procedure, quantum noise, and EI of 1660.

Because penetration and gray scale are sufficient on this image, the mAs needs to be adjusted by at least a factor of 2 to move the EI within acceptable parameters and closer to the 2000 ideal. If 10 mAs were used for this exposure, the image should be repeated using 20 mAs (10 multiplied by 2), raising the EI by 300 points to 1960.

When a gray image is produced with an exposure indicator reading that indicates excessive exposure, and there is no reason to suspect that a histogram analysis error occurred, the exposure indicator can be used to determine how the exposure should be adjusted to obtain an image with increased contrast and less radiation dose to the patient. Figure 2-9 displays an AP femur projection that demonstrates acceptable brightness, low contrast, and an EI of 2490. As long as the contrast scale is such that all aspects of the anatomic structure can be evaluated, it is not necessary to repeat this image because windowing can be used to increase contrast, but it should be noted when exposures are excessive and technique charts should be adjusted to reduce exposure and radiation dose for the next similar examination. If the gray scale is inadequate to demonstrate details, the kVp and/or mAs should be adjusted the needed amount

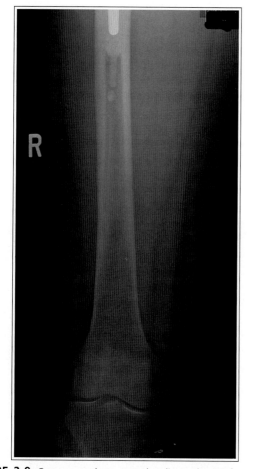

FIGURE 2-9 Overexposed computed radiography AP femur projection demonstrating acceptable brightness, proper procedure, low contrast, and EI of 2490.

to bring the exposure indicator within acceptable parameters (see Chapter 1).

Histogram Analysis Errors

When the image histogram includes brightness values in the VOI that should not be included, the histogram will be misshapen and will not match the LUT closely enough for the computer to rescale the image data accurately. Because the exposure indicator is derived from the histogram, anything that causes a histogram analysis error will also cause an erroneous exposure indicator. Figure 2-2 represents a PA chest histogram of a patient for whom the VOI was accurately identified. Figure 2-10 demonstrates the histogram of a PA chest projection in which collimation was such that a portion of the lead apron around the patient's waist was included on the image. The lead apron produced a digital value that was recorded on the histogram and included as part of the VOI, causing the histogram to widen. Compare the VOI (section between S1 and S2) on the histogram in Figure 2-2 with that in Figure 2-10. Note that the midpoint between the VOIs (where the exposure indicator is read) on each of these histograms is different. This difference is caused by the widening of the histogram, not because the exposure to the IP and patient itself was different between the images. Histogram analysis errors can result in the exposure indicator being falsely moved toward a lower or higher value, making its value erroneous and unreliable.

Images with histogram analysis errors will have the same image quality issues as images with exposure errors, but their causes will have less to do with the mAs and kVp set and more to do with the accuracy of the positioning procedures. For example, Figure 2-11 demonstrates an AP shoulder projection that was obtained using the Kodak CR system, optimal kVp, and the center automatic exposure control (AEC) ionization chamber. The image demonstrates adequate brightness, low contrast, poor collimation (excessive background included), poor centering beneath the chamber, and quantum mottle, and has an EI of 2410. Even though the EI indicates that excessive exposure was used, the potential for this reading being erroneous is very high. We know that when a portion of the chamber is exposed by part of the beam that does not go through the patient, as is the case with this image, the exposure terminates early and underexposure results, as indicated by the quantum noise. Also, because the image was not tightly collimated, excessive background radiation could have been included in the VOI, causing the EI to be read at a midpoint that indicated more exposure than was actually used. The procedural causes of this low-quality image clearly conflict with the exposure indicator value on the image. When a poor-quality image is produced, the effect of the positioning procedures on the amount of exposure that reaches the IP should be considered before deciding if the

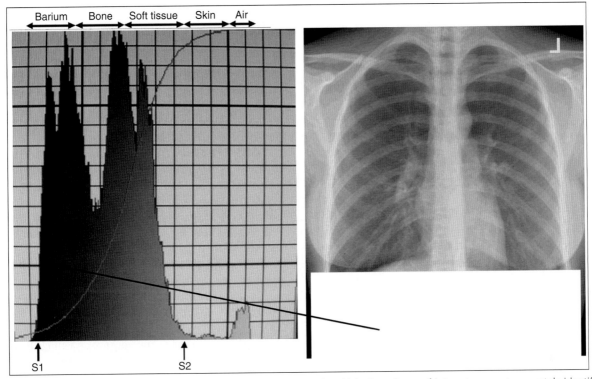

FIGURE 2-10 Computed radiography PA chest projection histogram in which the volume of interest was not accurately identified.

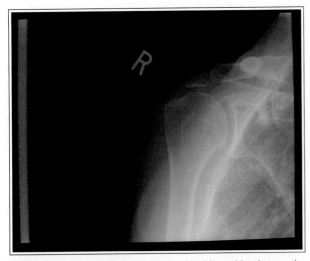

FIGURE 2-11 Computed radiography AP oblique (Grashey method) shoulder projection demonstrating a histogram analysis error.

exposures (Figure 2-12) are used and is most likely to occur when the technologist forgot to change the technique from the previous patient or the AEC ionization chamber(s) was poorly positioned in relation to the part of interest. Such an image must be repeated after the problem has been identified and corrected.

exposure factors (mAs, kVp) should be adjusted. Begin your evaluation by determining how accurately the positioning procedures listed in Box 2-1 were followed. Only if these are accurate should the mAs or kVp be adjusted.

Causes

Extremely High or Low Exposures. When the exposure range exceeds the range of the specified LUT, image information is lost as the automatic rescaling process fails and a bright, washed-out image results. This is most apparent when extremely high or low

FIGURE 2-12 Digital lateral chest projection demonstrating a histogram analysis error caused by using an extremely low exposure.

Part Selection From Workstation Menu. If the wrong body part or projection is selected on the workstation, the image will be rescaled using the wrong LUT. Because each body part has a specific LUT to use for each projection, rescaling to the incorrect one will cause a histogram analysis error as the computer tries to align the data histogram with the incorrect LUT. This error is easily detected because the study name is noted in the data field underneath each digital image; it may be corrected by reprocessing it under the correct LUT as long as the image has not yet been sent to the archiving system.

Central Ray Centering. If the central ray is not centered to the VOI, the exposure field needs to be expanded to include all the required anatomy. Increasing the exposure field size may result in additional anatomy or excessive background values being included on the image histogram and identified as part of the VOI. This misshapens and widens the histogram, causing a histogram analysis error. Figure 2-13 demonstrates an adult PA chest projection using the Kodak CR system. The image demonstrates adequate brightness, high contrast, and quantum noise, even though the resulting exposure index is 2300, which indicates excessive exposure. Improved central ray centering and tighter collimation is needed to improve this image. This problem occurs when excessive abdominal structures are included on chest or lateral lumbar vertebral images and/or excessive lung structures are included on abdominal images.

Collimation. Collimating to within 0.5 inch (2.5 cm) of the skin line prevents too much background density from being included within the exposure field. If excessive background density is inappropriately included in the VOI, a widening of the image histogram will result (Figure 2-14). Figure 2-15 demonstrates a PA hand projection taken of a 4-year-old child using the Kodak CR system. The image demonstrates adequate brightness, high contrast, and quantum noise, even though the resulting exposure index is 2430, which indicates excessive exposure. A histogram error resulted because the image was not tightly collimated and the background density was not excluded from the VOI.

Scatter Radiation Control. Reduce the scatter radiation fog reaching the IR through tight collimation, appropriate grid usage, and by placing a lead sheet along the edge of the exposure field when excessive scatter fogging is expected, such as on the posterior edge of lateral lumbar and thoracic vertebral images. When the amount of scatter radiation reaching the IR is high and the fog values outside the exposure field are included in the VOI, a widening of the histogram results (Figures 2-16 and 2-17).

Clearly Defining the Volume of Interest (For Computed Radiography Only). Clearly defining the VOI by using an IR size where the VOI will cover the entire IP, eliminating any exposure values from being recorded on the IP that are not of interest, will reduce the chance of histogram analysis errors. When it is necessary to collimate smaller than the IR, make certain to center the VOI in the center of the CR cassette and ideally have all four collimation borders showing and positioned at equal distances from the edges of the cassette. When only two collimation borders are present, as with an AP lumbar vertebral projection, they also should be equidistant from the edges of the cassette. It is not acceptable to have only one border showing without the opposite border also being present. In the exposure field recognition process, the computer identifies the difference between the brightness values that are outside from those inside the exposure field. When one of the collimation borders is missing, the computer may not distinguish the collimation border that is present as an actual border but instead include the area beyond it as part of the image, especially if there is any fogging present. Instead the computer will consider the area to be part of the VOI and include it in the histogram. When both borders are present, the computer can better identify the value differences at each end of the exposure field as being a collimation border. This often occurs on images of the axiolateral hip or inferosuperior (axial) shoulder, where the collimated field covers only the bottom two thirds of the cassette, demonstrating the upper collimation border but not the bottom one (Figure 2-18). To prevent this histogram analysis error, either build the patient up enough to collimate on each side equally, or tape a 1-inch lead strip to the bottom of the cassette to serve as the bottom collimation border and build the patient up enough to position the part above this lead strip to prevent clipping needed anatomic structures. Different CR system manufacturers also have suggestions specific to their system that can

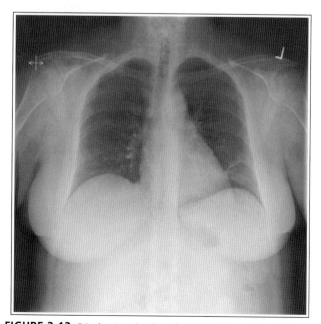

FIGURE 2-13 PA chest projection obtained with Kodak CR system that demonstrates a histogram analysis error caused by poor central ray centering and poor collimation.

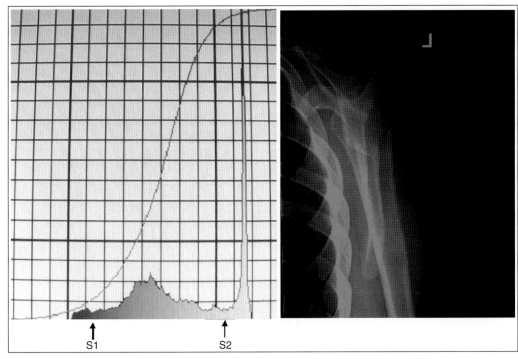

FIGURE 2-14 Computed radiography histogram that includes excessive background radiation values in the volume of interest.

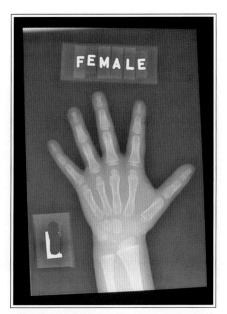

FIGURE 2-15 Digital PA hand projection demonstrating a histogram analysis error caused by poor collimation.

be used to obtain optimal images under these circumstances. For example, the image may be processed under a different scanning mode (Fuji), processed under a different anatomic specifier (Kodak), or you may be told to read only certain portions or sections of the IP.

Coverage of 30% (For Computed Radiography Only). It has been shown that exposure indicator errors are likely to occur in CR when less than 30% percent

of the IP is exposed. To ensure that at least 30% of the IP is exposed, the smallest possible IR size should be chosen, and when imaging parts that require tight collimation, such as the fingers or thumbs, it is recommended that two or three of the views be taken on one IP.

Multiple Images on One Imaging Plate (For Computed Radiography Only). When multiple exposures are taken on one IP, it is difficult for the computer to distinguish between the very bright areas between exposure fields and similar very light areas within the VOI when fog density is present between the collimated fields. To assist the exposure field recognition process, the body part should be centered within each exposure field, and all collimation should be parallel and equidistant from the edges of the IP (Figure 2-19). The farther apart the images are positioned from each other, the less chance that they will be mistaken for a single image. Also, use lead sheets over the areas of the IR that are not being used during exposures to protect them from scatter fogging.

Background Radiation Fogging (For Computed Radiography Only). CR plates are extrasensitive to scatter radiation. A fog density can accumulate across the plate from exposure to scatter fogging when the IP is left in the imaging room while other images are being exposed. Fog will decrease the brightness values of the pixels, resulting in histogram analysis errors. Figure 2-20 demonstrates an image of an AP abdomen that was exposed and left in the room while a second x-ray was performed. The image demonstrates low contrast caused by scatter fogging. The brighter streak that

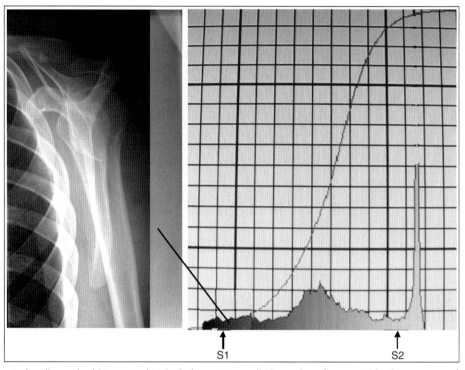

FIGURE 2-16 Computed radiography histogram that includes scatter radiation values from outside the exposure field in the volume of interest.

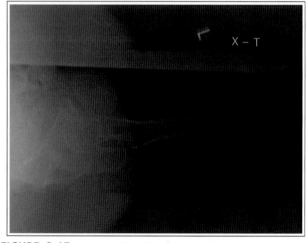

FIGURE 2-17 Computed radiography axiolateral hip projection demonstrating a histogram analysis error caused by including scatter radiation values from outside the exposure field in the volume of interest.

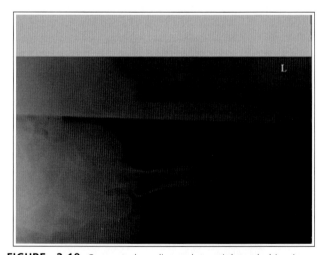

FIGURE 2-18 Computed radiography axiolateral hip image demonstrating a histogram analysis error caused by poor exposure field recognition.

runs through the center of the image is part of the wheelchair that the IR was resting against. The abdominal structures included in the brighter area demonstrate acceptable quality and suggests how the image would have looked if the scatter fogging had not occurred.

CR plates are also more sensitive than screen-film IR systems to accumulated background radiation during long periods of storage. Excessive background radiation

fogging will result in decreased pixel brightness values across the image, similar to that demonstrated on the image in Figure 2-20. CR cassettes that have been in storage for more than 48 to 72 hours (time frame varies among system manufacturers) should be put through the reader's erase process before being used to ensure that background fogging does not affect the subsequent images.

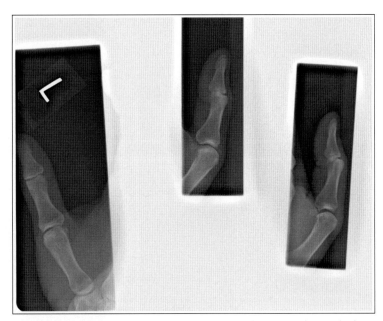

FIGURE 2-19 Computed radiography thumb images demonstrating poor image alignment when multiple images are placed on one imaging plate.

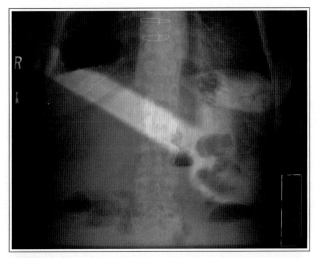

FIGURE 2-20 Computed radiography AP abdominal projection demonstrating a histogram analysis error caused by background radiation fogging.

Contrast Resolution

Contrast resolution refers to the ability of an imaging system to resolve low-contrast objects on an image. The higher the contrast resolution, the more distinct are adjacent structures of similar subject contrast. Digital radiography provides superior contrast resolution to screen-film radiography because of its ability to demonstrate an extensive gray scale or dynamic range.

Dynamic Range. The range of gray shades that the imaging system can display is referred to as the dynamic range. The higher this range, the more gray shades that are available for the pixels to display, resulting in better contrast resolution. The dynamic range is measured by

the bit capacity for each pixel. Digital radiography systems have a 14-bit dynamic range, allowing 16,384 shades of gray to be demonstrated. This is superior to screen-film systems that can demonstrate an optical density of 0 to 3.0, which represents a dynamic range of only 1000 shades of gray.

Quantum Noise. Quantum noise is generally characterized by graininess or a random pattern superimposed on the image. Noise can obscure borders, affecting edge discrimination, and can obscure underlying differences in shading, affecting contrast resolution. The *signal-to-noise ratio* (SNR) is the term used to describe the ratio of the desired signals to those that are undesirable. An increase in the SNR means that there has been a decrease in the noise signal in comparison to the desired signal, whereas a decrease in the SNR means that there has been an increase in the noise signal in comparison to the desired signal. Quantum noise is the most common noise seen in digital radiography and is present when photon flux (number of photons striking a specific area per unit of time) is insufficient. The technologist can increase photon flux and decrease quantum noise by making any change that will increase the number of photons that reach the IR, with the most common choice being to increase the technique factors of mAs or kVp. As noise decreases, the contrast on the object becomes more perceptible. The drawback of obtaining a higher SNR and increased contrast resolution is that the patient will receive a higher radiation dose.

Windowing. Digital radiography also allows for postprocessing manipulation of the image's brightness and contrast to demonstrate an area of interest more accurately. This process, called windowing, occurs after the image is displayed on the monitor. Adjusting the

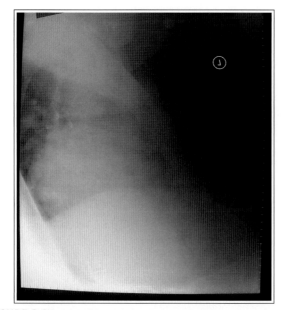

FIGURE 2-21 Digital lateral chest projection with narrow dynamic range caused by saving window settings to the PACS system.

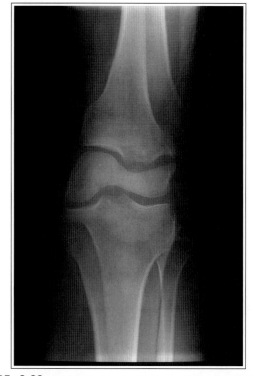

FIGURE 2-22 Double-exposed AP knee projections obtained using digital radiography.

window level allows the viewer to increase or decrease the brightness of the overall image, and adjusting the window width allows the viewer to increase or decrease the contrast of the overall image.

Technologists should avoid adjusting the window and level to improve image quality and then saving the new window settings to the PACS system. Once windowing has been done and the image saved, the wide dynamic range from the original image is lost, leaving only the range that was saved. The reviewer is then left with a narrower range of settings to use when evaluating different aspects of the image. Figure 2-21 displays an image for which the technologist saved the window settings of window width at 2111 and window level at 1,696 to the PACS system. If a 14-bit digital system were used for this image, the dynamic range of 16,384 possible gray shades has been reduced to 2111 for this image.

Artifacts

Double Exposure. When digital radiography is used, a double-exposed image will not demonstrate low brightness (high density) as with screen-film radiography, because the image will be normalized during processing (Figure 2-22).

Grid Alignment Artifact. When conventional screen-film radiography is used, an image taken with a grid alignment artifact demonstrates a loss in density where the grid lines are shown. With digital radiography, images demonstrating grid cutoff will show the grid lines, but will not demonstrate an increase in brightness values where the grid lines are visible because the image will be automatically rescaled to the correct brightness, as long as there is grid cutoff across the entire image.

For digital images where grid cutoff is demonstrated only on portions of the image, such as when a focused grid is inverted or the SID is out of the grid's focusing range, the rescaling process will be unable to rescale the areas with and without grid cutoff, resulting in the grid cutoff areas appearing brighter than areas without grid cutoff. Lower contrast will be visualized on the areas in the image where there is grid cutoff because the grid's lead lines will work like a filter to increase the uniformity of the exposure (Figures 2-23 and 2-24).

Aliasing or Moiré Grid Artifact. The CR moiré grid artifact occurs when a stationary grid is used and the IP is placed in the plate reader so that the grid's lead strips are aligned parallel with the scanning direction, resulting in a wavy line pattern on the image (Figure 2-25). It is more common with grids that have a frequency below 60 lines/cm. The moiré grid artifact can be eliminated by using a moving grid to blur lines and a grid frequency of 60 lines/cm or higher and by processing the image so that the grid's lead strips are aligned perpendicular to the plate reader's laser scanning direction. When you scan a 10- × 12-inch or 14- × 17-inch IP, it is scanned across its short axis. To position the grid's lead strips perpendicular to the scanning direction, the grid's lead strips should be placed with the long axis of the IP. An 8- × 10-inch IP is scanned across its long axis. To position the grid's lead strips perpendicular to the scanning direction, the grid's lead strips should be aligned with the short axis of the IP.

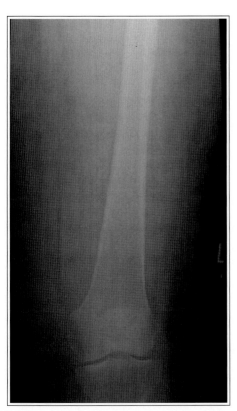

FIGURE 2-23 Digital AP femur projection demonstrating grid line artifacts.

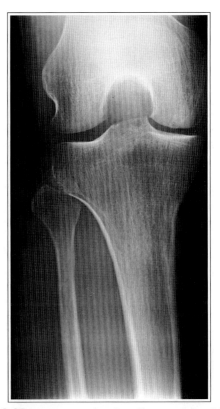

FIGURE 2-25 Equipment-related artifact—moiré grid artifact. *(Courtesy Cesar LJ, Schueler BA, Zink FE, et al. Artefacts found in computed radiography,* Br J Radiol *74:195–202, 2001.)*

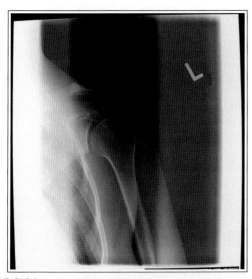

FIGURE 2-24 Digital AP oblique (Grashey method) shoulder projection demonstrating an inverted grid artifact.

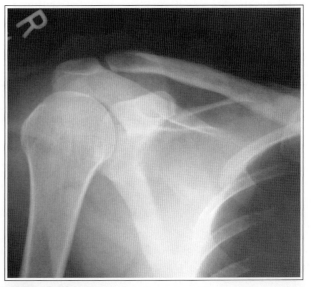

FIGURE 2-26 Computed radiography AP shoulder projection demonstrating a phantom image artifact.

Phantom Image Artifact. Phantom images are artifacts in CR that occur when the IP is not adequately erased before the next image is exposed on it. The resulting image is a light shadow of the image that was previously exposed onto the phosphors on the plate.

These images resemble a double exposure (Figure 2-26). After the exposure the IP is placed into the reader for processing. Information stored on the plate is released when it is exposed to a red laser light and then the plate goes to the erasing block, where it is exposed to a high-intensity light to release any remaining stored energy. The erasure block system is capable of erasing a phosphor plate that has received up to five times the normal exposure. If an exposure is more than this, stored energy in the form of a phantom image will remain on the plate and when reexposed and read may be seen on the new image, appearing similar to a double-exposed image. For this artifact to be prevented, the phosphor plate should be sent back to the erasure block for a second erasing when the exposure indicator indicates that an excessive exposure was used to create the image.

Scatter and Background Fogging. Phantom images may also be produced when the computed radiography IR is accidentally exposed to scatter radiation when left in the room during other exposures (see Figure 2-20) or has not been used for 48 to 72 hours and has collected a sufficient exposure from natural background radiation. Storing exposed and unexposed IR outside the x-ray room before and after exposures will prevent fogging caused by scatter radiation that occurs when an exposure is made. Completing a secondary erasure before using a phosphor plate that has not been used for some time will prevent background radiation fogging.

Back of Cassette Toward Source During Exposure. If the CR cassette is exposed with its back positioned toward the x-ray source, a faint white grid-type, honeycomb or square pattern will be overlaying the image (Figure 2-27). There will also be white areas that correspond to the hinges, if they are included within the exposure field.

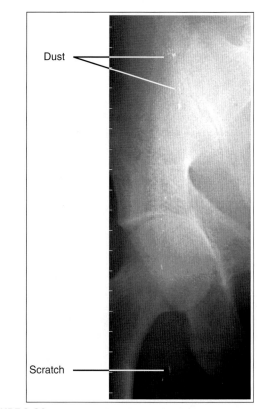

FIGURE 2-28 Equipment-handling artifact—phosphor plate scratches and dust on AP hip projection.

Phosphor Plate–Handling Artifacts. Dust or dirt particles and scratches on the surface of the phosphor plate produce small white dots or curved white lines, respectively (Figure 2-28). Dust or dirt artifacts can be corrected by cleaning the screen. Scratches are permanent, and replacement of the plate is required to eliminate them.

Digital System Artifacts. Occasionally, there are artifacts that appear on images that cannot be explained from a technologist's perspective and will require the system expert. Figure 2-29 has an orthopantomogram image that demonstrates a dark rectangular box in the lower left jaw area. Figure 2-30 shows an AP knee projection with bright spots in the knee joint. Both these artifacts were caused by problems with the digital system and were not a result of a technologist's error.

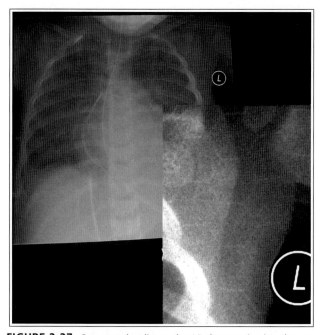

FIGURE 2-27 Computed radiography AP chest projection demonstrating honeycomb pattern overlying the image. This was caused by the back of the cassette being positioned toward the radiation source for the exposure.

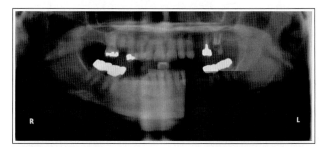

FIGURE 2-29 Digital orthopantomogram image with dark rectangular box in the lower left jaw from unknown cause.

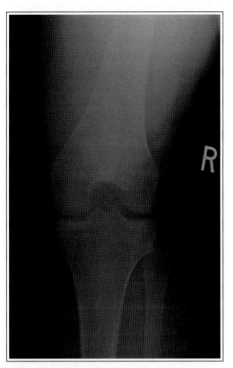

FIGURE 2-30 Digital AP knee projection with bright spots in the knee joint caused by poor detector elements.

BIBLIOGRAPHY

Bushberg JT, Seibert JA, Leidholdt EM, Boone JM: *The essential physics of medical imaging*, ed 2, Philadelphia, 2002, Lippincott Williams & Wilkins.

Carroll QB: *Practical radiographic imaging*, ed 8, Springfield, Ill, 2007, Charles C Thomas.

Fauber TL: *Radiographic imaging and exposure*, ed 3, St. Louis, 2009, Mosby Elsevier.

Chest and Abdomen

OBJECTIVES

After completion of this chapter, you should be able to do the following:

- Identify the required anatomy and describe the proper setup procedures for adult and pediatric chest and abdomen projections. Explain why each procedural step is required.
- State the technical data, marking and displaying requirements for chest and abdomen projections.
- List the image analysis requirements for accurately positioned adult and pediatric chest and abdomen images.
- State how to reposition the patient properly when chest and abdomen projections with poor positioning are produced.
- State how to position the patient and central ray to demonstrate air and fluid levels within the pleural cavity and when to expose chest images when the patient is unconscious or on a ventilator to obtain a fully aerated lung.
- State the purpose and proper location of the internal devices, tubes, and catheters demonstrated on adult and pediatric chest and abdomen images.

- Describe how the chest dimensions change when the patient breaths and discuss how to determine whether full lung expansion is obtained on chest images.
- Describe methods of identifying hemidiaphragms on chest images.
- State why the kilovoltage peak (kVp) level used for mobile chest images is lower than that for routine chest images. Discuss why a different kVp level is used when an image is taken to evaluate the patient's lung field versus the mediastinal region.
- Discuss how the patient is specifically positioned to rule out pneumothorax and pleural effusion on chest images.
- Explain how neonates' lungs develop and change as they grow.
- Discuss how technique is adjusted for imaging of the abdomen of patients with various abdominal conditions.

KEY TERMS

automatic implantable cardioverter defibrillator (ICD)
central venous catheter (CVC)
endotracheal tube (ETT)
intraperitoneal air
kyphosis

mammary line
pacemaker
pleural drainage tube
pleural effusion
pneumectomy
pneumothorax

pulmonary arterial catheter
scoliosis
umbilical artery catheter (UAC)
umbilical vein catheter (UVC)
vascular lung markings

The following image analysis criteria are used for all adult and pediatric chest projections and should be considered when completing the analysis for each chest projection presented in this chapter (Box 3-1).

Visibility of Chest Details

Beam penetration, contrast, and density are sufficient on chest images when the thoracic vertebrae and posterior ribs are faintly seen through the heart shadow and mediastinal structures, the vascular lung markings throughout the lung field and the soft tissue outlines of the air-filled trachea are visible, and fluid level or air within the pleural cavity and internal devices, tubes, and catheters, when present, are demonstrated.

An optimal kilovoltage peak (kVp) technique, as shown in Table 3-1, sufficiently penetrates the chest structures and provides the contrast scale necessary to visualize the lung details. To obtain optimal density, set milliampere-seconds (mAs) manually based on the patient's thorax thickness or choose the appropriate automatic exposure control (AEC) chamber when recommended (see Table 3-1). A grid is used in adult chest imaging, with the exception of mobile imaging, for which a grid is not commonly used because it is difficult to ensure that the grid and central ray are aligned accurately enough to prevent grid cutoff. When no grid is used, a lower kVp technique is needed to prevent excessive scatter radiation from reaching the IR and hindering contrast. Although the lower kVp will sufficiently penetrate the lung field, it seldom provides enough penetration to visualize structures within and behind the heart shadow fully.

Vascular Lung Markings

Vascular lung markings are scattered throughout the lungs and are evaluated for changes that may indicate pathology. To visualize these markings on chest images, the lungs must be fully expanded. To obtain maximum lung aeration in a patient who is able to follow instructions, take the exposure after the second full inspiration. For the unconscious patient, observe the chest moving and take the exposure after the patient takes a deep breath.

BOX 3-1	Chest Imaging Analysis Criteria

- Facility's identification requirements are visible.
- A right or left marker identifying the correct side of the patient is present on the image and is not superimposed over the anatomy of interest.
- Good radiation protection practices are evident.
- Lung markings, diaphragm, heart borders, hilum, greater vessels, and bony cortical outlines are sharply defined.
- Thoracic vertebrae and posterior ribs are seen through the heart and mediastinal structures.
- Vascular lung marking, and fluid-air levels and internal monitoring apparatus, when present, are demonstrated.
- There is no evidence of preventable artifacts, such as undergarments, necklaces, gown snaps, or removable external monitoring tubes or lines.

TABLE 3-1	Adult and Pediatric Chest Technical Data			
Projection	**kVp**	**Grid**	**AEC Chamber(s)**	**SID**
Adult Chest Technical Data				
PA	110	Grid	Both outside	72 inches (183 cm)
Lateral	125	Grid	Center	72 inches (183 cm)
AP mobile	80–95	Nongrid		48–50 inches (120 cm)
AP supine in Bucky	80–100	Grid	Both outside	48–50 inches (120 cm)
AP-PA (lateral decubitus)	125	Grid	Center	72 inches (183 cm)
AP axial (lordotic)	125	Grid	Both outside	72 inches (183 cm)
AP-PA oblique	125	Grid	Over lung of interest	72 inches (183 cm)
Pediatric Chest Technical Data				
Neonate: AP	65–70			40–48 inches (100–120 cm)
Infant: AP	70–75			40–48 inches (100–120 cm)
Child: PA	75–80	Grid (if measures 4 inches or larger)		72 inches (183 cm)
Child: AP	70–75			40–48 inches (100–120 cm)
Neonate: Cross-table lateral	65–70			40–48 inches (100–120 cm)
Infant: Cross-table lateral	75–80			40–48 inches (100–120 cm)
Child: Lateral	75–80	Grid (if measures 4 inches or larger)		72 inches (180 cm)
Neonate: AP (lateral decubitus)	65–70			40–48 inches (100–120 cm)
Infant: AP (lateral decubitus)	70–75			40–48 inches (100–120 cm)
Child: AP (lateral decubitus)	75–80			72 inches (183 cm)

AP, Anteroposterior; *kVp,* kilovoltage peak; *PA,* posteroanterior; *SID,* source–image receptor distance.

Ventilated Patient

For the patient who is being ventilated with a conventional ventilator, observe the ventilator's pressure manometer (Figure 3-1, *A*). The exposure should be taken when the manometer digital bar or analog needle moves to its highest position. If a high-frequency ventilator is being used, the exposure may be made at any time, because this ventilator maintains the lung expansion at a steady mean pressure without the bulk gas exchange of the conventional type (see Figure 3-1, *B*).

Lung Conditions Affecting Vascular Lung Marking Visualization

A pneumothorax (Figure 3-2) or pneumectomy (Figure 3-3) may be indicated if no lung markings are present, whereas excessive lung markings may suggest conditions such as fibrosis, interstitial or alveolar edema, or compression of the lung tissue. When selecting the technical factors (mAs and kVp) to be used for chest imaging, if a pneumothorax is suspected, decrease the kVp 8% from the routinely used setting (see Table 3-1). When a pneumectomy is indicated, do not select the AEC chamber that is positioned beneath the removed lung or overexposure will result (see Image 1).

Fluid Levels and Air

To demonstrate precise fluid levels when a pleural effusion is suspected, chest images are taken with the patient upright and the x-ray beam horizontal. With this setup the air rises and the fluid gravitates to the lowest position, creating an air-fluid line or separation. This separation

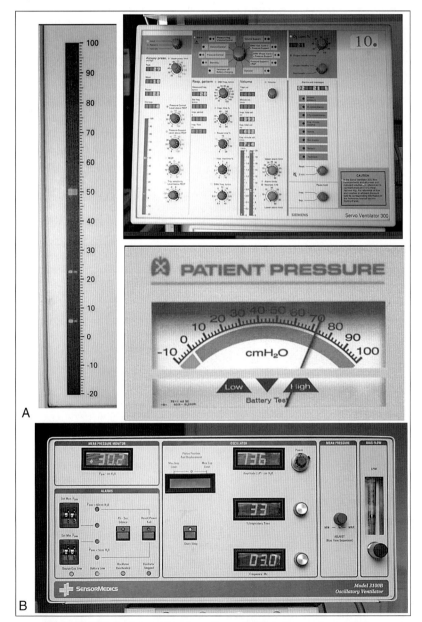

FIGURE 3-1   A, Conventional ventilator. **B**, High-frequency ventilator.

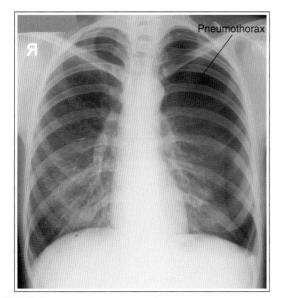

FIGURE 3-2 PA chest projection demonstrating a pneumothorax.

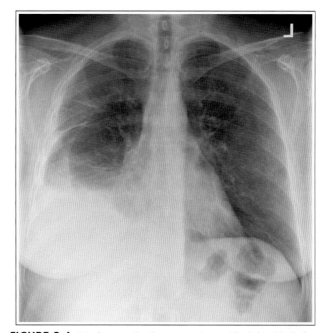

FIGURE 3-4 PA chest projection on patient with right-sided pleural effusion.

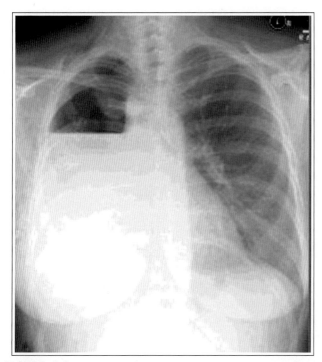

FIGURE 3-3 PA chest projection on patient with right-sided pneumectomy.

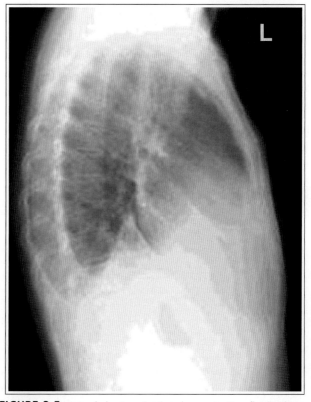

FIGURE 3-5 Lateral chest projection demonstrating fluid in lower lung field.

can be identified as a decrease in density on the image wherever the denser fluid is present in the lung field (Figures 3-4 and 3-5). If the patient is positioned only partially upright, the fluid line will slant, like water in a tilted jar. To demonstrate the true fluid line in a slanted position, the central ray must remain horizontal, which will result in foreshortening of the chest structures in the AP and PA projections. If the central ray is angled with the patient for a true AP-PA projection, the true amount of fluid cannot be discerned. When the patient

is supine, the fluid is evenly spread throughout the lung field, preventing visualization of fluid levels in the AP projection because a horizontal beam cannot be used. If pleural effusion is suspected, increase the mAs by 35% over the routinely used setting (see Table 1-3).

Free Intraperitoneal Air

The erect chest image is also an excellent method of discerning the presence of free intraperitoneal (within abdominal cavity) air because it will closely outline the diaphragm (Figure 3-6). As noted, the central ray must remain horizontal for the air to be demonstrated.

Internal Devices, Lines, and Catheters

Familiarizing yourself with the accurate placement of the devices, lines, and catheters that are seen on chest images will provide the information needed to identify when proper technique was used to visualize them and when poor placement is suspected (Table 3-2). Figure 3-7

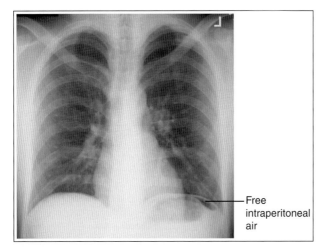

FIGURE 3-6 PA chest projection demonstrating free intraperitoneal air.

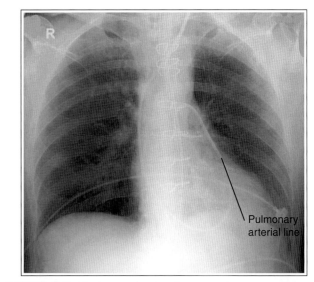

FIGURE 3-7 AP chest projection demonstrating poor pulmonary arterial line placement.

demonstrates poor placement of the pulmonary arterial line, because it was not advanced to the pulmonary artery. When a chest image is taken to determine the accuracy of line placement, it is within the technologist's scope of practice to inform the radiologist or attending physician immediately when a mispositioned device, line, or catheter is suspected.

Endotracheal Tube

The endotracheal tube (ETT) is a stiff, thick-walled tube used to inflate the lungs. For adults the distal tip of the ETT should be positioned 1 to 2 inches (3 to 5 cm)

TABLE 3-2	Chest Devices, Tubes, and Catheters	
Device, Tube, or Catheter	**Desired Location**	**Image Density and Penetration to Visualize**
Endotracheal tube (ETT)	Distal tip is placed 1–2 inches superior to carina when patient's neck is in neutral position	Upper mediastinal region
Pleural drainage tube (chest tube)	Fluid drainage–located laterally within pleural space at level of the fifth or sixth intercostal space Air drainage—located anteriorly within pleural space at level of midclavicle	Radiopaque identification line and side hole interruption
Central venous catheter (CVC)	Inserted into subclavian or jugular vein and extends to superior vena cava, about 2.5 cm above right atrial junction	CVC within heart shadow
Umbilical artery catheter (umbilical artery catheter [UAC])	Inserted into umbilicus and coursed to midthoracic aorta (T6 to T9) or below level of renal arteries, at approximately L1 to L2	UAC on lateral chest image adjacent to vertebral bodies
Umbilical vein catheter (UVC)	Inserted into umbilicus and advanced to junction of right atrium and inferior vena cava	UVC from umbilicus to heart
Pulmonary arterial catheter	Inserted into subclavian, internal or external jugular, or femoral vein and advanced through right atrium into pulmonary artery	Catheter within heart shadow
Pacemaker	Internal pacemaker implanted in subcutaneous fat in anterior chest wall and catheter tip(s) directed to right atrium or right ventricle	Pacemaker in lateral thorax and catheter tip(s) within heart shadow
Automatic implantable cardioverter defibrillator (ICD)	ICD is implanted in subcutaneous fat in anterior chest wall and catheter tip(s) directed to right atrium or right ventricle	ICD in lateral thorax and catheter tip(s) within heart shadow

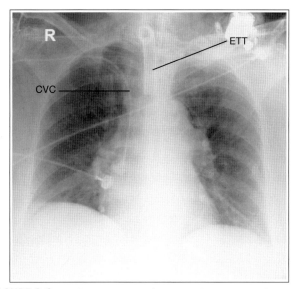

FIGURE 3-8 AP chest projection demonstrating accurate placement of an endotracheal tube (*ETT*) and central venous catheter (*CVC*).

superior to the tracheal bifurcation (carina) when the neck is in a neutral position (Figure 3-8). For neonates, the ETT should reside between the thoracic inlet and carina, which is at the level of T4 on the neonate (Figure 3-9). With the distance from the thoracic inlet to the carina being minimal on a neonate, the position of this tube is critical to within a few millimeters.

When imaging for ETT placement, the patient's face should be facing forward and the cervical vertebrae in a neutral position. With head rotation and cervical vertebrae flexion and extension, the ETT tip can move superiorly and inferiorly, respectively, making it more uncertain whether the tube is positioned in the correct location. Too superior positioning of the tube may place it in the esophagus, and too inferior placement may

place the tube in the right main bronchus, causing hyperinflation of the right lung and collapse of the left lung. Images taken for ETT placement should demonstrate penetration of the upper mediastinal region, and the longitudinal collimation should remain open to the bottom of the lip to include the upper airway.

Pleural Drainage Tube

The pleural drainage tube is a 1.25-cm diameter thick-walled tube used to remove fluid or air from the pleural space that could result in collapse of the lung. For drainage of air, the tube is placed anteriorly within the pleural space at the level of the midclavicle (Figures 3-10 and 3-11). For drainage of fluid, the tube is placed laterally

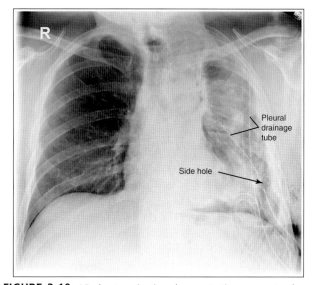

FIGURE 3-10 AP chest projection demonstrating accurate placement of two pleural drainage tubes.

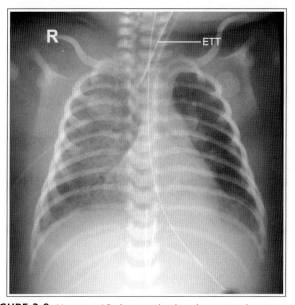

FIGURE 3-9 Neonate AP chest projection demonstrating accurate placement of an endotracheal tube (*ETT*).

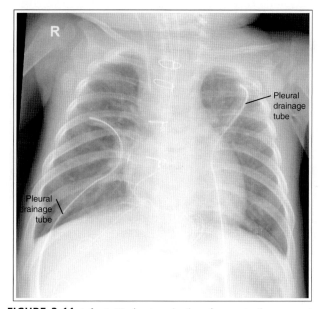

FIGURE 3-11 Infant AP chest projection demonstrating accurate placement of a pleural drainage tube in each lung.

within the pleural space at the level of the fifth or sixth intercostal space. The side hole of the tube is marked by an interruption of the radiopaque identification line. Images taken for pleural drainage tube placement should visualize the radiopaque identification line interruption at the side hole.

Central Venous Catheter

The central venous catheter (CVC) is a small (2- to 3-mm) radiopaque catheter used to allow infusion of substances that are too toxic for peripheral infusion, such as for chemotherapy, total parenteral nutrition, dialysis, or blood transfusions. The CVC is commonly inserted into the subclavian or jugular vein and extends to the superior vena cava, about 2.5 cm above the right atrial junction (Figures 3-12 and 3-13). Images taken for CVC placement should visualize the CVC and any lung condition that might result if tissue perforation occurred during line insertion, such as pneumothorax or hemothorax.

Pulmonary Arterial Catheter (Swan-Ganz Catheter)

The pulmonary arterial catheter is similar to the CVC catheter but it is longer. It is used to measure atrial pressures, pulmonary artery pressure, and cardiac output. The measurements obtained are used to diagnose ventricular failure and monitor the effects of specific medication, exercise, and stress on heart function. The pulmonary arterial catheter is inserted into the subclavian, internal or external jugular, or femoral vein and is advanced through the right atrium into the pulmonary artery (Figure 3-14). Images taken for pulmonary

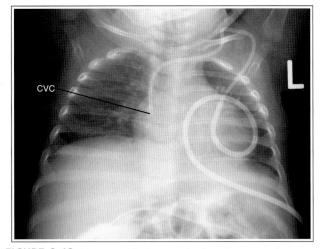

FIGURE 3-13 Neonate AP chest projection demonstrating accurate central venous catheter (*CVC*) placement.

arterial catheter placement should visualize the catheter and mediastinal structures to determine adequate placement.

Umbilical Artery Catheter

The umbilical artery catheter (UAC) is found only in neonates, because the cord has dried up and fallen off in older infants. The UAC is used to measure oxygen saturation. Optimal location for the UAC is in the midthoracic aorta (T6 to T9) or below the level of the renal arteries, at approximately L1 to L2. On a lateral chest image, the UAC is seen to lie posteriorly adjacent to the vertebral bodies because it courses in the aorta.

Umbilical Vein Catheter

The umbilical vein catheter (UVC) is found only in neonates, because the cord has dried up and fallen off in older infants. The UVC is used to deliver fluids and medications. The UVC courses anteriorly and superiorly to the level of the heart. The ideal location of the UVC is at the junction of the right atrium and inferior vena cava (Figure 3-15).

Pacemaker

The pacemaker is used to regulate the heart rate by supplying electrical stimulation to the heart. This electrical signal will stimulate the heart the needed amount to maintain an effective rate and rhythm. The internal pacemaker is surgically implanted in the subcutaneous fat in the patient's anterior chest wall and the catheter tip(s) directed to the right atrium or the right ventricle. On a PA-AP chest projection the pacemaker is typically seen laterally and the catheter tip(s) is seen in the heart shadow (Figure 3-16). Because the pacemaker is inserted

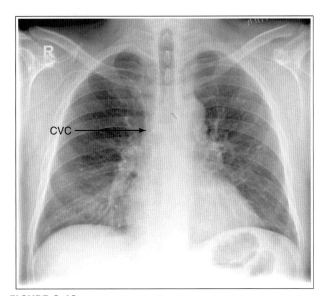

FIGURE 3-12 AP chest projection demonstrating accurate placement of a central venous catheter (*CVC*).

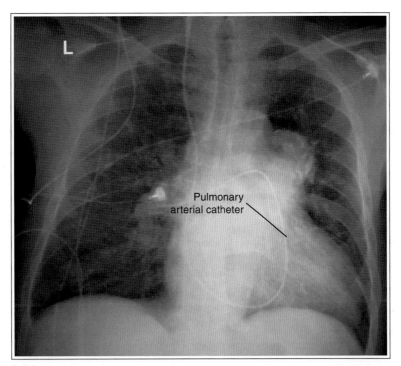

FIGURE 3-14 AP chest projection demonstrating accurate pulmonary arterial catheter placement.

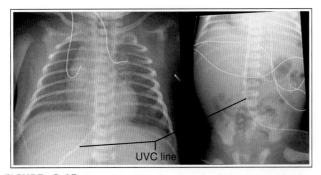

FIGURE 3-15 Neonate AP chest and abdomen projections demonstrating accurate placement of an umbilical vein catheter (*UVC*).

in the patient's upper thorax, care should be taken when lifting the patient's arm whose pacemaker was inserted within 24 hours of the examination, because elevation may dislodge the pacemaker and catheter.

Automatic Implantable Cardioverter Defibrillator

The implantable cardioverter defibrillator (ICD) is implanted in the anterior chest wall, as with the pacemaker, and the catheter tip(s) directed to the right atrium or the right ventricle. It is used to detect heart arrhythmias and then deliver an electrical shock to the heart to convert it to a normal rhythm. On a PA-AP chest projection the ICD is typically seen laterally and the catheter tip(s) is seen in the heart shadow (Figure 3-17).

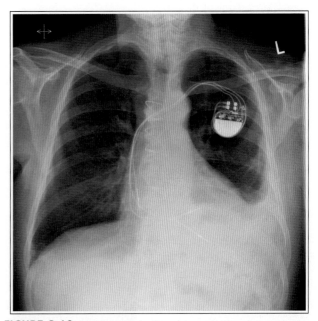

FIGURE 3-16 AP chest projection demonstrating accurate pacemaker placement.

External Monitoring Tubes and Lines

All external monitoring tubes or lines that can be removed or shifted out of the lung field should be. This includes oxygen tubing, electrocardiographic leads, external portions of nasogastric tubes, enteral feeding tubes, temporary pacemakers, and telemetry devices. Leaving these tubes and lines overlaying the lung field may result in obscuring important lung details (Figure 3-18).

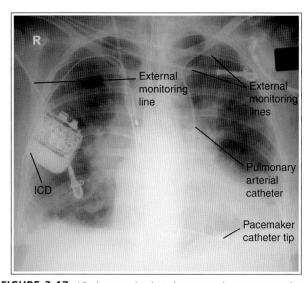

FIGURE 3-17 AP chest projection demonstrating accurate placement of implanted cardioverter defibrillator (*ICD*) and pulmonary arterial catheter.

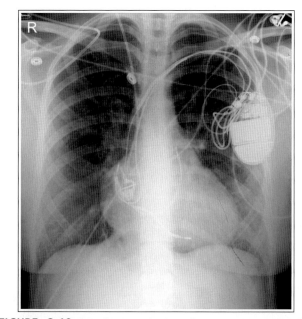

FIGURE 3-18 AP chest projection demonstrating removable external monitoring lines obscuring lung details.

CHEST: POSTEROANTERIOR PROJECTION

See Figure 3-19 and Box 3-2.

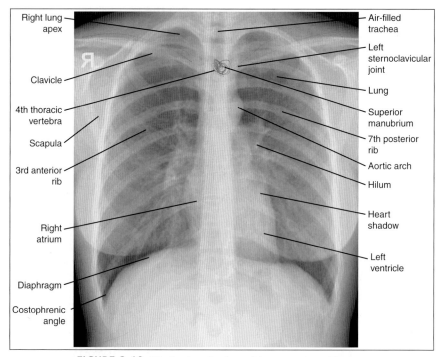

FIGURE 3-19 PA chest projection with accurate positioning.

The seventh thoracic vertebra is at the center of the exposure field. Both lungs, from the apices to costophrenic angles, are included within the collimated field.

- Centering a perpendicular central ray to the midsagittal plane, at a level approximately 7.5 inches

(18 cm) inferior to the vertebra prominens (seventh cervical spinous process), places the seventh thoracic vertebra in the center of the image. The seventh thoracic vertebra is identified on the image by counting down the vertebral column from the first thoracic vertebra, which is located just

BOX 3-2	**Posteroanterior Chest Projection Analysis Criteria**

- The seventh thoracic vertebra is at the center of the exposure field.
- Both lungs, from apices to costophrenic angles, are included within the collimated field.
- Distances from the vertebral column to the sternal clavicular ends are equal, and lengths of the right and left corresponding posterior ribs are equal.
- Clavicles are positioned on the same horizontal plane.
- Scapulae are located outside the lung field.
- Manubrium is superimposed by the fourth thoracic vertebra, with 1 inch (2.5 cm) of apical lung field visible above the clavicles.
- Ten or 11 posterior ribs are visualized above the diaphragm.

superior to the lung field and is the first vertebra that demonstrates rib attachment. This central ray placement also centers the lung field on the image. Center the image receptor (IR) to the central ray. Open the transversely collimated field to within 0.5 inch (2.5 cm) of the patient's lateral skin line. For most adult PA chest projections, the full IR length is needed, although you should collimate longitudinally on small patients.

- *IR size and direction.* A 14- × 17-inch (35- × 43-cm) IR should be large enough to include all the required anatomic structures. The direction of IR placement (crosswise versus lengthwise) must also be considered to ensure full lung coverage. For the average sthenic patient and hyposthenic and asthenic patients, whose lung fields are long and narrow, position the IR lengthwise. For the hypersthenic patient, whose lung fields are short and wide, position the IR crosswise.

- *Change in lung dimensions on inspiration.* Along with body type, consider how the lung expands on deep inspiration when choosing IR placement (crosswise, lengthwise). On inspiration, the lungs expand in three dimensions—transversely, anteroposteriorly, and vertically. Evaluate the transverse and vertical dimensions to determine how the IR should be placed. When a patient takes a deep breath, will the costophrenic angles still be included on the image? Determine this by placing a hand along the patient's side at the level of the costophrenic angles, and then asking the patient to inhale. If your hands remain within the IR's boundaries on inspiration, the IR is wide enough to accommodate the patient. If your hands move outside the IR's boundaries on inspiration, consider placing the IR crosswise. It is the vertical dimension that will demonstrate the greatest expansion. During high levels of breathing, as when we coax a patient into deep inspiration for a chest image, the vertical dimension can increase by as much as 4 inches (10 cm). This full vertical lung expansion is necessary to demonstrate the entire lung

field. Imaging the patient in an upright position and encouraging a deep inspiration by taking the exposure at the end of the second full inspiration allow demonstration of the greatest amount of vertical lung field. Circumstances that may prevent full lung expansion include disease processes, advanced pregnancy, excessive obesity, being seated in a slouching position, and confining abdominal clothing.

A PA projection is demonstrated. The distances from the vertebral column to the sternal (medial) ends of the clavicles are equal, and the lengths of the right and left corresponding posterior ribs are equal.

- To avoid chest rotation, position the patient's shoulders and arms at equal distances from the IR and instruct the patient to distribute body weight evenly on both feet and to face forward (Figure 3-20). Special attention should be given to female patients who have had one breast removed. The side of the patient on which the breast was removed may need to be placed at a greater object–image receptor distance (OID) than the opposite side to prevent rotation. A rotated chest image demonstrates distorted mediastinal structures and may create an uneven density between the lateral borders of the chest. This density difference occurs because the x-ray beam traveled through less tissue on the chest side positioned away from the IR than on the side positioned closer to the IR. It may be detected when the chest has been rotated as little as 2 or 3 degrees. Because any variation in structural relationships or density may represent a pathologic condition, the importance of providing nonrotated PA chest projections cannot be overemphasized.

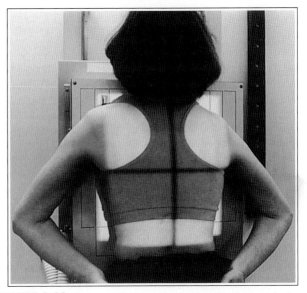

FIGURE 3-20 Proper patient positioning for PA chest projection.

- *Detecting rotation.* Rotation is readily detected on a PA chest projection by evaluating the distances between the vertebral column and the sternal ends of the clavicles and by comparing the lengths of the posterior ribs. On a nonrotated PA chest projection, these distances and lengths should be equal, respectively. On a rotated PA projection, the sternal clavicular end that demonstrates the least vertebral column superimposition and the side of the chest with the greatest posterior rib length represents the side of the chest positioned farthest from the IR (see Image 2).

- *Distinguishing scoliosis from rotation.* Scoliosis is a condition of the spine that results in the vertebral column's curving laterally instead of remaining straight. Scoliosis can be distinguished from rotation by comparing the distance from the vertebral column to the lateral lung edges down the length of the lungs. On images of a rotated patient, the distances are uniform down the length of the lung field, although when both lungs are compared, the distance is shorter on one side. If the patient has scoliosis, the vertebral column to lateral lung edge distances vary down the length of each lung and between each lung (see Image 3). The amount of distance variation increases with the severity of the scoliosis.

Clavicles are positioned on the same horizontal plane.

- The lateral ends of the clavicles are positioned on the same horizontal plane as the medial clavicle ends by depressing the patient's shoulders. Accurate clavicle positioning lowers the lateral clavicles, positioning the middle and lateral clavicles away from the apical chest region and providing better visualization of the apical lung field. When a PA chest projection is taken without depression of the shoulders, the lateral ends of the clavicles are elevated, causing the middle and lateral clavicles to be demonstrated within the apical chest region (see Image 4).

The humeri are abducted away from the chest, and the scapulae are located outside the lung field.

- Placing the back of the patient's hands on the hips draws the humeri away from the chest. This positioning also allows the patient easily to rotate the elbows and shoulders anteriorly to place the scapulae outside the lung field. When the scapulae are accurately positioned, the superolateral portion of the lungs is better visualized. If a chest image is taken without anterior rotation of the elbows and shoulders, the scapulae are seen superimposing the superolateral lung field (see Image 5).

- Scapular densities may prevent detection of abnormalities in the periphery of the lungs. Many dedicated chest units provide holding bars for the patient's arms. When using these units, make certain that the shoulders are protracted. If the patient is unable to protract the shoulders while using the bars, position the patient's arms as described earlier.

The manubrium is superimposed by the fourth thoracic vertebra, with approximately 1 inch (2.5 cm) of the apical lung field visible above the clavicles, and the lungs and heart are demonstrated without foreshortening.

- The tilt of the midcoronal plane determines the relationship of the manubrium to the thoracic vertebrae, the amount of apical lung field seen above the clavicles, and the degree of lung and heart foreshortening. When the midcoronal plane is vertical, the manubrium is projected at the level of the fourth thoracic vertebra, approximately 1 inch (2.5 cm) of the apices is visible above the clavicles, and the lungs and heart are demonstrated without foreshortening. If the superior midcoronal plane is tilted anteriorly (forward), however, as demonstrated in Figure 3-21, the lungs and heart are foreshortened, the manubrium is situated at the level of the fifth thoracic vertebra or lower, and more than 1 inch (2.5 cm) of the apices is demonstrated above the clavicles (see Image 6). This positioning error most often occurs during imaging of women with pendulous breasts and patients with protruding abdomens. Conversely, if the superior midcoronal plane is tilted posteriorly (backward), as demonstrated in Figure 3-22, the lungs and heart

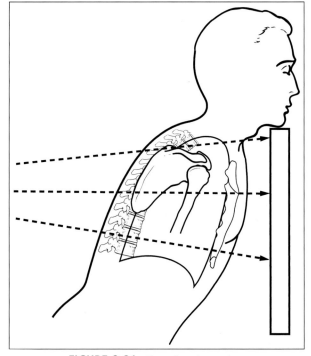

FIGURE 3-21 Chest foreshortening.

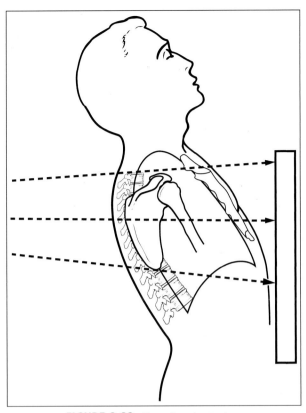

FIGURE 3-22 Chest foreshortening.

are foreshortened, the manubrium is situated at a level between the first and third thoracic vertebrae, and less than 1 inch (2.5 cm) of the apices is demonstrated above the clavicles (see Image 7).

• *Poor midcoronal plane versus poor shoulder positioning.* When a PA chest projection is taken with the patient's upper midcoronal plane tilted toward the IR, the clavicles are not always demonstrated horizontally but may be seen vertically (see Image 6). Distinguish poor shoulder positioning from poor midcoronal plane positioning by measuring the amount of lung field visualized superior to the clavicles and determining which vertebrae are superimposed over the manubrium. An image with poor shoulder positioning demonstrates decreased lung field superior to the clavicles and the manubrium at the level of the fourth vertebra. An image with the upper midcoronal plane tilting anteriorly demonstrates increased lung field superior to the clavicles and the manubrium at a level inferior to the fourth vertebra.

Ten or 11 posterior ribs are demonstrated above the diaphragm, indicating full lung aeration.

• To obtain maximum lung aeration, take the exposure with the patient in an upright position and after the second full inspiration. When the patient is positioned upright, the abdominal organs and diaphragm shift inferiorly, providing more space

for maximum vertical lung expansion. If fewer than 10 posterior ribs are demonstrated, the lungs were not fully inflated. Before repeating the procedure, attempt to obtain a deeper inspiration and determine whether a patient's condition might have caused the poor inhalation. Chest images that are taken with inadequate inspiration may demonstrate a decrease in image density, because a decrease in air volume increases the concentration of pulmonary tissues and the heart shadow may appear larger than it actually is.

• *Expiration chest image.* Abnormalities such as a pneumothorax or foreign body may indicate the need for an expiration chest image. For such an image, all evaluation requirements listed for a PA chest projection should be met except the number of ribs demonstrated above the diaphragm. On an expiration chest image, as few as nine posterior ribs may be demonstrated, the lungs are denser, and the heart shadow is broader and shorter (see Image 8). When manually setting technique, it may be necessary to increase the exposure (mAs) when a PA chest projection is taken on expiration and lung details are of interest.

Posteroanterior Chest Projection Analysis

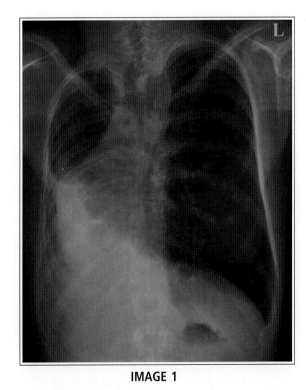

IMAGE 1

Analysis. The patient has a right-sided pneumectomy. The left lung was overexposed because the right AEC chamber was activated.

Correction. Repeat the image choosing the AEC chamber beneath the left lung field.

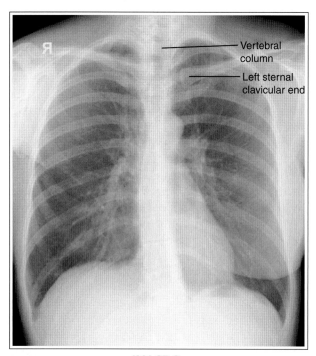

IMAGE 2

Analysis. The distances from the vertebral column to the lateral rib edges down the length of lungs vary, indicating that the patient has scoliosis.

Correction. No correction movement is required.

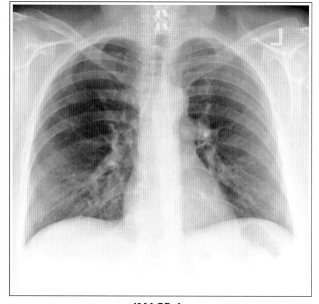

IMAGE 4

Analysis. The left sternal clavicular end is visualized without vertebral column superimposition, and the left posterior ribs demonstrate greater length than the right posterior ribs. The patient was slightly rotated, with the right side of the chest positioned closer to the IR than the left.

Correction. To offset chest rotation, position the left shoulder closer to the IR. The shoulders should be at equal distances from the IR.

Analysis. The clavicles are not horizontal, and the lateral ends of the clavicles are elevated, obscuring the apices. The manubrium is situated at the level of the fourth thoracic vertebra, and approximately 1 inch (2.5 cm) of the apices is demonstrated superior to the clavicles, indicating that the midcoronal plane was adequately positioned. The patient's shoulders were not depressed.

Correction. Depress the patient's shoulders.

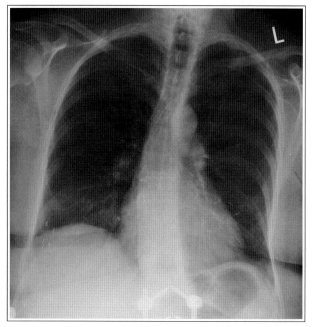

IMAGE 3

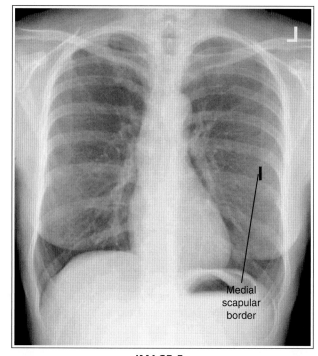

IMAGE 5

Analysis. The medial borders of the scapulae are demonstrated within the superolateral lung field; the shoulders and elbows were not anteriorly rotated.

Correction. Rotate the elbows and shoulders anteriorly, to draw the scapulae out of the lung field.

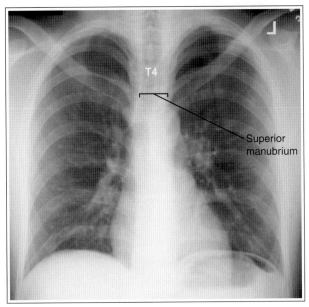

IMAGE 6

Analysis. The manubrium is situated at the level of the fifth thoracic vertebra, and more than 1 inch (2.5 cm) of the apices is demonstrated superior to the clavicles. The upper midcoronal plane was tilted anteriorly (see Figure 3-21).

Correction. Move the patient's upper thorax posteriorly until the midcoronal plane is vertical.

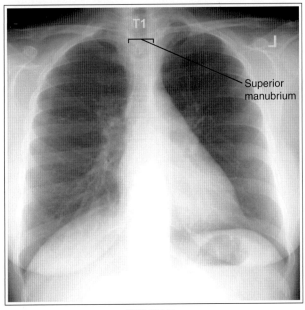

IMAGE 7

Analysis. The manubrium is situated at the level of the second thoracic vertebra, and less than 1 inch (2.5 cm) of the apices is demonstrated superior to the clavicles. The upper midcoronal plane was tilted away from the IR (see Figure 3-22).

Correction. Move the patient's upper thorax toward the IR until the midcoronal plane is vertical.

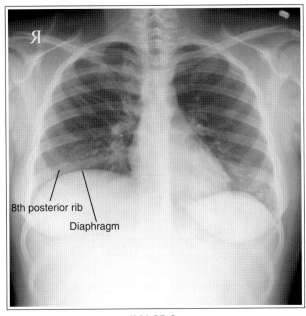

IMAGE 8

Analysis. Only the first through eighth posterior ribs are demonstrated above the diaphragm; the image was taken at the end of expiration.

Correction. If an expiration PA chest projection is desired, no change in respiration is required. If an inspiration PA chest projection is desired, repeat the image, making the exposure after the second full inspiration.

CHEST: LATERAL PROJECTION (LEFT LATERAL POSITION)

See Figure 3-23 and Box 3-3.

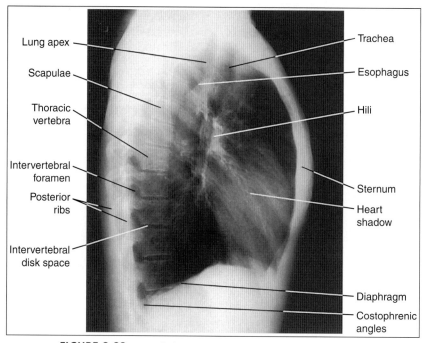

FIGURE 3-23 Lateral chest projection with accurate positioning.

The midcoronal plane, at the level of the eighth thoracic vertebra, is at the center of the exposure field. The entire lung field, including apices, costophrenic angles, and posterior ribs, is included within the collimated field.

- Centering a perpendicular central ray to the midcoronal plane, at a level approximately 8.5 inches (21.25 cm) inferior to the vertebra prominens places the central ray at the level of the eighth thoracic vertebra. This lower centering, compared with that for the PA chest projection, is needed to include the right costophrenic angle on the image. Because the right costophrenic angle is positioned at a long OID and the central ray is centered

---

BOX 3-3 | **Lateral Chest Projection Analysis Criteria**

- The midcoronal plane, at the level of the eighth thoracic vertebra, is at the center of the exposure field.
- The entire lung field, including apices, costophrenic angles, and posterior ribs, is included within the collimated field.
- The right and left posterior ribs are almost superimposed, demonstrating no more than a 0.5 inch (1 cm) of space between them, and the sternum is in profile.
- The lungs are demonstrated without foreshortening, with almost superimposed hemidiaphragms.
- No humeral soft tissue is seen superimposing the anterior lung apices.
- The anteroinferior lung and heart shadow are well defined.
- Hemidiaphragms demonstrate a gentle, cephalically bowed contour and are inferior to the eleventh thoracic vertebra.

---

superiorly to it, the costophrenic angle is projected inferiorly. Center the IR to the central ray.

- Positioning the midcoronal plane vertically prevents forward or backward leaning, which may result in clipping of the sternum or posterior ribs. Open the transversely collimated field to within 0.5 inch (1.25 cm) of the lateral skin line. For most adult lateral chest images, the full IR length is needed, although you should collimate longitudinally on small patients.
- A 14- × 17-inch (35- × 43-cm) lengthwise IR should be adequate to include all the required anatomic structures.

A lateral chest projection is demonstrated. The right and left posterior ribs are almost superimposed, demonstrating no more than a 0.5-inch (1-cm) space between them, and the sternum is in profile.

- To avoid chest rotation, align the shoulders, posterior ribs, and posterior pelvic wings perpendicular to the IR (Figure 3-24). This alignment is accomplished by resting an extended flat hand against each, respectively, and then adjusting the patient's rotation until the hand is positioned perpendicularly to the IR. Because the right lung field and ribs are positioned at a greater OID than the left lung field and ribs, the right lung field and ribs are more magnified. This magnification prevents the right and left ribs from being directly superimposed. Routinely, approximately a 0.5-inch (1-cm) separation is demonstrated between the right and left posterior

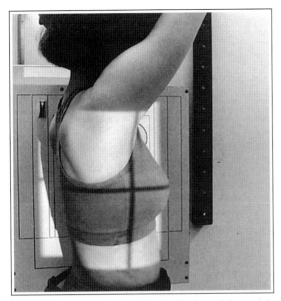

FIGURE 3-24 Proper patient positioning for lateral chest projection.

ribs, with the right posterior ribs projecting behind the left. When the posterior ribs are directly superimposed, this separation is demonstrated between the anterior ribs, but it is more difficult to distinguish (see Image 9).

- *Detecting chest rotation.* Chest rotation is effectively detected on a lateral chest projection by evaluating the degree of superimposition of the posterior ribs and anterior ribs. When more than 0.5 inch (1.25 cm) of space exists between the right and left posterior ribs, the chest was rotated for the image. A rotated lateral chest projection obscures portions of the lung field and distorts the heart and hilum shadows.
- *Distinguishing the right and left lungs.* When a rotated lateral chest projection has been obtained, determine how to reposition the patient by identifying the hemidiaphragms and therefore the lungs. The first and easiest method of discerning the hemidiaphragm is to identify the gastric air bubble. On an upright patient, gas in the stomach rises to the fundus (superior section of stomach), which is located just beneath the left hemidiaphragm (see Images 9 and 11). If this gastric bubble is visible on the image, you know that the left hemidiaphragm is located directly above it. The second method of distinguishing one lung from the other uses the heart shadow. Because the heart shadow is located in the left chest cavity and extends anteroinferiorly to the left hemidiaphragm, outlining the superior heart shadow enables you to recognize the left lung. As demonstrated in Figure 3-25, if the left lung is positioned anteriorly, the outline of the superior heart shadow continues beyond the sternum and into the anterior lung (see Image 10). Figure 3-26 demonstrates the opposite rotation; the right lung is positioned anteriorly. Note how the superior heart shadow does not extend into the anterior situated lung but ends at the sternum (see Image 11).

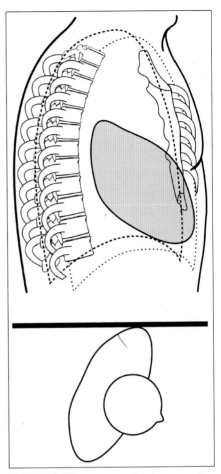

FIGURE 3-25 Rotation—left lung anterior.

It is most common on rotated lateral chest projections for the left lung to be rotated anteriorly and the right lung to be rotated posteriorly.

- *Repositioning the rotated patient.* Once the lungs have been identified, reposition the patient by rotating the thorax. When the left lung was anteriorly positioned on the original image, rotate the left thorax posteriorly, and when the right lung was anteriorly positioned, rotate the right thorax posteriorly. Because both lungs move simultaneously, the amount of adjustment should be only half of the distance demonstrated between the posterior ribs.
- *Distinguishing scoliosis from rotation.* On images of patients with spinal scoliosis, the lung field may appear rotated because of the lateral deviation of the vertebral column (see Image 12). The anterior ribs are superimposed, but the posterior ribs demonstrate differing degrees of separation, depending on the severity of scoliosis. View the accompanying PA chest projection to confirm this patient condition. Although the separation between the posterior ribs is not acceptable beyond 0.5 inch (1.25 cm) on a patient without scoliosis, it is acceptable on a patient with the condition.

The lungs are demonstrated without foreshortening, with almost superimposed hemidiaphragms.

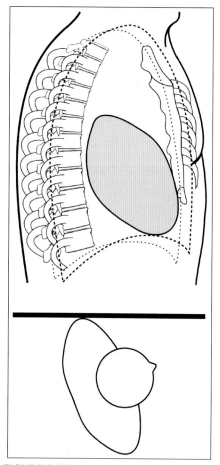

FIGURE 3-26 Rotation—right lung anterior.

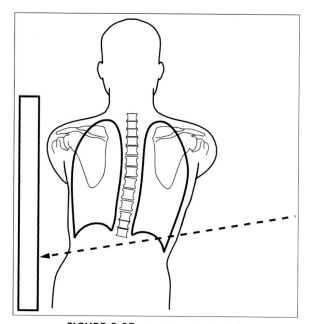

FIGURE 3-27 Chest foreshortening.

- *Lung foreshortening*. To obtain a lateral chest projection without lung foreshortening, position the midsagittal plane parallel with the IR. When imaging a patient with broad shoulders and narrow hips, it is essential to place the hips away from the IR to maintain a parallel midsagittal plane. In 90% of persons the right lung and diaphragm are situated at a slightly higher elevation than the left lung and diaphragm. This elevation is caused by the liver, which is situated directly below the right diaphragm. Because the right diaphragm is elevated, one might expect it to be demonstrated above the left diaphragm when the patient is imaged from the side, but this is not true when the midsagittal plane is correctly positioned. Because the anatomic part positioned farthest from the IR diverges and magnifies the most, the right lung will be projected and magnified more than the left lung. The resulting image demonstrates near superimposition of the two hemidiaphragms. When the midsagittal plane has not been positioned parallel with the IR, lung foreshortening and poor hemidiaphragm positioning occur.
- *Poor midsagittal plane positioning*. Figure 3-27 demonstrates a lateral chest projection obtained with the patient's shoulders and hips resting against the IR, causing the inferior midsagittal plane to tilt

toward the IR. This positioning projects the right hemidiaphragm inferior to the left on the image (see Image 13). When such an image has been obtained, determine how the patient was mispositioned by using one of the methods described earlier to distinguish the right lung from the left lung. Before retaking a lateral chest projection because of foreshortening, scrutinize the patient's accompanying PA projection to determine whether the patient is one of the 10% of those whose hemidiaphragms are at the same height or whether a pathologic condition is causing the left hemidiaphragm to be projected above the right (Figure 3-28).

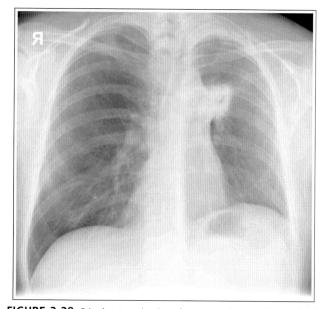

FIGURE 3-28 PA chest projection demonstrating an elevated left hemidiaphragm.

- *Right versus left position.* A lateral chest projection obtained with the left side versus the right side of the chest positioned against the IR will demonstrate two distinct differences, the size of the heart shadow and the superimposition of the hemidiaphragms. Both differences are a result of a change in OID and magnification. A lateral chest projection taken with the right thorax positioned closer to the IR will demonstrate the anatomic structures located in the left thorax with greater magnification than structures located in the right thorax. Radiographically, the heart shadow will be more magnified and the left hemidiaphragm will project lower than the right hemidiaphragm (see Image 14). One advantage of obtaining the lateral chest projection with the right thorax closer to the IR is that it will demonstrate increased right lung radiographic detail.

No superimposition of humeral soft tissue over the anterior lung apices is present.

- *Humeral positioning.* Placing the humeri in an upright vertical position and instructing the patient to cross the forearms above the head prevent superimposition of the humeral soft tissue over the anterior lung apices (see Image 15). Many dedicated chest units provide holding bars for the patient's arms. When they are used, make sure that the humeri are placed high enough to prevent this soft tissue overlap. If the holding bars cannot be raised high enough and the patient is able to prevent motion, position the patient's arms as just described.

The anteroinferior lung and the heart shadow are well defined.

- This area is most clearly defined when the patient is imaged in a standing position. If the patient is seated and leaning forward, the anterior abdominal tissue is compressed, obscuring the anteroinferior lung and the heart shadow; this is especially true in an obese patient (see Image 16). Consideration of patient condition dictates how the image will be taken. To best demonstrate this region on the seated patient, have the patient lean back slightly, allowing the anterior abdominal tissue to relax. Do not lean the patient so far back, however, that the posterior lungs are not on the image.

The hemidiaphragms demonstrate a gentle, cephalically bowed contour, and the eleventh thoracic vertebra is entirely superimposed by the lung field, with the hemidiaphragms visible inferior to it, indicating full lung aeration.

- *Maximum lung aeration.* When a lateral chest projection demonstrates the hemidiaphragms with an exaggerated cephalic bow, in addition to a portion of the eleventh thoracic vertebra inferior to

the hemidiaphragms in a patient with no condition to have caused such an image, full lung aeration has not been accomplished (see Image 17). Repeat the procedure with a deeper patient inspiration. The lungs must be fully inflated for lung markings to be evaluated. Chest images taken on expiration may also demonstrate a decrease in image density, because a decrease in air volume increases the concentration of pulmonary tissues.

When the patient is in an upright position and fluid is present in the inferior lungs, the hemidiaphragms are not clearly identifiable (see Figure 3-5).

- *Identifying the eleventh thoracic vertebra.* The eleventh thoracic vertebra can be identified by locating the twelfth thoracic vertebra, which has the last rib attached to it, and counting up one. To confirm this finding, evaluate the curvature of the posterior aspect of the thoracic and lumbar bodies. The thoracic curvature is kyphotic (forward curvature) and the lumbar curvature is lordotic (backward curvature). Follow the posterior vertebral bodies of the lower thoracic and upper lumbar vertebrae, watching for the subtle change in curvature from kyphotic to lordotic. The twelfth thoracic vertebra is located just above this change (Figure 3-29). On most fully aerated adult lateral chest images, the diaphragms are demonstrated dividing the body of the twelfth thoracic vertebra.

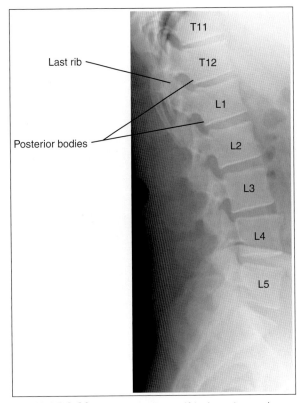

FIGURE 3-29 Identifying the twelfth thoracic vertebra.

Lateral Chest Image Analysis

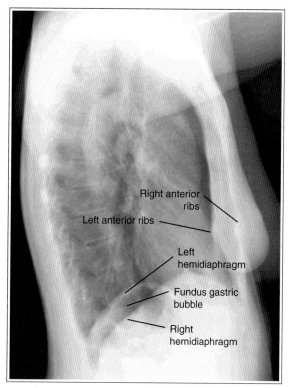

IMAGE 9

Right anterior ribs

Left anterior ribs

Left hemidiaphragm

Fundus gastric bubble

Right hemidiaphragm

Analysis. Posterior ribs are directly superimposed, and approximately 0.5 inch (1.25 cm) of space is present between the right and left anterior ribs.

Correction. No correction movement is required. The superimposition is a result of the increased magnification of the right lung over the left lung as a result of the greater OID.

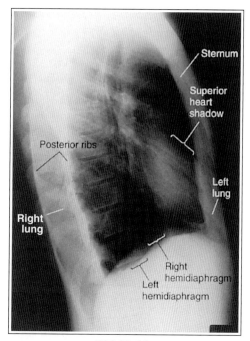

IMAGE 10

Sternum

Superior heart shadow

Posterior ribs

Left lung

Right lung

Right hemidiaphragm

Left hemidiaphragm

Analysis. The right and left posterior ribs are separated by more than 0.5 inch (1.25 cm), indicating that the chest was rotated. The gastric bubble has not been demonstrated, but the superior heart shadow is seen extending beyond the sternum and into the anteriorly situated lung, verifying that it is the left lung. The patient was positioned with the left thorax rotated anteriorly and the right thorax rotated posteriorly.

Correction. Position the right thorax slightly anteriorly. The amount of movement should be only half the distance between the posterior ribs. For this patient, the movement should be approximately 1 inch (2.5 cm).

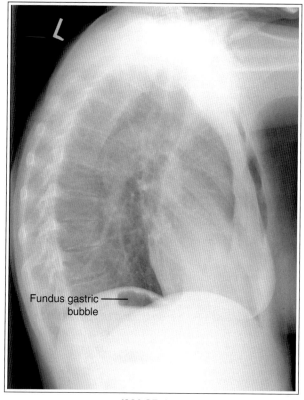

IMAGE 11

Fundus gastric bubble

Analysis. The right and left posterior ribs are separated by more than 0.5 inch (1.25 cm), indicating that the chest was rotated. The superior heart shadow does not extend beyond the sternum and the gastric air bubble is demonstrated adjacent to the posteriorly situated lung, verifying that the right lung is situated anterior to the sternum, and the left lung posteriorly. The patient was positioned with the right thorax rotated anteriorly and the left thorax rotated posteriorly.

Correction. Position the right thorax posteriorly.

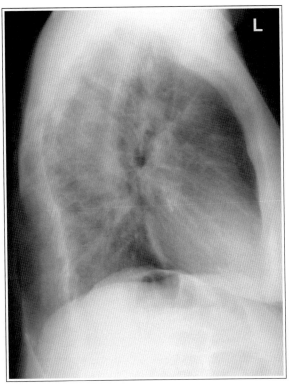

IMAGE 12

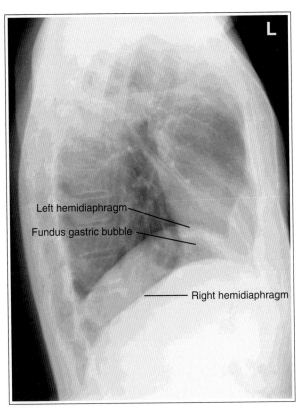

Left hemidiaphragm

Fundus gastric bubble

Right hemidiaphragm

IMAGE 13

Analysis. The right and left posterior ribs demonstrate differing degrees of separation. The patient has scoliosis. Evaluate the patient's accompanying PA projection to confirm this finding.

Correction. No correction movement is required. A lateral chest projection of a patient with scoliosis demonstrates uneven posterior rib separation.

Analysis. The left hemidiaphragm is superior to the right hemidiaphragm. This is verified by the visualization of the gastric bubble below the left hemidiaphragm. The patient's lower thorax was situated closer to the IR than the upper thorax (see Figure 3-27).

Correction. Before repeating the image, scrutinize the patient's accompanying PA projection carefully. Determine whether the hemidiaphragms are at the same height or whether a pathologic condition might have caused the left diaphragm to be projected above the right (see Figure 3-18). If no such condition is evident, repeat the procedure; shift the patient's hips away from the IR until the midsagittal plane is parallel with the IR.

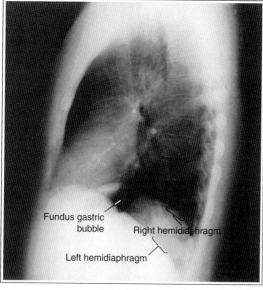

IMAGE 14

Analysis. This is a lateral chest projection obtained with the patient in a right lateral projection. The right hemidiaphragm is situated superior to the left hemi-diaphragm, and the heart shadow is enlarged.

Correction. If a right lateral projection is desired, no correction is needed. Otherwise, a lateral chest projection should be taken with the patient placed in a left lateral projection.

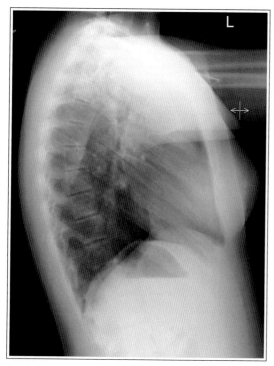

IMAGE 15

Analysis. The humeral soft tissue shadows are obscuring the anterior lung apices.

Correction. Have the patient raise the arms until the humeri are vertical, removing them from the field.

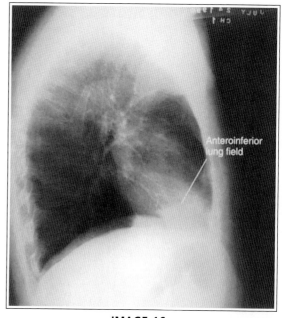

IMAGE 16

Analysis. The anterior abdominal tissue is pressing against the anteroinferior lung and heart shadows, pre-venting their clear visualization. The patient was leaning forward in a seated position.

Correction. Allow the patient to lean back slightly, relaxing the abdominal tissue. Do not lean the patient so far back, however, that the posterior lungs are not on the image.

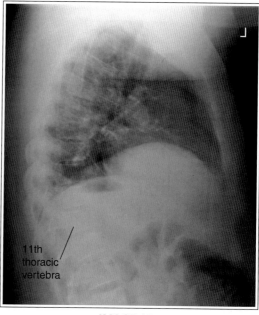

IMAGE 17

Analysis. The eleventh thoracic vertebra is demon-strated inferior to the hemidiaphragms. The image was not taken after full inspiration.

Correction. Coax the patient into taking a deeper inspiration.

CHEST: ANTEROPOSTERIOR PROJECTION (SUPINE OR WITH MOBILE X-RAY UNIT)

See Figure 3-30 and Box 3-4.

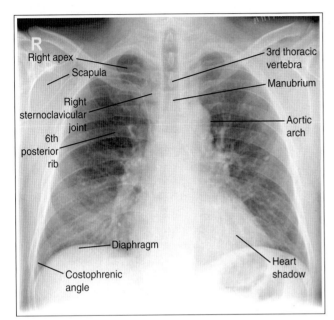

FIGURE 3-30 AP chest projection with accurate positioning.

The date and time of examination, SID used, degree of patient elevation, and technical factors used are recorded on image.

- Patients in an intensive care unit (ICU) often have mobile chest images taken on a daily basis that are compared for subtle changes. Consistent positioning is important to ensure that the subtle

changes are not caused by poor positioning, but is difficult to obtain when follow-up images are performed by multiple technologists. Consistency can best be accomplished through proper documentation. To do this, radiology departments use a sticker to record the information directly on the radiograph or, with digital radiography, the information is electronically annotated on the image. At a minimum, the information should include the date and time of examination, the SID used, the degree of patient elevation, and the technical factors used. The technologists should review this information prior to obtaining a subsequent chest image.

The heart demonstrates increased magnification when the images are compared with routine chest images.

- A 40- to 48-inch (102- to 120-cm) SID is used. This SID is lower than that used for routine chest images and demonstrates greater heart magnification because of the increase in x-ray divergence. The SID is often estimated during mobile procedures, but if available, a tape measure should be used to maintain appropriate SID, providing consistency in magnification and reducing the need to adjust technical factors.

The seventh thoracic vertebra is at the center of the exposure field. Both lungs, from the apices to costophrenic angles, are included within the collimated field.

- Centering the central ray to the midsagittal plane at a level approximately 4 inches (10 cm) inferior to the jugular notch places the seventh thoracic vertebra in the center of the image. This central ray placement also centers the lung field on the image. Center the IR to the central ray. Open the longitudinally collimated field to within 0.5 inch (2.5 cm) of the lateral skin line. For most adult AP chest projections, the full 14-inch (35-cm) length is needed. A 14- × 17-inch (35- × 43-cm) IR should be adequate to include all the required anatomic structures.

- *IR size and direction for mobile chest image.* The direction of IR placement (crosswise versus lengthwise) must also be considered to ensure full lung coverage. For the asthenic or hypersthenic patient, position the IR crosswise. For the sthenic patient, whose lung field is long and narrow, position the IR lengthwise. On inspiration, the lungs expand in three dimensions: transversely, anteroposteriorly, and vertically. Evaluate the transverse dimension to determine the direction in which the IR should be placed. View the lateral sides of the chest during the patient's deep inspiration to determine whether the lateral margins of the chest will remain within the IR boundaries. If the lateral chest margins move outside the IR boundaries during inspiration, consider placing the IR crosswise. It is safe to position

---

BOX 3-4 | **Anteroposterior Chest Projection (Supine or Mobile) Analysis Criteria**

- Date and time of examination, SID used, degree of patient elevation, and technical factors used are recorded on the image.
- The seventh thoracic vertebra is at the center of the exposure field.
- Both lungs, from apices to costophrenic angles, are included within the collimated field.
- The distances from the vertebral column to sternal clavicular ends are equal, and the lengths of the right and left corresponding posterior ribs are equal.
- The manubrium is superimposed by the fourth thoracic vertebra, with 1 inch (2.5 cm) of apical lung field visible above the clavicles.
- The clavicles are positioned on the same horizontal plane, when possible.
- The scapulae are located outside the lung field, when possible.
- The posterior ribs demonstrate a gentle cephalically bowed contour.
- Nine or 10 posterior ribs are visualized above the diaphragm.

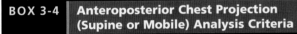

SID, Source–image receptor distance.

the IR crosswise on most patients for portable chest imaging because the vertical dimension does not fully expand in a recumbent or seated patient.

The chest demonstrates an AP projection when the distances from the vertebral column to the sternal ends of the clavicles and lengths of the right and left corresponding posterior ribs are equal.

- The patient, IR, and central ray must be accurately aligned to avoid chest rotation. The mobile light field provides a means of centering the central ray to the patient, but it does not indicate off-angling. This must be visually estimated by the technologist to avoid distortion. To align the patient and IR, place the patient's shoulders and pelvis on a straight plane and position the IR parallel with the bed (Figure 3-31). On beds with special padding, it may be necessary to place sponges beneath different aspects of the IR to keep it level and parallel in both the transverse and longitudinal axes. Because the patient's chest and IR move simultaneously, if the IR is not level, the chest is rotated. To align the central ray with the patient and IR, adjust the central ray position until it is perpendicular to the midcoronal plane and IR. If the central ray is angled to the right or left side of the patient instead of being perpendicular, the anatomic structures farthest from the IR (manubrium and clavicles) will be projected in the direction toward which the central ray is angled. Once the procedure has been set up, the technologist needs to evaluate the x-ray tube and patient relationship from two perspectives—side to side angle as observed from behind the x-ray tube, and cephalic-caudal angulation as observed from the side of the patient and the x-ray beam. When doing so the technologist should stand as far away from the mobile unit as possible because misalignment is easier to see from a distance.

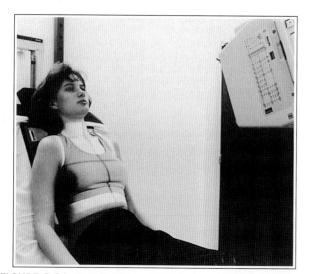

FIGURE 3-31 Proper patient positioning for AP chest projection.

- *Detecting chest rotation on a mobile image.* You can detect poor IR balance or poor central ray alignment and, consequently, chest rotation by evaluating the distances between the vertebral column and the sternal ends of the clavicles and by comparing the lengths of the posterior ribs. When the right sternal clavicular end demonstrates less superimposition of the vertebral column and the right posterior ribs demonstrate greater length than the left, the patient's right side was placed closer to the bed (see Image 18). When the left sternal clavicular end is seen without superimposition of the vertebral column and the left side demonstrates greater posterior rib length than the right, the patient's left side was placed closer to the bed (see Image 19). If the cause of this rotation was poor central ray alignment with the patient and IR, the sternal clavicular end that is superimposed over the least amount of the vertebral column and the posterior ribs that demonstrate the greatest length represent the side of the chest toward which the central ray angle was directed. Off-angling the central ray toward the right side of the chest will result in the right sternal clavicular end being seen at a greater distance from the vertebral column and greater right side posterior rib length (see Image 18), whereas angling the central ray toward the left side of the chest will result in the left sternal clavicular end being seen at a greater distance from the vertebral column and greater left side posterior rib length (see Image 19). It will be necessary to evaluate the positioning setup on rotated AP chest projections carefully to determine whether rotation was caused by poor alignment of the patient and IR with the central ray.

The manubrium is superimposed over the fourth thoracic vertebra with approximately 1 inch (2.5 cm) of the apices demonstrated above the clavicles, and the posterior ribs demonstrate a gentle cephalically bowed contour.

- The alignment of the central ray with respect to the patient determines the relationship of the manubrium to the thoracic vertebrae, the amount of apical lung field seen above the clavicles, and the contour of the posterior ribs. For accurate alignment of this anatomy, position the central ray perpendicular to the patient's midcoronal plane. Inaccurate central ray angulation misaligns this anatomy and elongates or foreshortens the heart and lung structures. The anatomic structures positioned farthest from the IR will move the greatest distance when the central ray is angled; angling the central ray caudally for an AP chest projection projects the manubrium inferior to the fourth thoracic vertebra, demonstrating more than 1 inch (2.5 cm) of lung apices superior to the clavicles, and changes the posterior rib contour to vertical. A caudal angle also elongates the heart and lung structures (see Image 20). Angling the central ray cephalically projects the manubrium superior to the fourth thoracic vertebra, demonstrating less than 1 inch (2.5 cm) of lung apices superior to the clavicles, and changes the posterior rib contour to horizontal. A cephalic angle also foreshortens the heart and lung structures (see Image 21). The more the angulation is mispositioned, either caudally or cephalically, the more distorted the anatomy.

- *Patient with spinal kyphosis.* On the supine or mobile chest image of a patient with spinal kyphosis (excess posterior convexity of the thoracic vertebrae), the position of the manubrium and clavicles and the contour of the posterior ribs may appear similar to those on a chest image for which the central ray was angled caudally. Also, if the patient is unable to elevate the chin, it may be superimposed over the apical chest region (Figure 3-32); compensate for this patient condition by using a slight (5- to 10-degree) cephalic angulation.

- *Supine patient.* For the supine AP chest projection, the patient's kyphotic upper vertebral column is forced to straighten because of the gravitational pull on it. This straightening causes the manubrium and clavicles to move superiorly and results in the image demonstrating less than 1 inch (2.5 cm) of apical lung field superior to the clavicles. Placing a 5-degree caudal angle on the central ray can offset this.

The clavicles are positioned on the same horizontal plane.

- When the patient's condition allows, position the lateral ends of the clavicles on the same horizontal plane as the medial ends by depressing the patient's shoulders. Accurate positioning of the clavicles lowers the lateral ends of the clavicles, positioning the middle and lateral clavicles away

from the apical chest region and improving visualization of the apical lung field. If the patient is unable to depress his or her shoulders, the middle and lateral ends of the clavicles will be seen in the apical chest region.

The scapulae are demonstrated within the lung field. The distal humeri have been abducted out of the imaging field.

- To position most of the scapulae outside the lung field, place the back of the patient's hands on the hips and rotate the elbows and shoulders anteriorly. Most patients who require mobile or supine chest images are incapable of positioning their arms in this manner, resulting in an image with the scapulae positioned in the lung field. In such a situation, abduct the patient's arms until they are placed outside the imaging field. Failure to do so will result in unnecessary exposure to the patient's arms (see Image 22).

Nine or 10 posterior ribs are demonstrated above the diaphragm, indicating full lung aeration for the nonerect chest image.

- In a supine or seated patient the diaphragm is unable to shift to its lowest position because the abdominal organs are compressed and push against the diaphragm. As a result, the lungs are not fully aerated, and only 9 or 10 posterior ribs are demonstrated above the diaphragm. If fewer than nine posterior ribs are demonstrated, then full lung expansion has not been obtained (see Image 23).

Anteroposterior Chest Projection Analysis

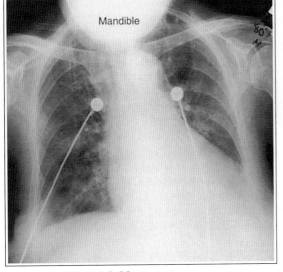

FIGURE 3-32 Kyphotic patient.

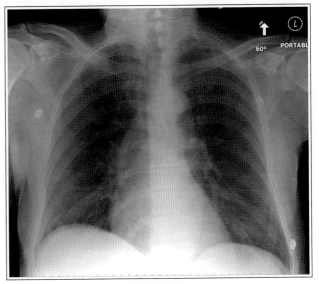

IMAGE 18

Analysis. The right sternal clavicular end is visualized away from the vertebral column, whereas the left sternal clavicular end is superimposed over the vertebral column and the right posterior ribs demonstrate greater length than the left. The IR was not positioned parallel with the bed but was positioned with the right side placed closer to the bed than the left, or the central ray was not aligned perpendicular to the IR but was off-angled toward the right side.

Correction. Place a sponge beneath the right IR border to position the IR parallel with the bed or slightly adjust the tube head and central ray toward the left side of the patient until it is aligned perpendicularly to the IR.

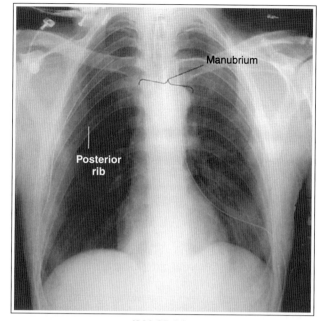

IMAGE 20

Analysis. The manubrium is superimposed over the fifth thoracic vertebra, more than 1 inch (2.5 cm) of apical lung field is visible above the clavicles, and the lateral clavicular ends are elevated. The posterior ribs demonstrate a vertical contour. All are indications that a caudal angulation was used.

Correction. For this image to be improved, the central ray needs to be adjusted in a cephalad direction until it is aligned perpendicularly to the midcoronal plane.

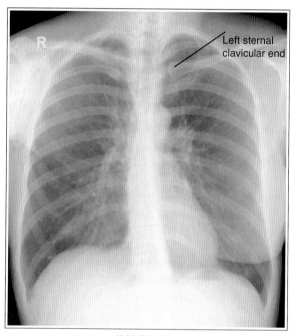

IMAGE 19

Analysis. The left sternal clavicular end is visualized away from the vertebral column, whereas the right sternal clavicular end is superimposed over the vertebral column, and the left posterior ribs demonstrate greater length than the right posterior ribs. The IR was not positioned parallel with the bed but was positioned with the left side placed closer to the bed than the right, or the central ray was not aligned perpendicularly to the IR but was off-angled toward the left side.

Correction. Place an elevating device beneath the left IR border to position the IR parallel with the bed or slightly adjust the tube head and central ray toward the right side of the patient until it is aligned perpendicularly to the IR.

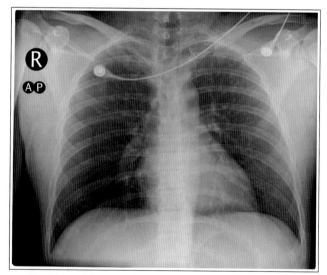

IMAGE 21

Analysis. The manubrium is superimposed over the second thoracic vertebra, and less than 1 inch (2.5 cm) of apical lung field is visible above the clavicles. The posterior ribs demonstrate a horizontal contour. The central ray was angled cephalically.

Correction. For this image to be improved, the central ray needs to be adjusted caudally until it is aligned perpendicularly to the midcoronal plane.

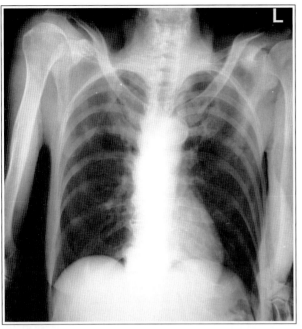

IMAGE 22

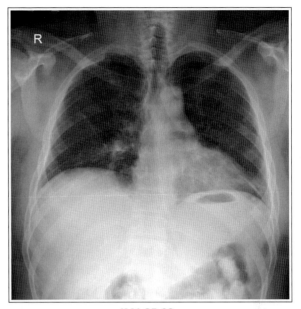

IMAGE 23

Analysis. The patient's arms were not abducted away from the chest region, unnecessarily exposing them.

Correction. Abduct the patient's arms until they are placed outside the collimated field. Increase the transverse collimation to within 0.5 inch (1.25 cm) of the patient's skin line.

Analysis. Eight posterior ribs are demonstrated above the diaphragm, indicating that the image was not taken with maximum lung aeration.

Correction. If the patient's condition allows, take the exposure after coaxing the patient into a deeper inspiration or at the point at which the ventilator indicates the greatest lung expansion.

CHEST: ANTEROPOSTERIOR OR POSTEROANTERIOR PROJECTION (RIGHT OR LEFT LATERAL DECUBITUS POSITION)

See Figure 3-33 and Box 3-5.

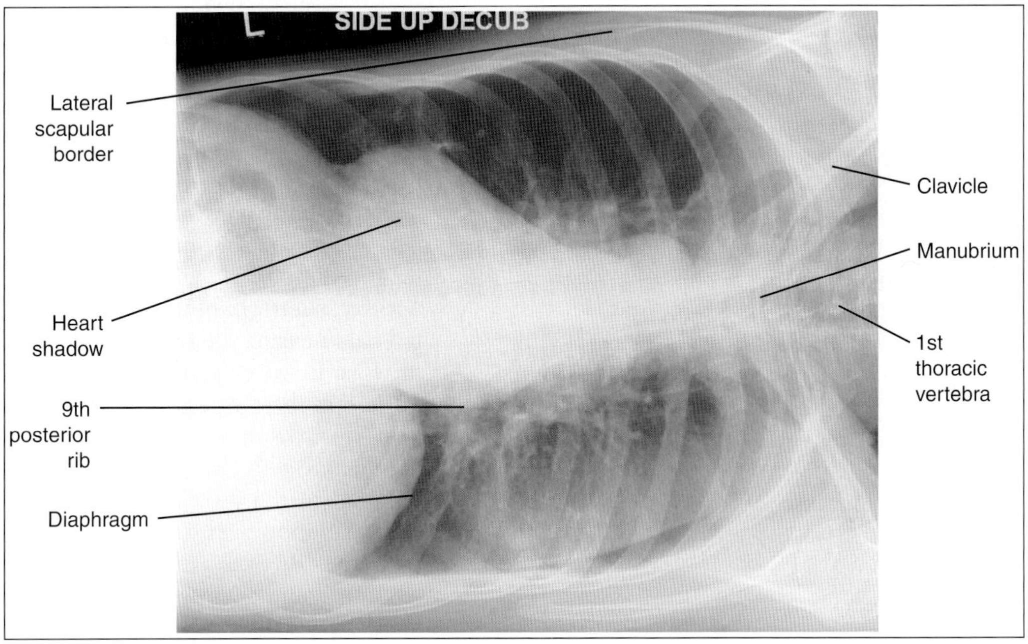

FIGURE 3-33 AP (lateral decubitus) chest projection with accurate positioning.

BOX 3-5	Anteroposterior-Posteroanterior (Lateral Decubitus) Chest Projection Analysis Criteria

- An arrow or "word" marker identifies the side of the patient positioned up and away from the imaging table or cart.
- The seventh thoracic vertebra is at the center of the exposure field.
- Both lungs, from apices to costophrenic angles, are included within the collimated field.
- The distances from the vertebral column to sternal clavicular ends are equal, and the lengths of the right and left corresponding posterior ribs are equal.
- The arms, mandible, and lateral borders of the scapulae are situated outside the lung field, and the lateral aspects of the clavicles are projected upward.
- The manubrium is superimposed by the fourth thoracic vertebra, with 1 inch (2.5 cm) of apical lung field visible above the clavicles.
- Nine or 10 posterior ribs are visualized above the diaphragm.
- The lung field adjacent to the cart is demonstrated without superimposition of the cart pad.

- *Positioning to demonstrate pleural air or fluid.* The AP or PA (lateral decubitus) projection is primarily used to confirm the presence of a pneumothorax or pleural effusion in the pleural cavity. To best demonstrate the presence of a pneumothorax, position the affected side of the thorax away from the tabletop or cart so that the air rises to the highest level in the pleural cavity. If the affected side were placed against the tabletop or cart, the air might be obscured by the mediastinal structures. To best demonstrate pleural effusion, position the affected side against the tabletop or cart. This positioning allows the fluid to gravitate to the lowest level of the pleural cavity, away from the mediastinal structures (Figure 3-34).

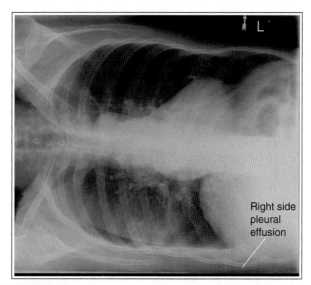

Right side pleural effusion

FIGURE 3-34 AP (lateral decubitus) chest projection demonstrating right-sided pleural effusion.

When imaging women with large pendulous breasts in the AP or PA (lateral decubitus) projection, it may be necessary to move and immobilize the overlapping breasts away from the areas where the air and fluid would collect (see Image 24). This will decrease the thickness of tissue in this region, providing more uniform density.

The seventh thoracic vertebra is at the center of the exposure field. Both lungs, from the apices to costophrenic angles, are included within the collimation field.

- Centering a perpendicular central ray to the midsagittal plane at a level approximately 7.5 inches (18 cm) inferior to the vertebra prominens for the PA projection and 4 inches (10 cm) inferior to the jugular notch for the AP projection places the seventh thoracic vertebra in the center of the image. This central ray placement also centers the lung field on the image. Center the IR to the central ray. Open the longitudinally collimated field to within 0.5 inch (2.5 cm) of the lateral skin line. For most adult AP chest projections, the full 14-inch (35-cm) length is needed. A 14- × 17-inch (35- × 43-cm) IR should be adequate to include all the required anatomic structures. For most patients, it is acceptable to use the dedicated chest unit, which will position the IR crosswise to the patient and still include the entire lung field on the image. In a recumbent patient, the diaphragm is unable to move to its lowest position on inspiration, preventing full vertical lung expansion. Because the lungs are unable to expand fully, a crosswise IR will provide adequate lung coverage. To be certain that the lateral borders are included on the image, center the IR and the central ray to the midsagittal plane.

The chest demonstrates an AP or PA projection. The distance from the lateral edges of the vertebral column to the sternal ends of the clavicles and the lengths of the right and left corresponding posterior ribs are equal.

- The decubitus chest image can be taken in an AP or a PA projection. In the AP projection, it is easier for the patient to maintain a true projection, without rotation, because the knees can be flexed. It is also easier for the patient to move closer to the IR and raise the arms when in an AP position. To avoid chest rotation, align the shoulders, the posterior ribs, and the posterior pelvic wings perpendicularly to the cart on which the patient is lying (Figure 3-35). This alignment positions the patient's shoulders and lungs at equal distances from the IR. Accomplish posterior rib and pelvic wing alignment by resting your extended flat hand against each, respectively, and then adjusting the patient's rotation until your hand is

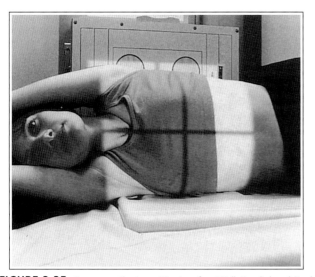

FIGURE 3-35 Proper patient positioning for AP (lateral decubitus) chest projection.

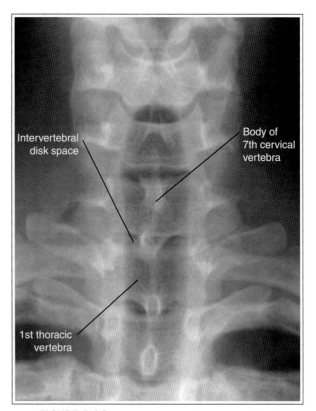

FIGURE 3-36 AP projection of cervical vertebrae.

positioned perpendicularly to the cart. It is most common for a patient to lean the elevated shoulder, lung, and pelvic wing anteriorly when rotated. A pillow or other support placed between the patient's knees may help eliminate this forward rotation.

- *Detecting chest rotation.* Rotation is readily detected on an AP or PA (lateral decubitus) chest projection by evaluating the distances between the vertebral column and the sternal ends of the clavicles and by comparing the lengths of the posterior ribs. On a nonrotated decubitus chest image, the distances and lengths, respectively, on each side of the patient should be equal. On a rotated AP projection, the sternal clavicular end that is superimposed over the lesser amount of the vertebral column, and the side on which the posterior ribs demonstrate the greatest length, is the side of the chest positioned closer to the IR (see Images 25 and 26). The opposite is true for a PA projection. For this projection, the sternal clavicular end that is superimposed over the least amount of the vertebral column and the posterior ribs that demonstrate the greatest length represent the side of the chest positioned farther from the IR.

- *AP versus PA chest images*: Determine whether a chest image was taken in an AP or PA projection by analyzing the appearance of the sixth and seventh cervical vertebrae and the first thoracic vertebra. In the AP projection, these vertebral bodies and their intervertebral disk spaces are demonstrated without distortion (Figure 3-36). In the PA projection, the vertebral bodies are distorted, the intervertebral disk spaces are closed, and the spinous processes and laminae of these three

vertebrae are well demonstrated (Figure 3-37). The reason for these variations is related to the divergence of the x-ray beam used to image these three vertebrae and the anterior convexity of the cervical and upper thoracic vertebrae.

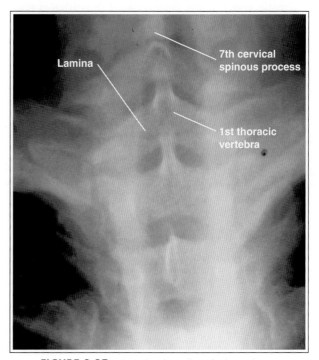

FIGURE 3-37 PA projection of cervical vertebrae.

The arms, mandible, and lateral borders of the scapulae are situated outside the lung field, and the lateral aspects of the clavicles are projected upward.

- The lateral borders of the scapulae are drawn away from the lung field when the patient's arms are positioned above the head. This positioning also draws the lateral ends of the clavicles superiorly. If the arms are not positioned in this manner, the arms and the lateral borders of the scapulae are demonstrated within the upper lung field (see Image 25).
- To prevent the chin from being superimposed over the lung apices on the image, position the patient with the chin elevated.

The manubrium and the fourth thoracic vertebra are superimposed, and the lungs and heart are demonstrated without foreshortening.

- The tilt of the midcoronal plane determines the degree of lung and heart foreshortening and the transverse level at which the manubrium is situated in comparison to the fourth thoracic vertebra. When the midcoronal plane is positioned parallel with the IR, the lungs and heart are demonstrated without foreshortening and the manubrium and fourth thoracic vertebra are superimposed over each other. If the image is taken in an AP projection and the superior midcoronal plane is tilted anteriorly (forward), the manubrium will move inferior to the fourth thoracic vertebra (see Image 27). Conversely, if the superior midcoronal plane is tilted posteriorly (backward), the manubrium will move superior to the fourth thoracic vertebra (see Image 28). If the image is taken in a PA projection and the superior midcoronal plane is tilted anteriorly, the manubrium will move inferior to the fourth thoracic vertebra. Conversely, if the superior midcoronal plane is tilted posteriorly, the manubrium will move superior to the fourth thoracic vertebra.

Nine or 10 posterior ribs are demonstrated above the diaphragm.

- In a recumbent position, the diaphragm is unable to shift to its lowest position because of pressure from the peritoneal cavity. As a result, the lungs are not fully aerated, and only 9 or 10 posterior ribs are demonstrated above the diaphragm.

The lung field positioned against the cart is demonstrated without superimposition of the cart pad.

- Elevating the patient on a radiolucent sponge or on a hard surface, such as a cardiac board, prevents the chest from sinking into the cart pad. When the patient's body is allowed to sink into the cart pad, artifact lines are seen superimposed over the lateral lung field of the side placed against the cart. Because fluid in the pleural cavity gravitates to the lowest level, it is in this area that the fluid will be demonstrated, and superimposition of the cart pad and the lower lung field may obscure fluid that has settled in the lowest level.

Anteroposterior and Posteroanterior (Lateral Decubitus) Chest Projection Analysis

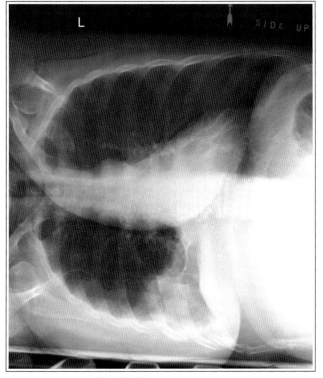

IMAGE 24 AP projection.

Analysis. The patient's breasts are obscuring the areas where fluid collects.

Correction. When imaging women with large pendulous breasts in the AP or PA (lateral decubitus) projection, it may be necessary to move and immobilize the overlapping breasts away from the areas where the air and fluid collect. This will decrease the thickness of tissue in this region, providing more uniform density.

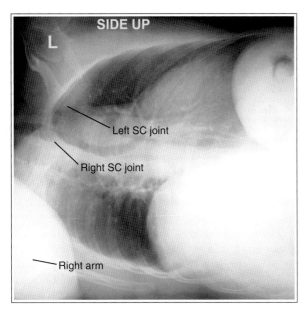

IMAGE 25 AP projection.

Analysis. The right sternal clavicular end is superimposed over the vertebral column, the posterior ribs on the left side demonstrate the greater length, and the arms are superimposed over the right lung apex. The patient's left side was rotated toward the IR, and the arm was positioned at a 90-degree angle to the body.

Correction. Rotate the patient's left side away from the IR until the patient's shoulders, posterior ribs, and posterior pelvic wing are aligned perpendicularly to the cart. Elevate the patient's right arm until it is positioned above the lung field.

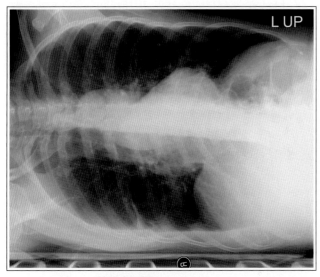

IMAGE 26 AP projection.

Analysis. The left sternal clavicular end is superimposed over the vertebral column, and the posterior ribs on the right side demonstrate the greater length. The patient's right side was rotated toward the IR.

Correction. Rotate the patient's right side away from the IR until the patient's shoulders, posterior ribs, and posterior pelvic wing are aligned perpendicularly to the cart.

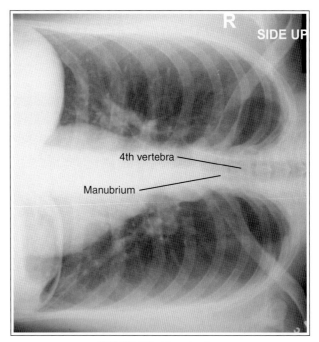

IMAGE 27 AP projection.

Analysis. The manubrium is superimposed over the fifth thoracic vertebra, indicating that the superior midcoronal plane was tilted anteriorly.

Correction. Move the superior midcoronal plane posteriorly until the midcoronal plane is parallel with the IR.

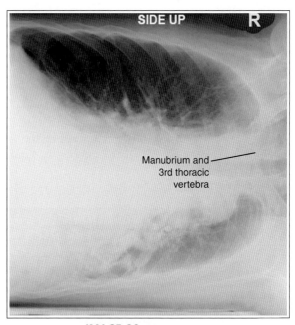

IMAGE 28 AP projection.

Analysis. The manubrium is superimposed over the third thoracic vertebra, indicating that the superior midcoronal plane was tilted posteriorly.

Correction. Move the superior midcoronal plane anteriorly until the midcoronal plane is parallel with the IR.

CHEST: ANTEROPOSTERIOR AXIAL PROJECTION (LORDOTIC POSITION)

See Figure 3-38.

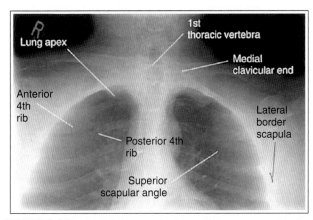

FIGURE 3-38 AP axial chest projection with accurate positioning.

Overlying soft tissues, clavicles, and upper ribs often obscure the apical lung markings on a PA projection of the chest. The anterior ends of the first ribs may also project a suspicious looking shadow in the apices. The AP axial projection is taken to demonstrate areas of the apical lungs obscured on the PA projection and to provide a different anatomic perspective that can be used to evaluate suspicious areas (Box 3-6).

The superior lung field is at the center of the exposure field. The clavicles, apices, and two thirds of the lung field are included within the collimated field.

- Centering the central ray to the midsagittal plane halfway between the manubrium and the xiphoid positions the superior lung field at the center of the image. Because the lung fields are foreshortened, this centering will include most of the lung fields on the image. A higher centering is required

if only the lung apices are desired. Lung foreshortening also creates the need for tight vertical collimation to prevent unnecessary exposure of abdominal and cervical vertebral tissue. Center the IR to the central ray.

- A 14- × 17-inch (35- × 43-cm), lengthwise IR should be adequate to include all the required anatomic structures. Longitudinally collimate to within 0.5 inch (1.25 cm) of shoulders and transversely collimate to 0.5 inch (1.25 cm) of lateral skin line.

The sternal ends of the clavicles are projected superiorly to the lung apices at the level of the first thoracic vertebra. The heart shadow can be outlined, although it is foreshortened and wider than on a corresponding PA chest projection. The posterior and anterior portions of the first through fourth ribs lie horizontally and are almost superimposed.

- The clavicles are projected above the apices, and the upper ribs are superimposed by positioning the patient using one of three methods. First, the patient's back can be arched, leaning the upper thorax and shoulders toward the IR, as demonstrated in Figure 3-39. The correct amount of arching is accomplished when the patient's feet are placed approximately 12 inches (30 cm) away from the IR before the back is arched. The angle formed between the midcoronal body plane and IR should be approximately 45 degrees. Second, the patient remains completely upright, and a 45-degree cephalic central ray angulation is used to shift the clavicles (Figure 3-40). Third, the patient's back is arched as much a possible and

---

BOX 3-6 | **Anteroposterior Axial (Lordotic) Chest Projection Analysis Criteria**

- The superior lung field is at the center of the exposure field.
- The clavicles, apices, and two thirds of the lungs are included within the collimated field.
- The sternoclavicular ends of clavicles are projected superior to the lung apices, and the first through fourth ribs lie horizontally and are almost superimposed.
- The lateral borders of the scapulae are drawn away from the lung field, and the superior angles of the scapulae are demonstrated away from lung apices.
- The distances from the vertebral column to sternal clavicular ends are equal.
- The clavicles are positioned on the same horizontal plane.

SC, Sternoclavicular.

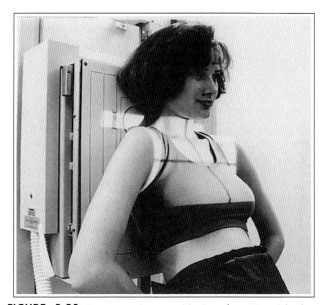

FIGURE 3-39 Proper patient positioning for AP axial chest projection—no central ray angle.

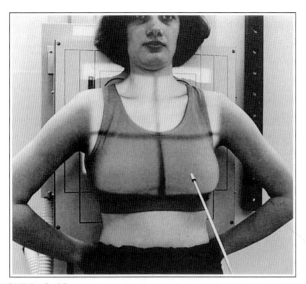

FIGURE 3-40 Proper patient positioning for AP axial chest projection—central ray angled.

the central ray is angled cephalically the amount necessary to equal a 45-degree angle. For example, if the patient is able to arch until the midcoronal plane is placed at a 30-degree angle to the IR, the needed central ray angle would be 15 degrees. With each of these methods, the clavicles are projected above the apices onto the first thoracic vertebra, and the anterior ribs are projected onto their corresponding posterior ribs.

- *Poor patient or central ray positioning.* Inadequate back extension or central ray angulation is identified on an image when the clavicles are not projected superiorly to the lung apices and when the anterior and posterior ribs are not superimposed. When the patient's back is not arched enough or when more cephalic angulation is needed, the clavicles superimpose the lung apices, and the anterior ribs are demonstrated inferior to their corresponding posterior rib (see Image 29). If an image is obtained in which lung fields have been so foreshortened that the apices are obscured and the posterior ribs are superimposed and cannot be distinguished, the patient's back was arched too much or the cephalic angle was too extreme (see Image 30).

The lateral borders of the scapulae are drawn away from the lung field, and the superior angles of the scapulae are demonstrated away from lung apices.

- The lateral borders and the superior angles of the scapulae are drawn away from the lung fields by placing the back of the patient's hands on the hips and rotating the elbows and shoulders anteriorly. This position allows visualization of the lung

apices without scapular obstruction. When the elbows and shoulders are not rotated anteriorly, the lateral borders of the scapulae are demonstrated in the lung fields, and the superior scapular angles are projected into the lung apices (see Image 31).

The chest demonstrates no signs of rotation when the distances from the vertebral column to the sternal ends of the clavicles are equal.

- The patient's shoulders should be equal distances from the IR to prevent rotation. Chest rotation can be identified on an AP axial projection by evaluating the distance between the vertebral column and the sternal ends of the clavicles or the sternoclavicular (SC) joints. When the distances between the sternal clavicles and the vertebral column are unequal, the SC joint that is superimposed over the smaller amount of the vertebral column is the side of the chest that was positioned closer to the IR.

Anteroposterior Axial Chest Projection Analysis

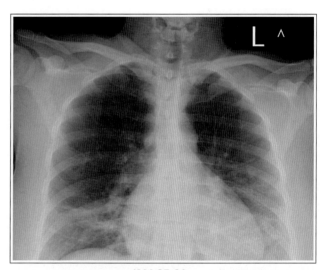

IMAGE 29

Analysis. The clavicles are superimposed over the lung apices, and the anterior ribs are demonstrated inferior to their corresponding posterior rib. Either the patient's back was not arched enough or the central ray was not angled cephalically enough to obtain a 45-degree angle between the midcoronal plane and central ray.

Correction. If the patient's back was arched to obtain this image, increase the amount of arch or add a cephalic angulation until the midcoronal plane and central ray form a 45-degree angle.

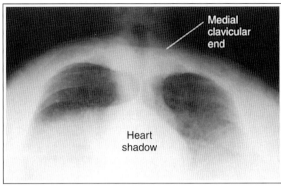

IMAGE 30

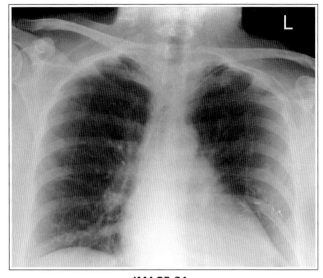

IMAGE 31

Analysis. The lung fields demonstrate excessive fore-shortening, and the individual ribs cannot be identified. Either the patient's back was arched too much or the central ray was angled too cephalically.

Correction. If the patient's back was arched to obtain this image, decrease the amount of arch. If this examination was obtained by using a cephalic angulation, decrease the degree of central ray angulation until the midcoronal plane and central ray form a 45-degree angle.

Analysis. The lateral borders of the scapulae are demonstrated within the lung fields, and the superior scapular angles are demonstrated within the apical region. The patient's elbows and shoulders were not rotated anteriorly.

Correction. Place the backs of the patient's hands on the hips, and rotate the elbows and shoulders anteriorly.

CHEST: POSTEROANTERIOR OBLIQUE PROJECTION (RIGHT ANTERIOR OBLIQUE AND LEFT ANTERIOR OBLIQUE POSITIONS)

See Figure 3-41 and Box 3-7.

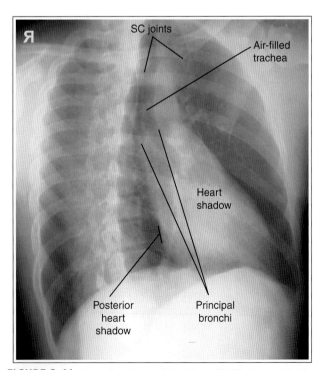

FIGURE 3-41 Forty-five-degree PA oblique (RAO) chest projection with accurate positioning.

The right and left principal bronchi are at the center of the exposure field. The apices, costophrenic angles, and lateral chest walls are included within the collimated field.

- Centering a perpendicular central ray at a level approximately 7.5 inches (18 cm) inferior to the vertebra prominens places the central ray at the level of the bronchi. Accurate transverse positioning is obtained when the same amount of IR distance is present on both sides of the patient. A 14- × 17-inch (35- × 43-cm) IR should be adequate to include all the required anatomic structures. Center the IR to the central ray. Open the transversely collimated field to within 0.5 inch (2.5 cm) of the lateral skin line. For

BOX 3-7	Posteroanterior Oblique Chest Projection Analysis Criteria

- The right and left principal bronchi are at the center of the exposure field.
- Both lungs, from the apices to costophrenic angles, are included within the collimated field.
- The SC joints are demonstrated without spinal superimposition, with approximately twice as much lung field demonstrated on one side of the thoracic vertebrae as on the other side.
- The manubrium is superimposed by the fourth thoracic vertebra, with 1 inch (2.5 cm) of apical lung field visible above the clavicles.
- Ten or 11 posterior ribs visualized above the diaphragm.

SC, Sternoclavicular.

most adult AP chest projections, the full 17-inch (43-cm) length is needed, although you should collimate on smaller patients.

Approximately twice as much lung field is demonstrated on one side of the thoracic vertebrae as on the other side, and the SC joints are demonstrated without spinal superimposition, indicating that a 45-degree obliquity has been obtained.

- Rotating the patient until the midcoronal plane is aligned 45 degrees to the IR (Figure 3-42) provides the reviewer with an additional perspective of the lungs, which will assist in the detection of pulmonary diseases or artifacts. The lung field better demonstrated on an AP projection is the one positioned farther from the IR. An RAO position demonstrates the left lung, whereas an LAO position demonstrates the right lung.
- *Verifying accuracy of obliquity.* When evaluating an image, you can be certain that a 45-degree obliquity has been obtained if (1) twice as much lung field is demonstrated on one side of the thoracic vertebrae as on the other side, and (2) the sternoclavicular (SC) joints, air-filled trachea, and principal bronchi are demonstrated without spinal superimposition. The heart shadow is also demonstrated without spinal superimposition on an RAO chest image, whereas a portion of the heart shadow is superimposed over the thoracic vertebrae on an LAO chest image. Because the heart is located more to the left of the thoracic vertebrae, a 60-degree patient obliquity is necessary to demonstrate the heart shadow without spinal superimposition on the LAO. Figure 3-43 demonstrates a 45-degree LAO chest image. Note that the lung field on one side is twice as large as on the other and that slight superimposition of the thoracic vertebrae and heart shadow is present. Compare this image with the 60-degree LAO chest image shown in Figure 3-44.

Note that more than twice as much lung field is present on one side of the thoracic vertebrae as on the other in Figure 3-44, and that the heart shadow and thoracic vertebrae are not superimposed. How much obliquity

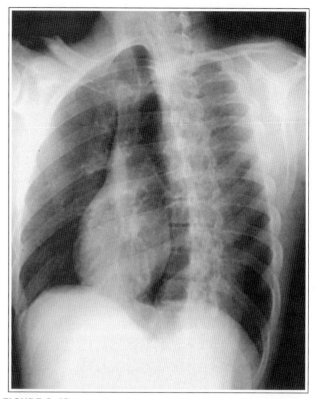

FIGURE 3-43 Forty-five-degree PA oblique (LAO) chest projection with proper positioning.

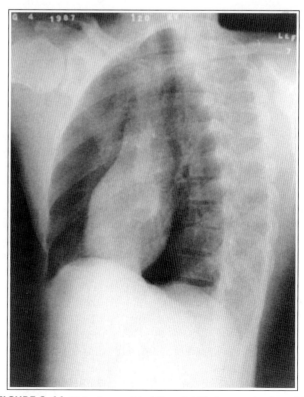

FIGURE 3-44 Sixty-degree PA oblique (LAO) chest projection with proper positioning.

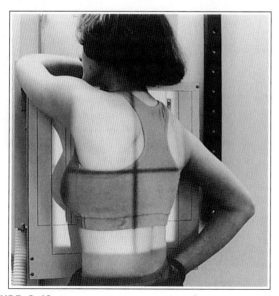

FIGURE 3-42 Proper patient positioning for PA oblique (RAO) chest projection.

should be obtained depends on the examination indications. When the examination is being performed to evaluate the lung field, a 45-degree oblique image is required; when the outline of the heart is of interest, a 60-degree oblique image is required.

- *Repositioning for improper patient rotation.* If the desired 45-degree obliquity is not obtained on a PA oblique chest projection, compare the amount of lung field demonstrated on both sides of the thoracic vertebrae. If the image demonstrates more than twice the lung field on one side of the thoracic vertebrae as on the other side, the patient was rotated more than 45 degrees. If less than twice the lung field is demonstrated on one side of the thoracic vertebrae as on the opposite side, the patient was not rotated enough (see Image 32). To determine repositioning movements for the 60-degree LAO image, evaluate the heart shadow and thoracic vertebrae superimposition. With adequate obliquity, the heart shadow is positioned just to the right of the thoracic vertebrae. If the PA oblique projection is less than 60 degrees, the heart shadow is superimposed over the thoracic vertebrae, as on a 45-degree LAO chest image. Excess obliquity produces an image similar to a rotated lateral chest projection.

- *AP oblique chest projections.* Routinely, PA oblique projections are performed for oblique chest images because they position the heart closer to the IR. When AP oblique projections are taken, however, the preceding evaluation corresponds in the following way. The LPO position demonstrates the lung situated closer to the IR, which is the left lung. To review this position, use the RAO evaluation previously described. For the RPO position, the right lung is of interest and the LAO evaluation should be followed. A 45-degree obliquity is required in the LPO image to rotate the heart away from the thoracic vertebrae, but a 60-degree obliquity is needed for the RPO position.

The manubrium is situated at the same level as the fourth thoracic vertebra, with approximately 1 inch (2.5 cm) of the apical lung field visible above the clavicles, and the lungs and heart are demonstrated without foreshortening.

- The tilt of the midcoronal plane determines the relationship of the manubrium to the thoracic vertebrae, the amount of apical lung field seen superior to the clavicles, and the degree of lung and heart foreshortening. When the midcoronal plane is vertical, the manubrium is projected at the level of the fourth thoracic vertebra, approximately 1 inch (2.5 cm) of the apices are visible above the clavicles, and the lungs and heart are demonstrated without foreshortening. In a PA oblique projection, if the superior midcoronal plane is tilted anteriorly (forward), as demonstrated in Figure 3-21, the lungs and heart are foreshortened, the manubrium is situated at a transverse level inferior to the fourth thoracic vertebra or lower, and more than 1

inch (2.5 cm) of apices is demonstrated above the clavicles (see Image 6). Conversely, if the superior midcoronal plane is tilted posteriorly (backward), as demonstrated in Figure 3-22, the lungs and heart are foreshortened, the manubrium is situated at a transverse level above the fourth thoracic vertebrae, and less than 1 inch (2.5 cm) of apices is demonstrated superior to the clavicles (see Image 7). The opposite is true for an AP oblique projection. Anterior tilt of the superior midcoronal plane will result in the manubrium projecting inferior to the fourth thoracic vertebra, and posterior tilt of the superior midcoronal plane will result in the manubrium projecting superior to the fourth thoracic vertebra.

Ten or 11 posterior ribs are demonstrated above the hemidiaphragms, indicating full lung aeration.

- If fewer than 10 posterior ribs are demonstrated, the lungs were not fully inflated. Determine whether a patient condition hindered full aeration. If not, repeat the image after full inspiration.

Posteroanterior Oblique Chest Projection Analysis

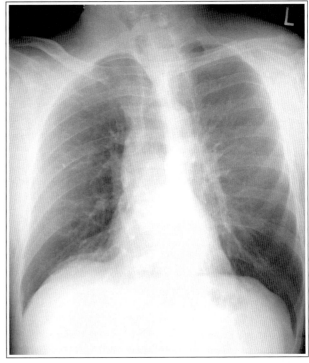

IMAGE 32

Analysis. This image was taken with the patient in an LAO position. Less than twice the lung field is demonstrated on the left side of the thoracic vertebrae as on the right side. The thoracic vertebrae are superimposed over a portion of the heart shadow and the air-filled trachea. The obliquity was less than 45 degrees.

Correction. Increase the degree of patient obliquity until the midcoronal plane is placed at a 45-degree angle with the IR.

PEDIATRIC CHEST

The lungs of the neonate continue to grow for at least 8 years after birth. The growth results mainly from an increase in the number of respiratory bronchioles and alveoli. Only from one eighth to one sixth of the number of alveoli in adults are present in newborn infants, causing the lungs to be denser. Therefore on neonate and infant chest images, the lungs demonstrate less image contrast within them and between them and the surrounding soft tissue than on adult chest images.

NEONATE AND INFANT CHEST: ANTEROPOSTERIOR PROJECTION

See Figure 3-45 and Box 3-8.

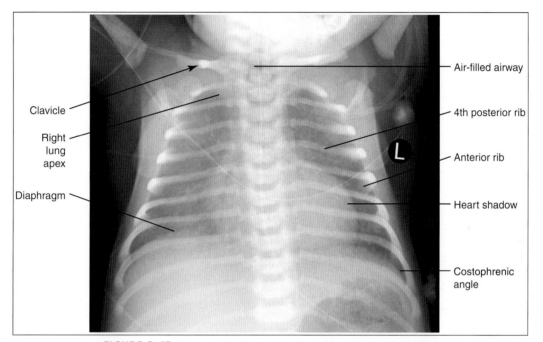

Clavicle

Right lung apex

Diaphragm

Air-filled airway

4th posterior rib

Anterior rib

Heart shadow

Costophrenic angle

FIGURE 3-45 Neonate AP chest projection with accurate positioning.

The fourth thoracic vertebra is at the center of the exposure field. The upper airway, lungs, mediastinal structures, and costophrenic angles are included within the collimated field.

- Center the neonate or infant's chest to the center of an 8- × 10-inch (18- × 24-cm), lengthwise IR, and center a perpendicular central ray to the midsagittal plane at the level of the mammary line (imaginary line connecting the nipples) for neonates and small infants. A larger IR and slightly inferior centering may be needed for larger infants. This IR and central ray placement centers the lung field on the image, permitting tight collimation on all sides of the lungs. Open the longitudinal collimation to include the upper airway (infant's bottom lip) and costophrenic angles (tenth posterior rib) and transversely collimate to within 0.5 inch (1.25 cm) of the lateral skin line.

BOX 3-8	Neonate and Infant Anteroposterior Chest Projection Analysis Criteria

- The fourth thoracic vertebra is at the center of the exposure field.
- The upper airway, lungs, mediastinal structures, and costophrenic angles are included within the collimated field.
- The distances from the vertebral column to the sternal ends of the clavicles are equal, and the lengths of the right and left corresponding posterior ribs are equal.
- The anterior ribs are projecting downward and the posterior ribs demonstrate a gentle, cephalically bowed contour.
- Neonate: Eight posterior ribs are demonstrated above the diaphragm, and the lungs demonstrate a fluffy appearance, with linear-appearing connecting tissue.
- Infant: Nine posterior ribs are demonstrated above the diaphragm.
- The chin does not obscure the airway or apical lung field.

- As the lungs grow, the shape of the thoracic cavity changes from the neonate and infant's short, wide shape to the older child and adult's longer, narrower shape. The technologist must adjust the central ray centering point to accommodate the changing shape to avoid distortion and clipping lung structures when tightly collimating.

The chest demonstrates an AP projection. The distances from the vertebral column to the sternal ends of the clavicles are equal, and the lengths of the right and left corresponding posterior ribs are equal.

- Rotation on a supine or mobile chest image is caused by poor patient positioning or central ray alignment. To position the infant without rotation accurately, immobilize the child using the immobilization equipment (Figure 3-46) or have an attendant use two hands for restraint (Figure 3-47). The thumb, forefinger, and middle finger of one hand are used to clasp the infant's wrists above his or her head, and the same digits of the other hand clasp the infant's ankles. The head and toes are positioned straight up. Head rotation is the most

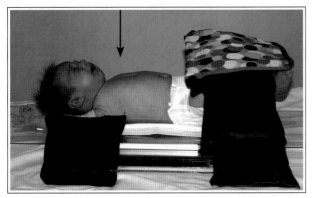

FIGURE 3-46 Proper patient positioning for neonate AP chest projection.

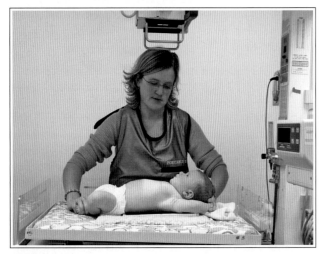

FIGURE 3-47 Proper patient positioning for infant AP chest projection using immobilization equipment.

common cause of chest rotation in neonates and infants. The chest will rotate in the same direction in which the infant's head is rotated. Align the central ray perpendicularly to the midsagittal plane and IR. To avoid rotation caused by poor central ray alignment, make certain that the central ray is not off-angled toward the right or left lateral side of the infant instead of being perpendicular. If the central ray is off-angled toward the lateral side of the infant, the anatomic structures farthest from the IR (clavicles and anterior ribs) will be projected in the direction toward which the central ray is off-angled.

- *Detecting chest rotation.* Chest rotation is detected by evaluating the distance between the vertebral column and the sternal ends of the clavicles and by comparing the length of the right and left inferior posterior ribs. The sternal clavicular end that is demonstrated farther from the vertebral column and the side of the chest that demonstrates the longer posterior ribs represents the side of the chest toward which the infant is rotated (see Images 33, 34, and 35). If the cause of the rotation is poor central ray alignment, the sternal clavicular end demonstrated farther from the vertebral column and the side of the chest with the longer posterior ribs represents the side of the chest toward which the central ray off-angled.

The anterior ribs are projecting downward and the posterior ribs demonstrate a gentle, cephalically bowed contour.

- The neonate or infant supine AP chest projection tends to have a lordotic appearance because of the lack of kyphotic thoracic curvature that is seen in adults. Some facilities offset this appearance by angling the central ray 5 degrees caudally or by tilting the foot end of the bed 5 degrees lower than the head end. Proper central ray centering will also help to reduce this lordotic appearance. Because the chest in neonates and infants is shorter than in adults, a common error is to center the central ray too inferiorly, resulting in an increase in the lordotic appearance.

  A neonate or infant chest projection that demonstrates an excessively lordotic appearance will demonstrate cephalically projected anterior ribs and posterior ribs without the gentle, cephalically bowed contour (see Image 36). Such distortion foreshortens the lungs and mediastinal structures, causing the cardiac apex to appear uptilted and the main pulmonary artery to be concealed beneath the cardiac silhouette.

Neonate: Eight posterior ribs are demonstrated above the diaphragm, and the lungs demonstrate a fluffy appearance with linear-appearing connecting tissue, indicating full lung aeration for the neonatal chest image.

Infant: Nine posterior ribs are demonstrated above the diaphragm.

- The appearance of the neonate's lungs may change with even one rib's difference in inflation. With dense substances such as blood, pus, protein, and cells filling the alveoli, it is the addition of the less dense air that will give the image the fluffy appearance, because the air is demonstrated on the image as a darker density among the lighter densities of blood, pus, protein, and cells. A lung that demonstrates a white-out appearance, even though the diaphragm is below the eighth rib, is filled with dense substances that do not allow air to fill the alveoli.

  For neonates and infants breathing without a respirator, observe the chest movement and expose the image after the infant takes a deep breath. Chest images that are taken on expiration may demonstrate a decrease in image density because a decrease in air volume increases the concentration of pulmonary tissues (see Images 37 and 38).

The chin does not obscure the airway or apical lung field.

- To prevent the chin from being superimposed on the airway and apical lung field, lift the neonate or infant's chin until the neck is in a neutral position. When the chin is superimposed on the airway and apical lung field, ETT placement cannot be evaluated (see Image 39).

Neonate and Infant Anteroposterior Chest Projection Analysis

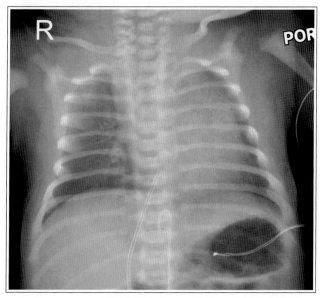

IMAGE 33 Neonate.

Analysis. The left sternal clavicular end is demonstrated farther from the vertebral column than the right sternal clavicular end, and the left lower posterior ribs are longer than the right.

Correction. Rotate the thorax toward the right side until the midcoronal plane is parallel with the IR and perpendicular to the central ray. Make certain that the patient's face is facing forward.

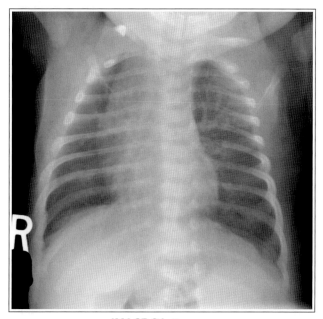

IMAGE 34 Neonate.

Analysis. The right sternal clavicular end is demonstrated farther from the vertebral column than the left sternal clavicular end, and the right lower posterior ribs are longer than the left.

Correction. Rotate the thorax toward the left side until the midcoronal plane is parallel with the IR and perpendicular to the central ray.

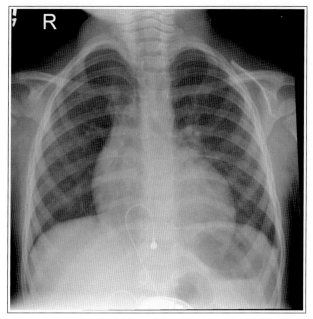

IMAGE 35 Infant.

Analysis. The right sternal clavicular end is demonstrated farther from the vertebral column than the left sternal clavicular end, and the right lower posterior ribs are longer than the left.

Correction. Rotate the thorax toward the left side until the midcoronal plane is parallel with the IR and perpendicular to the central ray.

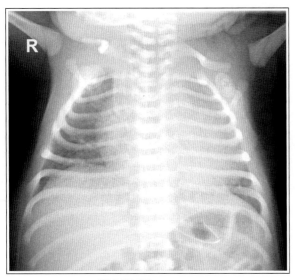

IMAGE 36 Neonate.

Analysis. The chest demonstrates an excessively lordotic appearance. The anterior ribs are projecting upwardly, and the posterior ribs do not demonstrate the slight upwardly bowed appearance, but are horizontal. The central ray was centered inferior to T4.

Correction. Move the central ray superiorly to align it better with the upper thorax. A 5-degree caudal angle may also be added to help align the central ray and thorax better.

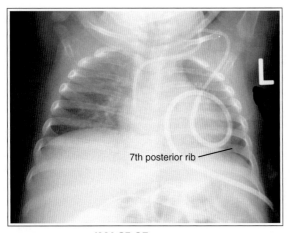

IMAGE 37 Neonate.

Analysis. Six posterior ribs are demonstrated above the diaphragm. Neonates should have at least eight and infants at least nine posterior ribs visible above the diaphragm. The lungs were not fully aerated.

Correction. If possible, take the exposure after the patient takes a deeper inspiration. If the patient is on a conventional ventilator, expose the image when the manometer is at its highest level, indicating a deep inspiration.

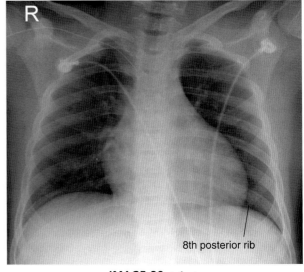

IMAGE 38 Infant.

Analysis. Eight posterior ribs are demonstrated above the diaphragm. Infants should have at least nine posterior ribs visible above the diaphragm. The lungs were not fully aerated.

Correction. If possible, take the exposure after the patient takes a deeper inspiration.

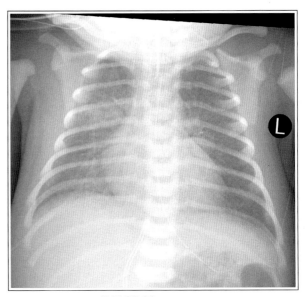

IMAGE 39 Neonate.

Analysis. The patient's chin is superimposed over the airway and apical lung field. The chin was not elevated to bring the neck into a neutral position.

Correction. Lift the chin until the patient's face is forward and the neck is in a neutral position.

CHILD CHEST: POSTEROANTERIOR AND ANTEROPOSTERIOR PROJECTIONS

See Figures 3-48 and 49.

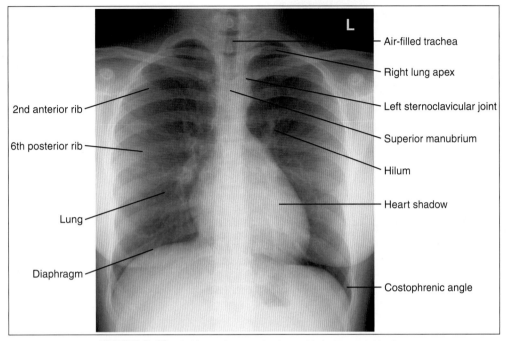

FIGURE 3-48 Child AP chest projection with proper positioning.

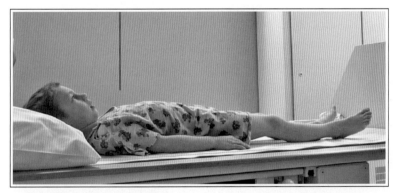

FIGURE 3-49 Proper patient positioning for a child AP chest projection.

The analysis of the child PA and AP chest projections is the same as that for the infant or adult PA or AP chest, already discussed. The size of the child determines which criterion best meets the situation.

For a discussion on topics needed to analyze Images 40 through 44 that follow, refer to the PA-AP adult or infant chest discussions earlier in this chapter.

Child Chest Posteroanterior and Anteroposterior Chest Projection Analysis

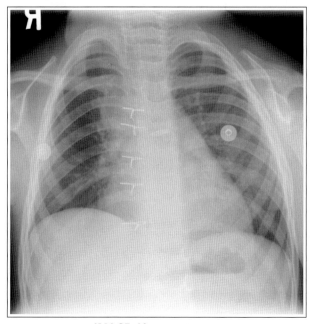

IMAGE 40 PA projection.

Analysis. The right sternal clavicular end is visible without superimposing the vertebral column, and the left sternal clavicular end superimposes the vertebral column. The patient was rotated toward the left side.

Correction. Rotate the right side of the patient's thorax toward the IR until the shoulders are at equal distances from the IR.

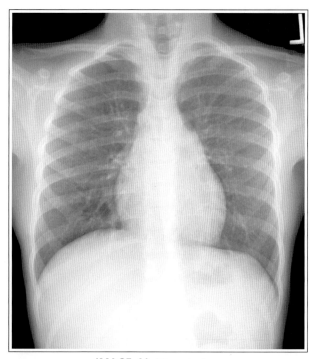

IMAGE 41 PA projection.

Analysis. The manubrium is at the level of the second thoracic vertebra, and less than 0.5 inch (1.25 cm) of apical lung field is demonstrated superior to the clavicles. The patient's upper midcoronal plane was tilted posteriorly.

Correction. Anteriorly tilt the upper midcoronal plane until it is aligned parallel with the IR.

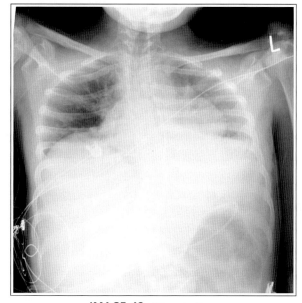

IMAGE 42 AP projection.

Analysis. Only six posterior ribs are demonstrated above the diaphragm. The manubrium is superimposed over the second thoracic vertebra, the posterior ribs demonstrate a horizontal contour, and less than 1 inch (2.5 cm) of apical lung field is visible above the clavicles. The image was taken on expiration, and the central ray was angled too cephalically.

Correction. If the patient's condition allows, take the exposure after coaxing the patient into a deeper inspiration and adjust the central ray caudally until it is aligned perpendicularly to the patient's midcoronal plane.

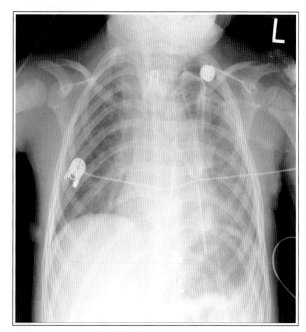

IMAGE 43 AP projection.

Analysis. The manubrium is superimposed over the fifth thoracic vertebra, the posterior ribs demonstrate a vertical contour, and more than 1 inch (2.5 cm) of apical lung field is visible above the clavicles. The central ray was angled too caudally.

Correction. Adjust the central ray cephalically until it is aligned perpendicular to the patient's midcoronal plane.

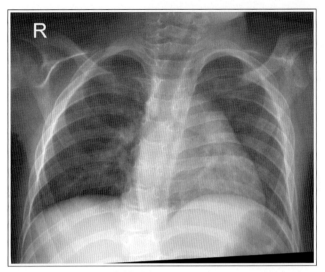

IMAGE 44 AP projection.

Analysis. The left sternal clavicular end is visible without superimposing the vertebral column, and the right sternal clavicular end superimposes the vertebral column. The patient was rotated toward the left side. Only eight posterior ribs are demonstrated above the diaphragm.

Correction. Rotate the right side of the patient's thorax toward the IR until the shoulders are at equal distances from the IR. Coax the patient into a deeper inspiration.

NEONATE AND INFANT CHEST: CROSS-TABLE LATERAL PROJECTION (LEFT LATERAL POSITION)

See Figure 3-50 and Box 3-9.

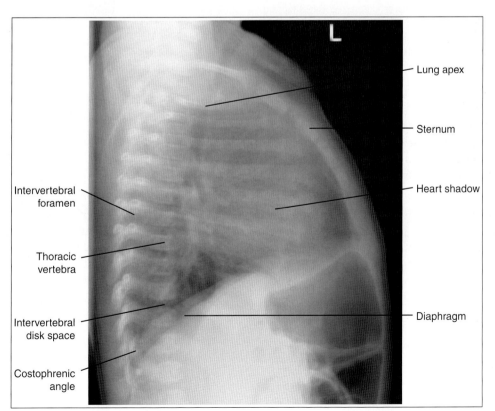

FIGURE 3-50 Neonatal cross-table lateral chest projection with accurate positioning.

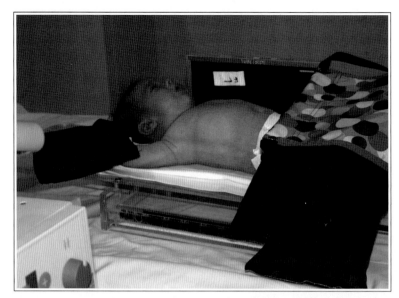

FIGURE 3-51 Proper patient positioning for an infant cross-table lateral chest projection using immobilization equipment.

BOX 3-9	**Neonate and Infant Lateral Chest Projection Analysis Criteria**

- The midcoronal plane, at the level of the fifth thoracic vertebra, is at the center of the exposure field.
- Both lung fields, including the apices and costophrenic angles, and the posterior ribs and airway are demonstrated within the collimated field.
- The posterior ribs are superimposed and the sternum is in profile.
- The humeral soft tissue is not superimposed over the anterior lung apices.
- The chin is not in the exposure field.
- The hemidiaphragms form a gentle cephalic curve.

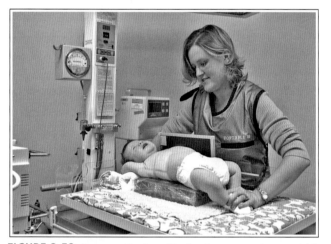

FIGURE 3-52 Proper patient positioning for a neonate cross-table lateral chest projection.

The midcoronal plane, at the level of the fifth thoracic vertebra, is at the center of the exposure field. The entire lung field, including the apices and costophrenic angles, and the posterior ribs and airway are included within the collimated field.

- Lateral chest projections are useful for assessing the degree of inflation, permit confident recognition of cardiomegaly, and provide the clearest view of the thoracic vertebrae and sternum. The needed anatomic structures are placed on a lateral chest projection when the neonate or infant is supine, and an 8- × 10-inch (18- × 24-cm), lengthwise IR is positioned against the neonate or infant's left lateral surface. The chest is placed in the middle of the IR by elevating the patient on a radiolucent sponge, and a horizontal central ray is positioned to the midcoronal plane at a level just inferior to

the mammary line. To position the infant without rotation accurately, immobilize the child using immobilization equipment (Figure 3-51) or have an attendant use two hands for restraint (Figure 3-52). A larger IR and slightly inferior centering may be needed for larger infants. This IR and central ray placement centers the lung field on the image, permitting tight collimation on all sides of the lungs. Open the longitudinal collimation to include the midcervical vertebrae and costophrenic angles, and transversely collimate to within 0.5 inch (1.25 cm) of the lateral skin line.

- *Cross-table versus overhead lateral projections.* Neonates are very sensitive. Performing a cross-table lateral projection on the neonate instead of the overhead lateral will reduce the amount of disturbance. Also, on overhead lateral projections, the lung adjacent to the IR tends to collapse, whereas the superior lung tends to overinflate.

The chest demonstrates no rotation when the posterior ribs are superimposed and the sternum is in profile.

- To avoid chest rotation, align an imaginary line connecting the shoulders, the posterior ribs, and the posterior pelvic wings perpendicular to the IR. Because the OID difference between the right and left lung fields is minimal on neonates and small infants, the posterior ribs on lateral chest projections do not demonstrate the 0.5-inch (1.25-cm) separation that is seen on adult lateral chest projections, but instead are directly superimposed.

- *Detecting chest rotation.* Chest rotation is effectively detected on a lateral chest projection by evaluating the degree of superimposition of the posterior ribs. When the posterior ribs are demonstrated without superimposition, the chest was rotated for the image (see Images 45 and 46). One means of identifying the lung that is positioned posteriorly is to locate the most inferiorly demonstrated right and left corresponding ribs. The rib on the right side will be projected slightly more inferiorly than the rib on the left side because it is positioned farthest from the IR. The heart shadow and gastric bubble may also be used, as described in the earlier discussion of the adult lateral chest projection.

Humeral soft tissue is not superimposed over the anterior lung apices.

- Positioning the humeri upward, near the patient's head, prevents superimposition of the humeral soft tissue over the anterior lung apices (see Image 46).

The chin is not in the exposure field.

- Good radiation protection practices dictate that anatomic structures that are not evaluated on an image should not be included, whenever possible. To prevent the chin from being included in the exposure field, lift it upward above the collimation field (see Image 47).

The hemidiaphragms form a gentle cephalic curve.

- *Respiration.* For neonates and infants breathing without a respirator, observe the chest movement and take the exposure after the infant takes a deep breath. Chest images that are taken on expiration may demonstrate a decrease in image density, because a decrease in air volume increases the concentration of pulmonary tissues. With underaeration, the cephalic curve of the hemidiaphragms is exaggerated and their position is higher in the thorax (see Image 48).

Neonate and Infant Lateral Chest Projection Analysis

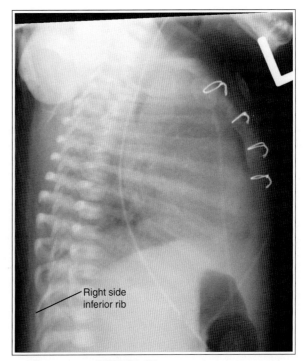

Right side inferior rib

IMAGE 45 Neonate.

Analysis. The posterior ribs are demonstrated without superimposition. The right lung is posterior to the left lung, as identified by the more inferior projection of the posterior rib on the right side compared with the left.

Correction. Rotate the right side of the thorax away from the bed or cart until the shoulders and posterior ribs are aligned perpendicular to the IR.

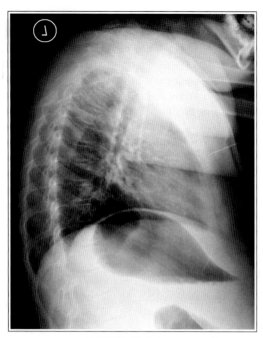

IMAGE 46 Infant.

Analysis. The humeral soft tissue is superimposed over the anterior lung apices. The patient's arms were not elevated. The left lung is anterior to the right lung, as identified by the gastric air bubble seen beneath the left hemidiaphragm.

Correction. Raise the patient's arms until the humeri are next to the patient's head. Rotate the left side of the thorax posteriorly until the shoulders and posterior ribs are aligned perpendicularly to the IR.

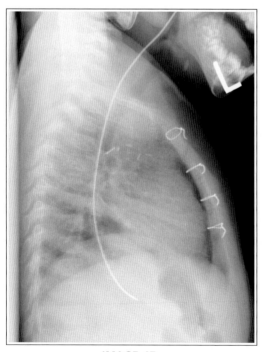

IMAGE 47

Analysis. The patient's chin is demonstrated within the collimated field. The chin was depressed.

Correction. Elevate the chin, outside the collimated field.

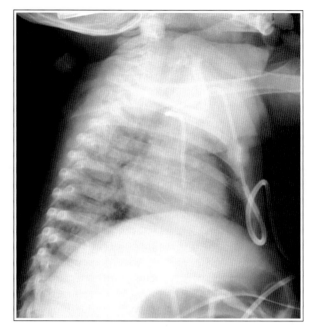

IMAGE 48

Analysis. The hemidiaphragms demonstrate an exaggerated cephalic curvature, and the humeral soft tissue is superimposed over the apical lung field. The lungs were not fully expanded, and the arms were not elevated to a position near the patient's head.

Correction. Expose the image after full inhalation, and raise the arms until they are adjacent to the patient's head.

CHILD CHEST: LATERAL PROJECTION (LEFT LATERAL POSITION)

See Figures 3-53 and 3-54.

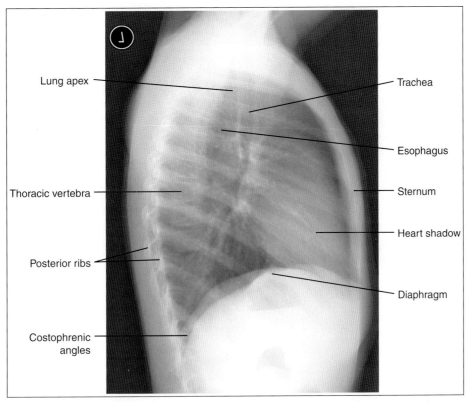

FIGURE 3-53 Child lateral chest projection with accurate positioning.

The analysis of the child lateral chest projection is the same as that of the infant or adult lateral chest projection (see earlier). The size of the child determines which criterion best meets the situation. For a discussion on the topics needed to analyze Images 49 through 51 that follow, see the lateral adult or infant chest discussions earlier in this chapter.

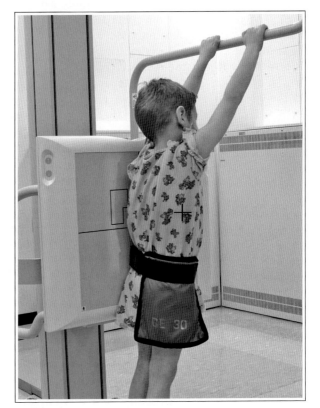

FIGURE 3-54 Proper positioning for a child lateral chest projection.

Child Lateral Chest Projection Analysis

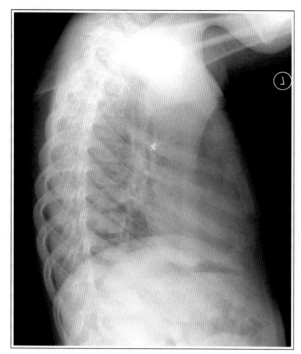

IMAGE 49

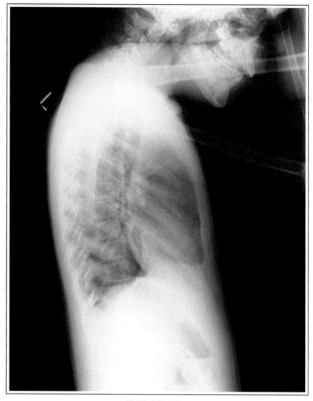

IMAGE 50

Analysis. More than 0.5 inch (1.25 cm) of separation is demonstrated between the posterior ribs. The gastric air bubble is adjacent to the anteriorly located lung, indicating that the left lung is anteriorly positioned. The chin is within the collimated field, and the humeral soft tissue is superimposed over the superior lung field. The chin and the humeri were not elevated.

Correction. Rotate the right side of the thorax anteriorly and the left side posteriorly until the shoulders and the posterior ribs are aligned perpendicularly to the IR. Elevate the chin outside the collimated field, and raise the humeri next to the patient's head.

Analysis. Anatomic artifacts (patient's arms and mandible) are demonstrated on this image. Poor radiation protection practices are demonstrated.

Correction. Raise the patient's chin to bring it above the level of the chest and out of a properly collimated field. Increase the transverse collimation to within 0.5 inch (1.25 cm) of thorax skin line.

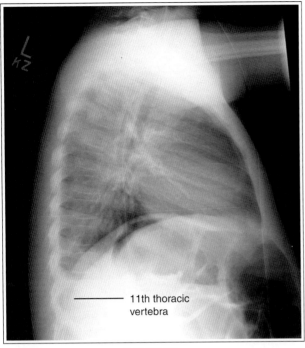

11th thoracic
vertebra

IMAGE 51

Analysis. The hemidiaphragms demonstrate an exaggerated cephalic curve, and they do not cover the entire eleventh thoracic vertebra. Full lung aeration is not demonstrated. The humeri are not elevated.

Correction. Coax the patient into taking a deeper inspiration. Elevate the humeri next to the patient's head.

NEONATE AND INFANT CHEST: ANTEROPOSTERIOR PROJECTION (RIGHT OR LEFT LATERAL DECUBITUS POSITION)

See Figure 3-55 and Box 3-10.

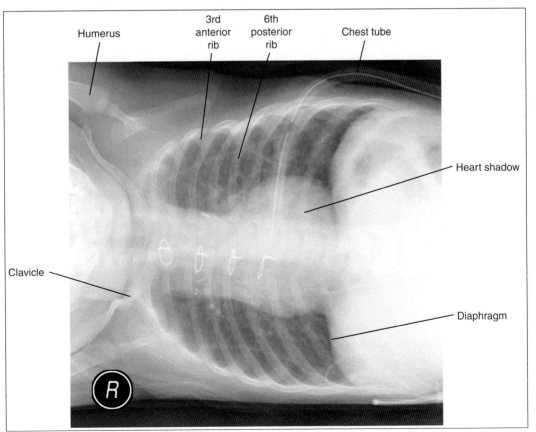

FIGURE 3-55 AP (lateral decubitus) chest projection with accurate positioning.

BOX 3-10	Neonate and Infant Anteroposterior (Lateral Decubitus) Chest Projection Analysis Criteria

- The fourth thoracic vertebra is at the center of the exposure field.
- The upper airway, lungs, mediastinal structures, and costophrenic angles are included within the collimated field.
- The distances from the vertebral column to the sternal ends of the clavicles are equal, and the lengths of the right and left corresponding posterior ribs are equal.
- The chin and arms are situated outside the lung field, and the lateral aspects of the clavicles are projected upward.
- The anterior ribs are projecting downward and the posterior ribs demonstrate a gentle, cephalically bowed contour.
- Eight posterior ribs are demonstrated above the diaphragm, and the lungs demonstrate a fluffy appearance, with linear-appearing connecting tissue.
- The lung field positioned against the bed or cart is demonstrated without superimposition of the bed or cart pad.
- The midsagittal plane is seen without lateral tilting.

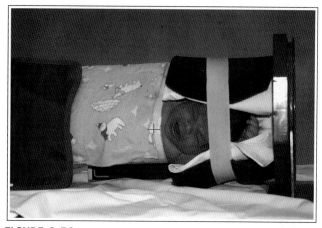

FIGURE 3-56 Proper patient positioning for neonate and infant AP (lateral decubitus) chest projection.

Contrast and density are adequate to visualize fluid levels or the presence of air within the pleural cavity.

- *Positioning to demonstrate pleural air or fluid.* The AP (lateral decubitus) projection is primarily used to confirm the presence of a pneumothorax or pleural effusion in the pleural cavity. To demonstrate the presence of air best, position the affected side of the thorax away from the bed or cart so that the air rises to the highest level in the pleural cavity. To demonstrate fluid in the pleural cavity best, position the affected side against the bed or cart. This positioning allows the fluid to move to the lowest level of the pleural cavity, away from the mediastinal structures (see Image 55).

The fourth thoracic vertebra is at the center of the exposure field. The upper airway, lungs, mediastinal structures, and costophrenic angles are included within the collimated field.

- With the neonate or infant positioned on the lateral side that best demonstrates the condition of interest, place an 8- × 10-inch (18- × 24-cm) lengthwise IR against the patient's posterior surface and position the chest in the middle of the IR by elevating the patient on a radiolucent sponge. Center a horizontal central ray to the midsagittal plane at the level of the mammary line for neonates and small infants (Figure 3-56). A larger IR and slightly inferior centering may be needed for larger infants. This IR and central ray placement centers the lung field on the image, permitting tight collimation on all sides of the lungs. Open the longitudinal collimation to include the upper airway (infant's bottom lip) and costophrenic angles (tenth posterior rib), and transversely collimate to within 0.5 inch (1.25 cm) of the lateral skin line.

The chest demonstrates an AP projection. The distances from the vertebral column to the sternal ends of the

clavicles are equal, and the lengths of the corresponding right and left posterior ribs are equal.

- To avoid chest rotation, align the shoulders, the posterior ribs, and the posterior pelvic wings perpendicularly to the bed or cart on which the neonate or infant is lying. This alignment positions the patient's shoulders and lungs at equal distances from the IR. Position the head straight ahead without rotation. The chest typically rotates in the same direction as the infant's head.
- *Detecting chest rotation.* Chest rotation is detected by evaluating the distance between the vertebral column and the sternal ends of the clavicles and by comparing the length of the right and left inferior posterior ribs. The sternal clavicular end that is superimposed over the least amount of the vertebral column, along with the side of the chest that demonstrates the longest inferior posterior ribs, represents the side of the chest toward which the infant is rotated (see Image 52).

The chin and arms are situated outside the lung field, and the lateral aspects of the clavicles are projected upward.

- To prevent the chin from being superimposed over the lung apices on the image, elevate the chin until the face is facing forward and the neck is in a neutral position (see Image 53). Placing the arms upward toward the patient's head positions them away from the lung field and projects the lateral clavicles in an upward position (see Image 54).

The anterior ribs are projecting downward, and the posterior ribs demonstrate a gentle, bowed downward contour.

- The neonate or infant AP (lateral decubitus) chest projection tends to have a lordotic appearance because of the lack of kyphotic thoracic curvature seen in adults. To reduce this lordotic appearance, align the central ray perpendicularly to the midcoronal plane and center the central ray at the level of the mammary line. Because the chest in neonates and infants is shorter than in adults, a common error is to center the central ray too inferiorly, resulting in an increase in the lordotic appearance.

- A neonate or infant AP (lateral decubitus) chest projection that demonstrates an excessively lordotic appearance will demonstrate cephalically projected anterior ribs and posterior ribs without their gentle, cephalically bowed appearance (see Image 53).

Eight posterior ribs are demonstrated above the diaphragm and the lungs demonstrate a fluffy appearance, with linear-appearing connecting tissue, indicating full lung aeration for the neonate or infant chest image.

- Observe the patient during quiet breathing, and expose the image when the lungs show expansion.

The lung field positioned against the bed or cart is demonstrated without superimposition of the bed or cart pad. The midsagittal plane is demonstrated without lateral tilting.

- Elevating the neonate or infant on a radiolucent sponge prevents the chest from sinking into the cart pad. When the body is allowed to sink into the cart pad, artifact lines are seen superimposed over the lateral lung field of the side adjacent to the cart. Because fluid in the pleural cavity gravitates to the lowest level, it is in this area that the fluid will be demonstrated, and superimposition of the cart pad and lower lung field may obscure fluid that has settled in the lowest level. Position the neonate or infant's entire body on the radiolucent sponge to align the midsagittal plane parallel with the bed or cart, preventing lateral tilting (see Image 55).

Neonate and Infant Anteroposterior (Lateral Decubitus) Chest Projection Analysis

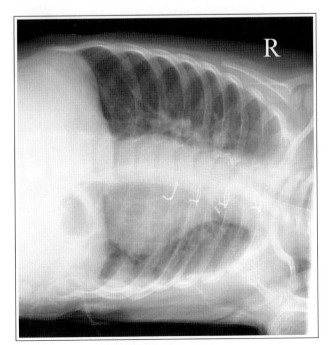

IMAGE 52 AP projection.

Analysis. The left sternal clavicular end is demonstrated farther from the vertebral column than the right sternal clavicular end, and the left posterior ribs are longer than the right. The patient's head is turned, and the thorax is rotated toward the left side.

Correction. Rotate the patient's face to a forward position, and rotate the thorax toward the right side until the midcoronal plane is parallel with the IR and perpendicular to the central ray.

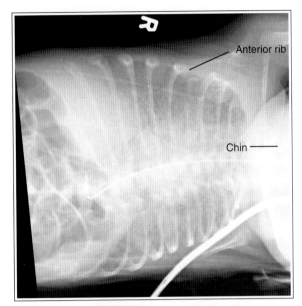

IMAGE 53 AP projection.

Analysis. The chest demonstrates an excessively lordotic appearance. The anterior ribs are projecting cephalically, and the posterior ribs do not demonstrate the slight cephalically bowed contour but are horizontal. The central ray was centered inferiorly to T6. The right inferior ribs are longer than the left posterior ribs. The patient was rotated toward the right side. The chin is superimposed over the apices and upper airway.

Correction. Move the central ray superiorly to align it with the upper thorax better. A 5-degree caudal angle may also be added to help align the central ray and thorax better. Rotate the patient toward the left side until the shoulders and the posterior ribs are at equal distances to the IR. Elevate the chin until it is positioned outside the collimated field.

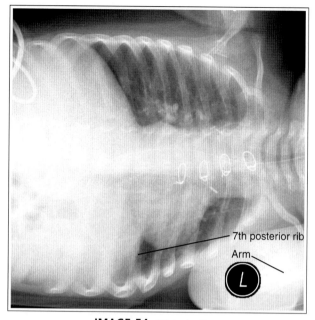

IMAGE 54 AP projection.

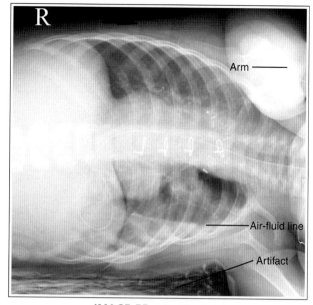

IMAGE 55 AP projection.

Analysis. Seven posterior ribs are demonstrated above the diaphragm. Full lung aeration was not accomplished. The left arm is superimposed over a small portion of the left lateral lung field. The right clavicle is horizontal. The arms were not brought upward by the patient's head.

Correction. If possible, take the exposure after the patient takes a deep inspiration. If the patient is on a conventional ventilator, expose the image when the manometer is at it highest level, indicating a deep inspiration. Raise the patient's arms; bring them next to the patient's head.

Analysis. The device on which the patient is elevated is demonstrated adjacent to the left lateral lung field. Because the patient has not sunk into this device, it is not superimposed over the lateral lung field and is acceptable. The patient's upper midsagittal plane is laterally tilted toward the left side. The patient's upper thorax was allowed to hang over the elevating device. The patient's right arm is obscuring the lateral apical area. The right arm was not elevated to a position near the patient's head.

Correction. Place the entire thorax on the elevating device, positioning the midsagittal plane parallel with the bed or cart. Elevate the right arm so it is positioned next to the patient's head.

CHILD CHEST: ANTEROPOSTERIOR AND POSTEROANTERIOR PROJECTION (RIGHT OR LEFT LATERAL DECUBITUS POSITION)

See Figures 3-57 and 3-58.

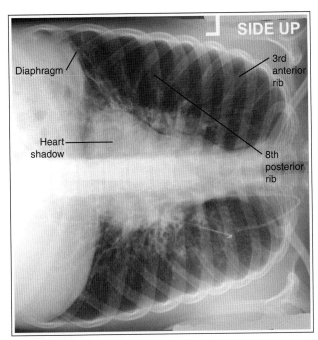

FIGURE 3-57 Child PA (lateral decubitus) chest projection with accurate positioning.

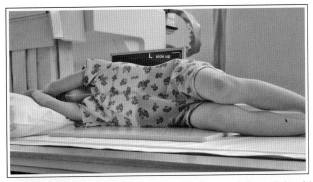

FIGURE 3-58 Proper patient positioning for an AP (lateral decubitus) chest projection.

The analysis of AP (lateral decubitus) chest projections in children is the same as that of infant or adult AP (lateral decubitus) chest projections (see earlier). The size of the child determines the criterion that best meets the situation. For a discussion on the topics needed to analyze Image 56, refer to the discussion of AP-PA (lateral decubitus) chest projections earlier in this chapter.

Child Anteroposterior-Posteroanterior (Lateral Decubitus) Chest Projection Analysis

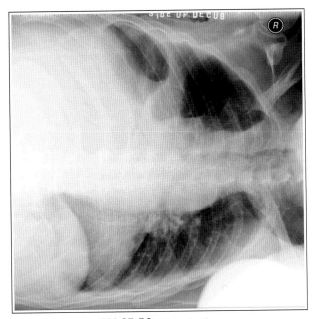

IMAGE 56 AP projection.

Analysis. The left sternal clavicular end is superimposed over the vertebral column, the posterior ribs on the right side demonstrate the greater length, and the arms are superimposed over the left lateral lung apex. The patient was rotated toward the right side, and the left arm was at a 90-degree angle with thorax.

Correction. Rotate the patient's right side away from the IR, and elevate the left arm until it is positioned next to the patent's head.

ABDOMEN

The following image analysis criteria are used for all adult and pediatric abdomen projections and should be considered when completing the analysis for each abdominal projection presented in this chapter (Box 3-11).

Voluntary and Involuntary Motion

Two types of motion may be evident on an abdominal image, voluntary and involuntary. Voluntary motion is caused by breathing or moving during the exposure. It can be controlled by explaining to the patient the importance of holding still, making the patient as comfortable as possible on the imaging table, and using the shortest possible exposure time. On an image, voluntary motion can be identified as blurred bony cortices and gastric and intestinal gases (see Image 57). Involuntary motion is caused by the peristaltic activity of the stomach or small or large intestine. This movement is considered

<table>
<tr><td colspan="2">

BOX 3-11　　**Abdomen Imaging Analysis Criteria**

- The facility's identification requirements are visible.
- A right or left marker identifying the correct side of the patient is present on the image and is not superimposed over the anatomy of interest.
- Good radiation protection practices are evident.
- The cortical outlines of the posterior ribs, lumbar vertebrae, and pelvis and the gases within the stomach and intestines are sharply defined.
- Adult: Collections of fat that outline the psoas muscles and kidneys, and the bony structures of the inferior ribs and transverse processes of the lumbar vertebrae, are demonstrated.
- Children: The diaphragm, bowel gas pattern, and faint outline of bony structures are demonstrated.
- Density is uniform across the abdomen.
- There is no evidence of preventable artifacts, such as undergarments, gown snaps, or removable external monitoring tubes or lines.

</td></tr>
</table>

involuntary because the patient cannot control this movement, as with breathing. The only means of decreasing the blur caused by involuntary motion is to use the shortest possible exposure time and, in some cases, this is not good enough. Involuntary motion can be identified on abdominal images as sharp bony cortices and blurry gastric and intestinal gases (see Image 58).

Visibility of Details

Beam penetration, contrast, and density are adequate on adult abdominal images when the collections of fat that outline the psoas major muscles and kidney as well as the bony structures of the inferior ribs and transverse processes of the lumbar vertebrae are demonstrated.

An optimal kVp technique, as shown in Table 3-3, sufficiently penetrates the soft tissue and bony structures of the abdomen. This kVp setting enhances the subtle radiation absorption differences among the fat, gas, muscles, and solid organs, which mainly consist of water. Because soft tissue abdominal structures are

similar in atomic number and density, whether two soft tissue structures that border each other are visible or not depends on their arrangement with respect to the gas and fat collections that lie next to them, around them, or within them. These same gas and fat collections are used to identify diseases and masses within the abdomen. The presence or absence of gas, as well as its amount and location within the intestinal system, may indicate a functional, metabolic, or mechanical disease, whereas routinely seen collections of fat may be displaced or obscured with organ enlargement or mass invasion. Use a high-ratio grid to reduce the scatter radiation that reaches the IR, thereby reducing fog, increasing the visibility of the recorded details, and providing a higher contrast image. To obtain optimal density, set a manual mAs based on the patient's abdominal thickness or choose all three AEC chambers.

The soft tissue structures that can be outlined if appropriate image density and contrast have been obtained on an AP abdominal projection are the psoas major muscles and kidneys. The psoas major muscles are located laterally to the lumbar vertebrae. They originate at the first lumbar vertebra on each side and extend to the corresponding lesser trochanter. On an AP abdominal projection, the psoas major muscles are visible as long, triangular, soft tissue shadows on each side of the vertebral bodies. The kidneys are found in the posterior abdomen and are identified on the image as bean-shaped densities located on each side of the vertebral column 3 inches (7.5 cm) from the midline. The upper poles of the kidney lie on the same transverse level as the spinous process of the eleventh thoracic vertebra, and the lower poles lie on the same transverse level as the spinous process of the third lumbar vertebra. The right kidney is usually demonstrated approximately 1 inch (2.5 cm) inferior to the left kidney because of its location beneath the liver. Occasionally a kidney may be displaced inferiorly (nephroptosis) to this location, because it is not held in place by adjacent organs or its fat covering; this condition is most often seen in thin patients.

TABLE 3-3　　**Adult and Pediatric Abdomen Technical Data**				
Projection	**kVp**	**Grid**	**AEC Chamber(s)**	**SID**
Adult Abdomen Technical Data				
AP	70–80	Grid	All	40–48 inches (100–120 cm)
AP (lateral decubitus)	70–80	Grid	Center	40–48 inches (100–120 cm)
Pediatric Abdomen Technical Data				
Neonate: AP	65–75			40–48 inches (100–120 cm)
Infant: AP	65–75			40–48 inches (100–120 cm)
Child: AP	70–80	Grid (if measures 4 inches (10 cm) or larger)		40–48 inches (100–120 cm)
Neonate: AP (lateral decubitus)	65–75			40–48 inches (100–120 cm)
Infant: AP (lateral decubitus)	65–75			40–48 inches (100–120 cm)
Child: AP (lateral decubitus)	70–80	Grid (if measures 4 inches (10 cm) or larger)		40–48 inches (100–120 cm)

AP, Anteroposterior; *kVp*, kilovoltage peak; *PA*, posteroanterior; *SID*, source–image receptor distance.

Adjusting Technique for Specific Patient Conditions

The routine manually set exposure factors obtained from the AP body measurement of patients with suspected large amounts of bowel gas may overexpose areas of the abdomen that are overlaid with gas (see Image 59). (The patient measures the same whether gas or dense soft tissue causes the thickness.) This increased image density results from the low density (number of atoms per given area) characteristic of gas. As the radiation passes through the patient's body, fewer photons are absorbed where gas is located than where dense soft tissue is present. To compensate for this situation, decrease the exposure (mAs) 30% to 50% or the kVp 5% to 8% from the routinely used manual technique before the image is taken. An underexposed image may result when patients have ascites, obesity, bowel obstructions, or soft tissue masses. This is because sections of the abdomen that nor-mally contain gas or fat do not, resulting in an increase in the density of the soft tissue. To compensate for this situation, increase the exposure (mAs) 30% to 50% or the kVp 5% to 8% from the routinely used technique before the image is taken.

Pediatric Abdomen

For the pediatric patient contrast, density, and penetration should be adequate to demonstrate the diaphragm, bowel gas pattern, and faint outline of bony structures. An optimal kVp technique, as shown in Table 3-3, sufficiently penetrates the bowel gas pattern and faintly outlines the bony structures. In infants and young children, it is difficult to differentiate between the small and large bowels. The gas loops tend to look the same. Because little intrinsic fat is present, the abdominal organs (such as kidneys) are not well defined.

ABDOMEN: AP PROJECTION (SUPINE AND UPRIGHT)

See Figures 3-59 and 3-60 and Box 3-12.

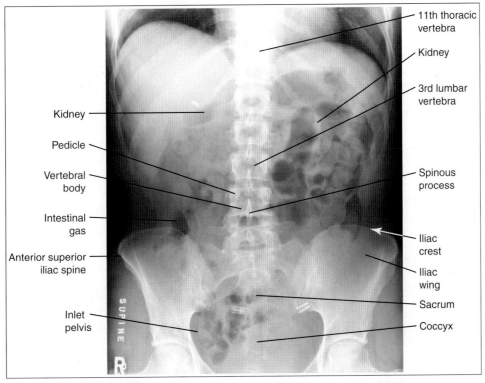

FIGURE 3-59 Supine AP abdomen projection with accurate positioning.

Density is uniform across the abdomen.

- *Excessive abdominal soft tissue.* When an upright AP abdomen projection is taken on a patient with excessive abdominal soft tissue, the soft tissue often drops down and forward. This movement results in a larger AP measurement at the lower abdominal level than at the upper abdominal level. For such patients, use two crosswise IRs to include all the abdominal structures, and take measurements of the lower and upper abdominal areas to ensure that accurate image density of each area will be obtained.

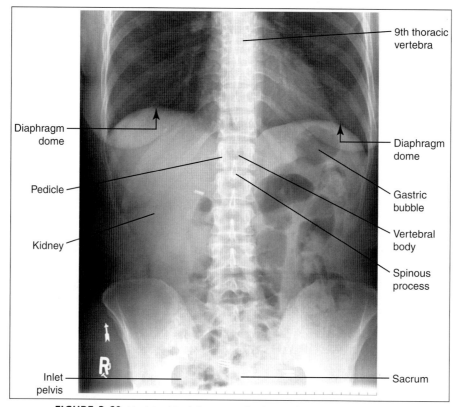

FIGURE 3-60 Upright AP abdomen projection with accurate positioning.

BOX 3-12	Anteroposterior Abdomen Projection Analysis Criteria

- Density is uniform across the abdomen.
- Spinous processes are aligned with the midline of the vertebral bodies, and the distance from the pedicles to the spinous processes is the same on both sides. The sacrum is centered within the inlet of pelvis and is aligned with the symphysis pubis.
- The long axis of the lumbar vertebral column is aligned with the long axis of the collimated field.
- Diaphragm domes are located superior to the ninth posterior ribs.
- Supine: The fourth lumbar vertebra is at the center of the exposure field.
- Supine: The eleventh thoracic vertebra, the lateral body soft tissues, the iliac wings, and the symphysis pubis are included within the collimated field.
- Upright: The third lumbar vertebra is at the center of the exposure field.
- Upright: The ninth thoracic vertebra, lateral body soft tissue, and iliac wings are included within the collimated field.

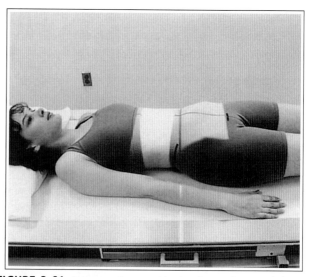

FIGURE 3-61 Proper patient positioning for supine AP abdomen projection.

The abdomen image demonstrates an AP projection. The spinous processes are aligned with the midline of the vertebral bodies, and the distance from the pedicles to the spinous processes is the same on both sides. The sacrum is centered within the inlet of pelvis and is aligned with the symphysis pubis.

- To obtain a supine abdomen projection, place the patient supine on the radiographic table. Position the shoulders and anterosuperior iliac spines at equal distances from the tabletop to prevent rotation, and draw the patient's arms away from the abdominal area to prevent them from being superimposed on the abdominal region (Figure 3-61).
- An upright abdomen projection is obtained by placing the patient against an upright imaging tabletop. Position the shoulders and anterosuperior iliac spines at equal distances from the tabletop to prevent rotation, and draw the patient's arms away from the

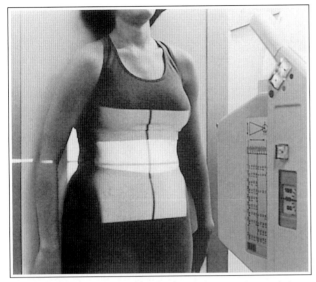

FIGURE 3-62 Proper patient positioning for upright AP abdomen projection.

abdominal area to prevent them from being superimposed on the abdominal region (Figure 3-62).

- *Demonstrating intraperitoneal air:* For intraperitoneal air to be demonstrated best, the patient should be positioned upright for 5 to 20 minutes before the image is taken. This allows enough time for the air to move away from the soft tissue abdominal structures and rise to the level of the diaphragms (Figure 3-63). If a patient has come to the imaging department for a supine and upright abdominal series, begin with the upright image if the patient is ambulatory (able to walk) or transported by wheelchair. An ambulatory or wheelchair-using patient has been upright long enough for the air to rise, so it is not necessary to wait to take the image.

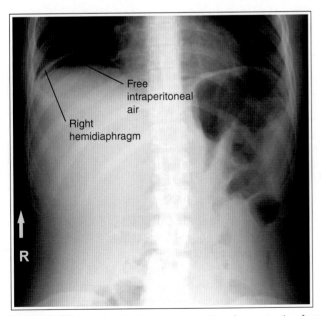

FIGURE 3-63 Upright AP abdomen projection demonstrating free air under the right hemidiaphragm.

- *Detecting abdominal rotation:* Rotation of an AP abdomen projection can decrease the visualization of fat lines that surround abdominal structures. For example, the psoas lateral muscles are outlined because of the fat that lies next to them. When the patient is rotated to one side, this fat shifts from lateral to anterior or posterior with respect to the muscle. The shift eliminates the subject contrast difference that exists when the muscle and fat are separated, hindering the usefulness of the psoas major muscles as diagnostic indicators. The upper and lower lumbar vertebrae can demonstrate rotation independently or simultaneously, depending on which section of the body is rotated. If the patient's thorax was rotated but the pelvis remained in an AP projection, the upper lumbar vertebrae and abdominal cavity demonstrate rotation. If the patient's pelvis was rotated but the thorax remained in an AP projection, the lower vertebrae and abdominal cavity demonstrate rotation. If the patient's thorax and pelvis were rotated simultaneously, the entire lumbar column and abdominal cavity demonstrate rotation. Rotation is effectively detected on an AP abdomen projection by comparing the distance from the pedicles to the spinous processes on each side and by evaluating the centering of the sacrum within the inlet pelvis. If the distance from the pedicles to the spinous processes is greater on one side of the vertebrae than on the other, or if the sacrum is rotated toward one side of the inlet, pelvic rotation is present (see Images 60 and 61). The side with the smaller distance between the pedicles and spinous processes and toward which the sacrum is rotated is the side of the patient positioned farther from the tabletop and IR.

- *Distinguishing abdominal rotation from scoliosis.* In patients with scoliosis, the lumbar bodies may appear rotated because of the lateral twisting of the vertebrae. Scoliosis of the vertebral column can be very severe, demonstrating a large degree of lateral deviation, or it can be subtle, demonstrating only a small degree of deviation. Severe scoliosis is very obvious and is seldom mistaken for patient rotation, whereas subtle scoliotic changes can be easily mistaken for patient rotation (see Image 62). Although both demonstrate unequal distances between the pedicles and spinous processes, clues that can be used to distinguish subtle scoliosis from rotation are present. The long axis of a rotated vertebral column remains straight, whereas the scoliotic vertebral column demonstrates lateral deviation. When the lumbar vertebrae demonstrate rotation, it has been caused by the rotation of the upper or lower torso. The middle lumbar vertebrae (L3 and L4) cannot rotate unless the lower thoracic vertebrae or upper or lower lumbar vertebrae are also rotated. On the scoliotic image, the middle lumbar vertebrae may demonstrate rotation without corresponding upper or lower vertebral rotation. This constitutes an acceptable image for a patient with this condition.

The long axis of the lumbar vertebral column is aligned with the long axis of the collimated field.

- Aligning the long axis of the lumbar vertebral column with the long axis of the collimated field ensures that the lateral abdominal cavity will not be clipped. To obtain proper upper abdominal alignment, align the xiphoid with the collimator's longitudinal light line. To obtain proper lower abdominal alignment, find the point midway between the patient's palpable anterior superior iliac spines (ASISs); then align this point with the collimator's longitudinal light line. Do not assume that the patient's navel is positioned directly above the vertebral column. Often it is shifted to one side.

The image was taken on expiration, and the diaphragm dome is located superior to the ninth posterior ribs.

- From full inspiration to expiration, the diaphragm position moves from an inferior to a superior position. This movement also changes the pressure placed on the abdominal structures. On full expiration, the right side of the diaphragm dome is at the same transverse level as the eighth or ninth thoracic vertebra, whereas on inspiration, it may be found at the same transverse level as the ninth posterior rib (see Image 63). If the abdominal image is taken on inspiration, the inferior placement of the diaphragm places pressure on the abdominal organs, resulting in less space in the peritoneal cavity and greater abdominal density. Underexposed images may also result with full inspiration on the upper abdomen image when two crosswise images are needed and the three AEC chambers are chosen, because the outside AEC chambers will be positioned beneath the lungs instead of abdominal structures.

Supine position: The fourth lumbar vertebra is at the center of the exposure field. The spinous process of the eleventh thoracic vertebra, the lateral body soft tissues, the iliac wings, and the symphysis pubis are included within the collimated field.

- Including the spinous process of the eleventh thoracic vertebra ensures that the kidneys, tip of liver, and spleen, all of which lie inferior to it, will be present on the image. The symphysis pubis ensures that the inferior border of the peritoneal cavity is included on the image (see Image 64). To position the fourth lumbar vertebra in the center of the collimated field, use a 40- to 48-inch (102- to 120-cm) SID. Center a perpendicular central ray with the patient's midsagittal plane at the level of the iliac crest for female patients and at a level 1 inch (2.5 cm) inferior to the iliac crest for male patients to

allow for the difference in size and longitudinal dimension between the female and male pelves.

- *Centering the central ray in males and females.* The centering determination measurements for male patients were taken from several male and female pelvic images, because of the following: (1) the patient is positioned in the same manner for a pelvic image as for an AP abdomen projection; (2) the magnification factors (SID and OID) are identical to those used for an AP abdominal image; and (3) all pelvic anatomy was included and could be easily measured. The only difference in setup procedure between AP pelvis and AP abdomen projections is the centering of the central ray. Although the superior centering used for the AP abdomen projection projects the anteriorly located pelvic structures slightly more inferiorly than they appear on an AP pelvis projection, the influence is the same on all abdominal IRs and affects the male and female pelves in the same manner. A measurement of each pelvic image was taken from the most superiorly located surface of the right iliac crest to the most inferior aspect of the right obturator foramen. Although slight variations of approximately 0.25 inch (0.6 cm) did exist in each gender, the average female measurement was 8.5 inches (21.25 cm) and the average male measurement was 9.5 inches (24 cm). Because the IR length used for AP abdomen projections is 17 inches (43 cm) and the pelvis is to fit on the lower half, or 8.5 inches (21.25 cm), one can understand why accurate central ray placement is important to include the needed structures.

- *IR size and direction.* A 14- × 17-inch (35- × 43-cm) lengthwise IR should be adequate to include all the required anatomic structures on sthenic and asthenic patients, as long as the transverse abdominal measurement is less than 14 inches (35 cm).

  If the spinous process of the eleventh thoracic vertebra is not included on this image, take a second image using an 11- × 14-inch (28- × 35-cm) crosswise IR. It is necessary for the second image to include approximately 2 to 3 inches (5 to 7.5 cm) of the same transverse section of the peritoneal cavity imaged on the first image to ensure that no middle peritoneal information has been excluded. The top of the IR should extend to the patient's xiphoid, which is at the level of the tenth thoracic vertebra, to make sure that the spinous process of the eleventh thoracic vertebra is included. The longitudinal collimated field should remain fully open for both IRs. Transversely, collimate to within 0.5 inch (1.25 cm) of the patient's lateral skin line.

  Use two 14- × 17-inch (35- × 43-cm) crosswise IRs on hypersthenic patients, and on patients who have a transverse abdominal measurement of 14 inches (35 cm) or greater, to include all the necessary anatomic structures. Take the first image with the central ray centered to the midsagittal plane at a level halfway between the symphysis pubis and ASIS. Position the bottom of the second IR so that it includes 2 to 3 inches (5 to 7.5 cm) of the same transverse section of the peritoneal cavity imaged on the first image to ensure that no middle peritoneal information has been excluded. The top of the IR should extend to the patient's xiphoid, which is at the level of the tenth thoracic vertebra, to make sure that the spinous process of the eleventh thoracic vertebra is included.

- *Gonadal shielding*: Use gonadal shielding for supine images on all male patients and on female patients if two IRs are required and the upper abdomen is being imaged. Do not shield female patients if the lower abdomen is being imaged, because the shield may obscure needed information.

Upright position: **The third lumbar vertebra is at the center of the exposure field. The diaphragm, the ninth thoracic vertebra, the lateral body soft tissue, and the iliac wings are included within the collimated field.**

- *Positioning and central ray.* The upright AP abdomen projection is most often used to evaluate the peritoneal cavity for intraperitoneal air. For intraperitoneal air to be demonstrated, the diaphragm must be included in its entirety, because the air would be located directly inferior to the domes of the diaphragm (see Figure 3-63). When the image is taken on expiration, including the ninth thoracic vertebra will ensure demonstration of the diaphragm. To include the ninth thoracic vertebra at the top of the image and to center the third thoracic vertebra to the center of the collimated field, place the top of the IR (not the top of the collimator's light field) at a level of the axilla for the sthenic patient, slightly higher for the hypersthenic patient, and slightly lower for the asthenic patient. Use a 40- to 48-inch (102- to 120-cm) SID. Center a perpendicular central ray with the midsagittal plane and IR center. An upright AP abdomen projection that does not include the entire diaphragm should be retaken (see Image 65).
- *IR size and direction*: A 14- × 17-inch (35- × 43-cm) lengthwise IR is adequate to include all the required anatomic structures on the sthenic or asthenic patient, as long as the patient's transverse abdominal measurement is less than 14 inches (35 cm). Open the longitudinal collimated field the full 17-inch (43-cm) field size and transversely collimate to within 0.5 inch (1.25 cm) of the lateral skin line. Use two 14- × 17-inch (35- × 43-cm) crosswise IRs on hypersthenic patients, and on sthenic and asthenic patients who have transverse abdominal measurement of 14 inches (35 cm) or greater, to include all the necessary anatomic structures. Take the first

image with the top of the IR positioned as described earlier. Place the top of the second IR so that it will include 2 to 3 inches (5 to 7.5 cm) of the same transverse section of the peritoneal cavity imaged on the first image to ensure that no middle peritoneal information has been excluded. Center the central ray to the midsagittal plane for both images.

- *Gonadal shielding*: Use gonadal shielding for upright images on all male abdomen projections and female patients if two IRs are required and the upper abdomen is being imaged. Do not shield female patients when the lower abdomen is imaged because the shield may obscure needed information.

Anteroposterior Abdomen Projection Analysis

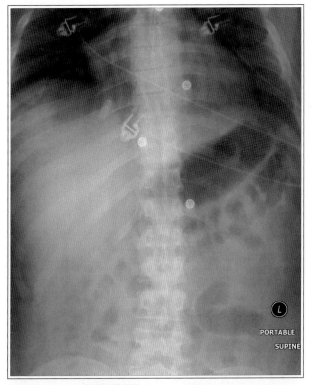

IMAGE 57 Supine abdomen.

Analysis. The ribs and intestines are blurred, indicating that the patient moved and/or breathed during the exposure. The symphysis pubis is not included on the image. The central ray was positioned too superiorly. The lateral soft tissue is not entirely included on the image. Two crosswise images should have been taken.

Correction. Instruct the patient to halt respiration during the exposure. Using a short exposure time will also help if the patient has difficulty holding still. Repeat the examination using two crosswise IRs, making certain that the lower image includes the inferior peritoneal cavity.

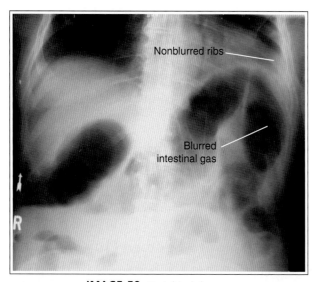

IMAGE 58 Upright abdomen.

Analysis. This is the upper image of a crosswise AP abdomen projection. The cortical outlines of the ribs and vertebral column are well defined without blur, whereas the intestinal structures demonstrate blur. This represents involuntary motion.

Correction. Repeat examination using the shortest possible exposure time.

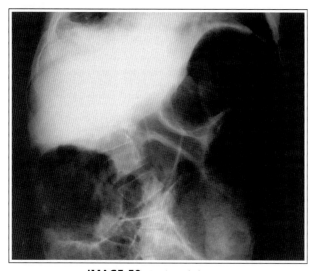

IMAGE 59 Supine abdomen.

Analysis. This abdomen projection is from a hypersthenic patient who had an excessive amount of bowel gas. In an attempt to demonstrate the areas superimposed with bowel gas, the exposure (mAs) was decreased. The decrease resulted in an underexposed area beneath the right diaphragm.

Correction. If this abdominal area is of importance, a second image should be taken with increased exposure. If the indication for the examination is to evaluate bowel gas, the image is acceptable.

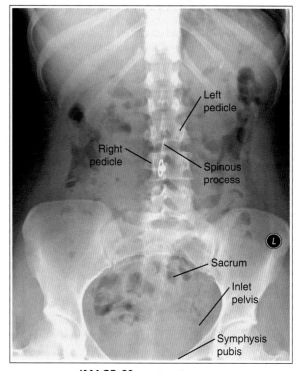

IMAGE 60 Supine abdomen.

Analysis. The sacrum is not aligned with the symphysis pubis but is situated closer to the right hip, and the distance from the right pedicles to the spinous processes is less than the distance from the left pedicles to the spinous processes. The patient was rotated toward the left side.

Correction. Rotate the patient toward the right side until the shoulders and ASISs are positioned at equal distances from the IR.

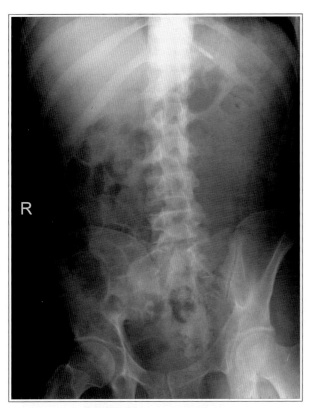

IMAGE 61 Supine abdomen.

Analysis. The sacrum is not aligned with the symphysis pubis but is situated closer to the left, and the distance from the left pedicles to the spinous processes is less than the distance from the right pedicles to the spinous processes. The patient was rotated toward the right side.

Correction. Rotate the patient toward the left side until the shoulders and ASISs are positioned at equal distances.

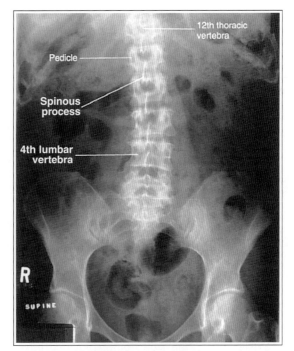

IMAGE 62 Supine abdomen.

Analysis. The vertebral column deviates laterally at the level of the second through fourth lumbar vertebrae, the sacrum is centered within the inlet pelvis, and the distances from the pedicles to the spinous processes of the twelfth thoracic vertebra and fifth lumbar vertebra are equal. The vertebral column demonstrates subtle spinal scoliosis.

Correction. No correction movement is required for scoliosis. An AP abdomen projection of a patient with scoliosis appears rotated.

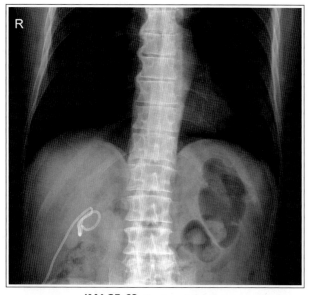

IMAGE 63 Supine abdomen.

Analysis. The diaphragm dome is located inferiorly to the ninth posterior ribs. The examination was taken on full inspiration.

Correction. Take the exposure after the patient exhales.

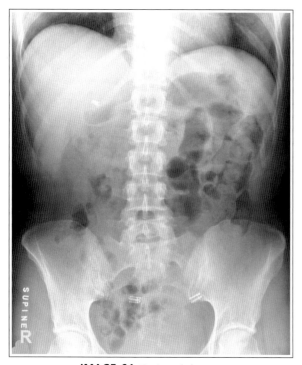

IMAGE 64 Supine abdomen.

Analysis. The symphysis pubis is not included on the image. The central ray was centered too superiorly.

Correction. Because this is a male patient, center the central ray 1 inch (2.5 cm) inferior to the iliac crest.

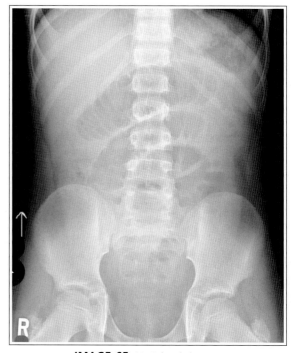

IMAGE 65 Upright abdomen.

Analysis. This is an upright AP abdomen projection. The domes of the diaphragm are not included on the image. The central ray was centered too inferiorly.

Correction. Center the central ray and IR approximately 2 inches (5 cm) superiorly.

ABDOMEN: ANTEROPOSTERIOR PROJECTION (LEFT LATERAL DECUBITUS POSITION)

See Figure 3-64 and Box 3-13.

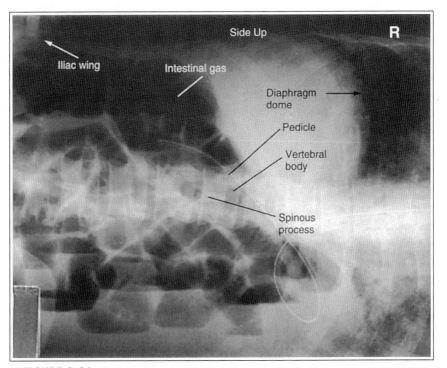

FIGURE 3-64 AP (lateral decubitus) abdomen projection with accurate positioning.

BOX 3-13	Anteroposterior (Lateral Decubitus) Abdomen Projection Analysis Criteria

- An arrow or "word" marker, indicating that the right side of the patient was positioned up and away from the imaging table or cart, is present.
- Density is uniform across the abdomen.
- The spinous processes are aligned with the midline of the vertebral bodies, and the distance from the pedicles to the spinous processes is the same on both sides. The sacrum is centered within the inlet of pelvis and is aligned with the symphysis pubis.
- The diaphragm domes are located superior to the ninth posterior ribs.
- The third lumbar vertebra is at the center of the exposure field.
- The right hemidiaphragm, ninth thoracic vertebra, right lateral body soft tissue, and iliac wings are included within the collimated field.

An arrow or "word" marker, indicating that the right side of the patient was positioned up and away from the imaging table or cart, is present on the image.

- Place an arrow or "word" marker indicating which side of the patient was positioned away from the tabletop or cart and in the collimated field.

Density is uniform across the abdomen.

- *Using a wedge-compensating filter.* When an AP (lateral decubitus) abdomen projection from a patient with excessive abdominal soft tissue is

taken, the soft tissue often drops toward the tabletop or cart. This movement results in a smaller AP measurement at the elevated right side than at the left side, which is positioned closer to the tabletop or cart. To compensate for this thickness difference, a wedge-compensating filter may be used. The wedge filter absorbs some of the x-ray photons before they reach the patient, thereby decreasing the number of photons exposing the IR where the filter is located. The thick end of the wedge filter absorbs more photons than the thin end. When a wedge-compensating filter is used, attach it to the x-ray collimator head, with the thick end positioned toward the patient's right side and the thin end toward the left side. The collimator light projects a shadow of the compensating filter onto the patient. Position the shadow of the thin end at the level of the thickest part of the abdomen, allowing the thick end to extend toward the right side. Then use a technique that will accurately expose the thickest abdominal region. The wedge-compensating filter should absorb the needed photons to prevent overexposure of the thinner abdominal region. When the filter has been accurately positioned, radiographic density is uniform throughout the abdominal structures. Positioning the filter too close to or too far away from the thickest part of the abdomen results in an overexposed or underexposed area on the image, respectively.

The abdomen demonstrates an AP projection. The spinous processes are aligned with the midline of the vertebral bodies, the distance from the pedicles to the spinous processes is the same on both sides, and the iliac wings are symmetrical.

- An AP (lateral decubitus) abdomen projection is obtained by placing the patient in a left lateral recumbent position on the tabletop or cart, with the back resting against a grid cassette or the upright IR holder. Because intraperitoneal air migrates to the highest position, which is typically the elevated diaphragm or iliac wing, the left lateral position is chosen to position the gastric bubble away from the elevated diaphragm. To avoid rotation, align the shoulders, the posterior ribs, and the posterior pelvic wings perpendicular to the tabletop or cart (Figure 3-65). Accomplish this alignment by resting your extended flat hand against each, respectively, and then adjusting the patient's rotation until your hand is positioned perpendicular to the tabletop or cart. It is most common for a patient to rotate the elevated thorax and pelvic wing anteriorly. A pillow or other support placed between the patient's knees may help eliminate this forward rotation.

- *Demonstrating intraperitoneal air.* The AP (lateral decubitus) projection is primarily used to confirm the presence of intraperitoneal air. For intraperitoneal air to be demonstrated best, the patient should be left in this position for 5 to 20 minutes before the image is taken, allowing enough time for the air to move away from the soft tissue abdominal structures and rise to the level of the right diaphragm or iliac wing (Figure 3-66). To eliminate long waiting periods for patients who are scheduled to have an AP (lateral decubitus) abdomen, have them transported to the imaging department in the left lateral decubitus position.

- *Detecting abdominal rotation.* The upper and lower lumbar vertebrae can demonstrate rotation

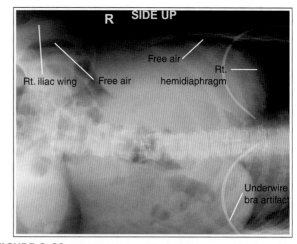

FIGURE 3-66 AP (lateral decubitus) abdomen projection demonstrating free intraperitoneal air under right hemidiaphragm and at right iliac wing.

independently or simultaneously, depending on which section of the body is rotated. If the patient's thorax is rotated but the pelvis remains in an AP projection, the upper lumbar vertebrae and abdominal cavity demonstrate rotation. If the patient's pelvis is rotated but the thorax remains in an AP projection, the lower vertebrae and abdominal cavity demonstrate rotation. If the patient's thorax and pelvis are rotated simultaneously, the entire lumbar column and abdominal cavity demonstrate rotation.

Rotation is effectively detected on an AP abdominal projection by comparing the distance from the pedicles to the spinous processes on each side and the symmetry of the iliac wings. If the distance from the pedicles to the spinous processes is greater on one side of the vertebrae than on the other side, the side with the smaller distance between the pedicles and spinous processes was the side of the patient positioned farther from the IR. If the iliac wings are not symmetrical, the wing demonstrating the smallest area is on the side of the patient positioned farther from the IR (see Image 66).

- *Distinguishing rotation from scoliosis.* In images from patients with spinal scoliosis the lumbar bodies may appear rotated because of the lateral twisting of the vertebrae. An image on a patient with spinal scoliosis and a rotated decubitus abdomen demonstrates unequal distances between the pedicles and spinous processes. Clues are present that can be used to distinguish scoliosis from rotation. The long axis of a rotated vertebral column remains straight, whereas the scoliotic vertebral column demonstrates lateral deviation. When the lumbar vertebrae demonstrate rotation, it has been caused by the rotation of the upper or lower torso. The middle lumbar vertebrae (L3 and L4) cannot rotate unless the lower thoracic vertebrae or the upper or lower lumbar vertebrae are also rotated. On the scoliotic decubitus

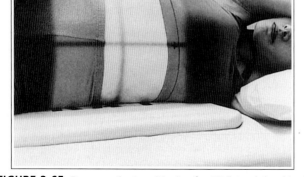

FIGURE 3-65 Proper patient positioning for AP (lateral decubitus) abdomen projection.

abdominal image, the middle lumbar vertebrae may demonstrate rotation without corresponding upper or lower vertebral rotation.

The image was taken on expiration. The diaphragm domes are located superiorly to the ninth posterior rib.

- From full inspiration to expiration, the diaphragm moves from an inferior to a superior position. This movement also changes the pressure exerted on the abdominal structures. On full expiration the superior portion of the right upper diaphragm dome is at the same transverse level as the eighth or ninth thoracic vertebrae, whereas on inspiration it may be found at the same transverse level as the ninth posterior rib. The left diaphragm is approximately 0.5 inch (1.25 cm) lower than the right diaphragm on both inspiration and expiration. When the AP (lateral decubitus) abdomen projection is taken on expiration, less pressure is exerted on the peritoneal contents and greater space exists in the peritoneal cavity. If the AP (lateral decubitus) abdomen projection is taken on inspiration, the inferior placement of the diaphragm puts pressure on the abdominal organs, resulting in less space in the peritoneal cavity and greater abdominal density.

The third lumbar vertebra is at the center of the exposure field. The right hemidiaphragm, ninth thoracic vertebra, right lateral body soft tissue, and iliac wing are included within the collimated field.

- The AP (lateral decubitus) abdomen projection is most often used to evaluate the peritoneal cavity for intraperitoneal air. To demonstrate intraperitoneal air, the right hemidiaphragm and iliac wing must be included. In the left lateral decubitus position, intraperitoneal air will rise to the highest level. In most patients the intraperitoneal air moves to the right upper quadrant just below the diaphragm, between the liver and abdominal wall. One exception to this placement of intraperitoneal air occurs in women with wide hips, whose highest level within the peritoneal cavity is just over the iliac bone (see Figure 3-66). Failure to include the right hemidiaphragm and iliac wing on the image will compromise an intraperitoneal air diagnosis (see Image 67).
- *IR size and direction.* A 14- × 17-inch (35- × 43-cm) IR positioned lengthwise with respect to the patient should be adequate to include all the anatomic structures in asthenic and sthenic patients, as long as the transverse abdominal measurement is less than 14 inches (35 cm). To place the ninth thoracic vertebra at the top of the image and to center the third thoracic vertebra within the center of the collimated field, place the top of the IR at a level 2.5 inches (6.25 cm) superior to the xiphoid (see Image 39). Use a 40- to 48-inch (102- to 120-cm) SID, and center a horizontal central ray with the midsagittal

plane. Open the longitudinally and transversely collimated fields to the full 14- × 17-inch (35- × 43-cm) size. If the right lateral soft tissue does not appear to be included with this positioning, use two crosswise IRs instead of one lengthwise IR.

Use two 14- × 17-inch (35- × -43-cm) IRs positioned crosswise with respect to the patient to include all the necessary anatomic structures in the hypersthenic patient and in sthenic and asthenic patients who have transverse abdominal measurements of 14 inches (35 cm) or greater. Take the first image with the top of the IR placed at a level 2.5 inches (6.25 cm) superior to the xiphoid. Position the top of the second IR such that it includes approximately 2 to 3 inches (5 to 7.5 cm) of the same transverse section of the peritoneal cavity imaged on the first image to ensure that no middle peritoneal information has been excluded. For both images, center a horizontal central ray with the midsagittal plane.

- *Gonadal shielding.* Use gonadal shielding on all male abdominal images and on female patients if two IRs are required and the upper abdomen is being imaged. Do not shield a female patient if the lower abdomen is imaged because the shield may obscure needed information.

AP (Lateral Decubitus) Abdomen Projection Analysis

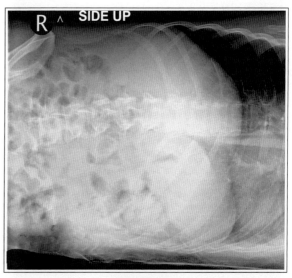

IMAGE 66

Analysis. The right iliac wing is narrower than the left iliac wing, and the distance from the right pedicles to the spinous processes is less than the distance from the left pedicles to the spinous processes. The patient's right side was positioned farther from the IR than the left side.

Correction. Rotate the patient's right side toward the IR until the shoulders and the ASISs are positioned at equal distances from the IR.

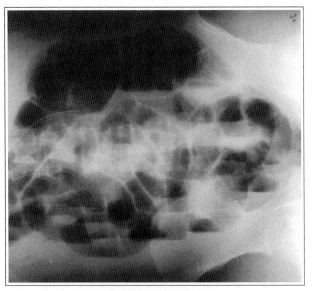

IMAGE 67

Analysis. The right hemidiaphragm is not included in the image. The IR and central ray were positioned too inferiorly.

Correction. Move the IR and central ray superiorly. Place the top of the IR at a level 2.5 inches (6.25 cm) superior to the xiphoid, and center the central ray with the midsagittal plane and IR center.

NEONATE AND INFANT ABDOMEN: ANTEROPOSTERIOR PROJECTION (SUPINE)

See Figure 3-67 and Box 3-14.

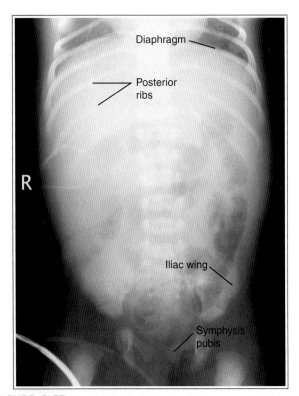

FIGURE 3-67 Neonatal AP abdomen projection with accurate positioning.

The abdomen demonstrates an AP projection. The right and left inferior posterior ribs and the iliac wings are symmetrical.

BOX 3-14	Anteroposterior Abdomen Projection Analysis Criteria

- The right and left inferior posterior ribs and the iliac wings are symmetrical.
- The diaphragm domes are superior to the eighth posterior rib.
- The long axis of the lumbar vertebral column is aligned with the long axis of the collimated field.
- The fourth lumbar vertebra is at the center of the exposure field.
- The diaphragm, abdominal structures, and symphysis pubis are included in the collimation field.

- An AP abdomen projection is obtained by placing the neonate or infant in a supine position with the IR centered beneath the abdomen. To avoid rotation, align the shoulders and the posterior pelvic wings at equal distances from the IR (Figure 3-68).
- *Detecting abdominal rotation.* The upper and lower lumbar vertebrae can demonstrate rotation independently or simultaneously, depending on which section of the body is rotated. If the patient's thorax is rotated but the pelvis remains in an AP projection, the upper lumbar vertebrae and abdominal cavity demonstrate rotation. If the patient's pelvis is rotated but the thorax remains in an AP projection, the lower vertebrae and abdominal cavity demonstrate rotation. If the patient's thorax and pelvis are rotated simultaneously, the entire lumbar column and abdominal cavity demonstrate rotation.

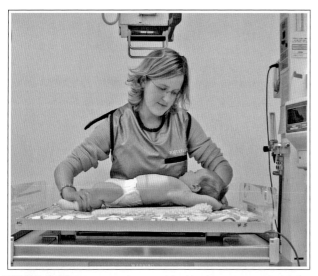

FIGURE 3-68 Proper patient positioning for neonate and infant AP abdomen projection.

Rotation is effectively detected on an AP abdominal projection by comparing the symmetry of the inferior posterior ribs and the iliac wings (see Image 68). The ribs that demonstrate the longer length and the iliac wing demonstrating the greater width are on the side toward which the patient is rotated.

The image was taken on expiration. The diaphragm domes are superior to the eighth posterior rib.

- From full inspiration to expiration, the diaphragm moves from an inferior to a superior position. This movement also changes the pressure placed on the abdominal structures. On full expiration the diaphragm dome is above the eighth posterior rib. When the AP abdomen projection is taken on expiration, less pressure is exerted on the peritoneal contents and the space in the peritoneal cavity is greater. If the AP projection is taken on inspiration, the inferior placement of the diaphragm puts pressure on the abdominal organs, resulting in less space in the peritoneal cavity and greater abdominal density (see Image 68).
- For neonates or infants being ventilated with a conventional ventilator, observe the ventilator's pressure manometer. The exposure should be taken when the manometer digital bar or analog needle moves to its highest position. If a high-frequency ventilator is being used, the exposure may be made at any time, because this ventilator maintains the lung expansion at a steady mean pressure without the bulk gas exchange of the conventional type.

The long axis of the lumbar vertebral column is aligned with the long axis of the collimated field.

- Aligning the long axis of the lumbar vertebral column with the long axis of the collimated field allows for tight transverse collimation (see Image 69).

The fourth lumbar vertebra is at the center of the exposure field. The diaphragm, abdominal structures, and symphysis pubis are included within the collimated field.

- *IR size and centering.* With the neonate or infant positioned in supine AP projection, center an 8- × 10-inch (18- ×24-cm), lengthwise IR beneath the neonate or infant. Center a perpendicular central ray to the midsagittal plane at a transverse level approximately 2 inches (5 cm) superior to the iliac crest. A larger IR and slightly inferior centering may be needed for larger infants. This IR and central ray placement centers the abdomen on the image, permitting tight collimation on all sides of the lungs. Open the longitudinal collimation to include the diaphragm (1 inch [2.5 cm] inferior to mammary line) and symphysis pubis, and transversely collimate to within 0.5 inch (1.25 cm) of the lateral skin line (see Image 70).
- *Gonadal shielding.* Use gonadal shielding on all male abdominal images. Do not shield a female patient, because the shield may obscure needed information.

Neonate and Infant: Anteroposterior Abdomen Projection Analysis

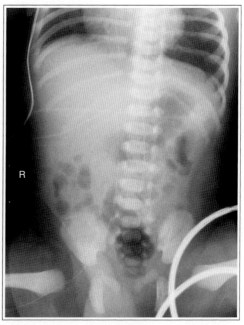

IMAGE 68

Analysis. The posterior ribs are longer on the right side than on the left, and the right iliac wing is wider than the left side posterior ribs. The diaphragm is at the level of the eighth posterior rib. The patient was rotated toward the right side, and the exposure was taken on inspiration.

Correction. Rotate the patient toward the left side until the shoulders and iliac wings are at equal distances to the IR, and expose the image after the patient exhales or the manometer is at its lowest level for conventional ventilators.

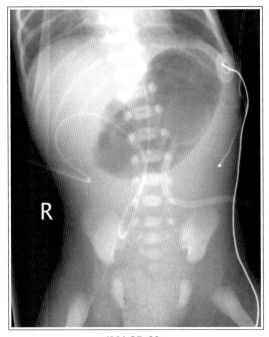

IMAGE 69

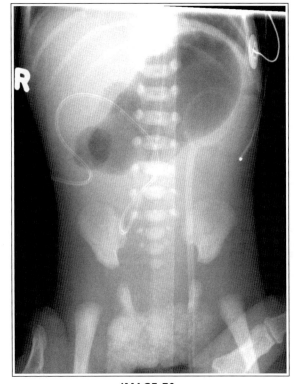

IMAGE 70

Analysis. The patient's upper vertebral column is tilted toward the right side. Tight collimation practices could not be followed.

Correction. Tilt the upper vertebral column toward the left side until the vertebral column is straight and aligned with the collimator's longitudinal light line. Increase transverse collimation to within 0.5 inch (1.25 cm) from skin line.

Analysis. The diaphragm is not included on the image, and anatomic artifacts (positioning attendant's fingers) are demonstrated on the image.

Correction. Move the central ray and IR 1 inch (2.5 cm) superiorly, and move the attendant's hands inferiorly outside of the collimated field.

CHILD ABDOMEN: AP PROJECTION

See Figures 3-69 to 3-72.

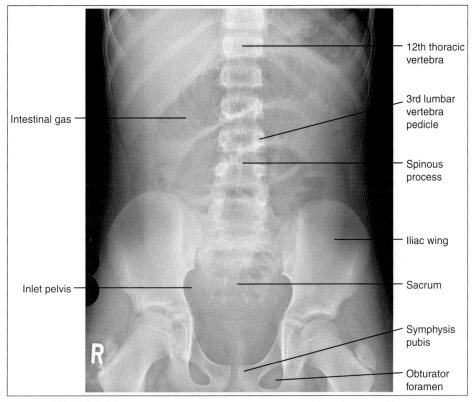

Labels: 12th thoracic vertebra · 3rd lumbar vertebra pedicle · Spinous process · Iliac wing · Sacrum · Symphysis pubis · Obturator foramen · Intestinal gas · Inlet pelvis · R

FIGURE 3-69 Child supine AP abdomen projection with accurate positioning.

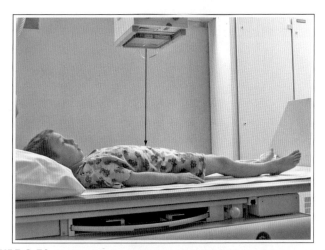

FIGURE 3-70 Proper positioning for a child supine AP abdomen projection.

The analysis of child AP abdomen projections is the same as that of infant or adult AP abdomen projections (see earlier). The size of the child determines which criterion best meets the situation. For a discussion on topics needed to analyze Images 71 and 72 that follow, refer to the adult or infant abdominal discussion earlier in this chapter.

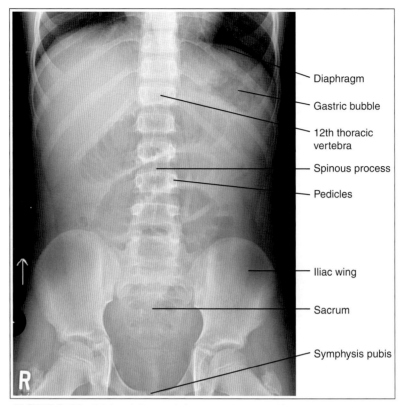

Diaphragm

Gastric bubble

12th thoracic vertebra

Spinous process

Pedicles

Iliac wing

Sacrum

Symphysis pubis

FIGURE 3-71 Child upright AP abdomen projection with accurate positioning.

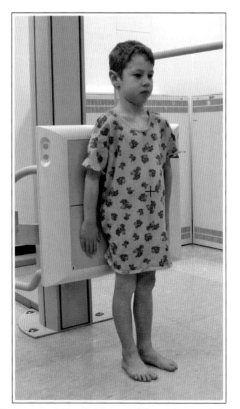

FIGURE 3-72 Proper positioning for a child upright AP abdomen projection.

Child Anteroposterior Abdomen Projection Analysis

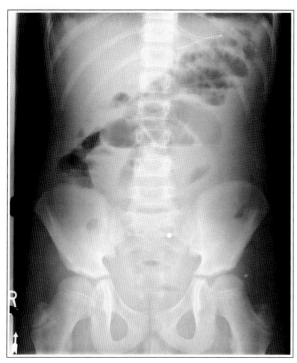

IMAGE 71 Upright abdomen.

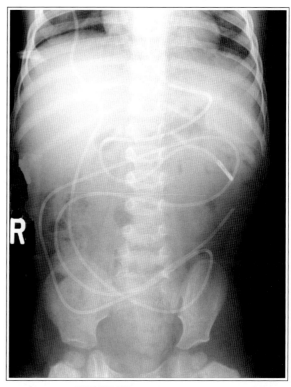

IMAGE 72 Supine abdomen.

Analysis. The diaphragm is not included on this image. The central ray and IR are positioned too inferiorly.

Correction. The central ray and IR should be moved 2 inches (5 cm) superiorly.

Analysis. The right posterior ribs are longer than the left, and the right iliac wing is wider than the left, indicating that the patient was rotated toward the right side.

Correction. Rotate the patient toward the left side until the shoulders and ASISs are at equal distances from the imaging table.

NEONATE AND INFANT ABDOMEN: ANTEROPOSTERIOR PROJECTION (LEFT LATERAL DECUBITUS POSITION)

See Figure 3-73 and Box 3-15.

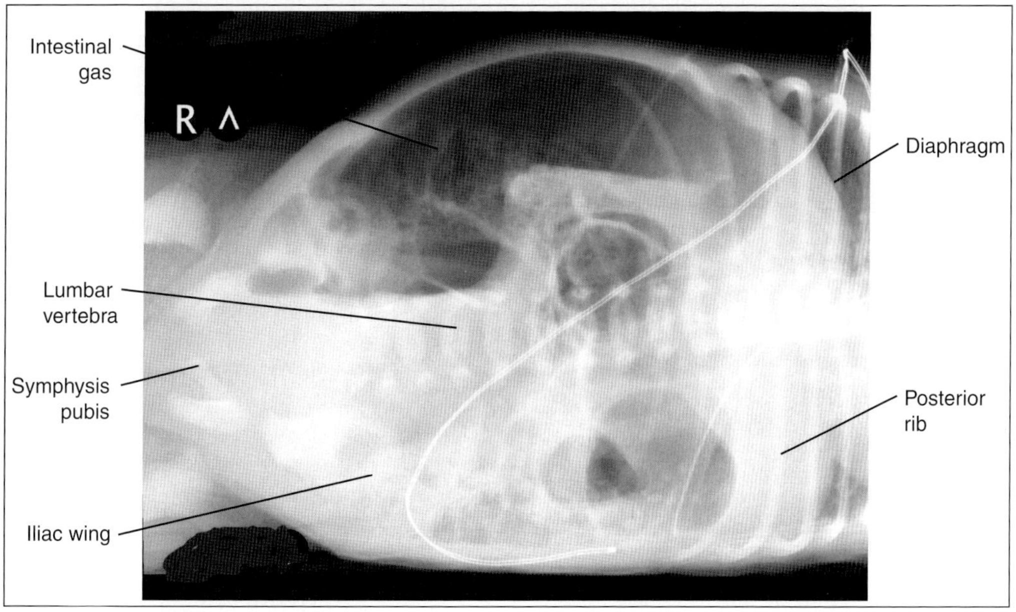

Intestinal gas

Diaphragm

Lumbar vertebra

Symphysis pubis

Posterior rib

Iliac wing

FIGURE 3-73 Neonatal AP (lateral decubitus) abdomen projection with accurate positioning.

BOX 3-15	Neonate and Infant Anteroposterior (Lateral Decubitus) Abdomen Projection Analysis Criteria

- An arrow or "word" marker, indicating that the right side of the patient was positioned up and away from the imaging table or cart, is present.
- The right and left corresponding posterior ribs and the iliac wings are symmetrical.
- The diaphragm domes are superior to the eighth posterior rib.
- The fourth lumbar vertebra is at the center of the exposure field.
- The diaphragm and abdominal structures are included within the collimation field.

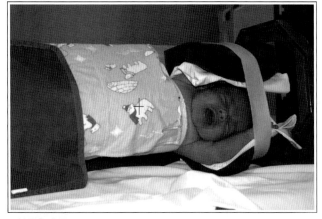

FIGURE 3-74 Proper patient positioning for neonate and infant AP (lateral decubitus) abdomen projection.

An arrow or "word" marker, indicating that the right side of the patient was positioned up and away from the bed or cart, is present on the image.

- Place an arrow or "word" marker indicating which side of the patient was positioned away from the tabletop or cart and in the collimated field.
- An AP (lateral decubitus) abdomen projection is obtained by placing the neonate or infant in a left lateral recumbent position on the bed or cart, with the posterior surface resting against a vertical IR. Because intraperitoneal air migrates to the highest position, which is typically the elevated diaphragm, the left lateral position is chosen to position the gastric bubble away from the elevated diaphragm. To avoid rotation, align the shoulders, the posterior ribs, and the posterior pelvic wings perpendicular to the bed or cart (Figure 3-74).
- *Demonstrating intraperitoneal air.* The left lateral decubitus position is primarily used to confirm the presence of intraperitoneal air. To demonstrate intraperitoneal air best, the patient should remain in this position for a few minutes to allow enough time for the air to move away from the soft tissue abdominal structures and rise to the level of the right diaphragm.
- *Detecting abdominal rotation.* The upper and lower lumbar vertebrae can demonstrate rotation independently or simultaneously, depending on which section of the body is rotated. If the patient's thorax is rotated but the pelvis remains in an AP projection, the upper lumbar vertebrae and abdominal cavity demonstrate rotation. If the patient's pelvis is rotated but the thorax remains in an AP projection, the lower vertebrae and abdominal cavity demonstrate rotation. If the patient's thorax and pelvis are rotated simultaneously, the entire lumbar column and abdominal cavity demonstrate rotation.

  Rotation is effectively detected on an AP (lateral decubitus) abdomen projection by comparing the symmetry of the posterior ribs and the iliac wings (see Image 73). The ribs that demonstrate the longer length and the iliac wing demonstrating the greater width are present on the side toward which the patient is rotated.

The image was taken on expiration. The diaphragm domes are superior to the eighth posterior rib.

- For neonates or infants being ventilated with a conventional ventilator, observe the ventilator's pressure manometer. The exposure should be taken when the manometer digital bar or analog needle moves to its highest position. If a high-frequency ventilator is being used, the exposure may be made at any time, because this ventilator maintains the lung expansion at a steady mean pressure without the bulk gas exchange of the conventional type.

  If the AP (lateral decubitus) projection is taken on inspiration, the inferior placement of the diaphragm puts pressure on the abdominal organs, resulting in less space in the peritoneal cavity and greater abdominal density.

The fourth lumbar vertebra is at the center of the exposure field. The diaphragm and abdominal structures are included within the collimated field.

- The AP (lateral decubitus) abdomen projection is most often used to evaluate the peritoneal cavity for intraperitoneal air. With the left lateral decubitus position, intraperitoneal air will rise to the highest level of the right hemidiaphragm, so it must be included (see Image 74).
- *IR size and centering.* With the neonate or infant positioned in a left lateral decubitus position, place an 8- × 10-inch (18- × 24-cm), lengthwise IR against the neonate or infant's posterior surface and position the abdomen in the middle of the IR. Center a horizontal central ray to the midsagittal plane at a transverse level 2 inches (5 cm) superior to the iliac crest. A larger IR and slightly inferior centering may be needed for larger infants. This IR and central ray placement centers the abdomen on the image, permitting tight collimation on all sides of

the lungs. Open the longitudinal collimation to include the diaphragm (1 inch [2.5 cm]) inferior to the mammary line, and transversely collimate to within 0.5 inch (1.25 cm) of the lateral skin line.

- *Gonadal shielding.* Use gonadal shielding on all male abdominal images. Do not shield a female patient because the shield may obscure needed information.

Analysis. The diaphragm is at the level of the eighth thoracic vertebra. The left posterior ribs are longer than the right, and the left iliac wing is wider than the right. The exposure was made after inspiration, and the patient was rotated toward the left side.

Correction. Take the exposure after the patient exhales or the manometer is at its lowest level, and rotate the patient toward the right side until the posterior ribs and the iliac wings are aligned perpendicular to the bed.

Neonate and Infant AP (Lateral Decubitus) Abdomen Projection Analysis

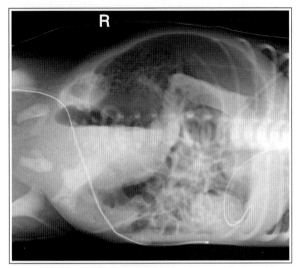

IMAGE 74

Analysis. The diaphragm is not included in its entirety. The central ray is positioned too inferiorly.

Correction. Move the central ray superiorly by 0.5 inch (1.25 cm).

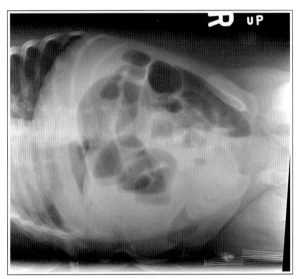

IMAGE 73

CHILD ABDOMEN: ANTEROPOSTERIOR PROJECTION (LEFT LATERAL DECUBITUS POSITION)

See Figures 3-75 and 3-76.

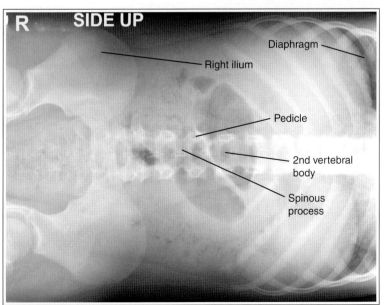

FIGURE 3-75 Child AP (lateral decubitus) abdomen projection with accurate positioning.

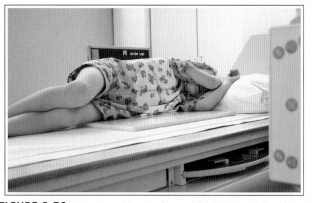

FIGURE 3-76 Proper positioning for a child AP (lateral decubitus) abdomen projection.

The analysis of the child AP (lateral decubitus) abdomen projection is the same as that of the infant or adult AP (lateral decubitus) abdomen projection (see earlier). The size of the child determines which criterion best meets the situation. For a discussion on topics needed to analyze Image 75, refer to the earlier discussion of adult or infant AP (lateral decubitus) abdomen projections.

Child AP (Lateral Decubitus) Abdomen Projection Analysis

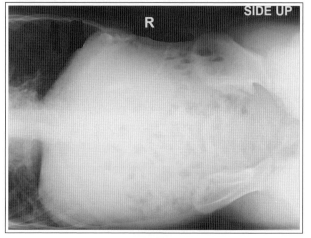

IMAGE 75

Analysis. The diaphragm is inferior to the 10th posterior rib, indicating that the examination was taken on inspiration.

Correction. Expose the image after the patient has exhaled.

BIBLIOGRAPHY

Carroll QB: *Practical radiographic imaging*, ed 8, Springfield, Ill, 2007, Charles C Thomas.

Hobbs DL: Chest radiography for radiologic technologists, *Radiol Technol* 78:494–516, 2007.

Jeffrey B, Ralls P, Leung A, Brant-Zawadzke M: *Emergency imaging*, Philadelphia, 1999, Lippincott Williams & Wilkins.

Upper Extremity

OBJECTIVES

- Identify the required anatomy on upper extremity projections.
- Describe how to properly position the patient, image receptor (IR), and central ray on upper extremity projections.
- List the image analysis requirements for upper extremity projections with accurate positioning.
- State how to reposition the patient properly when upper extremity projections with poor positioning are produced.
- State the kilovoltage that is routinely used for upper extremity projections, and describe which anatomic structures will be visible when the correct technique factors are used.
- Explain how a joint space is aligned with the central ray and IR to be demonstrated as an open space on an image.
- List the soft tissue structures that are of interest and should be demonstrated on upper extremity projections. State where they are located and describe why their visualization is important.
- Explain how wrist and elbow rotations affect the placement of the radial and ulnar styloids, and radial turberosity on upper extremity projections.

- Describe the slant of the distal radial articulating surface.
- Discuss how a patient with large, muscular, or thick proximal forearms should be positioned for good posteroanterior (PA) and lateral wrist projections to be obtained.
- State the carpal bone changes that occur when the wrist is extended, flexed, or ulnar- and radial-deviated in hand and wrist projections.
- Discuss how the degree of central ray angulation needs to be adjusted for the PA ulnar-deviated scaphoid position if a proximal or distal scaphoid fracture is in question.
- Describe what effect the anode heel effect has on forearm and humeral projections and discuss how to position the arm to take advantage of the anode heel effect.
- Explain how to position the patient to ensure that appropriate joints are included on forearm and humerus projections.
- State why the patient's humerus is never rotated if a humeral fracture is suspected.
- Explain when a grid is needed for humeral images and how the technique factors are adjusted when a grid is added.

KEY TERMS

articulate	concave	dorsiflex
bony trabeculae	convex	extension
carpal canal	distal	external rotation

fat pads	medial	radial deviation
flexion	palmar	scaphoid fat stripe
internal rotation	pronation	ulnar deviation
joint effusion	pronator fat stripe	
lateral	proximal	

The following image analysis criteria are used for all upper extremity images and should be considered when completing the analysis for each upper extremity projection presented in this chapter (Box 4-1).

BOX 4-1	**Upper Extremity Imaging Analysis Criteria**

- The facility's identification requirements are visible.
- A right or left marker identifying the correct side of the patient is present on the image and is not superimposed over the anatomy of interest.
- Good radiation protection practices are evident.
- Bony trabecular patterns and cortical outlines of the anatomic structures are sharply defined.
- Contrast and density are adequate to demonstrate the surrounding soft tissue and bony structures.
- Penetration is sufficient to visualize the bony trabecular patterns and cortical outlines of the upper extremity.
- No evidence of removable artifacts is present.

FINGER: POSTEROANTERIOR PROJECTION

See Figure 4-1 and Box 4-2.

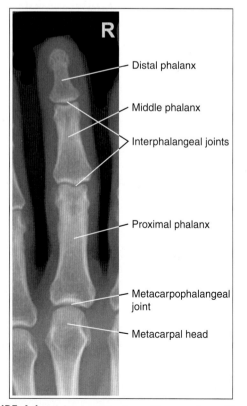

FIGURE 4-1 PA finger projection with accurate positioning.

An optimal kilovoltage peak (kVp) technique (Table 4-1) sufficiently penetrates the bony and soft tissue structures of the upper extremity and provides a contrast scale necessary to visualize the bony details. To obtain optimal density, set a manual milliampere-seconds (mAs) level based on the part thickness.

TABLE 4-1	**Upper Extremity Technical Data**	
Projection	**kVp**	**SID**
Finger	50–60	40–48 inches (100–120 cm)
Thumb	50–60	40–48 inches (100–120 cm)
PA hand	50–60	40–48 inches (100–120 cm)
PA oblique, hand	50–60	40–48 inches (100–120 cm)
Lateral hand	50–60	40–48 inches (100–120 cm)
Wrist	50–60	40–48 inches (100–120 cm)
Forearm	50–60	40–48 inches (100–120 cm)
Elbow	50–60	40–48 inches (100–120 cm)
Humerus	50–60	40–48 inches (100–120 cm)

SID, Source–image receptor distance.

BOX 4-2	**Posteroanterior Finger Projection Analysis Criteria**

- The long axis of the finger is aligned with the long axis of collimated field.
- The soft tissue width and midpoint concavity are equal on both sides of phalanges.
- There is no soft tissue overlap from adjacent digits.
- The IP and MP joints are demonstrated as open spaces, and the phalanges are not foreshortened.
- The PIP joint is at the center of the exposure field.
- The entire digit and half of the metacarpal are included within the collimated field.

IP, Interphalangeal; *MP,* metacarpophalangeal; *PIP,* proximal interphalangeal.

The finger demonstrates a PA projection. The soft tissue width and midpoint concavity are the same on both sides of the phalanges.

- Finger rotation is controlled by the amount of palm pronation. A PA projection is accomplished when the palm is positioned flat against the IR (Figure 4-2).
- *Detecting finger rotation.* Because the thumb prevents the hand from rotating laterally, medial rotation is the most common rotation error. Take a few minutes to study a finger skeleton, and note how

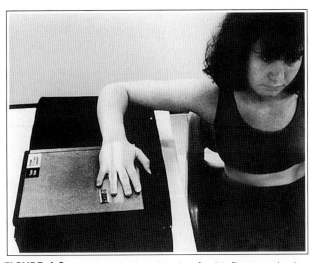

FIGURE 4-2 Proper patient positioning for PA finger projection.

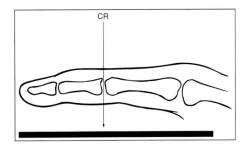

FIGURE 4-3 Accurate alignment of joint space and central ray (*CR*).

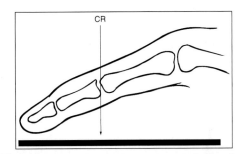

FIGURE 4-4 Poor alignment of joint space and central ray (*CR*).

the midpoints of the phalanges have equal side concavity when it is placed in a PA projection. Also, note that the anterior surface is concave, whereas the posterior surface is slightly convex. As the skeleton is rotated internally or externally, the amount of concavity increases on the side toward which the anterior surface is rotated, whereas the side toward which the posterior surface rotates demonstrates less concavity. The same observations can be made about the soft tissue that surrounds the phalanges. More soft tissue thickness is present on the anterior (palmar) hand surface than on the posterior surface, so the side demonstrating the greatest soft tissue width on an image is the side toward which the anterior surface was rotated. Look for this midpoint concavity and soft tissue width variation to indicate rotation on a PA finger projection (see Image 1). Note on a hand skeleton that the second metacarpal is the longest of the finger digits and that the length decreases with each adjacent metacarpal. This information can be used to determine whether the patient's finger was internally or externally rotated for a mispositioned PA finger image. If the finger was externally rotated, the aspect of the phalanges demonstrating the greater midpoint concavity faces the thumb or longer metacarpal (see Image 1). If the finger was internally rotated, the aspect of the phalanges demonstrating the greater midpoint concavity faces the shorter metacarpal.

No soft tissue overlap from adjacent digits is present.

- Spreading the fingers slightly prevents soft tissue overlapping from adjacent fingers. It is difficult to evaluate the soft tissue of an affected finger when superimposition of other soft tissue is present.

The interphalangeal (IP) and metacarpophalangeal (MP) joints are demonstrated as open spaces, and the phalanges are not foreshortened.

- Open IP and MP joint spaces and unforeshortened phalanges are demonstrated when the finger is fully extended and the central ray is perpendicular and centered to the proximal IP (PIP) joint. This finger positioning and central ray placement align the joint spaces parallel with the central ray and perpendicular to the IR, as shown in Figure 4-3, resulting in open joint spaces. It also prevents foreshortening of the phalanges, because their long axes are aligned parallel with the IR and perpendicular to the central ray. The alignment of the central ray and IR with the joint spaces and phalanges changes when the finger is flexed. In Figure 4-4, note how finger flexion causes the phalanges to foreshorten and be superimposed on the joint spaces (see Image 2).

- *Positioning the unextendable finger.* If the patient is unable to extend the finger, it may be necessary to use an anteroposterior (AP) projection to demonstrate open IP and MP joint spaces and to visualize the phalanges of greatest interest without foreshortening. In this case, carefully evaluate the requisition to determine the phalanx and joint space of interest. Then, supinate the patient's hand into an AP projection, elevating the proximal metacarpals until the phalanx of interest is parallel with the IR and the joint space of interest is perpendicular to the IR (Figure 4-5). Figures 4-6 and 4-7 demonstrate how patient positioning with respect to the central ray determines the anatomy

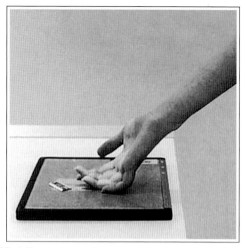

FIGURE 4-5 Patient positioning for AP flexed finger projection.

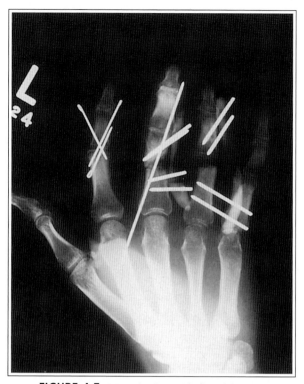

FIGURE 4-7 AP projection with flexed fingers.

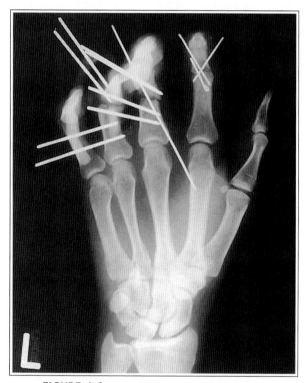

FIGURE 4-6 PA projection with flexed fingers.

The PIP joint is at the center of the exposure field. The distal, middle, and proximal phalanges and half of the metacarpal are included within the collimated field.

- Direct a perpendicular central ray to the PIP joint to place the joint in the center of the image. Open the longitudinal collimation to include the distal phalanx and the distal half of the metacarpal. Transverse collimation should be within 0.5 inch (1.25 cm) of the finger skin line.
- One third of an 8- × 10-inch (18- × 24-cm) detailed screen-film or computed radiography IR placed crosswise should be adequate to include all the required anatomic structures. Digital imaging requires tight collimation, lead masking, and no overlap of individual exposures to produce optimal images.
- Some facilities request that an unaffected adjacent digit be included on the image for comparison purposes. For a finger being imaged for the first time, some facilities want the entire metacarpal to be visualized on the image.

that is visible. For Figure 4-6, the patient was imaged in a PA projection with fingers flexed. For Figure 4-7, the same patient was imaged in an AP projection with the proximal metacarpals elevated to place the affected proximal phalanges parallel with the IR. Note the difference in demonstration of the joint spaces and proximal phalanx fractures.

Posteroanterior Finger Projection Analysis

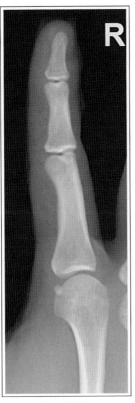

IMAGE 1

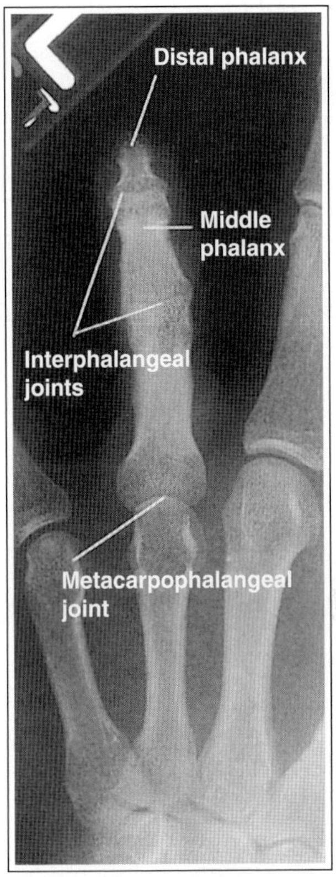

IMAGE 2

Analysis. The soft tissue width and the concavity of the phalangeal midshafts on either side of the phalanx are not equal; the finger was rotated for the image. Because the side of the phalanges with the greater concavity and soft tissue width is facing the thumb, the finger was rotated externally for the image.

Correction. Place the finger in a PA projection by rotating the finger slightly internally. The hand should be flat against the IR.

Analysis. The IP and MP joints are closed, and the distal and middle phalanges are foreshortened; the patient's finger was flexed.

Correction. Extend the patient's finger, and place the palm flat against the IR. If the patient is unable to extend the finger, image it in an AP projection, elevating the proximal metacarpals until the affected phalanx is parallel with the IR or the affected joint space is perpendicular to the IR (see Figure 4-5).

FINGER: POSTEROANTERIOR OBLIQUE PROJECTION

See Figure 4-8 and Box 4-3.

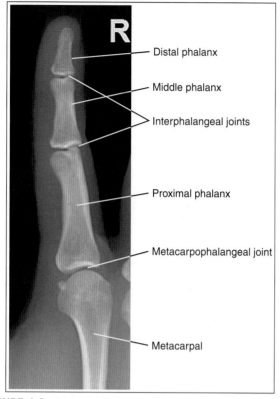

FIGURE 4-8 PA oblique finger projection with accurate positioning.

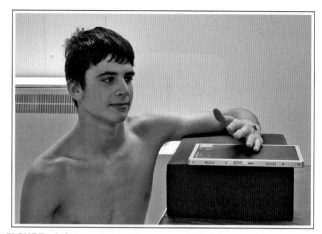

FIGURE 4-9 Proper patient positioning for PA oblique finger projection.

BOX 4-3	Oblique Finger Projection Analysis Criteria

- The long axis of the finger is aligned with the long axis of collimated field.
- Twice as much soft tissue width is demonstrated on one side of the digit as on the other side, and more concavity is seen on one aspect of the phalangeal midshafts than the others.
- There is no soft tissue overlap from adjacent digits.
- The IP and MP joints are demonstrated as open spaces, and the phalanges are not foreshortened.
- The PIP joint is at the center of the exposure field.
- The entire digit and half of the metacarpal are included within the collimated field.

IP, Interphalangeal; *MP,* metacarpophalangeal; *PIP,* proximal interphalangeal.

The digit has been placed in a 45-degree PA oblique projection. Twice as much soft tissue width is demonstrated on one side of the digit as on the other side, and more concavity is demonstrated on one aspect of the phalangeal midshafts than on the other.

- A PA oblique finger is accomplished by rotating the affected finger 45 degrees from the PA projection (Figure 4-9). It is most common and comfortable for a patient to rotate the finger and hand externally to obtain a PA oblique finger projection, although internal rotation may be used when the

second digit is imaged, to prevent a long object–image receptor distance (OID).

- *Assessing accuracy of PA oblique projection.* Study the amount of phalangeal midshaft concavity and soft tissue width demonstrated on PA oblique finger projections to verify the accuracy of rotation and to determine the proper repositioning movement needed when an oblique digit image shows too much or too little obliquity. A 45-degree oblique finger image demonstrates more phalangeal midshaft concavity and soft tissue width on the side positioned away from the IR. Use the soft tissue width to assess the degree of digital obliquity. If twice as much soft tissue width is present on one side of the digit as on the other, a 45-degree PA oblique projection has been obtained. If the phalangeal midshaft concavity and soft tissue width on both sides of the finger are more nearly equal, the finger was not rotated enough for the projection (see Image 3). If the soft tissue width on one side of the digit is more than twice as much as that on the other, and when one aspect of the phalangeal midshaft is concave but the other aspect is convex, the angle of obliquity was more than 45 degrees (see Image 4).

No soft tissue overlap from adjacent digits is present.

- Slightly spread the patient's fingers to prevent overlapping of the adjacent finger's soft tissue onto that of affected finger. Superimposition of these soft tissues makes it difficult to evaluate the soft tissue of the affected finger (see Image 5).

The IP and MP joints are visualized as open spaces, and the phalanges are not foreshortened.

- The IP and MP joint spaces are open and the phalanges are not foreshortened if the finger is fully extended and positioned parallel with the IR and perpendicular to the central ray. When the hand and fingers are positioned obliquely, some of the fingers are no longer placed against the IR but are positioned at varying OIDs. In this position the distal phalanges naturally tilt toward the IR. To keep the affected finger parallel with the IR and to maintain open joint spaces, it may be necessary to place an immobilization device beneath the distal phalanx. This is especially true when the second and third digits are imaged because they are at the greatest OID. It is also necessary to center a perpendicular central ray to the PIP joint to maintain open joint spaces. Failure to position the affected finger parallel with the IR and perpendicular to the central ray foreshortens the phalanges and closes the joint spaces (see Image 6).

The PIP joint is at the center of the exposure field. The distal, middle, and proximal phalanges and half of the metacarpal of the affected digit are included within the collimated field.

- Direct a perpendicular central ray to the PIP joint to place it in the center of the image. Open the longitudinal collimation to include the distal phalanx and the distal half of the metacarpal. Transversely collimate to within 0.5 inch (1.25 cm) of the finger skin line.
- One third of an 8- × 10-inch (18- × 24-cm) detailed screen-film or computed radiography IR placed crosswise should be adequate to include all the required anatomic structures.
- Some facilities require an unaffected adjacent digit to be included on the image for comparison purposes. Also, for a finger being imaged for the first time, some facilities want the entire metacarpal to be visualized on the image.

PA Oblique Finger Projection Analysis

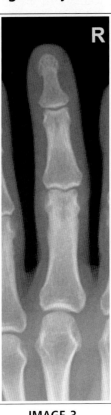

IMAGE 3

Analysis. On both sides of the phalanx the soft tissue width and midshaft concavity are almost equal; the patient's finger was positioned at less than 45 degrees of obliquity for the image.

Correction. Increase the finger obliquity to 45 degrees. Keep the finger parallel with the IR.

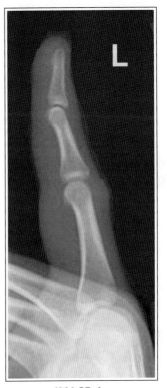

IMAGE 4

Analysis. More than twice as much soft tissue width is present on one side of the phalanges as on the other. One aspect of the midshafts of the phalanges is concave, and the other aspect is slightly convex. Obliquity was more than 45 degrees for this image.

Correction. Decrease the finger obliquity to 45 degrees.

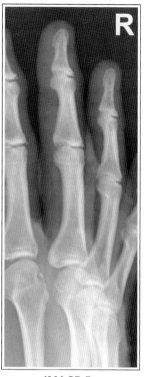

IMAGE 5

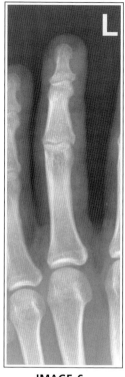

IMAGE 6

Analysis. Soft tissue from an adjacent finger is superimposed over the affected finger's soft tissue; the fingers were not spread apart.

Correction. Spread the fingers until the adjacent fingers are positioned away from the affected finger.

Analysis. The IP joint spaces are closed, and the distal and middle phalanges are foreshortened; the finger was not positioned parallel with the IR.

Correction. Position the finger parallel with the IR. It may be necessary to position an immobilization device beneath the distal phalanx to maintain accurate finger positioning. If the distal phalanx is of interest and the patient is unable to extend the finger, image it in an AP oblique projection, elevating the proximal metacarpals until the affected phalanx is aligned parallel with the IR and rotated 45 degrees.

FINGER: LATERAL PROJECTION

See Figure 4-10 and Box 4-4.

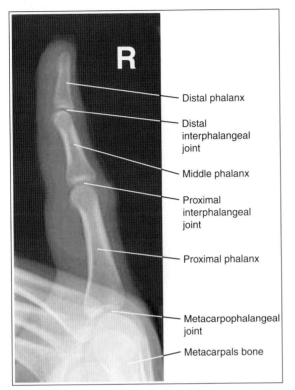

Distal phalanx

Distal interphalangeal joint

Middle phalanx

Proximal interphalangeal joint

Proximal phalanx

Metacarpophalangeal joint

Metacarpals bone

FIGURE 4-10 Lateral finger projection with accurate positioning.

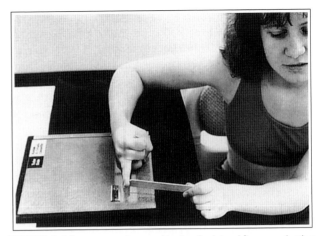

FIGURE 4-11 Proper patient positioning for lateral finger projection.

BOX 4-4	Lateral Finger Projection Analysis Criteria

- The long axis of the finger is aligned with the long axis of the collimated field.
- The anterior aspect of the middle and proximal phalanges demonstrate midshaft concavity, and the posterior aspects of the phalanges show slight convexity.
- There is no soft tissue overlap from adjacent digits.
- The IP joints are demonstrated as open spaces, and the phalanges are not foreshortened.
- The PIP joint is at the center of the exposure field.
- The entire digit and metacarpal head are included within the collimated field.

IP, Interphalangeal; *PIP,* proximal interphalangeal.

The digit of interest is in a lateral projection. The anterior aspect of the middle and proximal phalanges demonstrates midshaft concavity, and the posterior aspects of the phalanges show slight convexity.

- A lateral finger projection is accomplished by rotating the affected finger 90 degrees from the PA projection (Figure 4-11). Whether the hand is rotated internally or externally to obtain this goal depends on which direction will bring the finger closer to the IR. Typically, when the second and third fingers are imaged, the hand is rotated internally and, when the fourth and fifth fingers are imaged, the hand is rotated externally.

- *Distinguishing lateral projection from rotated projection.* To understand the difference between a truly lateral digit projection and a lateral projection that is rotated, study a finger skeleton in lateral and PA and AP oblique projections. Note how the midshaft concavity of the middle and proximal phalanges varies as the digit is rotated. In a lateral projection, the anterior aspect of these phalanges is concave, but the posterior aspect demonstrates slight convexity. In PA and AP oblique projections, both sides of the middle and proximal phalangeal midshafts demonstrate concavity, but the side toward which the anterior surface is rotated demonstrates a greater degree of concavity than the side toward which the posterior surface is rotated. The soft tissue width at either side of the phalanx also changes in the lateral and PA and AP oblique projections. More soft tissue is present on the side of the phalanges toward which the anterior surface is rotated (see Image 7).

No soft tissue overlap from adjacent digits is present.

- Flex the unaffected fingers into a tight fist, allowing the finger of interest to remain extended. To visualize the proximal phalanx, it may be necessary to extend the affected finger with an immobilization device or to tape the unaffected fingers away from the affected finger. If the unaffected fingers are not drawn away from the proximal phalanx of the affected finger, they will be superimposed on the area, preventing adequate visualization (see Image 8). *An immobilization device should not be used to extend the finger if a fracture is suspected and the device causes stress to the fractured area* (see Image 9).

The IP joints are visible as open spaces, and the phalanges are not foreshortened.

- The IP joints are open, and the phalanges are demonstrated without foreshortening as long as the finger was positioned parallel with the IR and the central ray was perpendicular to and centered with the PIP joint.
- When the third and fourth digits are imaged, they are positioned at a greater OID than the second and fifth digits. To keep the third and fourth digits parallel with the IR, it may be necessary to place an immobilization device beneath their distal phalanges. When a finger is not positioned parallel with the IR and perpendicular to the central ray, the IP joint spaces are closed and the phalanges are foreshortened.

The PIP joint is at the center of the exposure field. The distal, middle, and proximal phalanges and the metacarpal head of the affected digit are included within the collimated field.

- Center a perpendicular central ray to the PIP joint to place it in the center of the image. Open the longitudinal collimation to include the distal phalanx and the metacarpal head. Transversely collimate to within 0.5 inch (1.25 cm) of the finger skin line.
- One third of an 8- × 10-inch (18- × 24-cm) detailed screen-film or computed radiography IR placed crosswise should be adequate to include all the required anatomic structures.

LATERAL FINGER PROJECTION ANALYSIS

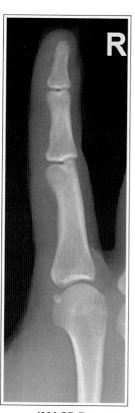

IMAGE 7

Analysis. Concavity is demonstrated on both sides of the middle and proximal phalangeal midshafts, indicating that the finger was not adequately rotated for this image.

Correction. Increase the degree of finger rotation until the finger is in a lateral projection.

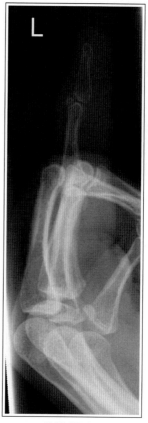

IMAGE 8

Analysis. The unaffected fingers were not flexed enough to prevent soft tissue or bony superimposition of the affected digit's proximal phalanx.

Correction. Tightly flex the unaffected fingers away from the affected finger. Hyperextending the affected finger with an immobilization prop may also help increase demonstration of the proximal phalanx if a fracture of this area is not suspected.

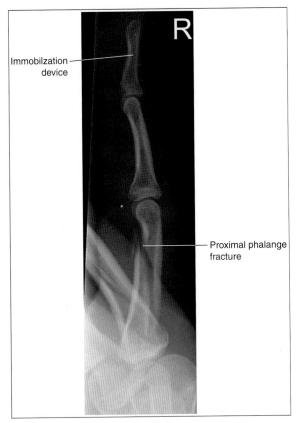

IMAGE 9

Immobilzation device

Proximal phalange fracture

Analysis. The finger demonstrates a fractured proximal phalanx that is being stressed because of the immobilization device that was used to extend the finger.

Correction. The immobilization device used to extend the finger should not be used when a fracture is suspected or evident.

THUMB: ANTEROPOSTERIOR PROJECTION

See Figures 4-12 and 4-13 and Box 4-5.

The first digit demonstrates an AP projection. The concavity on both sides of the phalangeal and metacarpal midshafts is equal, as is soft tissue width on both sides of the phalanges.

- An AP projection is accomplished by internally rotating the patient's hand until the thumb is positioned in an AP projection (Figure 4-14). The thumbnail can be used as a reference to determine when the thumb is truly placed in an AP projection. The nail should be positioned directly against the IR and should not be visible on either side of the thumb. A nonrotated AP thumb projection demonstrates equal concavity on both sides of the phalangeal and metacarpal midshafts, as well as equal soft tissue widths on both sides of the phalanges.

- *Detecting thumb rotation.* When the thumb is rotated away from an AP projection, the amount of midshaft concavity increases on the side of the thumb toward which the anterior surface rotates and decreases on the side toward which the posterior surface rotates. The same observation can be made about the soft tissue surrounding the phalanges when the thumb is rotated. More soft tissue

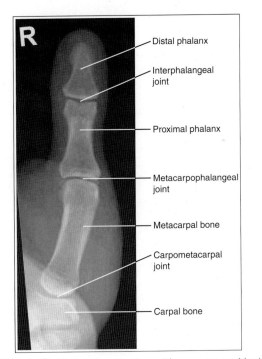

Distal phalanx

Interphalangeal joint

Proximal phalanx

Metacarpophalangeal joint

Metacarpal bone

Carpometacarpal joint

Carpal bone

FIGURE 4-12 AP thumb projection with accurate positioning.

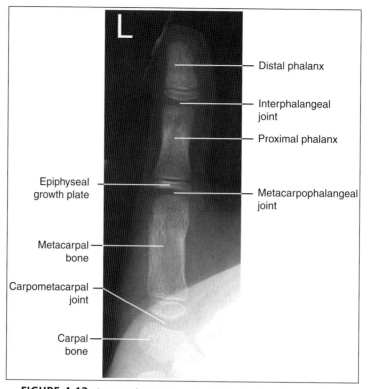

FIGURE 4-13 Accurately positioned pediatric PA thumb projection.

BOX 4-5	**Anteroposterior Thumb Projection Analysis Criteria**

- The concavity on both sides of the phalanges and metacarpal midshafts is equal. There is equal soft tissue width on each side of the phalanges.
- The long axis of the thumb is aligned with the long axis of the collimated field.
- There is no soft tissue overlap from adjacent digits.
- The IP, MP, and CM joints are demonstrated as open spaces and the phalanges are not foreshortened.
- Superimposition of the medial palm soft tissue over the proximal first metacarpal and the CM joint is minimal.
- The MP joint is at the center of the exposure field.
- The entire digit and CM joint are included within the collimated field.

CM, Carpometacarpal; *IP*, interphalangeal; *MP*, metacarpophalangeal.

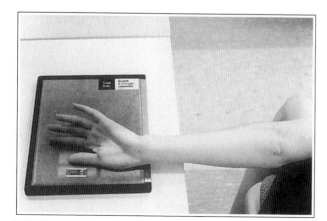

FIGURE 4-14 Proper patient positioning for AP thumb projection.

width is evident on the side toward which the anterior surface is rotated, and less soft tissue width is seen on the side toward which the posterior surface is rotated (see Image 10).

The long axis of the thumb is aligned with the long axis of the collimated field.

- Aligning the long axis of the thumb with the long axis of the collimator's longitudinal light line enables you to collimate tightly without clipping the distal phalanx or proximal metacarpal (see Image 11).

The IP, MP, and carpometacarpal (CM) joints are visible as open joint spaces, and the phalanges are not foreshortened.

- The IP, MP, and CM joint spaces are open, and the phalanges are demonstrated without foreshortening as long as the thumb is positioned flat against and placed parallel with the IR and the central ray was perpendicular to and centered with the MP joint space. This positioning aligns the joint spaces parallel with the central ray and perpendicular to the IR and positions the long axes of the phalanges perpendicular to the central ray and parallel with the IR. These relationships change when the thumb is flexed or posteriorly extended (hitchhiker's thumb) for the image. Thumb flexion and extension foreshorten the phalanges and superimpose them over the joint spaces (see Image 12).

Superimposition of the medial palm soft tissue over the proximal first metacarpal and the CM joint is minimal.

- Minimal soft tissue overlap occurs when the medial palm surface is drawn away from the thumb. It may be necessary to use the patient's other hand as an immobilization device to maintain good positioning of the medial palmar surface. If the medial surface of the palm is not drawn away from the thumb, the soft tissue and possibly the fourth and fifth metacarpals obscure the proximal first metacarpal and CM joint (see Image 13).
- *Evaluating a PA thumb projection.* The principles of AP thumb projection analysis can be used to evaluate a PA thumb projection (Figure 4-15), with the following modifications. First, the medial palm soft tissue does not overlap the proximal first metacarpal and CM joint. Second, on a PA projection, the CM joint is closed.

The MP joint is at the center of the exposure field. The distal and proximal phalanges, the metacarpal, and the CM joint are included within the collimated field.

- Center a perpendicular central ray to the MP joint, which is located where the palm's interconnecting skin attaches to the thumb, to place it in the center of the image. Open the longitudinal collimation to include the distal phalanx and CM joint. Transversely collimate to within 0.5 inch (1.25 cm) of the thumb skin line.
- One third of an 8- × 10-inch (18- × 24-cm) detailed screen-film or computed radiography IR placed crosswise should be adequate to include all the required anatomic structures. Digital imaging requires tight collimation, lead masking, and no overlap of individual exposures to produce optimal images.

Anteroposterior Thumb Projection Analysis

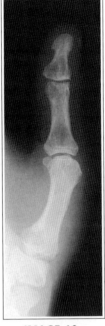

IMAGE 10

Analysis. The soft tissue width and the concavity of the phalangeal and metacarpal midshafts are not the same on both sides. The side next to the fingers demonstrates more concavity. The hand was internally rotated too far, demonstrating the thumb in an AP oblique projection.

Correction. Decrease the internal hand rotation until the thumb is in an AP projection. The thumbnail should be resting against the IR and should not be visible on either side of the thumb.

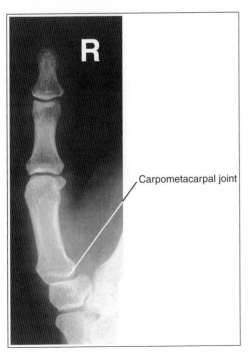

FIGURE 4-15 PA thumb projection with accurate positioning.

Carpometacarpal joint

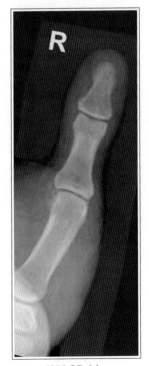

IMAGE 11

Analysis. The long axis of the thumb is not aligned with the long axis of the collimated field. Note that the proximal metacarpal and the CM joint are clipped.

Correction. Align the long axis of the thumb with the long axis of the collimated field.

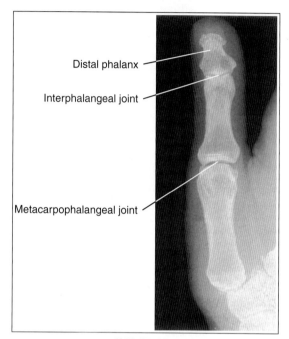

Distal phalanx

Interphalangeal joint

Metacarpophalangeal joint

IMAGE 12

Analysis. The distal phalanx is foreshortened, and the IP joint space is closed. The MP joint was elevated off the IR and the distal thumb was posteriorly extended (hitchhiker's thumb).

Correction. Position the thumb flat against and parallel with the IR.

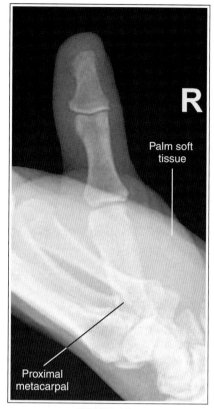

R

Palm soft tissue

Proximal metacarpal

IMAGE 13

Analysis. The fifth metacarpal and the medial palm soft tissue are superimposed over the proximal first metacarpal and CM joint. The medial metacarpal and palmar surface have not been drawn away from the thumb.

Correction. Using the patient's other hand or another immobilization device, draw the medial side of the hand and palmar surface away from the thumb. Make sure that the thumb does not rotate away from an AP projection with this movement and that the patient's opposite hand is not included in the exposure field.

THUMB: LATERAL PROJECTION

See Figures 4-16 and 4-17 and Box 4-6.

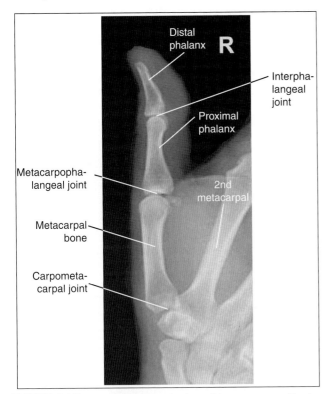

FIGURE 4-16 Lateral thumb projection with accurate positioning.

Distal phalanx R

Interphalangeal joint

Proximal phalanx

Metacarpopha-langeal joint

2nd metacarpal

Metacarpal bone

Carpometa-carpal joint

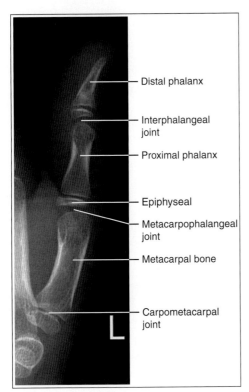

FIGURE 4-17 Accurately positioned pediatric lateral thumb projection.

Distal phalanx

Interphalangeal joint

Proximal phalanx

Epiphyseal

Metacarpophalangeal joint

Metacarpal bone

Carpometacarpal joint

L

The thumb demonstrates a lateral projection. The anterior aspect of the proximal phalanx and metacarpal demonstrates midshaft concavity, and the posterior

BOX 4-6 | **Lateral Thumb Projection Analysis Criteria**

- The anterior aspect of the proximal phalanx and metacarpal demonstrates midshaft concavity, and the posterior aspect of the proximal phalanx and metacarpal demonstrates slight convexity.
- The long axis of the thumb is aligned with the long axis of collimated field.
- There is no soft tissue overlap from adjacent digits.
- The IP, MP, and CM joints are demonstrated as open spaces, and the phalanges are not foreshortened.
- The proximal first metacarpal is only slightly superimposed by the proximal second metacarpal.
- The first MP joint is at the center of the exposure field.
- The entire digit and CM joint are included within the collimated field.

CM, Carpometacarpal; *IP*, interphalangeal; *MP*, metacarpophalangeal.

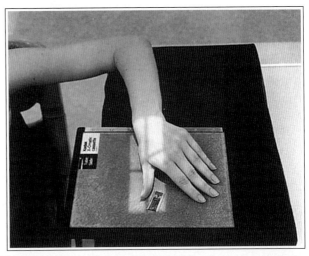

FIGURE 4-18 Proper patient positioning for lateral thumb projection.

aspect of the proximal phalanx and metacarpal demonstrates slight convexity.

- To accomplish a lateral thumb projection, place the patient's hand flat against the IR; then flex the hand and fingers only until the thumb naturally rolls into a lateral projection (Figure 4-18). Overflexion causes superimposition of the second and third proximal metacarpals onto the proximal first metacarpal, obscuring it (see Image 14). When the hand and fingers are accurately flexed and the thumb is in a lateral projection, the midshaft of the proximal phalanx and metacarpal demonstrates concavity on their anterior aspects and convexity on their posterior aspects. If the patient's hand is not rotated enough to place the thumb in a lateral projection, the posterior aspects of these midshafts show some degree of concavity (see Image 15).

The IP, MP, and CM joints are visible as open spaces, and the phalanges are not foreshortened.

- The IP, MP, and CM joints are open and the phalanges are visible without foreshortening if the entire thumb rests against and is positioned parallel with the IR and a perpendicular central ray is centered to the MP joint.

The proximal first metacarpal is only slightly superimposed by the proximal second metacarpal.

- Whenever possible, the anatomic part of interest should be demonstrated without superimposition. For a lateral thumb projection, the proximal metacarpal can be demonstrated with only a very small amount of superimposition if the thumb is abducted away from the palm. Failure to abduct the thumb results in a significant amount of first and second proximal metacarpal overlap and obstruction of the CM joint (see Image 16).

The first MP joint is at the center of the exposure field. The distal and proximal phalanges, the metacarpal, and the CM joint are included within the collimated field.

- Center a perpendicular central ray to the MP joint, which is located where the palm's interconnecting skin attaches to the thumb, to place it in the center of the image. Open the longitudinal collimation to include the distal phalanx and CM joint. Transversely collimate to within 0.5 inch (1.25 cm) of the thumb skin line.
- One third of an 8- × 10-inch (18- × 24-cm) detailed screen-film or computed radiography IR placed crosswise should be adequate to include all the required anatomic structures. Digital imaging requires tight collimation, lead masking, and no overlap of individual exposures to produce optimal images.

Lateral Thumb Projection Analysis

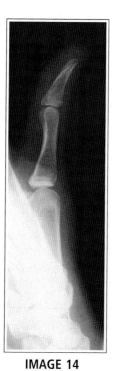

IMAGE 14

Analysis. The second and third proximal metacarpals are superimposed over the first proximal metacarpal. The hand was overflexed.

Correction. Abduct the thumb away from the hand, and decrease the amount of hand flexion while maintaining a lateral thumb projection.

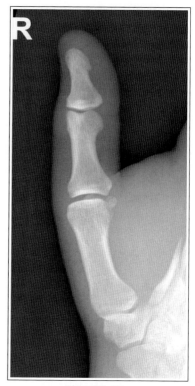

IMAGE 15

Analysis. The thumb is not in a lateral projection. The posterior aspect of the proximal phalanx and metacarpal midshafts demonstrates concavity, indicating that the hand was not adequately flexed.

Correction. Increase the degree of hand flexion until the thumb rolls into a lateral projection.

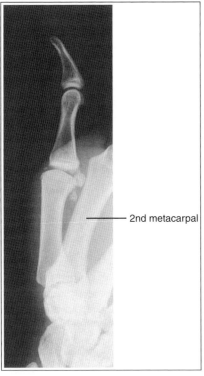

 2nd metacarpal

IMAGE 16

Analysis. The proximal metacarpal is superimposed by the proximal second metacarpal. The thumb was not abducted.

Correction. Abduct the thumb.

THUMB: POSTEROANTERIOR OBLIQUE PROJECTION

See Figures 4-19 and 4-20 and Box 4-7.

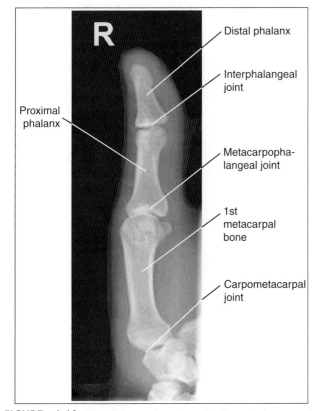

Distal phalanx

Interphalangeal joint

Proximal phalanx

Metacarpopha-langeal joint

1st metacarpal bone

Carpometacarpal joint

FIGURE 4-19 PA oblique thumb projection with accurate positioning.

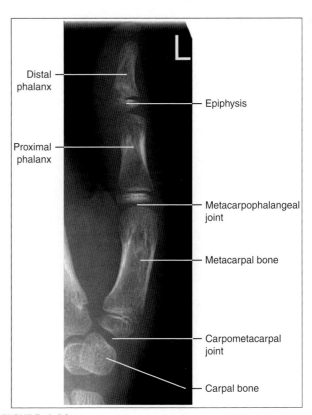

Distal phalanx

Proximal phalanx

Epiphysis

Metacarpophalangeal joint

Metacarpal bone

Carpometacarpal joint

Carpal bone

FIGURE 4-20 Accurately positioned pediatric PA oblique thumb projection.

BOX 4-7 | **Posteroanterior Oblique Thumb Projection Analysis Criteria**

- Twice as much soft tissue and more phalangeal and metacarpal midshaft concavity are present on the side of the thumb next to the fingers as on the other side.
- The long axis of the thumb is aligned with the long axis of collimated field.
- The IP, MP, and CM joints are demonstrated as open spaces, and the phalanges are not foreshortened.
- The first MP joint is at the center of the exposure field.
- The entire digit and CM joint are included within the collimated field.

CM, Carpometacarpal; *IP*, interphalangeal; *MP*, metacarpophalangeal.

The thumb is in a 45-degree PA oblique projection. Twice as much soft tissue and more phalangeal and metacarpal midshaft concavity are present on the side of the thumb next to the fingers as on the other side.

- When the hand is extended and the palmar surface is placed flat against the IR, the thumb is rotated into a 45-degree PA oblique projection (Figure 4-21). In this position, more midshaft concavity is present on one side of the phalanges and metacarpal than on the other side. If the hand is not placed flat against the IR, the thumb rolls toward a lateral projection. The more flexed the fingers, the closer the thumb is to a lateral projection. Such positioning can be identified on an image by noting the concavity of the anterior aspect and the convexity of the posterior aspect of the proximal phalanx and metacarpal (see Image 17).

The long axis of the thumb is aligned with the long axis of the collimated field.

- Aligning the long axis of the thumb with the long axis of the collimation light field enables you to

collimate tightly without clipping the distal phalanx or proximal metacarpal (see Image 18).

The IP, MP, and CM joints are visible as open joint spaces, and the phalanges are not foreshortened.

- The IP, MP, and CM joint spaces are open and the metacarpal and phalanges are visible without foreshortening when the first proximal metacarpal palmar surface remains flat against the IR. If the hand is medially rotated, the palmar surface is lifted off the IR, causing the thumb to tilt downward. The downward tilt closes the IP and MP joint spaces and foreshortens the phalanges (see Image 19).

The first MP joint is at the center of the exposure field. The distal and proximal phalanges, metacarpal, and CM joint are included within the collimated field.

- Center a perpendicular central ray to the MP joint, which is located where the palmar interconnecting skin attaches to the thumb, to place it in the center of the image. Open the longitudinal collimation to include the distal phalanx and CM joint. Transversely collimate to within 0.5 inch (1.25 cm) of the thumb skin line.
- One third of an 8- × 10-inch (18- × 24-cm) detailed screen-film or computed radiography IR placed crosswise should be adequate to include all the required anatomic structures.

PA Oblique Thumb Projection Analysis

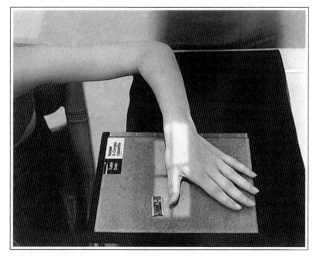

FIGURE 4-21 Proper patient positioning for PA oblique thumb projection.

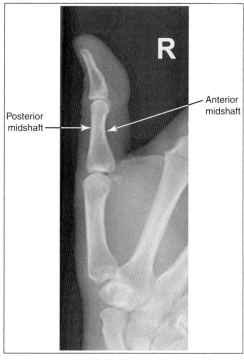

Posterior midshaft

Anterior midshaft

R

IMAGE 17

Analysis. The midshafts of the proximal phalanx and metacarpal demonstrate slight convexity on their posterior surfaces and concavity on their anterior surfaces. The thumb was positioned at more than 45 degrees of obliquity. The patient's palm was not placed flat against the IR.

Correction. Extend the patient's hand and place the palm flat against the IR.

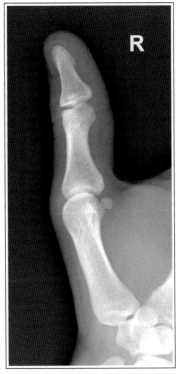

IMAGE 19

Analysis. The IP and MP joints are closed, and the phalanges are foreshortened. The lateral aspect of the palmar surface was not positioned against the IR, and the thumb was tilting down toward the IR.

Correction. Place the palmar surface and thumb against the IR.

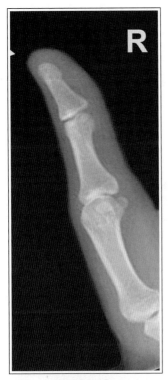

IMAGE 18

Analysis. The long axis of the thumb is not aligned with the long axis of the collimated field. Note that the proximal metacarpal and the CM joint are partially clipped.

Correction. Align the long axis of the thumb with the long axis of the collimation field.

HAND: POSTEROANTERIOR PROJECTION

See Figure 4-22 and Box 4-8.

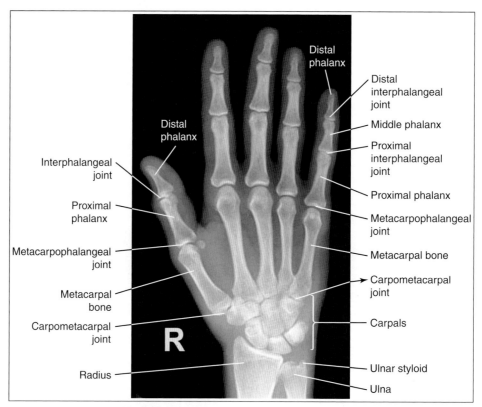

FIGURE 4-22 PA hand projection with accurate positioning.

BOX 4-8	**Posteroanterior Hand Projection Analysis Criteria**

- The soft tissue outlines of the second through fifth phalanges are uniform, the distance between the metacarpal heads is equal, and the same midshaft concavity is seen on both sides of the phalanges and metacarpals of the second through fifth digits.
- There is no soft tissue overlap from adjacent digits.
- The IP, MP, and CM joints are demonstrated as open spaces, and the phalanges are not foreshortened. The thumb demonstrates a 45-degree oblique projection.
- The third MP joint is at the center of the exposure field.
- The phalanges, metacarpals, carpals, and 1 inch (2.5 cm) of the distal radius and ulna are included within the collimated field.

CM, Carpometacarpal; *IP*, interphalangeal; *MP*, metacarpophalangeal.

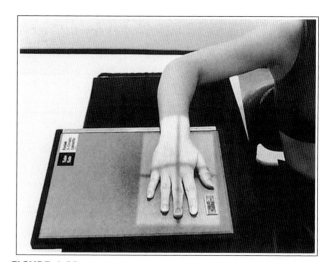

FIGURE 4-23 Proper patient positioning for PA hand projection.

The digits and metacarpals demonstrate a PA projection. The soft tissue outlines of the second through fifth phalanges are uniform, the distance between the metacarpal heads is equal, and the same midshaft concavity is demonstrated on both sides of the phalanges and metacarpals of the second through fifth digits.

- A PA projection of the hand is obtained when the patient fully extends the hand and rests the palmar surface flat against the IR (Figure 4-23).

- *PA versus external oblique hand position.* If the hand is not fully extended but is slightly flexed, it often relaxes into an external PA oblique projection when it is resting against the IR. A PA oblique hand projection is signified by slight superimposition of the third through fifth metacarpal heads and unequal soft tissue thickness and midshaft concavity on the sides of the phalanges. The metacarpals also show unequal midshaft concavity and spacing (see Image 20). Abducting the patient's arm and placing the forearm and humerus on the same horizontal plane, with the elbow flexed 90 degrees, assists in preventing an externally rotated PA oblique projection and will best demonstrate the wrist. This is important if a wrist condition is causing radiation hand pain. When the patient has been positioned in this manner, the ulnar styloid appears in profile on the image. Internal rotation of the hand is seldom a problem, because the thumb prevents this movement.

No soft tissue overlap of adjacent digits is present.

- Fingers should be spread slightly to prevent soft tissue overlapping.

The IP, MP, and CM joints are visible as open spaces, and the phalanges and metacarpals are not foreshortened. The thumb is demonstrated in a 45-degree PA oblique projection.

- When the hand and fingers are fully extended and a perpendicular central ray is centered to the third MP joint space, the IP, MP, and CM joints are demonstrated as open spaces and the phalanges and metacarpals are seen without foreshortening on the PA hand projection.
- Flexion of the hand causes poor alignment of the phalanges, metacarpals, and IP and CM joint spaces with the IR and central ray, resulting in closed joint spaces and foreshortening of the phalanges and metacarpals (see Image 21). The position of the first digit also changes when the image is taken with the hand flexed, because flexion rotates the first digit into a lateral projection.

The third MP joint is at the center of the exposure field. The distal, middle, and proximal phalanges, the metacarpals, the carpals, and approximately 1 inch (2.5 cm) of the distal radius and ulna are included within the collimated field.

- Center a perpendicular central ray to the third MP joint to place it in the center of the collimated light field. This MP joint is situated just slightly distal to the head of the third metacarpal. Once the central ray is centered, open the longitudinal collimation to include the distal phalanx and 1 inch (2.5 cm) of the distal forearm. Transversely collimate to within 0.5 inch (1.25 cm) of the first and fifth finger's skin line.
- Either half of a 10- × 12-inch (24- × 30-cm) detailed screen-film IR placed crosswise or a single 8- × 10-inch (18- × 24-cm) digital IR placed lengthwise should be adequate to include all the required anatomic structures.
- *Pediatric bone age assessment.* A bone age image is obtained to assess the skeletal versus the chronologic age of a child. Because bones develop in an orderly pattern, skeletal age may be assessed from infancy through adolescence. Illness, metabolic or endocrine dysfunction, and taking certain types of medications and therapies are all reasons why a pediatric patient's skeletal and chronologic age may not correspond. A left PA hand and wrist projection is typically the image of choice because bony developmental changes are readily visible and easily evaluated. For skeletal age to be evaluated, the phalanges, metacarpals, carpals, and distal radius and ulna must be included in their entirety (see Figure 1-130).

Posteroanterior Hand Projection Analysis

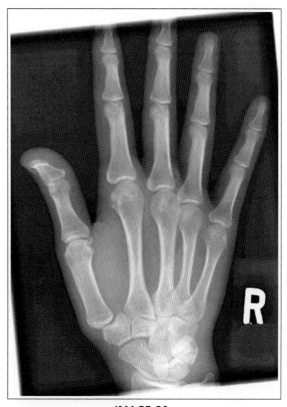

IMAGE 20

Analysis. The hand was externally rotated, as indicated by the superimposition of the third and fourth metacarpal heads, the unequal midshaft concavity on either side of the phalanges and metacarpals, and the uneven spacing of the metacarpal heads. The tip of the second and third fingers has been collimated off, and less than 1 inch (2.5 cm) of the distal radius and ulna is included.

Correction. Internally rotate the hand until the palm and fingers are placed flat against the IR, and open the longitudinally collimated field to include the second and third fingertips and 1 inch (2.5 cm) of the distal radius and ulna.

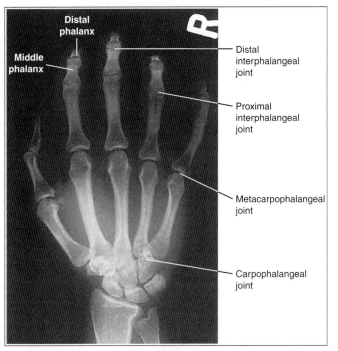

IMAGE 21

Analysis. The IP and CM joints are closed, and the phalanges and metacarpals are foreshortened. The first digit demonstrates a lateral projection. The hand and fingers were flexed for this image.

Correction. Fully extend the patient's hand and fingers, and then place them flat against the IR.

HAND: POSTEROANTERIOR OBLIQUE PROJECTION (EXTERNAL ROTATION)

See Figure 4-24 and Box 4-9.

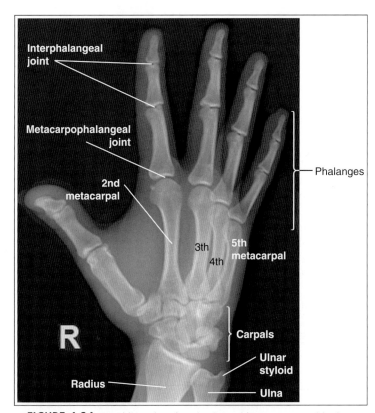

FIGURE 4-24 PA oblique hand projection with accurate positioning.

BOX 4-9 **Posteroanterior Oblique Hand Projection Analysis Criteria**

- Each of the second through fifth metacarpal midshafts demonstrate more concavity on one side than on the other and have varying amounts of space between them. The first and second metacarpal heads are not superimposed, the third through fifth metacarpal heads are slightly superimposed, and a slight space is present between the fourth and fifth metacarpal midshafts.
- There is no soft tissue overlap from adjacent digits.
- The IP and MP joints are demonstrated as open spaces, and the phalanges are not foreshortened. The thumb position may vary from a lateral to an oblique projection.
- The third MP joint is at the center of the exposure field.
- The phalanges, metacarpals, carpals, and one inch (2.5 cm) of the distal radius and ulna are included within the collimated field.

IP, Interphalangeal; *MP*, metacarpophalangeal.

The hand has been externally rotated 45 degrees. Each of the second through fifth metacarpal midshafts demonstrate more concavity on one side than on the other and have varying amounts of space between them. The first and second metacarpal heads are not superimposed, the third through fifth metacarpal heads are slightly superimposed, and a slight space is present between the fourth and fifth metacarpal midshafts.

- To accomplish a PA oblique hand projection, begin with the hand in a PA projection. Then, externally rotate the hand until it forms a 45-degree angle with the IR (Figure 4-25). To confirm the 45-degree angle, it is best to view the hand and not the wrist. The wrist will demonstrate more than 45 degrees of obliquity when the hand is in a 45-degree oblique projection, so using the wrist can result in a miscalculation of the amount of obliquity. This is especially true if the humerus and forearm have not been placed on the same horizontal plane. When the patient has been positioned with the arm on the same

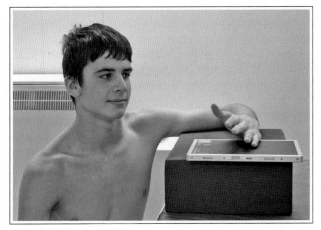

FIGURE 4-25 Proper patient positioning for PA oblique hand projection with extended fingers.

horizontal plane, the ulnar styloid is demonstrated in profile medially on the image. A radiolucent immobilization device can be used to help maintain this position.
- *Verifying PA oblique hand projection.* A 45-degree PA oblique hand projection can be recognized by the amount of metacarpal midshaft and metacarpal head superimposition. If the hand has not been rotated enough, the metacarpal relationship is similar to that demonstrated on a PA projection of the hand: The midshafts of the metacarpals are almost evenly spaced, and the metacarpal heads are not superimposed (see Image 22). On a 45-degree PA oblique hand projection, a space should be maintained between the fourth and fifth metacarpal midshafts. If the hand is rotated more than 45 degrees, this space is obscured and the fourth and fifth metacarpals demonstrate some degree of superimposition (see Image 23).

No soft tissue overlap of adjacent digits is present.

- Fingers should be spread slightly to prevent soft tissue overlapping (Images 24 and 25).

The IP and MP joints are visible as open spaces, and the phalanges are demonstrated without foreshortening. The thumb's position may vary from a lateral to a PA oblique projection.

- The IP and MP joint spaces are open and the phalanges are not foreshortened when the hand and fingers are fully extended and aligned parallel with the IR. An immobilization device should be used to help the patient maintain this positioning.
- *Disadvantages of using fingers as prop.* A common positioning error in PA oblique hand projection is to use the patient's fingers instead of an immobilization device to maintain the oblique position. For this positioning, the fingers are flexed until the fingertips touch the IR to prop the hand (Figure 4-26). Such positioning closes the IP joint spaces and foreshortens the phalanges (Images 23 and 25).

The third MP joint is at the center of the exposure field. The distal, middle, and proximal phalanges, the metacarpals, the carpals, and approximately 1 inch (2.5 cm) of the distal radius and ulna are included within the collimated field.

- Center a perpendicular central ray to the third MP joint to place it in the center of the collimated light field. The MP joint is situated just slightly distal to the head of the third metacarpal. Once the central ray is centered, open the longitudinal collimation to include the distal phalanges and the distal forearm. Transversely collimate to within 0.5 inch (1.25 cm) of the first and fifth finger's skin line.

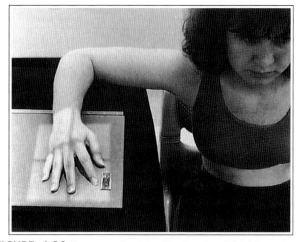

FIGURE 4-26 Proper patient positioning for PA oblique hand projection with flexed fingers.

- Either half of a 10- × 12-inch (24- × 30-cm) detailed screen-film IR placed crosswise or a single 8- ×10-inch (18- × 24-cm) digital IR placed lengthwise should be adequate to include all the required anatomic structures.

Posteroanterior Oblique Hand Projection Analysis

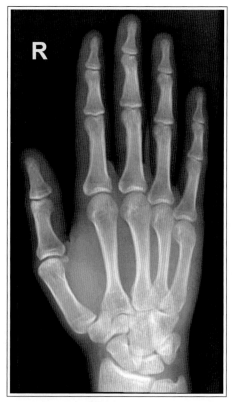

IMAGE 22

Analysis. The metacarpal heads demonstrate only slight superimposition, the metacarpal midshaft concavities are fairly uniform, and the spaces between the metacarpal midshafts are almost equal. The hand was not rotated enough. Open collimation includes 1 inch of radius and ulna.

Correction. Externally rotate the hand until the metacarpals and the IR form a 45-degree angle.

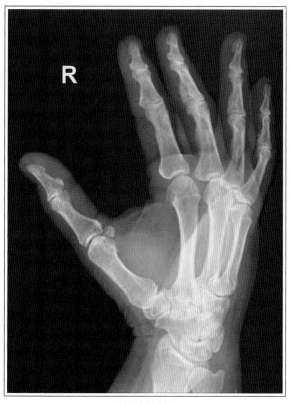

IMAGE 23

Analysis. The midshafts of the third through fifth metacarpals are superimposed. The patient's hand was placed at more than 45 degrees of obliquity. The phalanges are foreshortened, and the IP joints spaces are closed. The fingers were not positioned parallel with the IR, but instead were used to prop the hand (see Figure 4-26).

Correction. Internally rotate the hand until the metacarpals and the IR form a 45-degree angle and extend the fingers, placing them parallel with the IR.

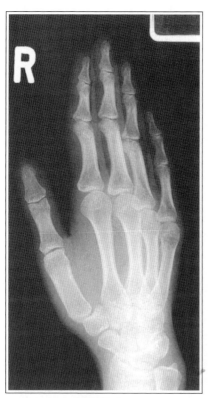

IMAGE 24

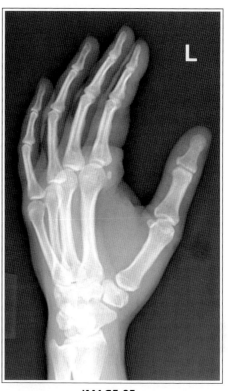

IMAGE 25

Analysis. Soft tissue and bony structure overlap of the digits is present. The fingers were not spread apart.

Correction. Spread all fingers enough to prevent soft tissue overlap.

Analysis. The distal and middle phalanges are fore-shortened, and the IP joint spaces are closed. The fingers were not positioned parallel with the IR, but were instead used to prop the hand (see Figure 4-26).

Correction. Extend the fingers and place them parallel with the IR. It may be necessary to situate an immobilization device beneath the fingers to maintain this positioning.

HAND: "FAN" LATERAL PROJECTION (LATEROMEDIAL)

See Figure 4-27 and Box 4-10.

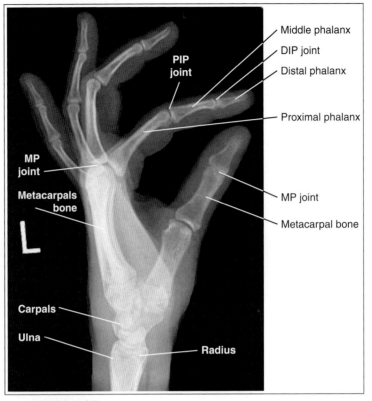

FIGURE 4-27 Lateral hand projection with accurate positioning.

BOX 4-10	Lateral Hand Projection Analysis Criteria

- The second through fifth digits are separated, demonstrating little superimposition of the proximal bony or soft tissue structures. The thumb is demonstrated without superimposition of the other digits and is in a PA to slight oblique position.
- The second through fifth metacarpals are superimposed.
- The IP joints are open, and the phalanges are not foreshortened.
- The MP joints are at the center of the exposure field.
- The phalanges, metacarpals, carpals, and 1 inch (2.5 cm) of the distal radius and ulna are included within the collimated field.

IP, Interphalangeal; *MP,* metacarpophalangeal.

Density is adequate to demonstrate the surrounding metacarpal soft tissue and bony structures of the hand.

- For the fan lateral hand projection, it is difficult to demonstrate the phalanges and the metacarpals with optimal density simultaneously because of the difference in thickness between the two body parts when the fingers are separated. Evaluate the requisition to determine which anatomy of the hand is of interest so that the mAs can be adjusted to obtain optimal density in that area.

The second through fifth digits are separated, demonstrating little superimposition of the proximal bony or

soft tissue structures. The thumb is demonstrated without superimposition of the other digits. Its position may vary from a PA projection to a slight PA oblique projection.

- For a lateral hand projection, place the medial hand surface resting against the IR; then fan or spread the fingers as far apart as possible without superimposing the thumb. The fingers are fanned most effectively by drawing the second and third fingers anteriorly and the fourth and fifth fingers posteriorly. The amount of finger separation obtained will depend on the patient's mobility (Figure 4-28). Immobilization devices are available to help maintain proper positioning. When the fingers are fanned, they can be individually studied. If the fingers are not adequately separated, they superimpose one another on the image (see Images 26 and 28).

The second through fifth metacarpals are superimposed.

- Superimpose the second through fifth metacarpals by palpating the patient's knuckles and placing them directly on top of one another.
- *Verifying a lateral hand projection.* On a lateral hand projection, a true lateral wrist position, represented by superimposition of the ulna and radius, is not always accomplished when the metacarpal midshafts are superimposed. Instead, the ulna is demonstrated

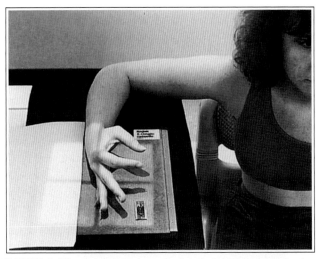

FIGURE 4-28 Proper patient positioning for lateral hand projection.

slightly posterior to the radius. Because of this variation, a true lateral projection of the hand should be determined by judging the degree of superimposition of the second through fifth metacarpal midshafts and not the degree of ulnar and radial superimposition. If the metacarpal midshafts are not superimposed and the fifth metacarpal is demonstrated anterior to the second through fourth metacarpals, the hand was slightly externally rotated or supinated (see Image 26). The fifth metacarpal can be identified by its length; it is the shortest of the second through fifth metacarpals. If the metacarpal midshafts are not superimposed and the second metacarpal is demonstrated anterior to the third through fifth metacarpals, the hand was slightly internally rotated or pronated (see Images 27 and 28). The second metacarpal can also be identified by its length; it is the longest.

The IP joints are open, and the phalanges are not foreshortened.

- The IP joint spaces are open and the phalanges are visible without foreshortening when the thumb is depressed and all the digits are positioned parallel with the IR.

The MP joints are at the center of the exposure field. The distal, middle, and proximal phalanges, the metacarpals, the carpals, and approximately 1 inch (2.5 cm) of the distal radius and ulna are included within the collimated field.

- Center a perpendicular central ray to the second MP joint to place it in the center of the collimated light field. Once the central ray is centered, open the longitudinal collimation to include the distal phalanges and the distal forearm. Transversely collimate to within 0.5 inch (1.25 cm) of the first and fifth finger's skin line.
- Either half of a 10- × 12-inch (24- × 30-cm) detailed screen-film IR placed crosswise or a single 8- × 10-inch (18- × 24-cm) screen-film or computed radiography IR placed lengthwise should be adequate to include all the required anatomic structures.

Optional Digit Positioning: Lateral Hand in Extension

The second through fifth digits are fully extended and superimposed (see Image 29). Density of the second through fifth digits and metacarpals is uniform, but the first metacarpal density is overexposed. The positioning analysis for the metacarpals is the same as for the fan lateral projection.

- Extending the hand and fingers until they are aligned on the same plane places the hand in extension. It has been suggested that foreign bodies of the palm can be better localized when the lateral hand projection is taken in extension.

Optional Digit Positioning: Lateral Hand in Flexion

The second through fifth digits are flexed and superimposed (see Image 30). Density of the second through fifth digits and metacarpals is uniform, but the first metacarpal density is overexposed. The positioning for the metacarpals is the same as for the fan lateral projection.

- Flex the second through fifth fingers until they meet the first finger but do not superimpose it. It has been suggested that this projection of the lateral hand is used to distinguish the degree of anterior or posterior displacement of a fractured metacarpal.

Lateral Hand Projection Analysis

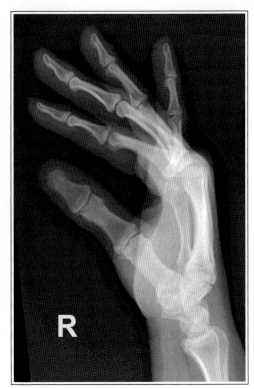

IMAGE 26

Analysis. The second through fifth metacarpal mid-shafts are not superimposed, and the shortest (fifth) metacarpal is anterior to the third through fourth metacarpals. The hand was externally rotated. This image may also result if the central ray was positioned anterior to the MP joints to increase transverse collimation.

Correction. Internally rotate the patient's hand until the metacarpals are superimposed. Center the central ray to the MP joints.

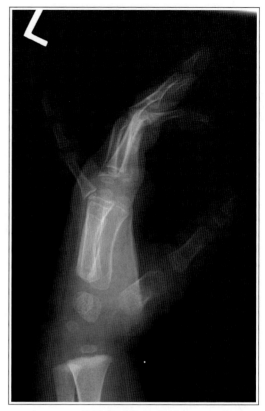

IMAGE 28 Pediatric.

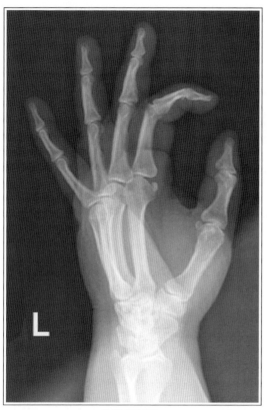

IMAGE 27

Analysis. The second through fifth metacarpal mid-shafts are not superimposed, and the longest (second) metacarpal is anterior to the third through fifth metacarpals. The hand was internally rotated.

Correction. Externally rotate the patient's hand until the metacarpals are superimposed.

Analysis. The second through fifth metacarpal mid-shafts are not superimposed, and the longest (second) metacarpal is anterior to the third through fifth metacarpals. The hand was internally rotated.

Correction. Externally rotate the patient's hand until the metacarpals are superimposed.

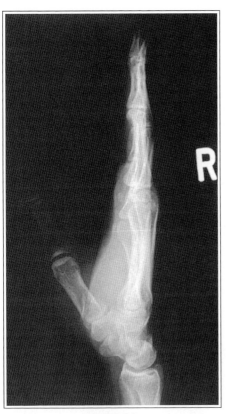

IMAGE 29

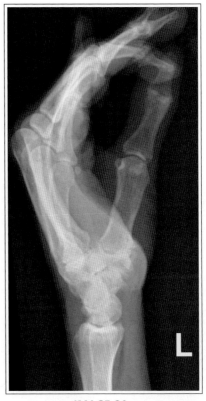

IMAGE 30

Analysis. The digits are superimposed. This image was taken with the hand and fingers in full extension.

Correction. If an extension lateral hand projection is desired, no correction is required. If a fan lateral hand projection is desired, fan or spread the fingers as far apart as possible by drawing the second and third fingers anteriorly and the fourth and fifth fingers posteriorly.

Analysis. The digits are superimposed. This image was taken with the hand and fingers flexed.

Correction. If a flexed lateral hand projection was desired, no correction is required. If a fan lateral hand projection was desired, fan or spread the fingers as far apart as possible by drawing the second and third fingers anteriorly and the fourth and fifth fingers posteriorly.

WRIST: POSTEROANTERIOR PROJECTION

See Figure 4-29 and Box 4-11.

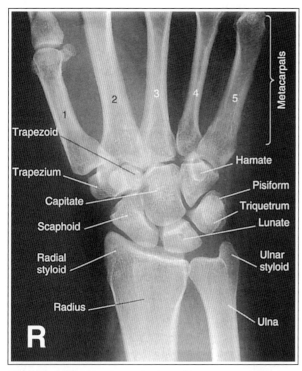

FIGURE 4-29 PA wrist projection with accurate positioning.

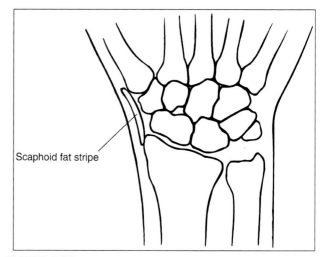

FIGURE 4-30 Location of scaphoid fat stripe. *(From Martensen K II: Radiographic positioning and analysis of the wrist,* In-Service Reviews in Radiologic Technology, *16[5], 1992.)*

BOX 4-11	**Posteroanterior Wrist Projection Analysis Criteria**

- The scaphoid fat stripe is demonstrated.
- The radial and ulnar styloids are at the extreme lateral and medial edges, respectively, of each bone. The radioulnar articulation is open, and superimposition of the metacarpal bases is limited.
- The anterior and posterior articulating margins of the radius are almost superimposed (within 0.25 inch or 0.6 cm).
- The second through fifth metacarpal joint spaces are open. The scaphoid is only slightly foreshortened, and the lunate is trapezoidal.
- The long axes of the third metacarpal and the midforearm are aligned with the long axis of the collimated field. The scaphoid and half of the lunate are positioned distal to the radius.
- The carpal bones are at the center of the exposure field.
- The carpal bones, one fourth of the distal ulna and radius, and half of the proximal metacarpals are included within the collimated field.

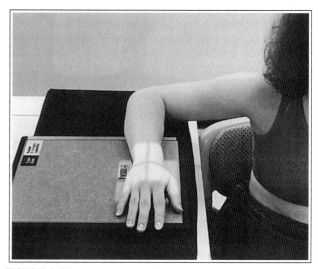

FIGURE 4-31 Proper patient positioning for PA wrist projection.

The wrist is positioned in a PA projection. The radial and ulnar styloids are at the extreme lateral and medial edges, respectively, of each bone. The radioulnar articulation is open, and superimposition of the metacarpal bases is limited.

Contrast and density are adequate to demonstrate the scaphoid fat stripe.

- *Significance of the scaphoid fat stripe.* The scaphoid fat stripe is one of the soft tissue structures that should be visible on all PA wrist projections (Figure 4-30). It is convex and located just lateral to the scaphoid in an uninjured wrist. A change in the convexity of this stripe may indicate to the reviewer the presence of joint effusion or of a radial side fracture of the scaphoid, radial styloid process, or proximal first metacarpal.

- Rotation of the wrist and forearm is controlled by the position of the hand, elbow, and humerus. A PA projection is accomplished by abducting the humerus until it is positioned parallel with the IR and the elbow is in a lateral projection. The hand is then pronated, placing the wrist in a PA projection (Figure 4-31).

- *Detecting wrist rotation and radial styloid position.* When the hand and wrist are rotated externally into an externally rotated PA oblique projection, the carpal bones and metacarpal bases located on the medial aspect of the wrist are superimposed, whereas those located laterally are not.

The lateral interconnecting carpal and metacarpal joint spaces are also demonstrated (see Image 31). Internal rotation of the hand and wrist causes the laterally located carpal bones and metacarpal bases to be superimposed and increases visibility of the pisiform and hamate hook (see Image 32).

- External and internal hand and wrist rotation also cause the radial styloid to rotate out of profile and closes the radioulnar articulation.
- *Humerus and elbow positioning and ulnar styloid visualization.* Humerus and elbow positioning determines the placement of the ulnar styloid. Abducting the humerus to position the elbow in a lateral projection with the humeral epicondyles aligned perpendicularly to the IR brings the ulnar styloid in profile and aligns the radius and ulna parallel with each other. The ulna and radius cross each other if the humerus is not abducted but is allowed to remain in a vertical position with the humeral epicondyles closer to parallel with the IR. This inaccurate positioning can be identified on a PA wrist projection by viewing the ulnar styloid, which is no longer demonstrated in profile (see Image 38).

The distal radius is demonstrated without foreshortening. The anterior and posterior articulating margins of the radius are nearly superimposed.

- The distal radial carpal articular surface is concave and slants approximately 11 degrees from posterior to anterior. Because the forearm is positioned parallel with the IR for a PA wrist projection, the slant of the distal radius causes the posterior radial margin to project slightly (0.25 inch or 0.6 cm) distal to the anterior radial margin, obscuring the radiocarpal joints.
- *Distal radius superimposition*: A PA wrist projection that demonstrates an excessive amount of the radial articulating surface, or if open radioscaphoid and radiolunate joint spaces are desired, view the distal radioulnar articulation to determine the correcting movement. The posterior edge of this surface is blunt, whereas the anterior edge is rounded. Study the distal end of a radial skeletal bone to familiarize yourself better with this difference. If a PA wrist projection is obtained that demonstrates the posterior radial margin distal to the anterior margin, the proximal forearm was elevated higher than the distal forearm (see Images 31 and 33). It should also be noted that when the wrist is medially rotated, the posterior radial surface is superimposed over the ulna. If the anterior radial margin is demonstrated distal to the posterior margin, the proximal forearm was positioned lower than the distal forearm. To superimpose the distal radial margins and to demonstrate radioscaphoid and radiolunate joints as open spaces (see Image 32), the proximal aspect of the forearm should be positioned slightly lower (5 to 6 degrees from horizontal) than the distal forearm.

- *Positioning patient with thick proximal forearm.* On a patient with a large muscular or thick proximal forearm, it may be necessary to allow the proximal forearm to extend off the IR or table to position the forearm parallel with the IR. If the patient is not positioned in this manner, the radius will be foreshortened, demonstrating an excessive amount of radial articular surface, and superimposition of the scaphoid and lunate onto the radius will be greater (see Image 33).

The second through fifth CM joint spaces are open. The scaphoid is only slightly foreshortened, and the lunate is trapezoidal.

- When the wrist is placed in a neutral nonflexed position, these three alignments are achieved. To place the wrist in a neutral position, flex the patient's fingers, flexing the hand until the metacarpals are angled to approximately 10 to 15 degrees with the IR.
- *Effect of flexion and extension on carpal bones.* View your own wrist in a PA projection with the hand extended flat against a hard surface. Note how the wrist is slightly flexed. Next, begin slowly flexing your hand and notice how the wrist moves from a flexed to an extended position with increased hand flexion. To understand how carpal bone position varies with wrist flexion and extension, study the drawings of the scaphoid, capitate, and lunate bones in Figure 4-32. Note how the positions of these carpals change with each movement. Also, study the position of the CM joint space in reference to a perpendicular central ray. Images 34 and 35 demonstrate PA wrist projections in flexion (the hand was extended) and extension (the hand was overflexed), respectively. Compare these images with the properly positioned wrist shown in Figure 4-29. Wrist flexion resulted in obscured third through fifth CM joint spaces, a severely foreshortened scaphoid that has taken a signet ring configuration (a large circle with a smaller circle within it), and a triangular lunate (see Image 34). Wrist extension has resulted in foreshortened metacarpals, closed second through third CM joint spaces, decreased scaphoid foreshortening, and a triangular lunate (see Image 35). Because the metacarpals are different lengths and may be positioned at different angles with the IR when the hand is flexed, it is necessary to position each metacarpal at a 10- to 15-degree angle to the IR to open all the CM joints.

The long axes of the third metacarpal and the midforearm are aligned with the long axis of the collimated light field. The scaphoid and half of the lunate are positioned distal to the radius.

- If the long axes of the third metacarpal and the midforearm are aligned with the long axis of the collimated light field, the patient's wrist has been placed in a neutral position. If a neutral position is

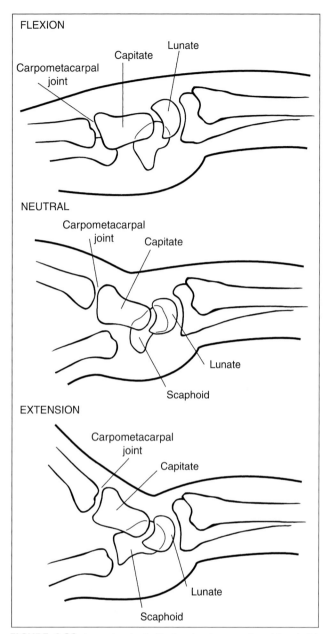

FIGURE 4-32 Lateral wrist in flexion (top), neutral position (middle), and extension (bottom). *(From Martensen K II: Radiographic positioning and analysis of the wrist,* In-Service Reviews in Radiologic Technology, *16[5], 1992.)*

The carpal bones are at the center of the exposure field. The carpal bones, one fourth of the distal ulna and radius, and half of the proximal metacarpals are included within the collimated field.

- The wrist joint is located at a level just distal to the palpable ulnar styloid. To obtain an image of the carpal bones with the least amount of distortion, place a perpendicular central ray at this level and centered to the midwrist area. Open the longitudinal collimation to include half of the metacarpals. Transversely collimate to within 0.5 inch (1.25 cm) of the wrist skin line.
- Either half of an 8- × 10-inch (18- × 24-cm) detailed screen-film or computed radiography IR or one third of a 10- × 12-inch (24- × 30-cm) detailed screen-film IR placed crosswise should be adequate to include all the required anatomic structures.
- *Wrist examination taken to include more than one fourth of the forearm.* When a wrist examination is requested to include more than one fourth of the distal forearm, the central ray should remain on the wrist joint, and the collimation field should be opened to demonstrate the desired amount of forearm. This method will result in an extended, unnecessary radiation field distal to the metacarpals. A lead strip placed over this extended radiation field protects the patient's phalanges and prevents backscatter from reaching the IR. The advantage of this method over centering the central ray proximal to the wrist joint is an undistorted demonstration of the carpal bones.

Effect of Upper Extremity Movements on Bony Components of the Wrist

The wrist is a very complex joint, with numerous bony components and movement possibilities. In an attempt to simplify the effect that different upper extremity movements have on the bony components, the following summary is offered. The positions of the elbow and hand affect forearm and wrist rotation and can be identified by the positions of the ulnar and radial styloid, respectively. When the elbow is in a lateral projection (humeral epicondyles aligned perpendicularly to IR), the ulnar styloid is in profile. When the hand is in a PA projection, the radial styloid is in profile.

It is the hand position that varies the shape of the scaphoid. If the wrist is flexed as a result of hand extension or is radially flexed, the scaphoid is foreshortened. If the wrist is extended as a result of hand flexion or is ulnar-flexed, the scaphoid is demonstrated with decreased foreshortening. The shape and location of the lunate also vary with the position of the wrist and hand. It becomes triangular with hand extension and flexion and changes position in reference to the distal radius with radial and ulnar flexion. In radial deviation the lunate is positioned distally to the radioulnar articulation, whereas in ulnar flexion it is positioned distally to the radius.

not maintained for a PA wrist projection, the shapes of the scaphoid and the position of the lunate are altered (Figure 4-33; see Images 36 and 37). Radial deviation of the wrist causes the distal scaphoid to shift anteriorly (toward the palmar surface) and to demonstrate increased foreshortening as it forms a signet ring configuration. The lunate will shift medially, toward the ulna. In ulnar deviation, the distal scaphoid tilts posteriorly and demonstrates decreased foreshortening, and the lunate shifts laterally, toward the radius. Radial and ulnar deviated PA wrist projections may be specifically requested to demonstrate wrist joint mobility.

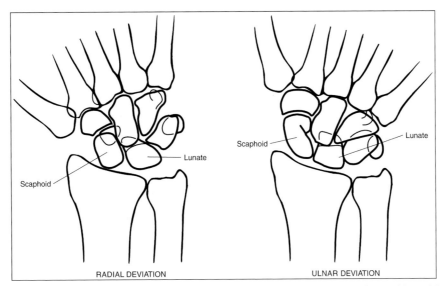

FIGURE 4-33 PA wrist in radial deviation (left) and ulnar deviation (right). *(From Martensen K II: Radiographic positioning and analysis of the wrist, In-Service Reviews in Radiologic Technology, 16[5], 1992.)*

Because the shapes of the scaphoid and lunate can be changed with more than one positioning movement, it is necessary to evaluate mispositioned images carefully to determine which movement is causing the misposition. It is also possible for two corrections to be needed simultaneously to obtain accurate positioning. The accuracy of hand flexion and extension are easily identified by evaluating the CM joints. Wrist ulnar or radial deviation is identified by evaluating the alignment of the third metacarpal with the radius.

Posteroanterior Wrist Projection Analysis

Analysis. The medially located carpal bones and metacarpals are superimposed, whereas the laterally located carpal and metacarpal joint spaces are open. The radioulnar articulation is closed, and the radial styloid is not in profile. The wrist was externally rotated. The posterior margin of the distal radius is too far distal to the anterior margin. The proximal forearm was slightly elevated. The ulnar styloid is in profile, indicating that the elbow and humerus were accurately positioned.

Correction. Internally rotate the hand until the wrist is in a PA projection, and depress the proximal forearm. For a patient with a thick proximal forearm, allow the proximal forearm to hang off the IR and/or the table.

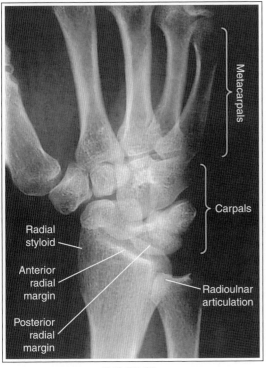

IMAGE 31

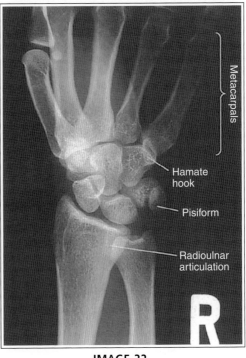

IMAGE 32

Analysis. The laterally located carpals and metacarpals are superimposed, and the pisiform and hamate hook are visualized. The radioulnar articulation is closed. The wrist was internally rotated. The ulnar styloid is in profile, indicating accurate elbow and humerus positioning, and the distal radial articular surfaces are directly superimposed over each other, demonstrating open radiolunate and radioscaphoid joint spaces. The proximal forearm was positioned slightly lower than the distal forearm.

Correction. Rotate the hand externally until the wrist is in a PA projection.

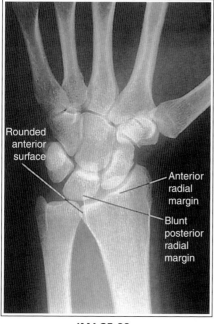

IMAGE 33

Analysis. The posterior margin of the distal radius is too far distal to the anterior margin. The posterior margin can be identified by the blunt, posterior ulnar articulating edge. The forearm was foreshortened, with the proximal forearm positioned higher than the distal forearm.

Correction. Lower the proximal forearm until it is parallel with the IR. If you desire a superimposed distal radial articular surface, which will demonstrate open radiolunate and radioscaphoid joint spaces, position the proximal forearm slightly lower (5 to 6 degrees from horizontal) than the distal forearm. For a patient with a thick proximal forearm, allow the proximal forearm to extend beyond the IR and/or table.

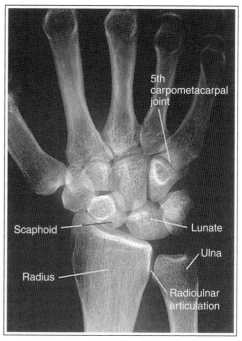

IMAGE 34

Analysis. The scaphoid demonstrates excessive foreshortening and has a signet ring configuration, the CM joints are obscured, and the lunate is triangular but is properly positioned distal to the radius. Two hand mispositions will cause this scaphoid shape—radial deviation and hand extension. Because the third metacarpal is aligned with the midforearm and the lunate is properly positioned distal to the radius, radial deviation can be eliminated as the positional problem. Hand extension (wrist flexion) is the cause of this mispositioning.

Correction. Curl the patient's fingers, flexing the hand until the second through fifth metacarpals are angled at approximately 10 to 15 degrees with the IR.

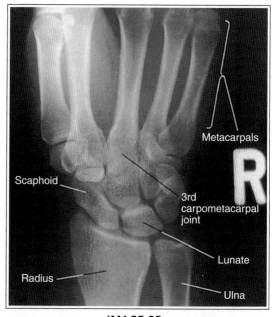

IMAGE 35

Analysis. The scaphoid is demonstrated with decreased foreshortening, and the second through third metacarpals are superimposed over the CM joints. The lunate is properly positioned distally to the radioulnar articulation. Two hand mispositions will cause this scaphoid shape, ulnar deviation and hand overflexion (metacarpals angled at more than 10 to 15 degrees with the IR). Because the third metacarpal is aligned with the midforearm and the lunate is properly positioned distally to the radioulnar articulation, ulnar deviation can be eliminated as the positional problem. Hand overflexion (wrist extension) is the cause of this misposition. The fifth CM joint is open because the fifth metacarpal is shorter and was placed at less of an angle to the IR than the other metacarpals when the hand was flexed.

Correction. Extend fingers and hand until the second through fifth metacarpals are angled at 10 to 15 degrees with the IR.

Correction. Ulnar-deviate the wrist until the third metacarpal and the midforearm are aligned, placing the hand and wrist in a neutral position. If a radial-deviated PA wrist projection is desired to evaluate patient mobility, no correction movement is required.

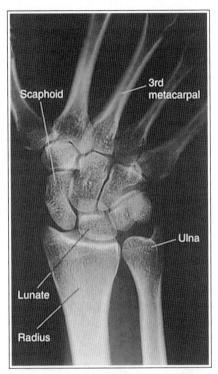

IMAGE 37

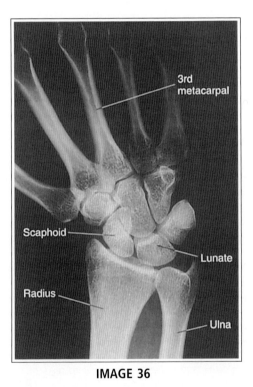

IMAGE 36

Analysis. The scaphoid demonstrates increased foreshortening, the lunate is positioned mostly distally to the ulna, and the third metacarpal is not aligned with the long axis of the midforearm. Because the scaphoid foreshortens with both hand extension and radial deviation, you can determine the correct repositioning movement for this image by evaluating the alignment of the third metacarpal with the midforearm and the openness of the CM joint spaces. The third metacarpal is not aligned with the midforearm and the scaphoid demonstrates increased foreshortening, so you can conclude that the patient was in radial deviation. Because the CM joint spaces are open, the hand was properly flexed.

Analysis. The scaphoid is demonstrated with decreased foreshortening, the lunate is entirely positioned distal to the radius, and the third metacarpal is not aligned with the midforearm. All these positioning points indicate that the wrist was in ulnar deviation for the image. Because the CM joint spaces are open, you can conclude that the hand was accurately flexed.

Correction. Radially deviate the wrist until the third metacarpal is aligned with the midforearm, placing the hand and wrist in a neutral position. If an ulnar-deviated PA wrist image is desired to evaluate patient mobility, no correcting movement is required.

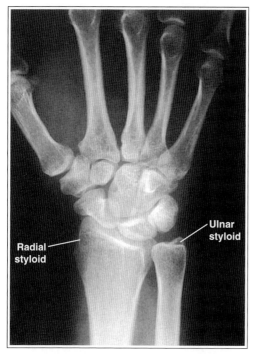

IMAGE 38

Analysis. This image has many positioning problems. First, the radioulnar articulation is closed and the lateral intercarpal joints are open while the medial intercarpal joints are closed, indicating that the hand and wrist were externally rotated. Second, the ulnar styloid is not in profile, indicating that the elbow and humerus were mispositioned. Next, the distal radius is foreshortened. Note how the articulating surface is demonstrated with the posterior margin far too distal to the anterior margin. The proximal forearm was positioned higher than the distal forearm. Finally, the scaphoid demonstrates excessive foreshortening, and the fourth and fifth CM joints are obscured. The image was taken with the wrist in slight external rotation, with the fourth and fifth metacarpals positioned at less than a 10- to 15-degree angle to the IR, although the second and third distal metacarpals were elevated accurately.

Correction. Flex the elbow and abduct the humerus 90 degrees, placing the entire arm on the same horizontal plane. Slightly depress the proximal forearm. Internally rotate the hand and wrist until they are positioned in a PA projection. Curl the fingers, flexing the hand until all the metacarpals are angled at 10 to 15 degrees to the IR.

WRIST: POSTEROANTERIOR OBLIQUE PROJECTION (EXTERNAL ROTATION)

See Figure 4-34 and Box 4-12.

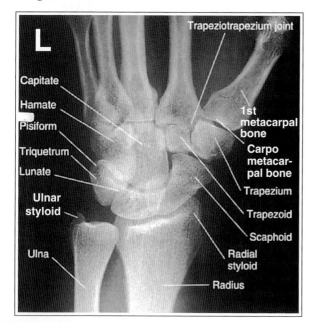

FIGURE 4-34 PA oblique wrist projection with accurate positioning.

Contrast and density are adequate to demonstrate the scaphoid fat stripe.

- The scaphoid fat stripe is one of the soft tissue structures that should be visible on all PA oblique wrist projections. It is convex and located just lateral to the scaphoid on an uninjured wrist (see

BOX 4-12	Posteroanterior Oblique Wrist Projection Analysis Criteria

- The scaphoid fat stripe is demonstrated.
- The trapezoid and trapezium are demonstrated without superimposition, and the trapeziotrapezoidal joint space is open.
- The scaphoid tuberosity and waist are demonstrated in profile. Only a small degree of trapezoid and capitate superimposition is present.
- The second carpometacarpal is demonstrated as an open space.
- The long axes of the third metacarpal and midforearm are aligned with the long axis of the collimated field. The scaphoid tuberosity and waist are demonstrated in profile and are not positioned directly next to the radius.
- The anterior and posterior articulating margins of the radius are nearly superimposed (within 0.25 inch [0.6 cm]).
- The ulnar styloid is in profile at the far medial edge.
- The carpal bones are at the center of the exposure field.
- The carpal bones, one fourth of the distal ulna and radius, and half of the proximal metacarpals are included within the collimated field.

Figure 4-30). A change in the shape of this fat stripe or in its proximity to the scaphoid may indicate joint effusion or a radial side fracture.

The wrist has been externally rotated to a 45-degree PA oblique projection. The trapezoid and trapezium are demonstrated without superimposition, and the trapeziotrapezoidal joint space is open. The scaphoid tuberosity and waist are demonstrated in profile. Only a

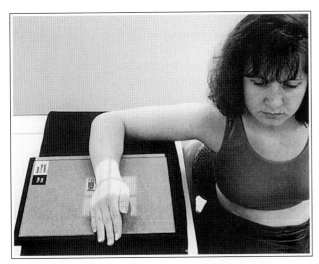

FIGURE 4-35 Proper patient positioning for PA oblique wrist projection.

small degree of trapezoid and capitate superimposition is present.

- To accomplish a PA oblique wrist projection, begin with the wrist in a PA projection, with the humerus and the forearm on the same horizontal plane. Externally rotate the hand and wrist until the wrist forms a 45-degree angle with the IR (Figure 4-35). When judging the degree of wrist obliquity, it is best to view the wrist and not the hand. The obliquity of the hand and wrist are not always equal when they are rotated, especially if the humerus and forearm are not positioned on the same horizontal plane for the image.
- *Determining the accuracy of wrist obliquity.* On a PA wrist projection (see Image 39), the trapezoid and trapezium are superimposed. Placing the wrist in a 45-degree externally rotated PA oblique projection draws the trapezium from beneath the trapezoid, providing clear visualization of both carpal bones and the joint space (trapeziotrapezoidal) between them. The PA oblique projection also rotates the scaphoid tuberosity and waist into profile. The relationships between the trapezoid and trapezium and the trapezoid and capitate are used to discern an accurate PA oblique wrist projection. If the wrist is underrotated, the trapezoid and trapezium are superimposed, the trapeziotrapezoidal joint space is obscured, and the trapezoid demonstrates minimal capitate superimposition (see Image 40). If wrist obliquity is more than 45 degrees, the trapezium demonstrates minimal trapezoidal superimposition, the capitate is superimposed by the trapezoid, and the trapeziotrapezoidal joint space is obscured (see Image 41).

The second CM and the scaphotrapezoidal joint spaces are demonstrated.

- For the PA wrist projection, the CM joints are opened by flexing the hand until the metacarpals are at a 10- to 15-degree angle to the IR. When the

hand and wrist are placed in obliquity, the same metacarpal tilt must be maintained to open the second CM and scaphotrapezoidal joint spaces. If the distal second metacarpal is positioned too far away from the IR, a portion of the metacarpal (MC) superimposes the trapezoid, closing the second CM and scaphotrapezoidal joints (see Image 40).

The long axes of the third metacarpal and midforearm are aligned with the long axis of the collimated field. The scaphoid tuberosity and waist are demonstrated in profile and are not positioned directly next to the radius.

- If the long axes of the third metacarpal and midforearm are aligned with the long axis of the collimation field, the patient's wrist is placed in a neutral position. Radial deviation increases the foreshortening of the scaphoid, preventing visualization of the scaphoid tuberosity and waist, and positions the scaphoid directly next to the radius (see Image 42). Ulnar deviation decreases scaphoid foreshortening (see Image 43).

The distal radius is demonstrated without foreshortening. The anterior and posterior margins of the radius are nearly superimposed.

- The distal radial carpal articular surface is concave and slants approximately 11 degrees from posterior to anterior when the radius and ulna are positioned parallel with the IR. Because the forearm is positioned parallel with the IR for a PA oblique wrist projection, the slant of the distal radius causes the posterior margin to be projected slightly (0.25 inch or 0.6 cm) distal to the anterior radial margin, obscuring the radiocarpal joints.

  If an image is obtained that demonstrates an excessive amount of the radial articulating surface, or if open radioscaphoid and radiolunate joint spaces are desired, you should view the distal radioulnar articulation to determine the correcting movement. The radial surface superimposed over the ulna is associated with the posterior radial margin.

- *Distal radius margin superimposition.* If a PA oblique projection is obtained that demonstrates the posterior radial margin too far distal to the anterior margin, the proximal forearm was elevated higher than the distal forearm (see Image 43). If the anterior radial margin is demonstrated distal to the posterior margin, the proximal forearm was positioned lower than the distal forearm. To demonstrate open radioscaphoid and radiolunate joint spaces (see Image 44), position the proximal forearm slightly (5 to 6 degrees) lower than the distal forearm.

- *Positioning patient with thick proximal forearm.* For the patient with a large muscular or thick proximal forearm, allow the proximal forearm to extend beyond the IR or table to position it parallel with the IR. If the patient is not positioned in this manner, the radius is foreshortened, demonstrating an excessive amount of radial articular surface, and superimposition of the scaphoid and lunate onto the radius is increased.

The ulnar styloid is in profile at the far medial edge.

- The position of the humerus and elbow determines the placement of the ulnar styloid. The ulnar styloid is demonstrated in profile when the patient's humerus is abducted to align the humeral epicondyles perpendicular to the IR and place the elbow in a lateral position. If the humerus is not abducted to this degree, the ulnar styloid is no longer demonstrated in profile.

The carpal bones are at the center of the exposure field. The carpal bones, one fourth of the distal ulna and radius, and half of the proximal metacarpals are included within the collimated field.

- The wrist joint is located at the base of the first proximal metacarpal. To obtain a PA oblique projection of the carpal bones with the least amount of distortion, place a perpendicular central ray at this level and centered with the midwrist area. Open longitudinal collimation to include half of the metacarpals. Transversely collimate to within 0.5 inch (1.25 cm) of the wrist skin line.
- Either half of an 8- ×10-inch (18- × 24-cm) detailed screen-film or computed radiography IR or one third of a 10- × 12-inch (24- × 30-cm) detailed screen-film IR placed crosswise should be adequate to include all the required anatomic structures.

Posteroanterior Oblique Wrist Projection Analysis

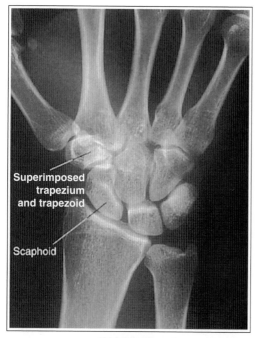

IMAGE 39

Analysis. The trapezoid and trapezium are superimposed, and the scaphoid tuberosity is not demonstrated in profile. This is a PA projection.

Correction. Externally rotate the wrist until it forms a 45-degree angle with the IR.

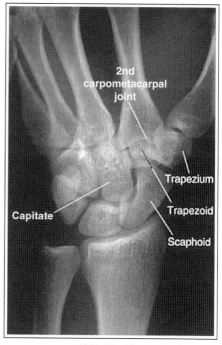

IMAGE 40

Analysis. The trapezoid and trapezium are partially superimposed, obscuring the trapeziotrapezoidal joint space. Trapezoid capitate superimposition is minimal. The wrist was rotated less than 45 degrees. The second CM and scaphotrapezoidal joint spaces are closed. The distal second metacarpal was positioned too far away from the IR.

Correction. Externally rotate the wrist until it forms a 45-degree angle with the IR. Depress the distal second metacarpal until it is positioned at a 10- to 15-degree angle to the IR.

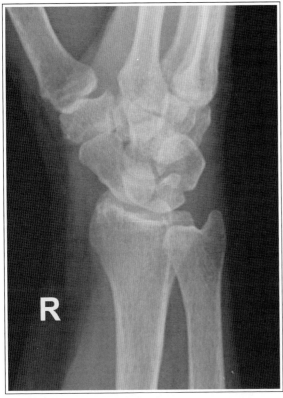

IMAGE 41

Analysis. Trapezoid and trapezium are partially superimposed, obscuring the trapeziotrapezoidal joint space. The trapezoid demonstrates excessive capitate superimposition. The wrist obliquity was more than 45 degrees.

Correction. Internally rotate the wrist until it forms a 45-degree angle with the IR.

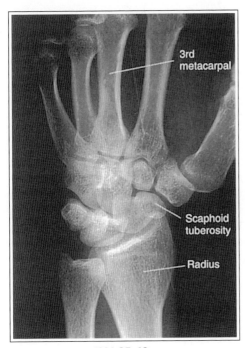

IMAGE 42

Analysis. The third metacarpal and midforearm are not aligned, the scaphoid is foreshortened, and the scaphoid tuberosity is situated next to the radius. The wrist was radially flexed.

Correction. Ulnar-deviate the wrist until the long axes of the third metacarpal and the midforearm are aligned.

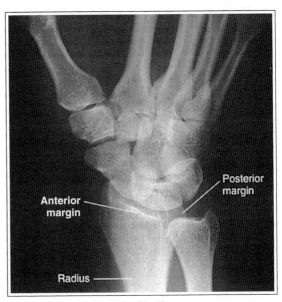

IMAGE 43

Analysis. The posterior margin of the distal radius is quite distal to the anterior margin, the third metacarpal and midforearm are not aligned, and the scaphoid demonstrates little foreshortening. The proximal forearm was elevated, and the wrist was ulnar-flexed.

Correction. Lower the proximal forearm until the forearm is parallel with the IR. For a patient with a muscular or thick proximal forearm, it may be necessary to allow the proximal forearm to hang off the IR or table to obtain a parallel forearm. Radial-deviate the wrist until the third metacarpal and midforearm are aligned.

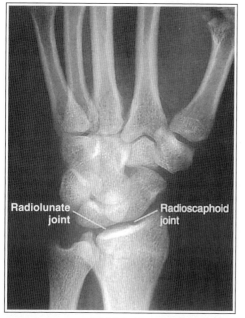

IMAGE 44

Analysis. The anterior and posterior margins of the distal radius are superimposed, demonstrating open radiolunate and radioscaphoid joint spaces. The proximal forearm was positioned slightly (5 to 6 degrees from horizontal) lower than the distal forearm.

Correction. This is an acceptable image. No correction movement is needed.

WRIST: LATERAL PROJECTION (LATEROMEDIAL)

See Figure 4-36 and Box 4-13.

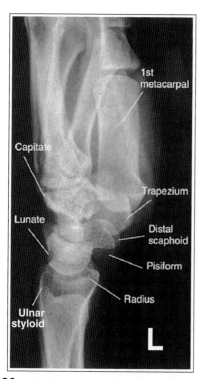

FIGURE 4-36 Lateral wrist projection with accurate positioning.

Contrast and density are adequate to demonstrate the pronator fat stripe and surrounding posterior wrist soft tissue.

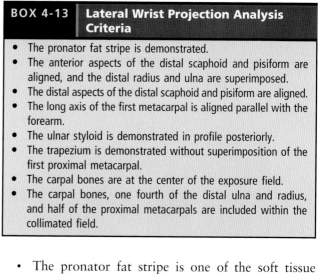

BOX 4-13	Lateral Wrist Projection Analysis Criteria

- The pronator fat stripe is demonstrated.
- The anterior aspects of the distal scaphoid and pisiform are aligned, and the distal radius and ulna are superimposed.
- The distal aspects of the distal scaphoid and pisiform are aligned.
- The long axis of the first metacarpal is aligned parallel with the forearm.
- The ulnar styloid is demonstrated in profile posteriorly.
- The trapezium is demonstrated without superimposition of the first proximal metacarpal.
- The carpal bones are at the center of the exposure field.
- The carpal bones, one fourth of the distal ulna and radius, and half of the proximal metacarpals are included within the collimated field.

- The pronator fat stripe is one of the soft tissue structures that should be demonstrated on all lateral wrist projections (Figure 4-37). It is located parallel to the anterior (volar) surface of the distal radius, is normally convex, and lies within 0.25 inch (0.6 cm) of the radial cortex. Bowing or obliteration of this fat stripe may be the only indication of a subtle radial fracture.
- The soft tissue that surrounds the posterior (dorsal) aspect of the wrist should also be visible. This posterior soft tissue is convex on the uninjured wrist. To the reviewer, a straightening or concave appearance of this surface may indicate swelling and injury.

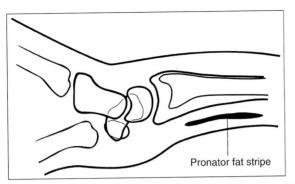

FIGURE 4-37 Location of pronator fat stripe. *(From Martensen K II: Radiographic positioning and analysis of the wrist,* In-Service Reviews in Radiologic Technology, *16[5], 1992.)*

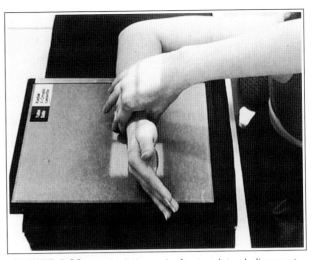

FIGURE 4-39 Manipulating wrist for true lateral alignment.

The wrist is in a lateral projection. The anterior aspect of the distal scaphoid and pisiform are aligned, and the radius and ulna are superimposed.

- A lateral projection of the wrist is accomplished by flexing the elbow 90 degrees and abducting the humerus until it is parallel with the IR, placing the entire arm on the same horizontal plane. Rotate the wrist into a lateral projection with its ulnar (medial) aspect against the IR (Figure 4-38). To ensure a true lateral projection, place the palmar aspect of your thumb and forefinger against the anterior and posterior aspects, respectively, of the patient's wrist joint, as shown in Figure 4-39. Adjust wrist rotation until your thumb and finger are aligned perpendicular to the IR.

- *Detecting wrist rotation.* The relationship between the pisiform and distal aspect of the scaphoid can best be used to discern whether a lateral wrist projection has been obtained. On a lateral projection, these two carpals should be superimposed, with their anterior aspects aligned. When the wrist is rotated, the anteroposterior relationship between the distal scaphoid and pisiform changes, and the pronator fat stripe is obscured. If the anterior aspect

of the distal scaphoid is positioned posterior to the anterior aspect of the pisiform, the patient's wrist was externally rotated (see Image 45). If the anterior aspect of the distal scaphoid is positioned anterior to the anterior aspect of the pisiform, the patient's wrist was internally rotated (see Images 46 and 47). A second method of determining how to reposition a rotated lateral wrist projection uses the radius and ulna. The ulna is positioned anterior to the radius when the wrist was externally rotated and the ulna is positioned posterior to the radius when the wrist was internally rotated. Because the exact amount of superimposition of the radius and ulna depends on the position of the humerus, and their poor positioning is not as sensitive, you should always view the pisiform and distal scaphoid relationship when determining whether the wrist is in a lateral projection.

- *Mediolateral wrist projection.* Routinely, the lateral wrist projection is taken with the ulnar side of the wrist against the IR. If, instead, the radial side of the wrist was placed against the IR (mediolateral projection), the ulna and pisiform are visualized anterior to the radius and scaphoid, respectively, and the ulnar styloid is demonstrated in profile anteriorly (see Image 48).

The carpal bones do not indicate radial or ulnar deviation. The distal aspect of the distal scaphoid is aligned with the distal aspect of the pisiform.

- To obtain a neutral lateral wrist projection, align the long axes of the third metacarpal and the midforearm parallel with the IR. When the proximal forearm is higher or lower than the distal forearm, the wrist is radial-deviated or ulnar-deviated, respectively. In radial and ulnar deviation the distal scaphoid moves but the pisiform's position remains relatively unchanged. Radial deviation of the wrist forces the distal scaphoid to move anteriorly and

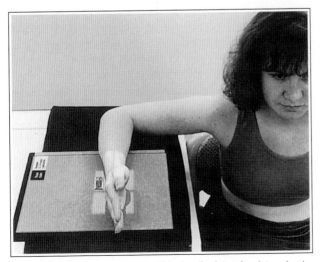

FIGURE 4-38 Proper patient positioning for lateral wrist projection.

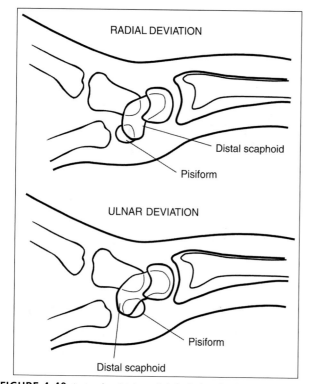

FIGURE 4-40 Lateral wrist in radial deviation *(top)* and ulnar deviation *(bottom).*

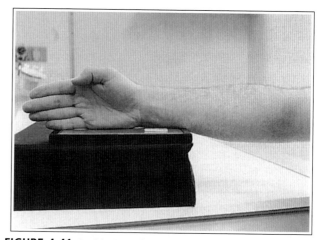

FIGURE 4-41 Positioning of patient with thick proximal forearm.

proximally (Figure 4-40), causing the distal aspect of the distal scaphoid to be positioned proximal to the distal aspect of the pisiform (see Image 49). Ulnar deviation shifts the distal scaphoid posteriorly and distally (see Figure 4-40), causing the distal aspect of the distal scaphoid to be positioned distal to the distal aspect of the pisiform (see Image 50). The degree of pisiform and distal scaphoid separation is usually very small, because you would be unlikely to position a patient in maximum wrist deviation without being aware of the positioning error. To obtain optimal lateral wrist projections, however, you must learn to eliminate even small degrees of deviation.

- *Positioning patient with thick proximal forearm.* For a patient with a large muscular or thick proximal forearm, it may be necessary to allow the proximal forearm to hang off the IR or table to maintain a neutral wrist position (Figure 4-41). If the patient is not positioned in this manner, radial deviation of the wrist will result. If the proximal forearm does not remain level but is allowed to depress lower than the distal forearm in this situation, ulnar deviation will result.

The long axis of the first metacarpal is aligned parallel with the forearm.

- If the long axis of the first metacarpal is positioned adjacent to the second metacarpal and aligned parallel with the forearm, the patient's wrist is placed in a neutral position.

- When the wrist is flexed or extended, the positions of the scaphoid and lunate are altered. In wrist flexion the lunate and distal scaphoid tilt anteriorly (see Image 51). In wrist extension the lunate and distal scaphoid tilt posteriorly (see Image 52). Flexion and extension, lateral wrist projections may be specifically requested to demonstrate wrist joint mobility.

The ulnar styloid is demonstrated in profile posteriorly.

- When the humerus and elbow are positioned, the placement of the ulna styloid changes. The ulnar styloid is demonstrated in profile when the patient's elbow is in a lateral projection, with the humerus abducted and the humeral epicondyles aligned perpendicularly to the IR. If the humerus is not abducted to this degree, the ulnar styloid will not be demonstrated in profile (Images 45 and 53).

- *Lateral wrist projection with no forearm rotation.* In contrast to positioning the forearm and humerus on the same horizontal plane for a lateral wrist projection, Epner and colleagues[1] have suggested that a lateral wrist projection be taken with zero forearm rotation. For this to be accomplished the humerus is not abducted and the elbow is placed in an AP projection (Figure 4-42). Such positioning rotates the ulnar styloid out of profile, demonstrating it distal to the midline of the ulnar head (see Images 45 and 53). Because forearm rotation has been eliminated, the ulnar head also shifts closer to the lunate. Epner and associates[1] have stated that this positioning allows for more accurate measuring of the ulnar length. Department policy determines which humerus positioning is performed in your facility.

The trapezium is demonstrated without superimposition of the first proximal metacarpal.

- To obtain optimal demonstration of the trapezium, lower the distal first metacarpal until it is at the same level as the second metacarpal. This positioning places the trapezium and metacarpal parallel with the IR, demonstrating them without

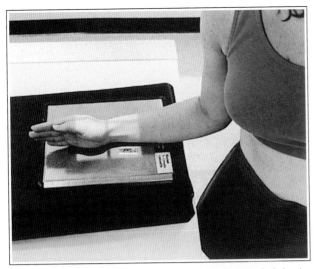

FIGURE 4-42 Lateral wrist projection without humeral abduction.

superimposition. If the distal first metacarpal is not lowered, it is foreshortened, and its proximal aspect is superimposed over the trapezium (see Image 54).

The carpal bones are at the center of the exposure field. The carpal bones, one fourth of the distal ulna and radius, and half of the proximal metacarpals are included within the collimated field.

- In a lateral projection the wrist joint is located just proximal to the first metacarpal base. To obtain an image of the carpal bones with the least amount of distortion, place a perpendicular central ray at this level and centered to the midwrist area. Open the longitudinal collimation to include half of the metacarpals. Transversely collimate to within 0.5 inch (1.25 cm) of the wrist skin line.
- Either half of an 8- × 10-inch (18- × 24-cm) detailed screen-film or computed radiography IR or one third of a 10- × 12-inch (24- × 30-cm) detailed screen-film IR placed crosswise should be adequate to include all the required anatomic structures.
- *Wrist examination that includes more than one fourth of the forearm.* When a wrist examination is requested to include more than one fourth of the distal forearm, the central ray should remain on the wrist joint, and the collimation field should be opened to demonstrate the desired amount of forearm. This method results in an extended, unnecessary radiation field distal to the metacarpals. A lead strip placed over this extended radiation field protects the patient's phalanges and prevents any possible backscatter from reaching the IR. The advantage of this method over centering the central ray proximal to the wrist joint is an undistorted demonstration of the carpal bones. A lateral wrist projection taken with the central ray positioned proximal to the wrist joint demonstrates the distal scaphoid projecting distal to the pisiform (see Image 50).

Lateral Wrist Projection Analysis

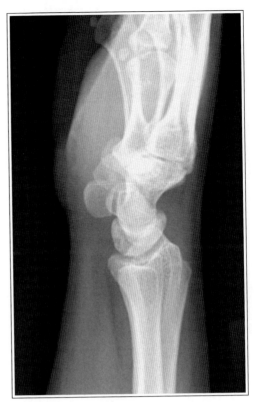

IMAGE 45

Analysis. The anterior aspect of the pisiform is shown anterior to the anterior aspect of the distal scaphoid. The wrist was externally rotated. The proximal first metacarpal is partially superimposed over the trapezium. The first metacarpal was not positioned parallel with the forearm. The ulnar styloid is not positioned in profile but is demonstrated projecting distally to the midline of the ulnar head. This ulnar positioning indicates that the humerus was positioned without abduction, as shown in Figure 4-42.

Correction. Internally rotate the wrist until the wrist is in a lateral position, and depress the distal metacarpal until the metacarpal is aligned parallel with the forearm. Adjust the patient's humerus to meet your department protocol. If the ulnar styloid is to be demonstrated in profile, abduct the humerus and flex the elbow 90 degrees, placing the forearm and humerus on the same horizontal plane. If department protocol requires that a lateral wrist image be taken without humeral abduction, no correction movement is needed. Consistency in arm position is important for evaluating ulnar length.

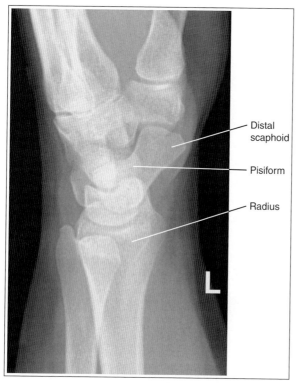

IMAGE 46

Analysis. The anterior aspect of the distal scaphoid is anterior to the anterior aspect of the pisiform, and the radius is anterior to the ulna. The wrist was internally rotated.

Correction. Externally rotate the wrist until the wrist is in a lateral projection.

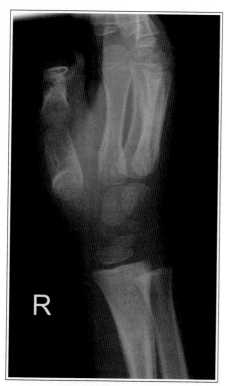

IMAGE 47 Pediatric.

Analysis. The radius is anterior to the ulna. The wrist was internally rotated.

Correction. Externally rotate the wrist until the wrist is in a true lateral position.

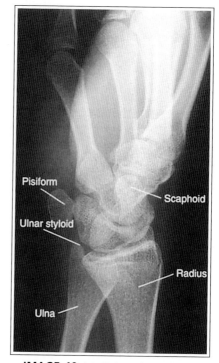

IMAGE 48 Mediolateral projection.

Analysis. The ulna and pisiform are demonstrated anterior to the radius and scaphoid, respectively, and the ulnar styloid is demonstrated in profile anteriorly. The radial side of the wrist was placed against the IR (mediolateral projection).

Correction. Externally rotate the hand and wrist until the ulnar side of the wrist is placed against the IR if a lateromedial projection is desired.

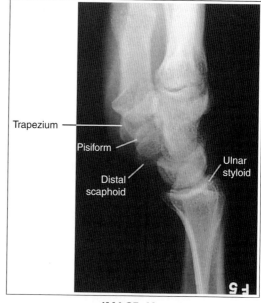

IMAGE 49

Analysis. The distal aspect of the pisiform is demonstrated distal to the distal aspect of the distal scaphoid. Two possible positioning errors cause such an image. Either the central ray was not centered with the wrist joint but was positioned distally, or the wrist was in radial deviation. Note that the ulnar styloid is not in profile but is projecting distally to the midline of the ulnar head. This ulnar positioning indicates that the patient was positioned without humerus abduction, as demonstrated in Figure 4-42. The proximal first metacarpal is partially superimposed over the trapezium. The metacarpal was not aligned parallel with the IR.

Correction. Center the central ray with the wrist joint, which is located just proximal to the trapezium. Position the wrist in a neutral position by aligning the long axes of the third metacarpal and midforearm parallel with the IR. Depress the distal metacarpal until the first metacarpal is aligned parallel with the IR.

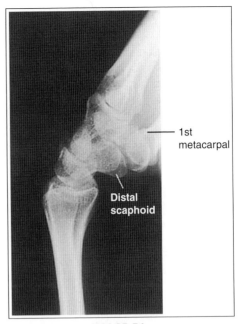

IMAGE 51

Analysis. The first metacarpal is not aligned parallel with the midforearm. The wrist was flexed anteriorly.

Correction. If a neutral position is desired, align the long axis of the first metacarpal parallel with the midforearm. If a wrist flexion image was taken to evaluate wrist mobility, no correction movement is required.

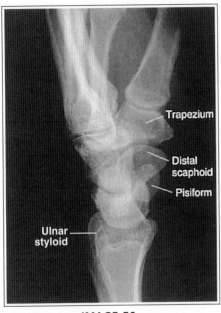

IMAGE 50

Analysis. The distal aspect of the distal scaphoid is demonstrated distal to the distal aspect of the pisiform. Two possible positioning errors cause such a problem. Either the wrist was in ulnar deviation or the central ray was not centered with the wrist joint but was positioned to the midforearm.

Correction. Place the wrist in a neutral position by aligning the long axes of the third metacarpal and the midforearm parallel with the IR. Center the central ray with the wrist joint, which is located just proximal to the trapezium.

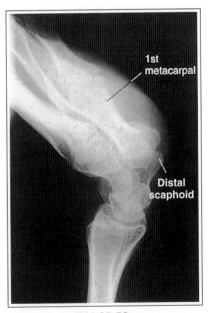

IMAGE 52

Analysis. The first metacarpal is not aligned parallel with the midforearm. The wrist is extended posteriorly.

Correction. If a neutral position is desired, align the first metacarpal parallel with the midforearm. If a wrist extension image was taken to evaluate wrist mobility, no correction movement is required.

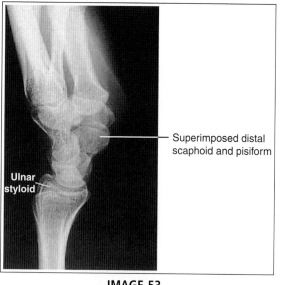

— Superimposed distal scaphoid and pisiform

Ulnar styloid

IMAGE 53

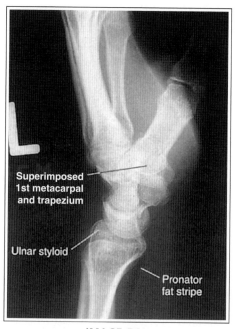

Superimposed 1st metacarpal and trapezium

Ulnar styloid

Pronator fat stripe

IMAGE 54

Analysis. The pisiform and the distal scaphoid are positioned accurately for a lateral wrist projection. The ulnar styloid is not positioned in profile but is demonstrated projecting distally to the midline of the ulnar head. This ulnar positioning indicates that the humerus was positioned without abduction, as shown in Figure 4-42.

Correction. Adjust the patient's humerus to meet your department protocol. If the ulnar styloid is to be demonstrated in profile, abduct the humerus and flex the elbow 90 degrees, placing the forearm and humerus on the same horizontal plane. If department protocol requires that a lateral wrist projection be taken without humeral abduction, no correction movement is needed. Consistency in arm position is important to evaluating ulnar length.

Analysis. The first proximal metacarpal is superimposed over the trapezium. The thumb was not positioned parallel with the midforearm but was pointing upward. The ulnar styloid is not in profile.

Correction. Depress the patient's distal thumb until the metacarpal is aligned parallel with the midforearm. Adjust the patient's humerus to meet your department protocol. If the ulnar styloid is to be demonstrated in profile, abduct the humerus and flex the elbow 90 degrees, placing the forearm and humerus on the same horizontal plane. If department protocol requires that a lateral wrist projection be taken without humeral abduction, no correction movement is needed.

WRIST: ULNAR DEVIATION, POSTEROANTERIOR AXIAL PROJECTION (SCAPHOID)

See Figure 4-43 and Box 4-14.

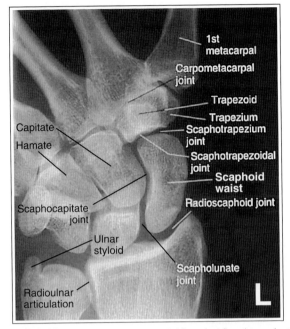

FIGURE 4-43 Ulnar-deviated, PA axial (scaphoid) wrist projection with accurate positioning.

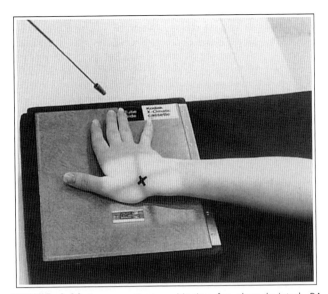

FIGURE 4-44 Proper patient positioning for ulnar-deviated, PA axial (scaphoid) wrist projection. X indicates location of the scaphoid.

BOX 4-14	Posteroanterior Axial (Scaphoid) Wrist Projection Analysis Criteria

- The scaphoid fat stripe is demonstrated.
- The scaphotrapezium and scaphotrapezoidal joint spaces are open.
- The long axis of the first metacarpal and the radius are aligned.
- The scaphocapitate and scapholunate joints are open. The ulnar styloid is in profile medially.
- The radioscaphoid joint space is open.
- The scaphoid is at the center of the exposure field.
- The carpal bones, radiolunar articulation, and proximal first through fourth metacarpals are included within the collimated field.

Contrast and density are adequate to demonstrate the scaphoid fat stripe.

- The scaphoid fat stripe is one of the soft tissue structures that should be visible on all scaphoid images (see Figure 4-30). It is convex and located just lateral to the scaphoid in an uninjured wrist.

The scaphotrapezium and scaphotrapezoidal joint spaces are open.

- To obtain an accurate PA axial (scaphoid) projection, abduct the humerus until it is positioned parallel with the IR and place the elbow in a flexed, lateral position. Then pronate the extended hand, place the wrist in ulnar deviation, and ensure the

wrist is rotated medially approximately 25 degrees (Figure 4-44).
- The scaphotrapezium and scaphotrapezoidal joints are aligned at a 15-degree angle to the IR when the patient's hand is in full extension. These joints will be open when a 15-degree proximally angled central ray is used. If the hand is not extended so that the palm is placed flat against the IR, but rather is flexed, the second metacarpal is superimposed over the trapezoid and trapezium and closes the scaphotrapezium and scaphotrapezoidal joint spaces (see Image 55).

The wrist is in maximum ulnar deviation, as demonstrated by the alignment of the long axis of the first metacarpal and the radius, and the position of the lunate distal to the radius. The scaphoid is demonstrated without foreshortening or excessive elongation. When a scaphoid fracture is indicated, the fracture line is demonstrated.

- To demonstrate the scaphoid without foreshortening, position the patient's wrist in maximum ulnar deviation; then direct a 15-degree proximal (toward the elbow) central ray angulation to the long axis of the scaphoid. Maximum ulnar deviation has been accomplished when the first metacarpal is aligned with the radius. In a neutral PA projection of the nondeviated wrist, the distal scaphoid tilts anteriorly approximately 20 degrees. This tilt results in foreshortening of the scaphoid on the PA axial projection (Figures 4-29 and 4-45). To offset some of this foreshortening and demonstrate more of the scaphoid, place the wrist in ulnar deviation. In ulnar deviation the distal scaphoid moves posteriorly, decreasing the degree of foreshortening by 5 degrees (see Figure 4-45).

Adequate ulnar deviation and central ray angulation place the central ray perpendicular to the long axis of the scaphoid (Figure 4-46). Because 70% of the fractures occur at the waist, most scaphoid fractures should be visualized with this positioning and angulation (see Image 56).

- *Compensating for inadequate ulnar deviation.* Many patients with suspected scaphoid fractures are unable to achieve maximum ulnar wrist deviation. Without adequate ulnar deviation, the distal scaphoid is titled more anteriorly. To compensate

for this increased anterior tilt, the central ray angulation should be increased to approximately 20 degrees to place the central ray and scaphoid long axis perpendicular to each other.

- *Scaphoid elongation.* The goal of the PA axial (scaphoid) projection is to demonstrate the scaphoid with the least amount of foreshortening or elongation. A slight amount of elongation of the scaphoid occurs on PA axial projections because the IR is not positioned parallel with the long axis of the scaphoid and the central ray is not aligned perpendicularly with the IR (Figure 4-46). Excessive elongation of the scaphoid results when the central ray is angled more than needed to align it perpendicularly to the long axis of the scaphoid.

- *Mechanics of scaphoid fracture.* The scaphoid is the most commonly fractured carpal bone. One reason for this is its location among the other carpal bones. Two rows of carpal bones exist, a distal row and a proximal row, with joint spaces between them that allow the wrist to flex. The long scaphoid bone, however, is aligned partially with both these rows, with no joint space. When an individual falls on an outstretched hand, the wrist is hyperextended, causing the proximal and distal carpal rows to flex at the joints, and a great deal of stress is placed on the narrow waist of the scaphoid. This stress may result in a fracture.

- Three areas of the scaphoid may be fractured: the waist, which sustains approximately 70% of the fractures; the distal end, which sustains 20% of the fractures; and the proximal end, which sustains 10% (Figure 4-47). Because scaphoid fractures can be at different locations on the scaphoid, precise

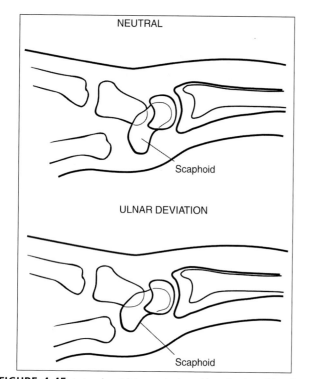

FIGURE 4-45 Lateral wrist in neutral position *(top)* and in ulnar flexion *(bottom)*.

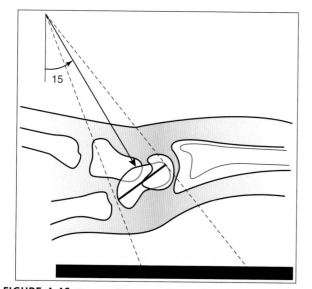

FIGURE 4-46 Proper alignment of central ray *(CR)* and fracture.

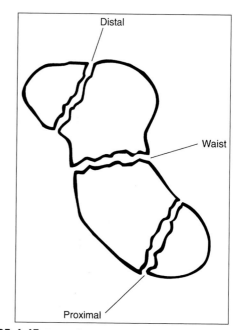

FIGURE 4-47 Poor alignment of central ray *(CR)* and fracture.

positioning and central ray angulation are essential to obtain the optimum demonstration of this bone.

- *Demonstrating fractures of distal and proximal scaphoid.* When a fracture is suspected because of persistent pain and obliteration of the fat stripe but has not been demonstrated on routine images, it may be necessary to use different angles to position the central ray parallel with these fractures sites (Figure 4-48). A decrease of 5 to 10 degrees in central ray angulation better demonstrates the proximal scaphoid. Compare Figures 4-49 and 4-50.

These PA axial projections demonstrate a proximal fracture. Figure 4-49 was taken with the typical 15-degree proximal angle, and Figure 4-50 was taken with a 5-degree proximal angle. Note the increase in fracture line visualization in Figure 4-50. Increase the central ray angle by 5 to 10 degrees, with a maximum of 25 degrees, to demonstrate a distal scaphoid fracture best (Figure 4-51). Angulations more than 25 degrees project the proximal second metacarpal onto the distal scaphoid, obscuring the area of interest (see Image 57).

The scaphocapitate and scapholunate joints are open. The ulnar styloid is in profile medially.

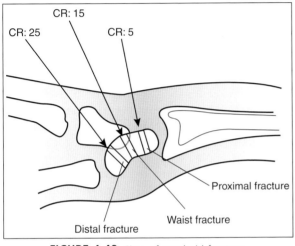

FIGURE 4-48 Sites of scaphoid fracture.

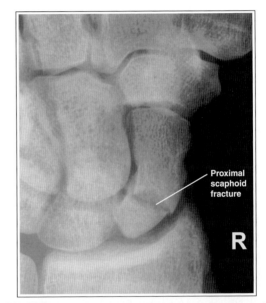

FIGURE 4-50 PA axial (scaphoid) projection taken with a 5-degree proximal central ray angle demonstrating a proximal scaphoid fracture.

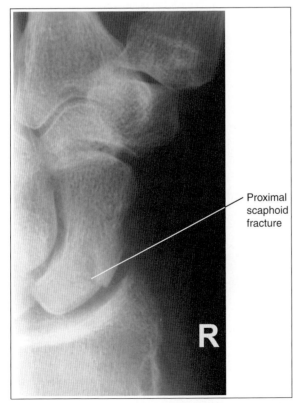

FIGURE 4-49 PA axial (scaphoid) projection taken with a 15-degree proximal central ray angle demonstrating a proximal scaphoid fracture.

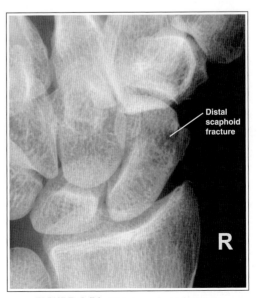

FIGURE 4-51 Distal scaphoid fracture.

- The scaphocapitate and scapholunate joints are open when the wrist is medially rotated approximately 25 degrees. This obliquity is accomplished somewhat naturally as the patient's wrist is ulnardeviated, with the humerus abducted and positioned parallel with the IR, and the elbow placed in a flexed lateral projection. If the scaphocapitate joint space is closed and the capitate and hamate are demonstrated without superimposition, the degree of obliquity was insufficient (see Image 58). If the scapholunate joint space is closed and the capitate and hamate demonstrate some degree of superimposition, the wrist was rotated more than needed (see Image 59). Excessive external wrist obliquity often occurs when the humerus and forearm are not positioned on the same horizontal plane and the elbow is not placed in a lateral projection. On a PA axial projection, one can judge accurate humerus, forearm, and elbow positioning by evaluating the ulnar styloid. Accurate positioning places the ulnar styloid in profile medially. If the arm is not positioned accurately, the ulnar styloid is demonstrated distal to the midline of the ulnar head (see Image 60).

The radioscaphoid joint space is open.

- The distal radial carpal articular surface is concave and slants approximately 11 degrees from posterior to anterior when the forearm is positioned parallel with the IR. On a PA projection without a central ray angulation, the posterior radial margin is demonstrated slightly distal to the anterior margin if the forearm is placed parallel with the IR. When a 15-degree proximal central ray angulation is used for the PA axial (scaphoid) projection, the posterior margin is projected slightly proximal to the anterior margin (Figure 4-52). To demonstrate an open radioscaphoid joint, the

anterior and posterior margins of the distal radius should be superimposed. This superimposition is accomplished by elevating the proximal forearm very slightly (2 degrees) above the distal forearm.

The scaphoid is at the center of the exposure field. The carpal bones, the radioulnar articulation, and the proximal first through fourth metacarpals are included within the collimated field.

- To place the scaphoid at the center of the collimated field, center the central ray with the scaphoid. In ulnar deviation, the scaphoid can be palpated halfway between the first metacarpal base and the radial styloid. After the central ray is centered, open the longitudinal collimation to include the first through fourth metacarpal bases and the distal radius. Transversely collimate to within 0.5 inch (1.25 cm) of the wrist skin line.

  Avoid collimating too tightly. It is difficult to determine how to reposition the patient when an image reveals poor positioning if key anatomic structures are not included.

- Half of an 8- × 10-inch (18- × 24-cm) detailed screen-film or computed radiography IR placed crosswise should be adequate to include all the required anatomic structures.

Posteroanterior Axial (Scaphoid) Projection Analysis

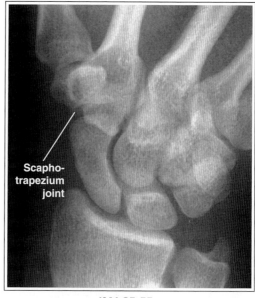

IMAGE 55

Analysis. The scaphotrapezium, scaphotrapezoidal, and CM joint spaces are closed. The hand and fingers were not positioned flat against the IR.

Correction. Extend the patient's fingers, placing the hand flat against the IR.

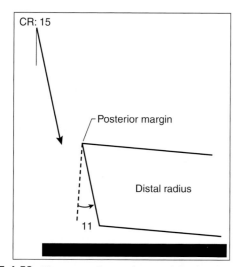

FIGURE 4-52 Alignment of central ray and distal radius to obtain open radioscaphoid joint.

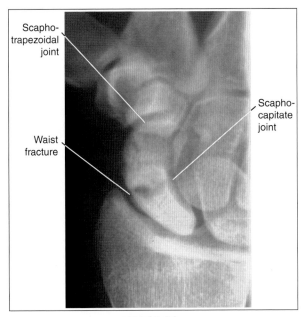

IMAGE 56

Analysis. This image demonstrates a scaphoid waist fracture. The scaphotrapezium, scaphotrapezoidal, and CM joint spaces are closed. The hand and fingers were not positioned flat against the IR. The scaphocapitate and radioscaphoid joints are closed, indicating that the degree of obliquity was inadequate and the proximal forearm was slightly depressed, respectively.

Correction. Extend the patient's fingers, placing the hand flat against the IR, and slightly increase the amount of external wrist obliquity and elevate the proximal forearm.

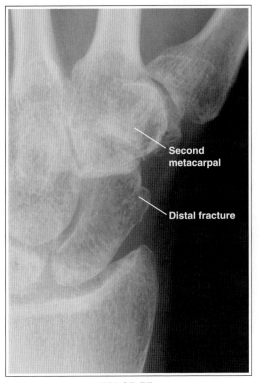

IMAGE 57

Analysis. A 30-degree proximal central ray angle was used, with the hand and fingers positioned flat against the IR. A distal scaphoid fracture is present. The proximal first metacarpal is superimposed over the distal scaphoid, and the radioscaphoid joint is closed. The central ray angulation was too great, and the proximal forearm was slightly depressed.

Correction. To demonstrate a distal scaphoid fracture best, decrease the amount of central ray angulation. A maximum 25-degree angle should be used to demonstrate a distal scaphoid fracture. Compare this image with one shown in Figure 4-51, which was taken on the same patient with a 25-degree angle. Slightly elevate the proximal forearm to open the radioscaphoid joint.

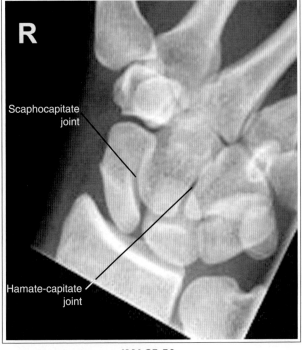

IMAGE 58

Analysis. The scaphocapitate joint is closed and the hamate-capitate joint is open. The wrist was not externally rotated enough.

Correction. Increase the degree of external wrist rotation.

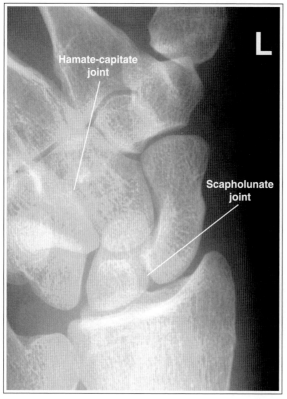

IMAGE 59

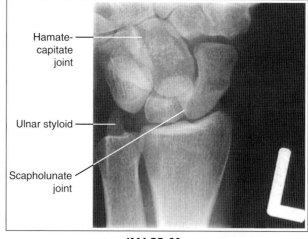

Correction. Decrease the amount of external wrist rotation.

IMAGE 60

Analysis. The scapholunate and hamate-capitate joints are closed. The wrist was externally rotated more than needed. The styloid process is demonstrated distal to the ulnar head midline. The humerus was not abducted with the elbow in a flexed lateral projection. The scaphoid is not in the center of the field, and the proximal metacarpals are not included on the image.

Correction. Decrease the amount of external wrist rotation and abduct the humerus, placing the elbow in a flexed lateral projection. Move the central ray 0.5 inch (1.25 cm) distally.

Analysis. The scapholunate and hamate-capitate joints are closed. The wrist was externally rotated more than needed.

WRIST CARPAL CANAL: TANGENTIAL, INFEROSUPERIOR PROJECTION

See Figure 4-53 and Box 4-15.

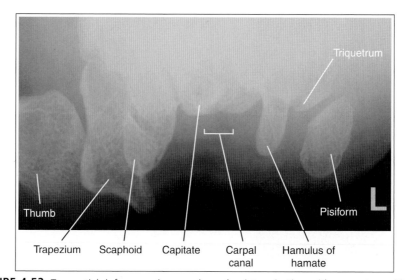

FIGURE 4-53 Tangential, inferosuperior carpal canal wrist projection with accurate positioning.

BOX 4-15 **Tangential, Inferosuperior Carpal Canal Wrist Projection Analysis Criteria**

- The pisiform is demonstrated without superimposition of the hamulus of the hamate, and the carpal canal is clearly demonstrated.
- The carpal canal is visualized in its entirety, and the carpal bones are demonstrated with only slight elongation.
- The carpal canal is at the center of the exposure field.
- The trapezium, distal scaphoid, pisiform and hamulus of the hamate are included within the collimated field.

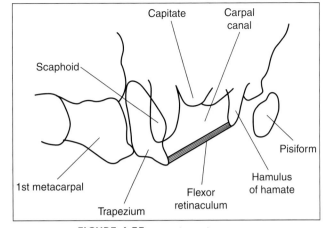

FIGURE 4-55 Carpal canal anatomy.

The pisiform is demonstrated without superimposition of the hamulus of the hamate, and the carpal canal is clearly demonstrated.

- The tangential, inferosuperior carpal canal wrist projection is accomplished by placing the distal forearm and wrist on the IR in a PA projection, and then hyperextending (dorsiflexing) the wrist until the long axis of the metacarpals are close to vertical while the wrist remains in contact with the IR. To obtain adequate wrist hyperextension, have the patient grasp his or her fingers with the opposite hand and gently pull them posteriorly (Figure 4-54).
- The tangential, inferosuperior carpal canal projection is used to evaluate the carpal canal for the narrowing that results in carpal canal syndrome and demonstrate fractures of the pisiform and hamulus of the hamate. The carpal canal is a passageway formed anteriorly by the flexor retinaculum, posteriorly by the capitate, laterally by the scaphoid and trapezium, and medially by the pisiform and hamate (Figure 4-55). Fractures of the pisiform and hamulus process are best demonstrated when they are seen without superimposition. This is accomplished by rotating the patient's

hand 10 degrees internally (toward the radial side) until the fifth metacarpal is aligned perpendicularly to the IR. If the hand is not internally rotated, the pisiform will be superimposed over the hamulus process on the resulting image (see Image 61).

The carpal canal is visualized in its entirety, and the carpal bones are demonstrated with only slight elongation.

- To show the carpal canal and demonstrate the carpals with only slight elongation, the patient's hand is positioned vertically, and the central ray is angled proximally (toward the palmar surface). The degree of central ray angulation that is needed will depend on how vertical the patient can bring the hand. To determine the angle to use, adjust the central ray proximally until it is aligned at a 15-degree angle with the palmar surface (Figure 4-56). The most common tube angle used is 25 to 30 degrees.
- *Immaculate angle.* If the angle between the central ray and palmar surface is too great, the carpal canal will not be fully demonstrated and the carpal bones will be foreshortened (see Image 62). If the angle between the central ray and palmar surface is too small, the bases of the hamulus process, pisiform, and scaphoid are obscured by the metacarpal bases (see Image 63).
- *Insufficient wrist extension.* When imaging a patient who is unable to extend the wrist enough to place the palmar surface even close to vertical, the resulting image will demonstrate adequate visualization of the carpal bones and carpal canal, although there will be increased elongation as the angle between the central ray and IR becomes more acute (see Image 64).

The carpal canal is at the center of the exposure field. The trapezium, distal scaphoid, pisiform, and hamulus of the hamate are included within the collimated field.

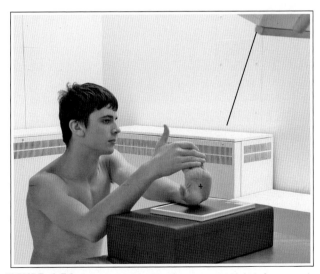

FIGURE 4-54 Proper positioning for a tangential, inferosuperior carpal canal wrist projection.

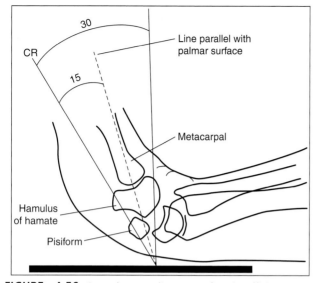

FIGURE 4-56 Central ray alignment for insufficient wrist extension.

- The carpal canal is positioned in the center of the collimated field by centering the central ray to center of the palm of the hand. After the central ray is centered, open the longitudinal and transverse collimations to within 0.5 inch (1.25 cm) of the wrist skin line.
- Half of an 8- × 10-inch (18- × 24-cm) detailed screen-film or computed IR placed crosswise should be adequate to include all the required anatomic structures.

Tangential, Inferosuperior Carpal Canal Wrist Projection Analysis

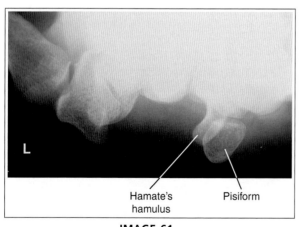

IMAGE 61

Analysis. The pisiform is superimposed over the hamulus of the hamate. The patient's wrist and distal forearm were either in a PA projection or in slight external (toward the ulnar side) rotation.

Correction. Rotate the hand internally (toward the radius) until the fifth metacarpal is vertical.

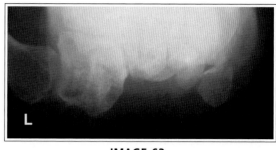

IMAGE 62

Analysis. The carpal canal is not demonstrated in its entirety, and the carpal bones are foreshortened. The angle between the central ray and palmar surface was too great.

Correction. Decrease the central ray angle until it is at a 15-degree angle with the palmar surface (Figure 4-56).

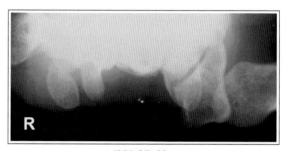

IMAGE 63

Analysis. The metacarpal bases obscure the bases of the hamate's hamulus process, pisiform, and scaphoid. The angle between the central ray and palmar surface was too small.

Correction. Increase the central ray angle until it is at a 15-degree angle with the palmar surface (Figure 4-56), or increase the amount of wrist hyperextension by pulling the fingers posteriorly until the metacarpals are vertical.

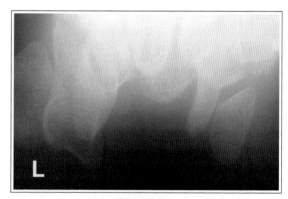

IMAGE 64

Analysis. The carpal bones and carpal canal demonstrate excessive elongation because the angle formed between the central ray and IR was too acute.

Correction. Increase the amount of wrist hyperextension by having the patient pull the fingers posteriorly until the palmar surface is as vertical as possible and then angle the central ray proximally until it is at a 15-degree angle with the palmar surface.

FOREARM: ANTEROPOSTERIOR PROJECTION

See Figure 4-57 and Box 4-16.

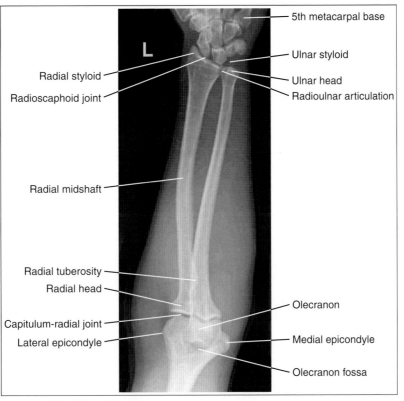

FIGURE 4-57 AP forearm projection with accurate positioning.

Image density is uniform across entire forearm.

- *Anode heel effect.* To use the anode heel effect to obtain uniform density across the forearm, position the thinner wrist (distal forearm) at the anode end of the tube and the thicker elbow (proximal forearm) at the cathode end. Set an exposure (mAs) that will adequately demonstrate the midpoint of the forearm.

The long axis of the forearm is aligned with the long axis of the collimated field.

- Aligning the long axis of the forearm with the long axis of the collimated field enables you to collimate tightly without clipping the distal or proximal forearm.

The forearm midpoint is at the center of the exposure field. The wrist and elbow joints and forearm soft tissue are included within the collimated field.

- A perpendicular central ray is centered to the midpoint of the forearm to place it in the center of the image.
- When the wrist and elbow joints are included on the image, the degree of radiation beam divergence used to image a long body part needs to be considered (Figure 4-58).

BOX 4-16	**Anteroposterior Forearm Projection Analysis Criteria**

- Image density is uniform across entire forearm.
- The long axis of the forearm is aligned with the long axis of collimated field.
- The forearm midpoint is at the center of the exposure field.
- The wrist and elbow joints and forearm soft tissue are included within the collimated field.
- The radial styloid is demonstrated in profile laterally, and superimposition of the metacarpal bases and of the radius and ulna is minimal.
- The ulnar styloid is projected distally to the midline of the ulnar head.
- The anterior and posterior carpal articulating surfaces of the distal radius are superimposed, and the radioscaphoid and radiolunate joint spaces are open.
- The radial head is superimposed over the lateral aspect of the proximal ulna by about 0.25 inch (0.6 cm).
- The capitulum-radius joint is either partially or completely closed, and the radial head articulating surface is demonstrated. Olecranon process is situated within the olecranon fossa, and the coronoid process is visible on end.
- The radial tuberosity is demonstrated in profile medially, and the radius and ulna appear parallel.

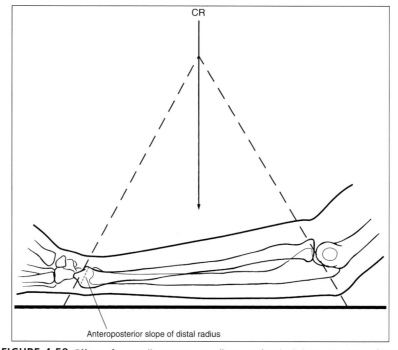

CR

Anteroposterior slope of distal radius

FIGURE 4-58 Effect of x-ray divergence on elbow and wrist joints. *CR*, Central ray.

- *IR length for the forearm.* Choose an IR that is long enough to allow at least 1 inch (2.5 cm) of IR to extend beyond each joint space; half of a 14- × 17-inch (35- × 44-cm) IR placed lengthwise should be adequate. To ensure that the IR extends beyond the elbow joint, palpate the medial epicondyle, which is located approximately 0.75 inch (2 cm) proximal to the elbow joint. To ensure that the IR extends beyond the wrist joint, palpate the base of the first metacarpal; the wrist joint is located just proximal to this base. Digital imaging requires tight collimation without overlapping of individual exposures.
- *Central ray centering and collimation.* Once the forearm is accurately positioned in relation to the IR, center the central ray with the midpoint of the forearm and open the longitudinal collimation field until it extends just beyond the elbow and the wrist. If the collimation does not extend beyond the joints, adjust the centering point of the central ray until both the elbow and the wrist joint are included within the collimated field without demonstrating an excessive field beyond them. Transverse collimation should be within 0.5 inch (1.25 cm) of the forearm skin line.

Distal Forearm Positioning

The distal and proximal forearm is positioned in an AP projection. The radial styloid is demonstrated in profile laterally, and superimposition of the metacarpal bases and of the radius and ulna is minimal.

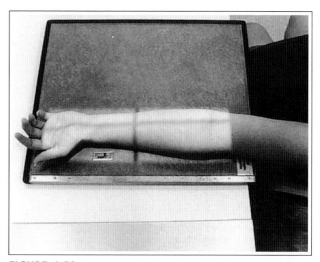

FIGURE 4-59 Proper positioning for an AP forearm projection.

- To obtain an AP projection of the distal forearm, supinate the hand and place the second through fifth metacarpal heads against the IR (Figure 4-59).
- *Detecting distal forearm rotation.* Rotation of the distal forearm results from inaccurate positioning of the hand and wrist. If the wrist and hand are not positioned in an AP projection but are rotated, the radial styloid is no longer in profile and the distal radius and ulna and metacarpal bases are superimposed. To identify which way the wrist is rotated, evaluate the metacarpal and carpal bones. When the wrist and hand are internally rotated, the laterally located first and second

metacarpal bases and carpal bones are superimposed, and the medially located metacarpals, pisiform, and hamate hook are better demonstrated (see Images 65 and 67). If the wrist and hand are externally rotated, the medially located fourth and fifth metacarpal bases and carpal bones will be superimposed, whereas the laterally located metacarpals and carpal bones will demonstrate less superimposition.

- *Distal forearm positioning for fracture.* Patients with known or suspected fractures may be unable to position both the wrist and elbow joints into an AP projection simultaneously. In such cases, position the joint closer to the fracture in a true position. When the fracture is situated closer to the wrist joint, the wrist joint and distal forearm should meet the requirements for an AP projection, but the elbow and proximal forearm may demonstrate an AP oblique or lateral projection. It may be necessary to position the distal forearm in a PA projection when an AP projection is difficult for the patient. The wrist joint and distal forearm should still be positioned as described earlier (see Image 66).

The ulnar styloid is projected distally to the midline of the ulnar head.

- The position of the ulnar styloid is determined by the position of the humerus and elbow. When the humerus and elbow positions are adjusted but the wrist position is maintained, it is the ulna that rotates and changes position. Positioning the humeral epicondyles parallel with the IR for the AP projection of the forearm places the ulnar styloid posterior to the head of the ulna. If the elbow is rotated internally and the wrist remains in an AP projection, the ulnar styloid is demonstrated laterally, next to the radius. If the elbow is rotated externally and the wrist remains in an AP projection, the ulnar styloid is demonstrated in profile medially.

The anterior and posterior carpal articulating surfaces of the distal radius are superimposed, and the radioscaphoid and radiolunate joint spaces are open.

- The distal radial carpal articular surface is concave and slants at approximately 11 degrees from posterior to anterior. When the forearm is placed parallel with the IR in an AP projection and the central ray is centered to the midforearm, diverged x-rays record the image much as if the central ray were angled toward the wrist joint. If this angle of divergence is parallel with the AP slant of the distal radius, the resulting image shows superimposed distal radial margins and open radioscaphoid and radiolunate joint spaces.

Proximal Forearm Positioning

The proximal forearm is positioned in an AP projection. The radial head is superimposed over the lateral aspect of the proximal ulna by approximately 0.25 inch (0.6 cm). If included on the IR, the medial and lateral humeral epicondyles are demonstrated in profile at the extreme medial and lateral edges of the distal humerus.

- An AP proximal forearm projection is obtained by palpating the humeral epicondyles and aligning them parallel with the IR, placing the proximal radius anterior to the ulna (see Figure 4-59).
- *Detecting proximal forearm rotation:* Proximal forearm rotation results when the humeral epicondyles are poorly positioned. Rotation can be identified on the image when the radial head demonstrates more or less than 0.25 inch (0.6 cm) superimposition on the ulna and when the humeral epicondyles are not visualized in profile. When more than 0.25 inch (0.6 cm) of the radial head is superimposed over the ulna, the elbow has been internally rotated (see Image 74). When less than 0.25 inch (0.6 cm) of radial head is superimposed over the ulna, the elbow has been externally rotated (see Image 67).
- *Proximal forearm positioning for fracture.* Patients with known or suspected fractures may be unable to position both the wrist and elbow joint into an AP projection simultaneously. In such cases, position the joint closer to the fracture in the truer position. When the fracture is situated closer to the elbow joint, the elbow joint and proximal forearm should meet the requirements for an AP projection, whereas the wrist and distal forearm may demonstrate obliquity.

The capitulum-radius joint is either partially or completely closed, and the radial head articulating surface is demonstrated. The olecranon process is situated within the olecranon fossa, and the coronoid process is visible on end.

- The anatomical relationships of the elbow on an AP forearm projection are slightly different from those on an AP elbow projection because of the difference in centering of the central ray. The central ray is placed directly over the elbow joint for an AP elbow projection but is centered distally to the elbow joint, at the midforearm, for an AP forearm projection. With distal centering, diverged rays record the elbow joint image instead of straight central rays, much the same as if the central ray were angled toward the elbow joint. Imaging the elbow with diverged rays projects the radial head into the capitulum-radius joint and causes the anterior margin of the radial head to

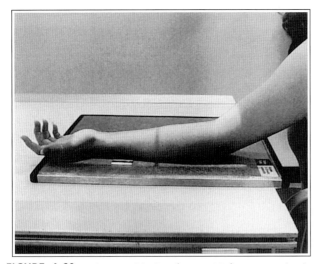

FIGURE 4-60 Patient positioning for an AP forearm projection with flexed humerus.

project beyond the posterior margin, demonstrating its articulating surface.

- *Effect of elbow flexion.* The positions of the olecranon process and fossa and the coronoid process are determined by the amount of elbow flexion. Accurate forearm positioning requires us to position the elbow in full extension, which places the olecranon process within the olecranon fossa and demonstrates the coronoid process on end. When a forearm image is taken with the elbow flexed and the proximal humerus elevated (Figure 4-60), the olecranon process moves away from the olecranon fossa and the coronoid process shifts proximally. How far the olecranon process is from the fossa depends on the degree of elbow flexion. The greater the elbow flexion, the farther the olecranon process is positioned away from the fossa and the more foreshortened is the distal humerus.

The radial tuberosity is demonstrated in profile medially, and the radius and ulna appear parallel.

- When the distal humerus is positioned with the epicondyles parallel with the IR, the relationship of the radius and ulna is controlled by wrist positioning. To place the radius and ulna parallel and the radial tuberosity in profile medially, position the wrist and hand in an AP projection. When the hand and wrist are pronated, the radius crosses over the ulna, and the radial tuberosity is rotated posteriorly, out of profile (see Image 68).

Anteroposterior Forearm Projection Analysis

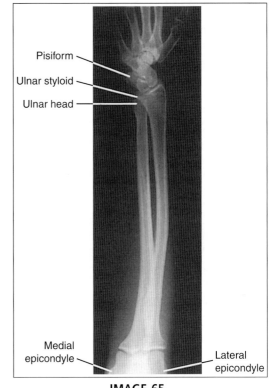

Pisiform

Ulnar styloid

Ulnar head

Medial epicondyle

Lateral epicondyle

IMAGE 65

Analysis. The humeral epicondyles are demonstrated in profile, and the ulnar styloid is demonstrated distal to the midline of the ulnar head. The elbow has been accurately positioned. The first and second metacarpal bases and the laterally located carpal bones are superimposed, and the medially located carpal bones and pisiform are well demonstrated. The radial styloid is not visible in profile. The wrist was internally rotated.

Correction. While maintaining the AP projection of the elbow, rotate the wrist and hand externally until the hand is supinated and the wrist is in an AP projection.

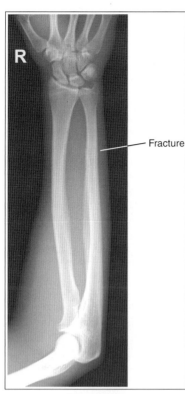

IMAGE 66

Analysis. A fracture is located at the distal forearm. The wrist demonstrates a PA projection, whereas the elbow is in a lateral projection.

Correction. Because the joint closer to the fracture is in the true projection, no repositioning movement is needed.

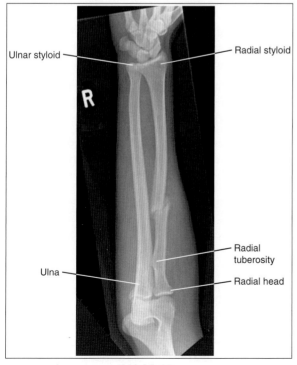

IMAGE 67

Analysis. The radial styloid is not demonstrated in profile, the laterally located first and second metacarpal bases and carpal bones are superimposed, and the medially located carpals are better demonstrated. The wrist was internally rotated. Less than 0.25 inch (0.6 cm) of the radial head is superimposed over the ulna. The elbow was externally rotated.

Correction. Rotate the wrist and hand externally until they are in an AP projection, and rotate the elbow internally until the humeral epicondyles are parallel with the IR.

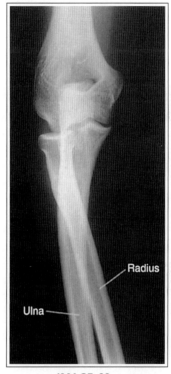

IMAGE 68

Analysis. The radius and ulna are not parallel. The radius is crossed over the ulna, and the radial tuberosity is not demonstrated in profile. For this image, the elbow is in an AP projection but the wrist and hand are positioned in a PA projection. The distal forearm and wrist joint were not included on the image.

Correction. While maintaining an AP projection of the elbow, externally rotate the wrist and hand until they are in an AP projection. Center the central ray more distally, and open the longitudinal collimation to include the wrist joint.

FOREARM: LATERAL PROJECTION (LATEROMEDIAL)

See Figure 4-61 and Box 4-17.

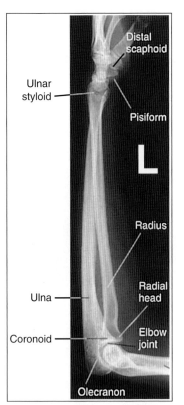

FIGURE 4-61 Lateral forearm projection with accurate positioning.

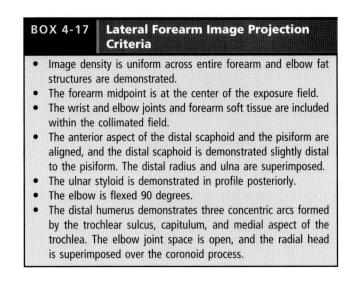

BOX 4-17	*Lateral Forearm Image Projection Criteria*

- Image density is uniform across entire forearm and elbow fat structures are demonstrated.
- The forearm midpoint is at the center of the exposure field.
- The wrist and elbow joints and forearm soft tissue are included within the collimated field.
- The anterior aspect of the distal scaphoid and the pisiform are aligned, and the distal scaphoid is demonstrated slightly distal to the pisiform. The distal radius and ulna are superimposed.
- The ulnar styloid is demonstrated in profile posteriorly.
- The elbow is flexed 90 degrees.
- The distal humerus demonstrates three concentric arcs formed by the trochlear sulcus, capitulum, and medial aspect of the trochlea. The elbow joint space is open, and the radial head is superimposed over the coronoid process.

Density is uniform across the entire forearm, and contrast and density are adequate to demonstrate the elbow fat structures.

- *Anode heel effect.* To use the anode heel effect to obtain uniform density across the forearm, position the thinner wrist (distal forearm) at the anode end of the tube and the thicker elbow (proximal forearm) at the cathode end. Set an exposure (mAs) that will adequately demonstrate the midpoint of the forearm.
- *Soft tissue structures on lateral forearm projection.* Soft tissue structures of interest are the anterior and posterior fat pads and the supinator fat stripe at the elbow and pronator fat stripe at the wrist (Figure 4-62). The elbow's anterior fat pad is situated anterior to the distal humerus, and the elbow's supinator fat stripe is visible parallel to the anterior aspect of the proximal radius. A change in the shape or placement of these fat structures indicates joint effusion and elbow injury. The elbow's posterior fat pad is normally obscured on a negative lateral forearm image because of its location within the olecranon fossa. On elbow injury, joint effusion pushes this pad out of the fossa, allowing it to be visualized proximally and posterior to the olecranon process. The wrist's pronator fat stripe is demonstrated parallel to the anterior surface of the distal radius. Bowing or obliteration of this fat stripe may be the only indication of subtle radial fractures.

The forearm midpoint is at the center of the exposure field. The radius and ulna, wrist and elbow joints, and forearm soft tissue are included within the collimated field.

- A perpendicular central ray is centered to the midpoint of the forearm to place the forearm in the center of the image.

When the wrist and elbow joints are included on the image, the degree of radiation beam divergence used to image a long body part needs to be considered (Figure 4-63).

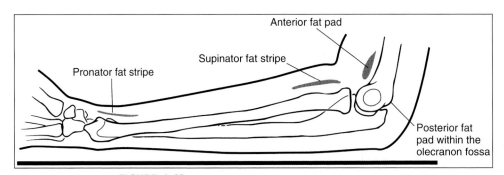

FIGURE 4-62 Placement of wrist and elbow soft tissue.

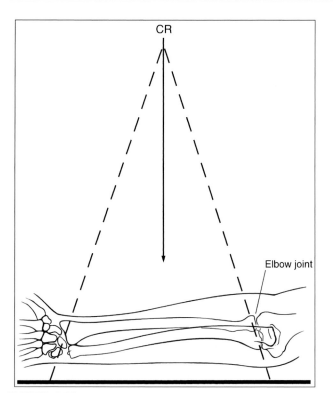

FIGURE 4-63 Alignment of x-ray divergence on distal forearm. *CR*, Central ray.

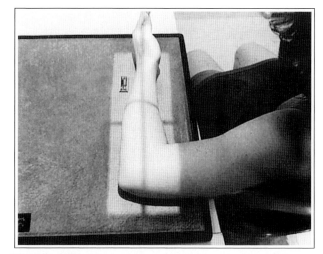

FIGURE 4-64 Proper patient positioning for lateral forearm projection.

- *IR length for the forearm.* Choose an IR that is long enough to allow at least 1 inch (2.5 cm) of IR to extend beyond each joint space; half of a 14- × 17-inch (35- × 44-cm) screen-film or computed radiography IR placed lengthwise should be adequate. To ensure that the IR extends beyond the elbow, palpate the medial epicondyle, which is located 0.75 inch (2 cm) proximal to the elbow joint. To ensure that the IR extends beyond the wrist joint, palpate the base of the first metacarpal; the wrist joint is located just proximal to this base.
- *Central ray centering and collimation.* Once the forearm is accurately positioned in relation to the IR, center the central ray to the midpoint of the forearm, and open the longitudinal collimation field until it extends just beyond the elbow and wrist joints. If collimation does not extend beyond the joints, adjust the centering point of the central ray until both the elbow and the wrist joint are included within the collimated field without demonstrating an excessive field beyond them. Transverse collimation should be within 0.5 inch (1.25 cm) of the forearm skin line.

Distal Forearm Positioning

The distal forearm is in a lateral projection. The anterior aspects of the distal scaphoid and pisiform are aligned with each other, and the distal scaphoid is demonstrated slightly distal to the pisiform. The distal radius and ulna are superimposed.

- A lateral wrist and distal forearm projection is obtained by externally rotating the wrist into a lateral projection with its ulnar aspect against the IR (Figure 4-64). To ensure true lateral positioning, place the palmar aspect of your thumb and forefinger against the anterior and posterior aspects of the patient's wrist joint. Then adjust the rotation until your thumb and finger are aligned perpendicularly to the IR.
- *Distal forearm positioning for fracture.* Patients with known or suspected fractures may be unable to position both the wrist and elbow joint into a lateral projection simultaneously. In such cases, position the joint closer to the fracture in a true position and position the other joint as close as possible to the true position (see Image 69).
- *Verifying a lateral forearm projection.* The pisiform and distal scaphoid relationship can be used to discern whether a true lateral wrist and distal forearm are demonstrated. On a lateral forearm projection with accurate positioning, these two bones should be visible anterior to the capitate and lunate, with their anterior aspects aligned and the distal scaphoid projecting distally to the pisiform. It is the diverged x-ray beams used to image the pisiform and scaphoid that cause the distal scaphoid to be projected distally to the pisiform. When the wrist and distal forearm are rotated, the anterior alignment of the scaphoid and pisiform, as well as of the radius and ulna, changes. If the wrist and distal forearm have been externally rotated, the pisiform is visible anterior to the distal scaphoid, and the ulna appears

anterior to the radius. The radial tuberosity will also be visible anteriorly if the elbow is placed in a true lateral projection (see Image 70). If the wrist and distal forearm have been internally rotated, the distal scaphoid is visible anterior to the pisiform and the radius appears anterior to the ulna (see Image 71).

The ulnar styloid is demonstrated in profile posteriorly.

- When the humerus and elbow are mispositioned, the placement of the ulna changes. The ulnar styloid is put in profile by placing the elbow in a lateral position and abducting the humerus until it is parallel with the IR, aligning the entire arm on the same horizontal plane. If the humerus is not abducted, nor the elbow positioned laterally, the ulnar styloid is positioned medially, out of profile.

Proximal Forearm and Distal Humerus Positioning

Elbow is flexed 90 degrees.

- When the elbow is flexed 90 degrees, displacement of the anterior or posterior fat pads can be used as a sign to determine diagnosis. Poor elbow positioning, however, also displaces these fat pads and consequently simulates joint pathology. When the elbow is extended, nonpathologic displacement of the anterior and posterior fat pads may result from intraarticular pressure and the olecranon's position within the olecranon fossa.

The distal humerus is in a lateral projection. The distal humerus demonstrates three concentric (having the same center) arcs, formed by the trochlear sulcus, capitulum, and medial aspect of the trochlea. The elbow joint space is open, and the radial head is superimposed over the coronoid process.

- A lateral proximal forearm projection is obtained by placing the elbow in a lateral projection and abducting the humerus until it is parallel with the IR, thereby putting the entire arm on the same horizontal plane. The wrist and hand are then placed in a lateral projection, and the medial (ulnar) aspect of the forearm rests against the IR (see Figure 4-64). Even though the capitulum is placed anterior to the medial trochlea and the humeral epicondyles are not superimposed for this position, an open joint space may still be obtained. Because the central ray is centered to the midforearm, the diverged x-rays used to image the distal humerus align parallel with the slant of the capitulum and medial trochlea (see Figure 4-63). The result of this parallelism is an open elbow joint space.
- *Effect of muscular or thick forearm.* Because the patient's forearm rests on its ulnar surface, the size

of the proximal and distal forearm affects the appearance of the elbow joint space. For a patient with a muscular or thick proximal forearm, which is therefore elevated higher than the distal forearm, the capitulum is positioned too far anteriorly and the medial trochlea too posteriorly to align with the x-ray beam divergence. The resulting image demonstrates a closed elbow joint space, and the radial head is positioned distal to the coronoid process (see Image 72).

- *Forearm and humeral positioning for fracture.* Patients with known or suspected fractures may be unable to position both the wrist and elbow joint into a lateral projection simultaneously. In such cases, position the joint closer to the fracture in the true position. When the fracture is situated closer to the elbow joint, the elbow joint and proximal forearm should meet the requirements for a lateral projection, whereas the wrist and distal forearm should be positioned as close as possible to a lateral projection.
- *Effect of poor humeral positioning.* Misalignment of the capitulum and medial trochlea, as well as of the radial head and coronoid process, is also the result of poor humeral positioning. When the distal surface of the capitulum appears quite distal to the distal surface of the medial trochlea and the radial head is positioned posterior to the coronoid process, the proximal humerus was elevated (Figure 4-65; see Image 73). When the distal surface of the capitulum appears proximal to the distal surface of the medial trochlea and the radial head is positioned too anteriorly on the coronoid process, the proximal humerus was positioned lower than the distal humerus.

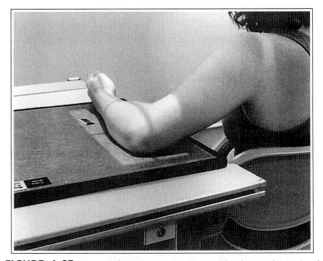

FIGURE 4-65 Lateral forearm projection with elevated proximal humerus.

Lateral Forearm Projection Analysis

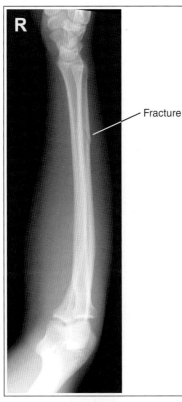

IMAGE 69

Analysis. A fracture is located at the distal forearm. The wrist demonstrates a lateral projection, but the elbow is rotated.

Correction. Because the joint closer to the fracture is in the true lateral projection, no repositioning movement is needed.

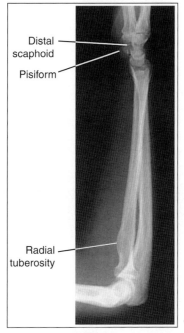

Distal scaphoid

Pisiform

Radial tuberosity

IMAGE 70

Analysis. On this image the elbow has been accurately positioned. The pisiform is demonstrated anterior to the scaphoid and the radial tuberosity is shown anteriorly in profile, indicating that the wrist and distal forearm were slightly externally rotated.

Correction. While maintaining accurate elbow positioning, internally rotate the wrist and distal forearm into a lateral position. This movement will rotate the scaphoid toward the pisiform, aligning their anterior aspects.

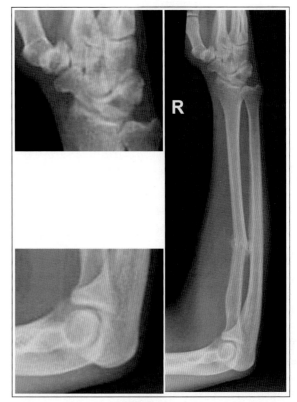

R

IMAGE 71

Analysis. The distal scaphoid is anterior to the pisiform and the radius is anterior to the ulna, indicating that the wrist and hand were internally rotated.

Correction. If the patient is able, externally rotate the hand and wrist until they are in a true lateral projection. This may not be possible because of the radial fracture.

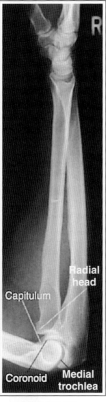

IMAGE 72

Analysis. The capitulum is positioned too far anterior to the medial trochlea, and the radial head is positioned distal to the coronoid process. The proximal forearm was elevated higher than the distal forearm, possibly because the patient has a muscular or thick proximal forearm.

Correction. Raise the distal forearm until the forearm is positioned parallel with the IR, or, if the patient's proximal forearm is muscular or thick, no positioning adjustment is needed.

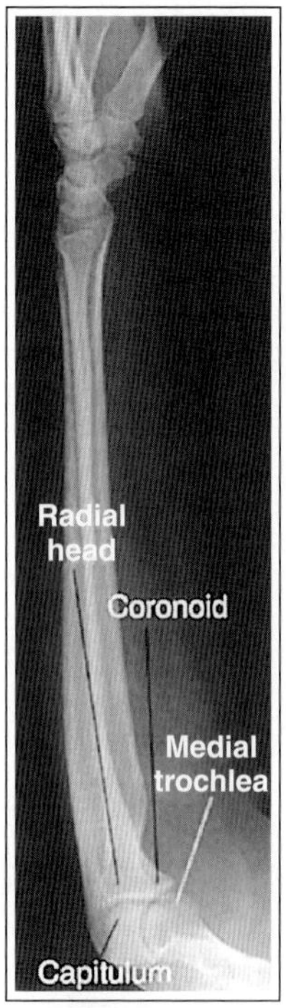

IMAGE 73

Analysis. The wrist is accurately positioned. The distal end of the capitulum is shown distal to the medial trochlea, and the radial head is posterior to the coronoid process. The proximal humerus was elevated as shown in Figure 4-65.

Correction. While maintaining accurate wrist positioning, depress the proximal humerus until the humerus is parallel with the IR.

ELBOW: ANTEROPOSTERIOR PROJECTION

See Figure 4-66 and Box 4-18.

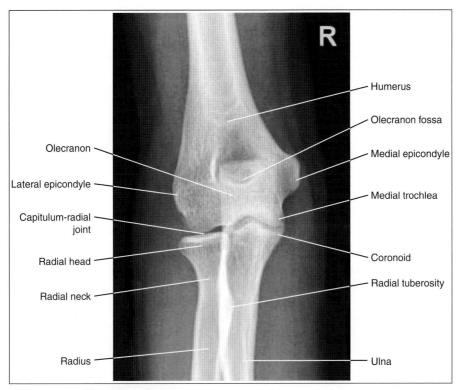

FIGURE 4-66 AP elbow projection with accurate positioning.

| BOX 4-18 | Anteroposterior Elbow Projection Analysis Criteria |

- The medial and lateral humeral epicondyles are demonstrated in profile at the extreme medial and lateral edges of the distal humerus, and the radial head is superimposed over the lateral aspect of the proximal ulna by 0.25 inch (0.6 cm). The coronoid process is demonstrated on end.
- The radial tuberosity is in profile medially, and the radius and ulna are parallel.
- The elbow joint is open, the radial head articulating surface is not demonstrated, and the olecranon process is situated within the olecranon fossa.
- The elbow joint is at the center of the exposure field.
- The elbow joint, one fourth of the proximal forearm and distal humerus, and the lateral soft tissue are included within the collimation field.

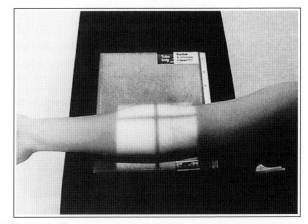

FIGURE 4-67 Proper patient positioning for AP elbow projection.

The elbow is positioned in an AP projection. The medial and lateral humeral epicondyles are demonstrated in profile at the extreme medial and lateral edges of the distal humerus, and the radial head is superimposed over the lateral aspect of the proximal ulna by approximately 0.25 inch (0.6 cm). The coronoid process is demonstrated on end.

- An AP projection of the elbow is obtained by supinating the patient's hand and externally rotating the forearm and humerus until an imaginary line drawn between the humeral epicondyles is parallel with the IR (Figure 4-67). This positioning places the proximal radius anterior to the ulna.
- *Detecting elbow rotation.* Rotation of the elbow is a result of poor humeral epicondyle positioning and can be identified on an image when (1) the

epicondyles are not visualized in profile, (2) the radial head is demonstrated with more or less than 0.25 inch (0.6 cm) superimposition of the ulna, and (3) the coronoid process is seen in profile. The smaller, lateral humeral epicondyle is more sensitive to rotation, moving out of profile with only a slight degree of elbow rotation. If the epicondyles are not demonstrated in profile, evaluate the degree of radial head superimposition of the ulna to determine how to reposition for an AP projection. If more than 0.25 inch (0.6 cm) of radial head is superimposed over the ulna, the elbow has been internally rotated (see Image 74). If less than 0.25 inch (0.6 cm) of the radial head is superimposed over the ulna, the elbow has been externally rotated (see Images 75 and 76).

The radial tuberosity is demonstrated in profile medially, and the radius and ulna are parallel.

- The alignment of the radius and ulna is determined by the position of the humerus and the wrist. When the humerus is positioned with the humeral epicondyles parallel with the IR, the radial and ulnar relationship can be adjusted with wrist rotation. For an AP projection of the elbow, the hand and wrist should also be positioned in an AP projection by supinating the hand. This positioning places the radial tuberosity medially in profile and eliminates crossing of the radius and ulna. As the hand and wrist are pronated, the radius crosses over the ulna, and the radial tuberosity is rotated posteriorly, out of profile (see Image 77).

The capitulum-radius joint is open, the radial head articulating surface is not demonstrated, the olecranon process is situated within the olecranon fossa, and the coronoid process is demonstrated on end.

- You must use accurate central ray placement and position the forearm parallel with the IR to obtain an open capitulum-radius joint space. When the central ray is centered proximal to the elbow joint space, the capitulum is projected into the joint; when the central ray is centered distal to the elbow joint, the radial head is projected into the joint space (see Image 78). Poor central ray placement also distorts the radial head, causing its articulating surface to be demonstrated. The degree of joint closure depends on how far the central ray is positioned from the elbow joint. The farther away from the joint the central ray is centered, the more the capitulum-radial joint space is obscured and the more the radial head articulating surface is demonstrated.
- *Effect of elbow flexion.* Flexion of the elbow joint also distorts the AP elbow projection. With elbow flexion, the capitulum-radial joint closes, the olecranon process moves away from the olecranon

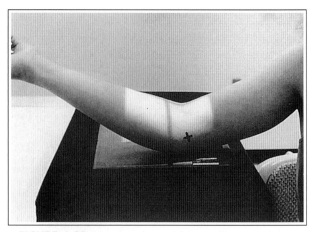

FIGURE 4-68 Proper nonextendable AP elbow projection.

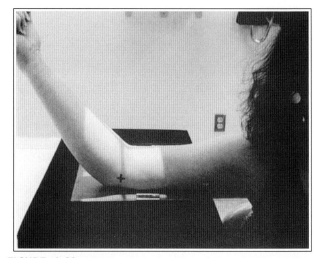

FIGURE 4-69 Patient positioning for nonextendable AP elbow projection—humerus parallel with image receptor.

fossa, and the coronoid process shifts proximally. How a flexed elbow is positioned with respect to the IR determines which elbow structures are distorted on the image. If a flexed elbow is resting on the posterior point of the olecranon, with the proximal humerus and the distal forearm elevated as shown in Figure 4-68, both the humerus and the forearm are foreshortened and the capitulum-radial joint is obscured (see Image 79). Foreshortening of the proximal humerus is indicated on the image by an oval olecranon fossa that is clearly demonstrated, without the olecranon within it. Foreshortening of the distal forearm is demonstrated if the radial head articulating surface is imaged partially on end. The severity of the distortion increases with increased elbow flexion.

- *Compensating for a nonextendable elbow.* An elbow that cannot be fully extended should be imaged using separate exposures to image the distal humerus and the proximal forearm. Figure 4-69

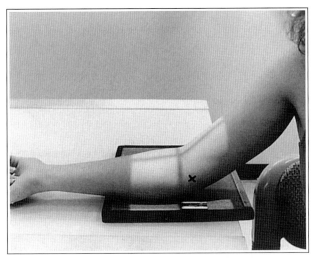

FIGURE 4-70 Patient positioning for nonextendable AP elbow projection—forearm parallel with image receptor.

Anteroposterior Elbow Projection Analysis

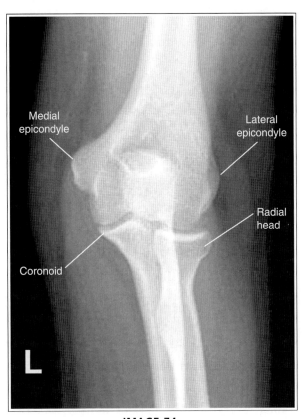

IMAGE 74

demonstrates how the patient should be positioned for an undistorted AP distal humerus image to be obtained. Note that the humerus is placed parallel with the IR. The resulting image demonstrates an undistorted image of the distal humerus, whereas the proximal forearm is severely distorted and the capitulum-radial joint space is obscured (see Image 80). Figure 4-70 demonstrates how the patient should be positioned for an undistorted AP proximal forearm projection to be obtained. Note that the forearm is placed parallel with the IR. The resulting image demonstrates an undistorted image of the proximal forearm and an open capitulum-radial joint, but the distal humerus is severely distorted (see Image 81). The capitulum-radial joint space is visible on the image only if the forearm is positioned parallel with the IR.

The elbow joint is at the center of the exposure field. The elbow joint, one fourth of the proximal forearm and distal humerus, and the lateral soft tissue are included within the collimated field.

- The elbow joint is located 0.75 inch (2 cm) distal to the easily palpable medial epicondyle. To obtain an image of the elbow joint with the least amount of distortion, place a perpendicular central ray at this level and centered to the midelbow. Open longitudinal collimation to include one fourth of the proximal forearm and distal humerus. Transverse collimation should be within 0.5 inch (1.25 cm) of the elbow skin line.
- Half of a 10- × 12-inch (24- × 30-cm) detailed screen-film IR placed crosswise or an 8- × 10-inch (18- × 24-cm) computed radiography IR placed lengthwise should be adequate to include all the required anatomic structures.

Analysis. The humeral epicondyles are not in profile. The radial head is superimposing more than 0.25 inch (0.6 cm) of the ulna, and the coronoid process is visible medially. The elbow was internally rotated. The capitulum-radial joint space is closed. The distal forearm was slightly elevated.

Correction. Rotate the elbow externally until the humeral epicondyles are parallel with the IR, and position the forearm parallel with the IR.

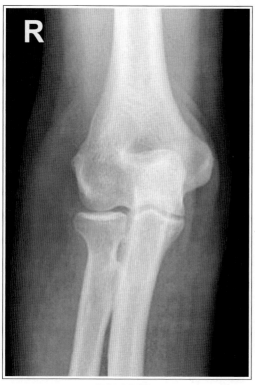

IMAGE 75

Analysis. The humeral epicondyles are not in profile, and less than 0.25 inch (0.6 cm) of the radial head is superimposing the ulna. The image was taken with the elbow in external rotation.

Correction. Rotate the elbow internally until the humeral epicondyles are parallel with the IR.

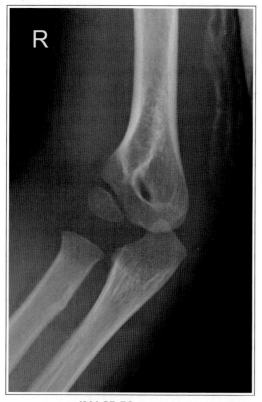

IMAGE 76 Pediatric.

Analysis. The humeral epicondyles are not in profile, and less than 0.25 inch (0.6 cm) of the radial head is superimposing the ulna. The image was taken with the elbow in external rotation. The olecranon is not situated in the olecranon fossa. The elbow was in slight flexion.

Correction. Rotate the elbow internally until the humeral epicondyles are parallel with the IR. If possible, fully extend the elbow. If the patient is unable to extend the elbow, this is an acceptable image of the distal humerus. A second AP projection of the elbow should be taken with the forearm positioned parallel with the IR.

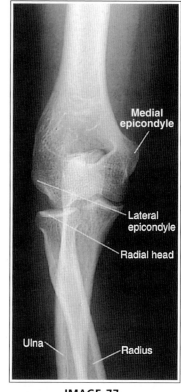

IMAGE 77

Analysis. The radius is crossed over the ulna, and the radial tuberosity is not demonstrated in profile. The hand and wrist were pronated for this image.

Correction. Supinate the hand and wrist into an AP projection.

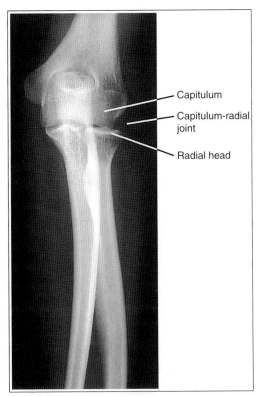

IMAGE 78

Analysis. The capitulum-radial joint space is closed, and the radial head articulating surface is demonstrated. The central ray was centered distal to the joint space.

Correction. Center the central ray to the midelbow at a level 0.75 inch (2 cm) distal to the medial epicondyle.

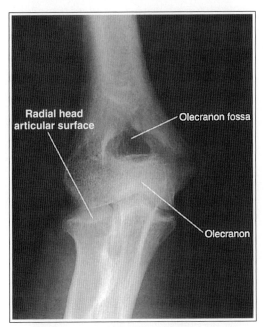

IMAGE 79

Analysis. The capitulum-radial joint space is closed, and the proximal forearm and distal humerus are foreshortened. The elbow was flexed (40 degrees), and the arm was resting on the posterior point of the elbow with the distal forearm and proximal humerus elevated.

Correction. If possible, fully extend the elbow. If the patient is unable to extend the elbow, take two nonextendable AP projections, one with the forearm and one with the humerus positioned parallel with the IR, as shown in Figures 4-69 and 4-70.

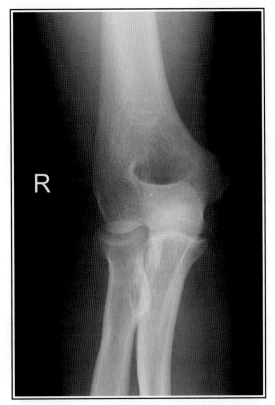

IMAGE 80

Analysis. The distal humerus is demonstrated without foreshortening, but the proximal forearm is severely distorted. The humerus was positioned parallel with the IR, but the distal forearm was elevated, as shown in Figure 4-69.

Correction. If possible, fully extend the elbow. If the patient is unable to extend the elbow, this is an acceptable image of the distal humerus. A second AP projection of the elbow should be taken with the forearm positioned parallel with the IR, as shown in Figure 4-70.

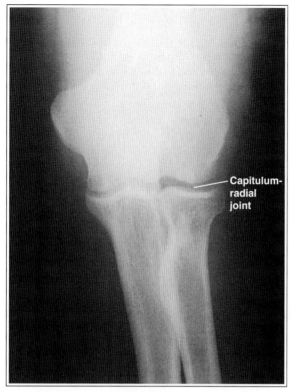

IMAGE 81

Analysis. The proximal forearm is demonstrated without foreshortening, and the capitulum-radial joint space is open, but the distal humerus is severely distorted. The forearm was positioned parallel with the IR, whereas the proximal humerus was elevated, as shown in Figure 4-70.

Correction. If possible, fully extend the elbow. If the patient is unable to extend the elbow, this is an acceptable image of the proximal forearm. A second AP projection of the elbow should be taken with the humerus positioned parallel with the IR, as shown in Figure 4-69.

ELBOW: ANTEROPOSTERIOR OBLIQUE PROJECTIONS (INTERNAL AND EXTERNAL ROTATION)

See Figures 4-71 and 4-72 and Box 4-19.

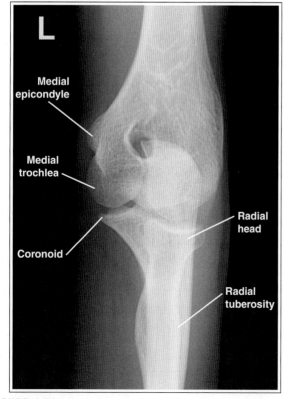

FIGURE 4-71 Internally rotated AP oblique elbow projection with accurate positioning.

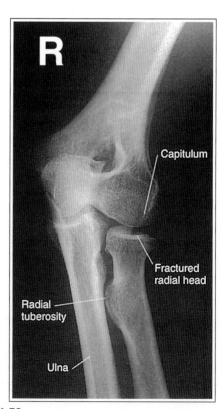

FIGURE 4-72 Externally rotated AP oblique elbow projection with accurate positioning.

BOX 4-19 | **Anteroposterior Oblique Elbow Projection Analysis Criteria**

- External oblique: The capitulum-radial joint is open, and the radial head articulating surface is not demonstrated.
- External oblique: The capitulum and radial tuberosity are seen in profile, the ulna is demonstrated without radial head, neck, and tuberosity superimposition, and the radioulnar articulation is open.
- Internal oblique: The trochlea-coronoid process joint is open, and the coronoid process articulating surface is not demonstrated.
- Internal oblique: The coronoid process, trochlear notch, and medial aspect of the trochlea are seen in profile. The trochlear-coronoid process articulation is open, and the radial head and neck are superimposed over the ulna.
- The elbow joint is at the center of the exposure field.
- The elbow joint, one fourth of the proximal forearm and distal humerus, and the lateral soft tissue are included within the collimation field.

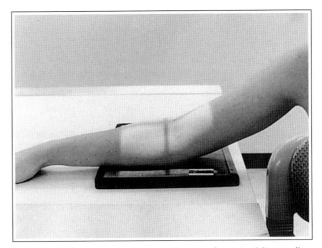

FIGURE 4-73 Proper patient positioning for AP oblique elbow projection with a flexed elbow.

External AP oblique projection: The capitulum-radial joint is open, and the radial head articulating surface is not demonstrated.

Internal AP oblique projection: The trochlea-coronoid process joint is open, and the coronoid process articulating surface is not demonstrated.

- To obtain open capitulum-radial and trochlear-coronoid process joint spaces, you must use accurate central ray placement and position the elbow with the forearm parallel with the IR. When the central ray is centered proximal to the elbow joint spaces, the structures of the distal humerus are projected into the joint; when the central ray is centered distal to the elbow joint, the structures of the proximal forearm are projected into the joint space. Poor central ray positioning also distorts the radial head and coronoid process, causing their articulating surface to be visualized. The degree of joint closure and radial head and coronoid process distortion depends on how far the central ray is positioned from the elbow joint. The farther away from the joint the central ray is centered, the more the joint spaces will be obscured, and the more the articulating surfaces of the radial head and coronoid process will be demonstrated.
- *Effect of elbow flexion.* Flexion of the elbow joint also distorts the AP oblique elbow projection. With elbow flexion, the olecranon process moves away from the olecranon fossa and the coronoid process shifts proximally. How the flexed elbow is positioned with respect to the IR determines which elbow structures are distorted on the image. If a flexed elbow is resting on the posterior point of the olecranon, with the proximal humerus and the distal forearm elevated, both the humerus and the forearm are foreshortened and the capitulum-radial and trochlear-coronoid process joints are obscured. Foreshortening of the proximal humerus is demonstrated on an image by an oval olecranon fossa that

is clearly shown but without the olecranon process within it. Foreshortening of the distal forearm is demonstrated on the image if the radial head and trochlear articulating surfaces are visualized.

The severity of the distortion depends on the degree of elbow flexion. If the humerus is positioned parallel with the IR and the distal forearm is elevated, the image shows an undistorted distal humerus, but the proximal forearm is severely distorted and the capitulum-radial joint is obscured (see Image 82). If the forearm is positioned parallel with the IR and the proximal humerus is elevated, the image shows an undistorted proximal forearm and open capitulum-radial and trochlear-coronoid process joints, but the distal humerus is severely distorted.

- *Positioning of the nonextendable elbow.* For AP oblique elbow projections, if the patient's condition prevents full elbow extension, the anatomic structure (forearm or humerus) of interest should be positioned parallel with the IR. If the radial head or coronoid process is of interest, position the forearm parallel with the IR (Figure 4-73). If the capitulum or medial trochlea is of interest, position the humerus parallel with the IR. The degree and direction of elbow obliquity are the same as those used for an extended elbow.

Internally Rotated AP Oblique Projection

The elbow has been internally rotated 45 degrees. The coronoid process, the trochlear notch, and the medial aspect of the trochlea are demonstrated in profile. The trochlear-coronoid process articulation is open, and the radial head and neck are superimposed over the ulna.

- An accurately positioned internally rotated AP oblique elbow projection is obtained by placing the arm in an AP elbow projection and then internally rotating the hand and humerus until the humeral epicondyles are at a 45-degree angle to the IR (Figure 4-74). When the elbow obliquity is correct, the

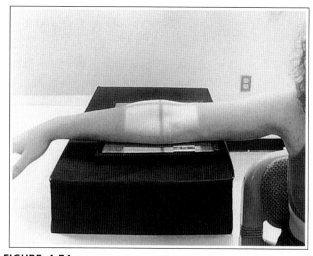

FIGURE 4-74 Proper patient positioning for internal AP oblique elbow projection.

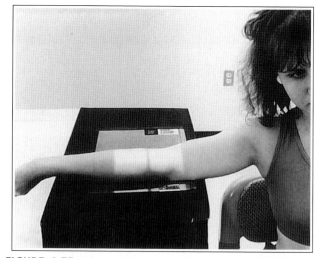

FIGURE 4-75 Proper patient positioning for external AP oblique elbow projection.

coronoid process is demonstrated in profile and the radial head and tuberosity are superimposed over the ulna. If the humeral epicondyles are at less than 45 degrees of obliquity, the radial head is demonstrated lateral to the coronoid process and does not entirely superimpose the ulna (see Image 83). If the humeral epicondyles are at more than 45 degrees of obliquity, the radial head is partially visualized anterior to the coronoid process (see Image 84).

Externally Rotated Oblique Projection

The elbow has been externally rotated 45 degrees. The capitulum and radial tuberosity are demonstrated in profile, the radial head, neck, and tuberosity are visualized without superimposing the ulna, and the radioulnar articulation is demonstrated.

- Accurate positioning for an externally rotated AP oblique elbow projection is achieved by positioning the arm in an AP projection and then externally rotating the humerus and forearm until the humeral epicondyles form a 45-degree angle with the IR (Figure 4-75). This positioning rotates the radius away from the ulna, demonstrating it without superimposition. If the humeral epicondyles are at less than 45 degrees of obliquity, the radial head and tuberosity still partially superimpose the ulna (see Image 85). If the humeral epicondyles are at more than 45 degrees of obliquity, the coronoid process is partially superimposed over the radial head, and the radial neck and tuberosity are free of superimposition; the radial tuberosity is no longer in profile (see Image 86).

The elbow joint is at the center of the exposure field. The elbow joint, one fourth of the proximal forearm and distal humerus, and surrounding soft tissue are included within the collimated field.

- The elbow joint is located 0.75 inch (2 cm) distal to the easily palpable medial humeral epicondyle.

To obtain an undistorted image of the elbow joint, place a perpendicular central ray at this level and centered to the midelbow. Open longitudinal collimation to include one fourth of the proximal forearm and distal humerus. Transverse collimation should be within 0.5 inch (1.25 cm) of the elbow skin line.

- Half of a 10- × 12-inch (24- × 30-cm) detailed screen-film IR placed crosswise or an 8- ×10-inch (18- × 24-cm) computed radiography IR placed lengthwise should be adequate to include all the required anatomic structures.

AP Oblique Elbow Projection Analysis

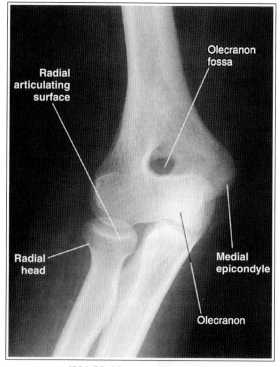

IMAGE 82 External rotation.

Analysis. The olecranon process is drawn slightly away from the olecranon fossa, the capitulum-radial joint space is closed, and the radial articulating surface is demonstrated. The forearm was not positioned parallel with the IR.

Correction. If possible, fully extend the elbow. If the patient is unable to fully extend the elbow and the radial head is of interest, position the forearm parallel with the IR and allow the proximal humerus to be elevated, as shown in Figure 4-73.

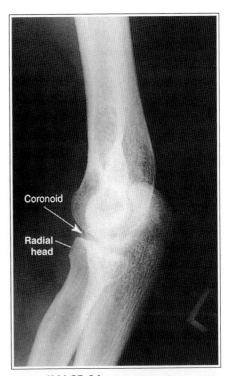

IMAGE 84 Internal rotation.

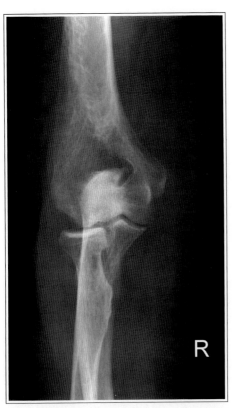

IMAGE 83 Internal rotation.

Analysis. The radial head is partially demonstrated anterior to the coronoid process, without complete superimposition of the ulna. The degree of elbow obliquity is more than 45 degrees.

Correction. Decrease the degree of internal obliquity until the humeral epicondyles are angled at 45 degrees with the IR.

Analysis. The radial head is demonstrated lateral to the coronoid process without complete superimposition of the ulna, and the most proximal aspect of the olecranon is not demonstrated in profile. The degree of elbow obliquity is less than 45 degrees.

Correction. Increase the degree of internal obliquity until the humeral epicondyles are angled at 45 degrees with the IR.

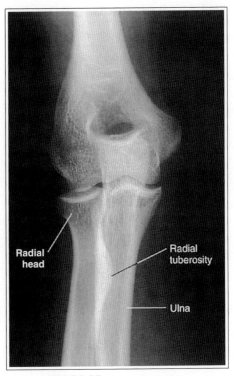

IMAGE 85 External rotation.

Analysis. The radial head and tuberosity are partially superimposed over the ulna, and the radioulnar articulation is obscured. The degree of elbow obliquity is less than 45 degrees. The forearm was not positioned parallel with the IR.

Correction. Increase the degree of external obliquity until the humeral epicondyles are angled at 45 degrees with the IR, and position the forearm parallel with the IR.

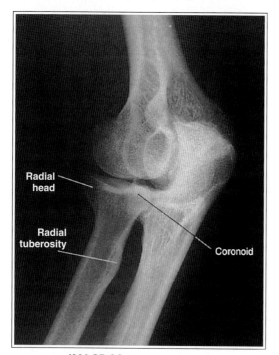

IMAGE 86 External rotation.

Analysis. The coronoid process is partially superimposed over the radial head, but the radial neck and tuberosity are free of superimposition. The radial tuberosity is not demonstrated in profile. The elbow was rotated more than 45 degrees.

Correction. Decrease the degree of lateral obliquity until the humeral epicondyles are angled at 45 degrees with the IR.

ELBOW: LATERAL PROJECTION (LATEROMEDIAL)

See Figure 4-76 and Box 4-20.

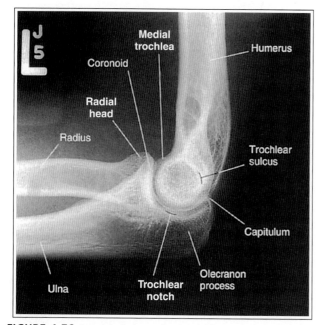

FIGURE 4-76 Lateral elbow projection with accurate positioning.

BOX 4-20	Lateral Elbow Projection Analysis Criteria

- Contrast and density are adequate to demonstrate the anterior, posterior, and supinator fat pads.
- The elbow is flexed 90 degrees.
- The distal humerus demonstrates three concentric arcs, which are formed by the trochlear sulcus, capitulum, and medial trochlea. The elbow joint is open, and the distal and anterior surfaces of the radial head and the coronoid process are aligned.
- The radial tuberosity is not demonstrated in profile.
- The elbow joint is at the center of the exposure field.
- The elbow joint, one fourth of the proximal forearm and distal humerus, and the lateral soft tissue are included within the collimation field.

Contrast and density are adequate to demonstrate the anterior, posterior, and supinator fat pads, surrounding soft tissue, and bony structures.

- *Fat pads on lateral elbow projection.* To evaluate a lateral elbow projection, the reviewer not only

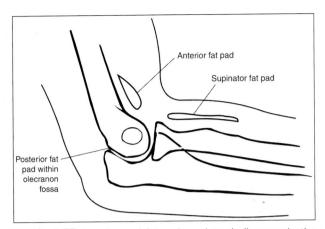

FIGURE 4-77 Locations of fat pads on lateral elbow projection. *(From Martensen K III: The elbow,* In-Service Reviews in Radiologic Technology, *14[11], 1992.)*

analyzes the bony structure, but also studies the placement of the soft tissue fat pads. Three fat pads of interest are present on a lateral elbow projection, the anterior and posterior fat pads and the supinator fat stripe. The anterior fat pad should routinely be seen on all lateral elbow projections when adequate exposure factors are used. This pad is formed by the superimposed coronoid process and radial pads and is situated immediately anterior to the distal humerus (Figure 4-77). A change in the shape or placement of the anterior fat pad may indicate joint effusion and elbow injury. The posterior fat pad is normally obscured on a negative lateral elbow projection because of its location within the olecranon fossa. When an injury occurs, joint effusion pushes this pad out of the fossa, allowing it to be visualized proximal and posterior to the olecranon fossa. The supinator fat stripe is visible parallel to the anterior aspect of the proximal radius (see Figure 4-77). Displacement of this fat stripe is useful for diagnosing fractures of the radial head and neck.

The elbow is flexed 90 degrees.

- When the elbow is flexed 90 degrees, the forearm can be elevated to align the anatomic structures of the distal humerus properly, and displacement of the anterior and posterior fat pads can be used as signs to determine diagnosis. If the elbow is not adequately flexed, these fat pads can be displaced by poor positioning instead of joint pathology, interfering with their diagnostic usefulness. When the arm is extended, nonpathologic displacement of the anterior fat pad results from intraarticular pressure placed on the joint. Nonpathologic displacement of the posterior fat pad is a result of positioning of the olecranon within the olecranon fossa, which causes proximal and posterior displacement of the pad (see Image 87).

The elbow is in a lateral projection. The distal humerus demonstrates three concentric arcs, which are formed by

the trochlear sulcus, capitulum, and medial trochlea. The elbow joint space is open, and the radial head is superimposed over the coronoid process.

- A lateral elbow projection is obtained when the humeral epicondyles are positioned directly on top of each other, placing an imaginary line drawn between them perpendicular to the IR. To obtain this humeral epicondyle positioning, place the humerus parallel with the IR and elevate the distal forearm until the palpable medial and lateral epicondyles are superimposed (Figure 4-78). This positioning aligns the trochlear sulcus, capitulum, and medial trochlea into three concentric (having the same center) arcs (Figure 4-79). The trochlear sulcus is the small center arc. It moves very little when a positional change is made and works like a pivoting point between the capitulum and medial aspect of the trochlea. The largest of the arcs is the medial aspect of the trochlea. It is demonstrated very close to and slightly superimposed on the curve of the trochlear notch. The intermediate-sized arc is the capitulum. When these three arcs are in accurate alignment, the elbow joint is visualized as an open space and the anterior and proximal surfaces of the radial head and coronoid process are aligned.

- *Importance of accurate positioning.* The distal humerus, radial head, and coronoid process are misaligned when the proximal humerus and distal forearm are inaccurately positioned. Proximal humerus positioning determines the alignment of the distal surfaces of the capitulum and medial trochlea, whereas distal forearm positioning determines the AP alignment of the capitulum and medial trochlea. Proximal humerus and distal forearm positioning also determines the alignment of the radial head and coronoid process. Depression or elevation of the proximal humerus moves the

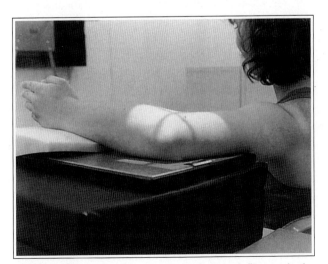

FIGURE 4-78 Proper patient positioning for lateral elbow projection.

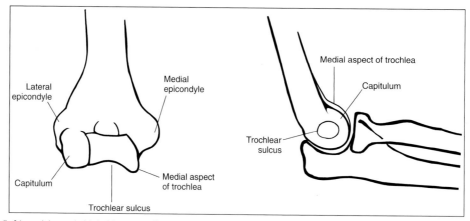

FIGURE 4-79 AP *(left)* and lateral *(right)* images showing anatomy of the distal humerus. *(From Martensen K III: The elbow,* In-Service Reviews in Radiologic Technology, *14[11], 1992.)*

radial head anteriorly or posteriorly on the coronoid process, respectively. Depression or elevation of the distal forearm shifts the radial head distally or proximally, respectively, to the coronoid process. To help understand how the distal humerus and radial head move together, remember that ligaments connect the capitulum and the radial head, so any movement in one causes an equal amount of movement in the other. Precise positioning is a must to obtain a true lateral elbow projection. It takes only a small amount of inaccurate positioning to misalign the distal humerus and close the elbow joint space.

- *Mispositioning of the proximal humerus.* If the proximal humerus is elevated (Figure 4-80), the radial head is positioned too far posteriorly on the coronoid process, and the distal capitulum surface is demonstrated too far distal to the distal surface of the medial trochlea (see Image 88). If the proximal humerus is positioned lower than the distal humerus (Figure 4-81), the radial head is positioned too far anteriorly on the coronoid process and the distal capitulum surface is demonstrated too far proximal to the distal medial trochlear surface (see Images 89, 90, and 96).

- *Mispositioning of the distal forearm.* When the distal forearm is positioned too low (Figure 4-82), the image shows the radial head distal to the coronoid process and the capitulum too far anterior to the

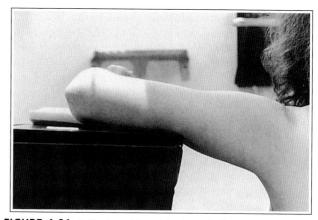

FIGURE 4-81 Patient positioned for lateral elbow projection with depressed proximal humerus.

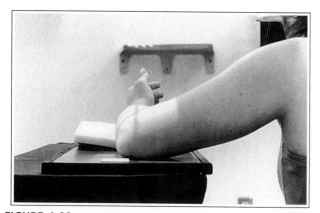

FIGURE 4-80 Patient positioned for lateral elbow projection with elevated proximal humerus.

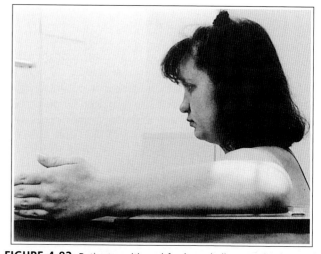

FIGURE 4-82 Patient positioned for lateral elbow projection with depressed distal forearm.

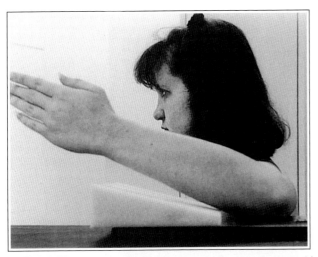

FIGURE 4-83 Patient positioned for lateral elbow projection with elevated distal forearm.

medial trochlea (Images 91 and 92). When the distal forearm is positioned too high (Figure 4-83), the image shows the radial head proximal to the coronoid process and the capitulum too far posterior to the medial trochlea (see Images 93 and 96). Carefully evaluate images that show poor positioning. Often, both forearm and humeral corrections are needed to obtain accurate positioning.

The radial tuberosity is superimposed by the radius and is not demonstrated in profile.

- Visibility of the radial tuberosity is determined by the position of the wrist and hand. When the wrist and hand are placed in a lateral position, the radial tuberosity is situated on the medial aspect of the radius. Because a lateral elbow projection is taken in a lateromedial projection, the radius is superimposed over the radial tuberosity. If the wrist and hand are not placed in a lateral position, placement of the radial tuberosity changes. When the wrist and hand are supinated (externally rotated), the radial tuberosity is demonstrated in profile anteriorly (see Image 94). Pronation (internal rotation) of the wrist and hand shows the radial tuberosity in profile posteriorly (see Image 95).
- Lateral elbow projections obtained with the different hand and wrist positions just described are often taken to study the circumference of the radial head and neck for fractures; they are referred to as radial head images.

The elbow joint is at the center of the exposure field. The elbow joint, one fourth of the proximal forearm and distal humerus, and the surrounding soft tissue are included within the collimated field.

- The elbow joint is located 0.75 inch (2 cm) distal to the lateral epicondyle. To obtain an undistorted image of the elbow joint, place a perpendicular

central ray at this level and centered to the midelbow. Open longitudinal collimation to include one fourth of the proximal forearm and distal humerus. Transverse collimation should be within 0.5 inch (1.25 cm) of the elbow skin line.

- Half of a 10- × 12-inch (24- × 30-cm) detailed screen-film IR placed crosswise or an 8- × 10-inch (18- × 24-cm) computed radiography IR placed lengthwise should be adequate to include all the required anatomic structures.

Lateral Elbow Projection Analysis

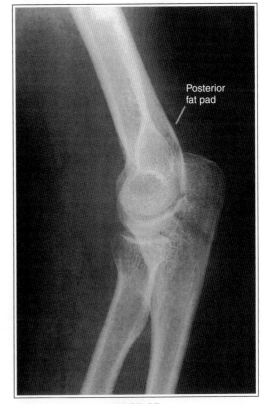

IMAGE 87

Analysis. The elbow is extended. The olecranon is positioned within the olecranon fossa, and the posterior fat pad is demonstrated proximal to the olecranon process. The radial tuberosity is demonstrated in profile posteriorly, indicating that the hand and wrist were pronated.

Correction. If possible, flex the elbow 90 degrees. Position the hand and wrist in a lateral position.

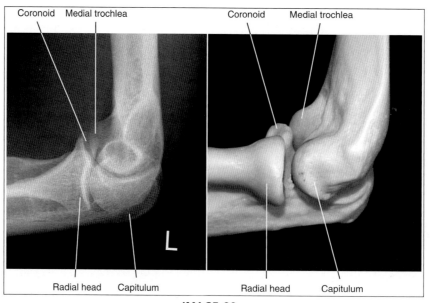

IMAGE 88

Analysis. The radial head is positioned too far posteriorly on the coronoid process and the distal surface of the capitulum is demonstrated too far distally to the distal surface of the medial trochlea. The patient was positioned with the proximal humerus elevated, as shown in Figure 4-80.

Correction. Lower the proximal humerus until the humeral epicondyles are superimposed and the humerus is positioned parallel with the IR. This change will move the capitulum proximally and the medial trochlea distally. Because the capitulum and the trochlea move simultaneously, the amount of adjustment needed is only half the distance demonstrated between where the two distal surfaces should be on a lateral elbow projection with accurate positioning and where they are on this image. On this image this distance is approximately 0.5 inch (1 cm), so the repositioning adjustment needed is only 0.25 inch (0.6 cm).

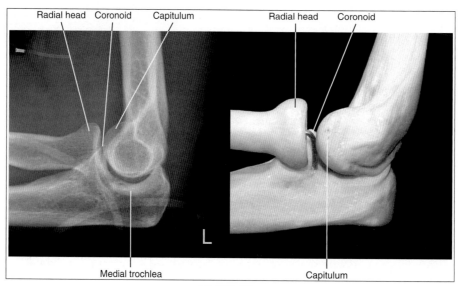

IMAGE 89

Analysis. The radial head is positioned anterior on the coronoid process, and the distal surface of the capitulum is too far proximal to the distal surface of the medial trochlea. The patient was positioned with the proximal humerus depressed, as shown in Figure 4-81.

Correction. Elevate the proximal humerus until the humeral epicondyles are superimposed and the humerus is positioned parallel with the IR. Because the radial head and coronoid process, the capitulum, and the trochlea move simultaneously, the amount of adjustment required is only half the distance demonstrated between the two anterior and distal surfaces, respectively.

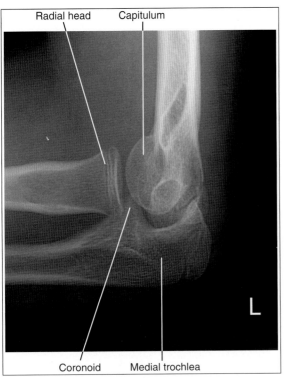

IMAGE 90 Pediatric.

Analysis. The radial head is positioned anterior and distal to the coronoid process, and the capitulum is too far proximal and anterior to the medial trochlea. The patient was placed with the proximal humerus and distal forearm positioned too low.

Correction. Elevate the proximal humerus and distal forearm until the humeral epicondyles are superimposed.

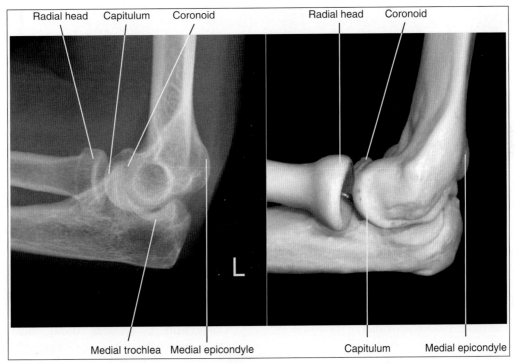

IMAGE 91

Analysis. The radial head is distal to the coronoid process, and the capitulum is too far anterior to the medial trochlea. The patient was placed with the distal forearm positioned too close to the IR, as shown in Figure 4-82.

Correction. Elevate the distal forearm until the humeral epicondyles are superimposed. This change will move the capitulum posteriorly and the medial trochlea anteriorly. Because the radial head and coronoid process, capitulum, and trochlea move simultaneously, the amount of adjustment required is only half the distance demonstrated between the two distal and anterior surfaces, respectively.

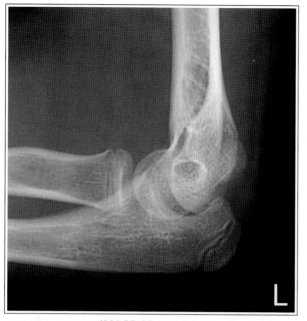

IMAGE 92 Pediatric.

Analysis. The radial head is distal to the coronoid process, and the capitulum is too far anterior to the medial trochlea. The patient was placed with the distal forearm positioned too close to the IR.

Correction. Elevate the distal forearm until the humeral epicondyles are superimposed.

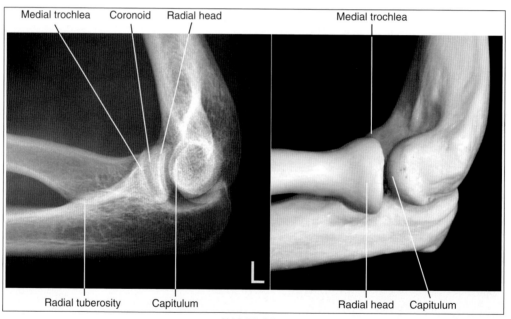

IMAGE 93

Analysis. The radial head is proximal to the coronoid process, and the capitulum appears too far posterior to the medial trochlea. The patient was positioned with the distal forearm placed too far away from the IR, as shown in Figure 4-83. The radial tuberosity is visible posteriorly. The distal forearm was internally rotated.

Correction. Lower the distal forearm until the humeral epicondyles are superimposed, and internally rotate the distal forearm until the wrist is in a lateral projection.

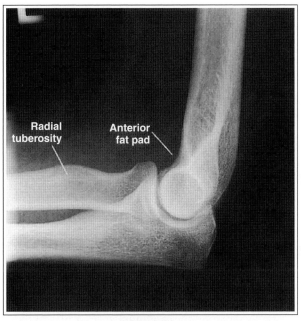

IMAGE 94

Analysis. The elbow joint space is open, and the distal humerus demonstrates accurate alignment. The radial tuberosity is demonstrated in profile anteriorly, indicating that the wrist and hand were supinated (externally rotated).

Correction. If the circumference of the radial head and neck is being evaluated and the medial aspect of the radial head in profile is desired, the radial tuberosity should be demonstrated in profile anteriorly and no repositioning movement is needed. If a true lateral elbow image is desired, the distal forearm should be internally rotated until the wrist is in a lateral projection.

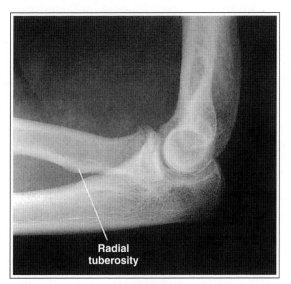

IMAGE 95

Analysis. The elbow joint space is open, and the distal humerus demonstrates accurate alignment. The radial tuberosity is demonstrated in profile posteriorly, indicating that the hand and wrist were pronated (internally rotated).

Correction. If the circumference of the radial head and neck is being evaluated and the medial aspect of the radial head in profile is desired, the radial tuberosity should be seen in profile anteriorly and no repositioning movement is needed. If a true lateral elbow projection is desired, the distal forearm should be externally rotated until the wrist is in a lateral projection.

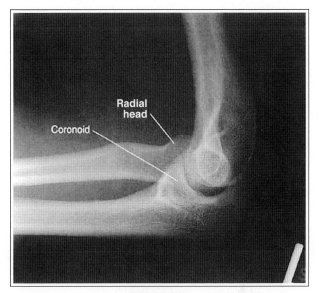

IMAGE 96

Analysis. Two positional problems on this image are preventing the distal humerus from demonstrating accurate alignment. The radial head is positioned anteriorly and proximally to the coronoid process, and the capitulum is positioned too far proximally and posteriorly to the medial trochlea. The proximal humerus was positioned too low, and the distal forearm was positioned too high, a combination of the errors shown in Figures 4-81 and 4-83.

Correction. Raise the proximal humerus and lower the distal forearm until the humeral epicondyles are superimposed.

ELBOW: AXIOLATERAL PROJECTION (COYLE METHOD)

The radial axiolateral elbow image is a special projection taken when a fracture of the radial head or capitulum is suspected (Figure 4-84 and Box 4-21).
The elbow is flexed 90 degrees.

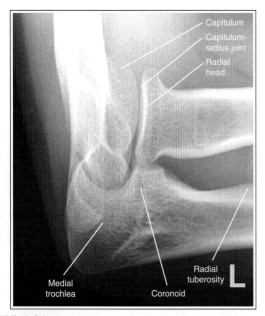

FIGURE 4-84 Axiolateral (Coyle method) elbow projection with accurate positioning.

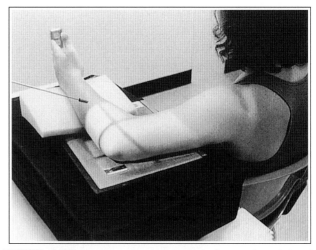

FIGURE 4-85 Proper patient positioning for axiolateral (Coyle method) elbow projection.

BOX 4-21	Axiolateral Elbow Projection Analysis Criteria

- The elbow is flexed 90 degrees.
- The capitulum and medial trochlea are demonstrated without superimposition, and the radial head is superimposed only on the anterior tip of the coronoid process.
- The capitulum-radial joint is open and the proximal radial head and coronoid process are aligned.
- The radial head surface of interest is demonstrated in profile.
- The radial head is at the center of the exposure field.
- One fourth of the proximal forearm and distal humerus and the lateral soft tissue are included within the collimation field.

- If the elbow is flexed 90 degrees, the forearm can be elevated to align the anatomic structures of the distal humerus properly.

The capitulum and medial trochlea are demonstrated without superimposition, and the radial head is superimposed on only the anterior tip of the coronoid process.

- The axiolateral elbow projection is obtained by placing the patient's elbow in a lateral projection, with the humeral epicondyles aligned perpendicular to the IR and placing a 45-degree proximal (toward the shoulder) angle on the central ray (Figure 4-85). It is

this humerus and central ray positioning that accurately separates the capitulum and trochlea of the distal humerus and positions the radial head anteriorly to the coronoid process. The combination of positioning and angulation projects the anatomic structures (radial head and capitulum) situated farther from the IR proximal to those structures (coronoid process and medial trochlea) situated closer to the IR.

- **Effects of errors in positioning or angulation.** If the central ray is angled accurately but the proximal humerus is depressed lower than the distal humerus, the medial trochlea and capitulum cortices are not clearly defined, the coronoid process is free of radial head superimposition, and the radial neck and tuberosity are superimposed by the ulnar supinator crest (a sharp, prominent ridge running along the lateral margin of the ulna that divides the ulna's anterior and posterior surfaces; see Image 97). The same image can result if the patient is accurately positioned but the central ray is angled more than 45 degrees.

  If the central ray is accurately angled but the proximal humerus is elevated, the medial trochlea demonstrates some capitular superimposition and the radial head is superimposed over a greater portion of the coronoid process (see Image 98). The same image can result if the patient is accurately positioned but the central ray is angled less than 45 degrees.

The capitulum-radial joint is open, and the proximal radial head and coronoid process are aligned.

- An accurately aligned radial head and coronoid process and an open capitulum-radial head joint is obtained when the elbow is in a lateral projection. A lateral elbow projection is accomplished when the humeral epicondyles are positioned directly on top of each other, placing them perpendicular to the IR (see Figure 4-85).

• *Effect of distal forearm mispositioning.* The alignment of the proximal surfaces of the radial head and coronoid process is affected when the distal forearm is positioned. Precise positioning is necessary to obtain accurate alignment. It takes only a small degree of inaccurate positioning to close the capitulum-radius joint. If the distal forearm is positioned too low, the image shows a closed capitulum-radius joint space and shows the capitulum too far anterior to the medial trochlea and the radial head distal to the coronoid process (see Image 99). If the distal forearm is positioned too high, the image shows the capitulum too far posterior to the medial trochlea and the radial head proximal to the coronoid process.

The radial head surface of interest is demonstrated in profile.

• The position of the wrist determines which surface of the radial head is placed in profile.
• *Effect of wrist position.* When the patient's elbow is placed in a lateral projection, wrist rotation causes the radius to rotate around the ulna. This rotation places different radial head surfaces in profile. To determine which surfaces are in profile, one should become familiar with the relationship between the wrist position and visualization of the radial tuberosity. The radial tuberosity is adjacent to the medial aspect of the radius. If the tuberosity is demonstrated, the medial aspect of the radial head is also shown on that same surface and the lateral aspect of the radial head is visible on the opposite surface. If the patient's wrist is positioned in a PA projection, the radial tuberosity and medial radial head are demonstrated posteriorly and the lateral radial head appears in profile anteriorly (see Image 98). If the wrist is in a lateral projection, the radial tuberosity is not demonstrated in profile but is superimposed by the radius. In this position, the anterior radial head is demonstrated in profile anteriorly and the posterior surface is shown in profile posteriorly (see Image 93).

The radial head is at the center of the exposure field. The proximal forearm, distal humerus, and surrounding soft tissue are included within the collimated field.

• To place the radial head in the center of the collimated field, center the central ray 0.75 inch (2 cm) distal (toward the wrist) to the lateral epicondyle. Open the longitudinally and transversely collimated fields to within 0.5 inch (1.25 cm) of the posterior elbow skin line.
• An 8- × 10-inch (18- × 24-cm) detailed screen-film or computed radiography IR placed lengthwise should be adequate to include all the required anatomic structures.

Axiolateral Elbow (Coyle Method) Projection Analysis

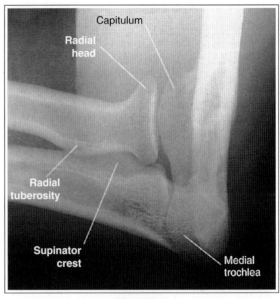

IMAGE 97

Analysis. The distal medial trochlea and capitulum cortices are not clearly defined, the coronoid process is free of radial head superimposition, and the radial neck and tuberosity are superimposed by the ulnar supinator crest. The proximal humerus was depressed lower than the distal humerus. The radial tuberosity is in partial profile, indicating that the wrist was in an oblique position. The radial tuberosity is in partial profile, indicating that the wrist was in an oblique position.

Correction. Elevate the proximal humerus until the humeral epicondyles are perpendicular to the image. If the image was to demonstrate the anterior and posterior surfaces of the radial head in profile, place the wrist in a lateral position. If it is desired that the anterior and posterior surfaces of the radiation head be demonstrated in profile, place the wrist in a lateral projection.

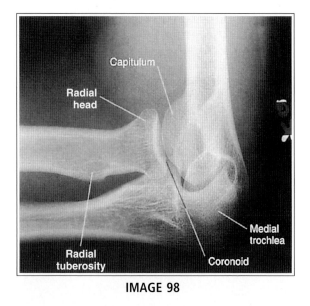

IMAGE 98

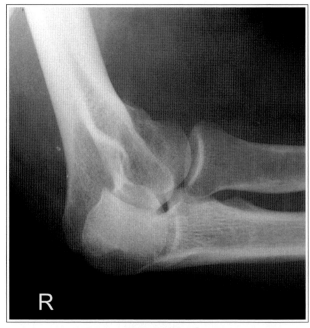

IMAGE 99

Analysis. The capitulum-radius joint space is closed, the radial head is demonstrated distal to the coronoid process, and the capitulum is demonstrated too far anterior to the medial trochlea, indicating that the distal forearm was depressed. The radial head is superimposed over more than just the tip of the coronoid process, and the medial trochlea and capitulum would demonstrate slight superimposition if the distal forearm had been accurately positioned; the proximal humerus was elevated. The radial tuberosity is demonstrated in profile posteriorly and the lateral surface of the radial head is demonstrated in profile anteriorly, whereas the medial surface is in profile posteriorly; the wrist was placed in a PA projection.

Correction. Elevate the distal forearm and depress the proximal humerus until the humeral epicondyles are aligned perpendicularly to the IR. If you want the anterior and posterior surfaces of the radial head to be demonstrated in profile, place the wrist in a lateral projection.

Analysis. The capitulum-radius joint space is closed, and the radial head is demonstrated distally to the coronoid process. The radial tuberosity is not demonstrated in profile, the anterior surface of the radial head is in profile anteriorly, and the posterior surface is in profile posteriorly; the wrist was placed in a lateral position.

Correction. Elevate the distal forearm until the humeral epicondyles are aligned perpendicularly to the IR. The amount of movement needed is half the difference between how close the anterior surfaces of the capitulum and medial trochlea should be on a radial head and capitulum image with accurate positioning and how close they are located on this image. If the lateral and medial surfaces of the radial head should be demonstrated in profile, the patient's wrist needs to be placed in a PA projection.

HUMERUS: ANTEROPOSTERIOR PROJECTION

See Figures 4-86 and 4-87 and Box 4-22.

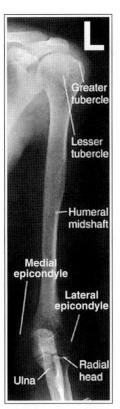

FIGURE 4-86 AP humerus projection with accurate positioning.

Scatter radiation is controlled. Image density is uniform across the humerus.

- If the patient's upper arm AP thickness measures less than 4 inches (10 cm), a grid is not required. For such a patient, a high-contrast, low-kVp (below 60) technique sufficiently penetrates the bony and soft tissue structures of the humerus without causing excessive scatter radiation to reach the IR and hinder image contrast. If the upper arm measures more than 4 inches (10 cm), a grid should be used, because this thickness would produce enough scatter radiation to affect the image contrast negatively. When a grid is used, increase the kVp to above 70 to penetrate the thicker humerus and provide an adequate scale of contrast. If the technique is manually set, increase the exposure (mAs) by the standard density conversion factor for the grid ratio (number used to express a grid's scatter-eliminating ability) being used to compensate for the scatter and the primary radiation that the grid will absorb.
- *Anode heel effect.* To take advantage of the anode heel effect, position the thinner elbow (distal humerus) at the anode end of the tube and the thicker (proximal humerus) at the cathode end. Set an exposure (mAs) that will adequately demonstrate the midpoint of the humerus.

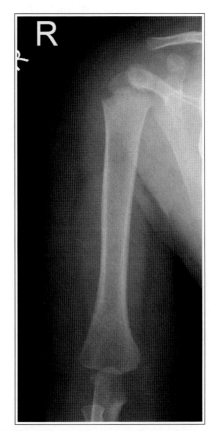

FIGURE 4-87 Pediatric AP humerus projection with accurate positioning.

BOX 4-22	Anteroposterior Humerus Projection Analysis Criteria

- Image density is uniform across the humerus.
- The medial and lateral humeral epicondyles are demonstrated in profile, and the radial head and tuberosity are superimposed over the lateral aspect of the proximal ulna by about 0.25 inch (0.6 cm).
- The greater tubercle is demonstrated in profile laterally, the humeral head is demonstrated medially in profile, and the vertical cortical margin of the lesser tubercle is visible about halfway between the greater tubercle and the humeral head.
- The long axis of the humerus is aligned with the long axis of the collimated field.
- The humeral midpoint is at the center of the exposure field.
- The shoulder and elbow joints and the lateral humeral soft tissue are included within the collimated field.

The humerus is in an AP projection. The medial and lateral humeral epicondyles are demonstrated in profile, and the radial head and tuberosity are superimposed over the lateral aspect of the proximal ulna by approximately 0.25 inch (0.6 cm). The greater tubercle is demonstrated in profile laterally, the humeral head is demonstrated medially in profile, and the vertical

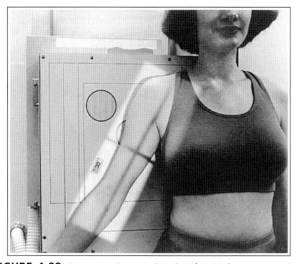

FIGURE 4-88 Proper patient positioning for AP humerus projection—collimator head rotated.

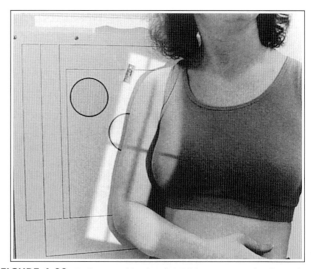

FIGURE 4-89 Patient positioning for AP humerus projection when fracture is located close to shoulder.

cortical margin of the lesser tubercle is visible approximately halfway between the greater tubercle and the humeral head.

- An AP projection is obtained by placing the patient in a supine or upright AP projection, with the affected arm extended. Supinate the hand and externally rotate the elbow until an imaginary line drawn between the palpable humeral epicondyles is aligned parallel with the IR (Figure 4-88). This positioning places the proximal radius anterior to the ulna, causing the radial head and tuberosity to be superimposed over the lateral ulna by approximately 0.25 inch (0.6 cm), and places the greater tuberosity in profile.

- *Detecting humeral rotation.* Rotation of the humerus is a result of poor humeral epicondyle positioning. When the humeral epicondyles and the greater tuberosity are not demonstrated in profile, measure the amount of radial head and tuberosity superimposition of the ulna to determine how the patient should be repositioned. If less than 0.25 inch (0.6 cm) of the radial head and tuberosity are superimposed over the ulna, the elbow and humerus have been excessively externally rotated (see Image 100). If more than 0.25 inch (0.6 cm) of the radial head and tubercle are superimposed over the ulna, the elbow and humerus have been internally rotated (see Image 101).

- *Positioning for humeral fracture.* When a fracture of the humerus is suspected or a follow-up image is being taken to assess healing of a humeral fracture, the patient's arm should not be externally rotated to obtain the AP projection because external rotation of the forearm increases the risk of radial nerve damage. For such an examination, the joint closer to the fracture should be aligned in the true AP projection. If the fracture site is

situated closer to the shoulder joint and the arm cannot be externally rotated, the greater tuberosity is placed in profile by rotating the patient's body toward the affected humerus 35 to 40 degrees (Figure 4-89). Depending on the amount of humeral rotation at the fracture site, the distal humerus may or may not be an AP projection (see Image 102). If the fracture is situated closer to the elbow joint, extend the arm and rotate the patient's body toward the affected humerus until the humeral epicondyles are aligned parallel with the IR. Depending on the amount of humeral rotation at the fracture site, the greater tubercle may or may not be in profile.

The long axis of the humerus is aligned with the long axis of the collimated field.

- If the humerus can remain aligned with the long axis of the IR while including the elbow and shoulder joints, align the long axis of the collimated light field with the long axis of the humerus to allow for tight transverse collimation.

- For many adult humeral projections, it may be necessary to position the humerus diagonally on the IR to include the elbow and shoulder joint. If using screen-film or DR systems for this positioning, the collimator head or tube column should be turned or rotated to align the long axis of the collimated light field with the long axis of the humerus. If a grid is used, the collimator head may be rotated, but do not rotate the tube column or grid cutoff will result. This is not recommended with computed radiography (CR) systems. If the collimator head or tube column cannot be adjusted for a diagonal positioning, leave the transversely collimated field open enough to include the shoulder joint and elbow. With this

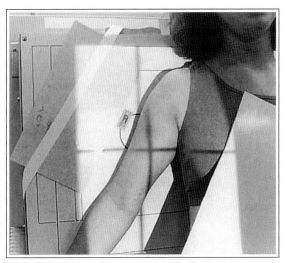

FIGURE 4-90 Proper patient positioning for AP humerus projection using shields when collimator head cannot be rotated.

setup the collimated field includes a large portion of the patient's thorax. Therefore the thorax is exposed to unnecessary radiation but can be protected by use of a contact shield across it. Remember to leave at least 3 inches (7.5 cm) of space between the humeral head and the shield to allow for magnification, so that the shoulder joint is not obscured by the shield (Figure 4-90).

The humeral midpoint is at the center of the exposure field. The shoulder and elbow joints and the lateral humeral soft tissue are included within the collimated field.

- To place the humeral midpoint in the center of the image, palpate the coracoid process and the medial epicondyle and position the central ray halfway between these two palpable landmarks. When the elbow and shoulder joints are included on the image, the degree of radiation beam divergence used for a long body part needs to be considered.
- *IR length and positioning:* Choose an IR that is long enough to allow at least 1 inch (2.5 cm) of IR to extend beyond each joint space; a 14- × 17-inch (35- × 44-cm) screen-film or computed radiography IR placed lengthwise should be adequate. For a patient with a long humerus, it may be necessary to position the humerus somewhat diagonally on the IR to obtain the needed IR length. For the computed radiography system, it is not advisable to position the part diagonally unless the system is set to handle this alignment. Palpate the two joints to ensure that the IR extends beyond them. The elbow is located approximately 0.75 inch (2 cm) proximal to the medial epicondyle. The shoulder joint is located at the same level as the palpable coracoid.
- *Central ray centering and collimation.* Once the humerus is accurately positioned with the IR,

center a perpendicular central ray to the humeral midpoint, and open the longitudinal collimated field until it extends 1 inch (2.5 cm) beyond the elbow and shoulder joint. If the collimation does not extend beyond both joints, adjust the centering point of the central ray until both the elbow and the shoulder joint are included within the collimated field without demonstrating an excessive light field beyond them. Transverse collimation should be to within 0.5 inch (1.25 cm) of the skin line laterally and the coracoid medially.

Anteroposterior Humeral Projection Analysis

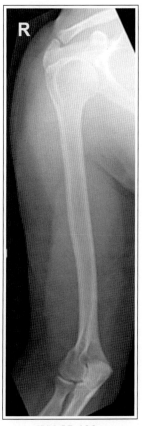

IMAGE 100

Analysis. The humeral epicondyles are not demonstrated in profile, the radial head and tuberosity do not superimpose the ulna, and the cortical margin of the lesser tubercle is not shown halfway between the greater tubercle and the humeral head. The arm was externally rotated more than the required amount.

Correction. Internally rotate the arm until the humeral epicondyles are positioned parallel with the IR.

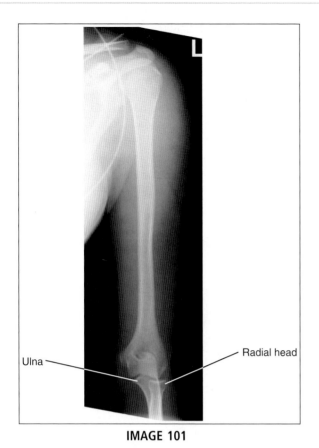

Ulna — — Radial head

IMAGE 101

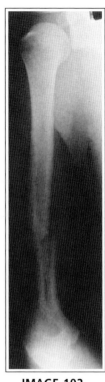

IMAGE 102

Analysis. Neither the humeral epicondyles nor the greater tubercle is demonstrated in profile, and the radial head and tuberosity are superimposed over more than 0.25 inch (0.6 cm) of the ulna. The arm was internally rotated.

Correction. Externally rotate the arm until the humeral epicondyles are positioned parallel with the IR.

Analysis. A fracture is present at the distal humerus. The glenohumeral joint space is demonstrated, indicating that this image was taken with the patient rotated toward the humerus.

Correction. Because the joint closer to the fracture is in a true projection, no repositioning movement is needed.

HUMERUS: LATERAL PROJECTION (LATEROMEDIAL AND MEDIOLATERAL)

See Figures 4-91 and 4-92 and Box 4-23.

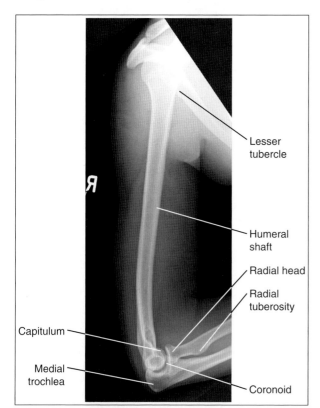

FIGURE 4-91 Mediolateral humerus projection with accurate positioning.

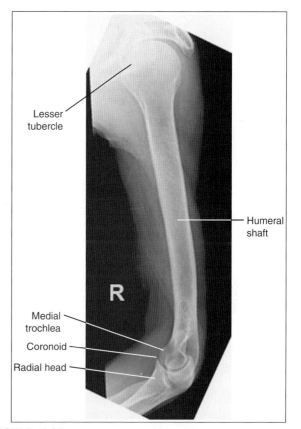

FIGURE 4-92 Lateromedial humerus projection with accurate positioning.

Scatter radiation is controlled. Image density is uniform across the humerus.

- If the patient's upper arm AP thickness measures less than 4 inches (10 cm), a grid is not required, but a grid is required if the patient's upper arm measures more than 4 inches (10 cm). When a grid is used, increase the penetration to above 60 kVp to penetrate the thicker humerus and provide an adequate scale of contrast. If the technique is manually set, increase the exposure (mAs) by the standard density conversion factor for the grid ratio used to compensate for the absorption of the scatter and primary radiation that occurs.

- *Anode heel effect.* To take advantage of the anode heel effect, position the thinner elbow (distal humerus) at the anode end of the tube and the thicker (proximal humerus) at the cathode end. Set an exposure (mAs) that will adequately demonstrate the midpoint of the humerus.

The humerus is in a lateral projection. The lesser tubercle is demonstrated in profile medially, and the humeral head and greater tubercle are superimposed. For a mediolateral projection, most of the radial head is demonstrated anterior to the coronoid process, the radial tuberosity is demonstrated in profile, and the capitulum is visualized

BOX 4-23	Lateral Humerus Projection Analysis Criteria

- Image density is uniform across the humerus.
- The lesser tubercle is demonstrated in profile medially, and the humeral head and greater tubercle are superimposed.
- Lateromedial: The radial head and coronoid process are superimposed, the radial tuberosity is not in profile, and the capitulum is visible distal to the medial trochlea.
- Mediolateral: Most of the radial head is demonstrated anterior to the coronoid process, the radial tuberosity is seen in profile, and the capitulum is visualized proximal to the medial trochlea.
- The long axis of the humerus is aligned with the long axis of the collimated field.
- The humeral midpoint is at the center of the exposure field.
- The shoulder and elbow joints and the lateral humeral soft tissue are included within the collimated field.

proximal to the medial trochlea (see Figure 4-91). For a lateromedial projection, the radial head and coronoid process are superimposed, the radial tuberosity is not demonstrated in profile, and the capitulum is visible distal to the medial trochlea (see Figure 4-92).

- Two methods can be used to position the patient for a lateral humerus projection, mediolateral and lateromedial. The first method positions the

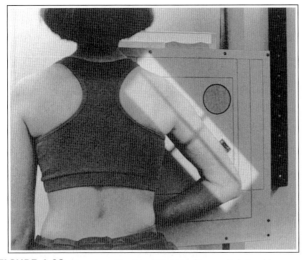

FIGURE 4-93 Proper patient positioning for mediolateral humerus projection.

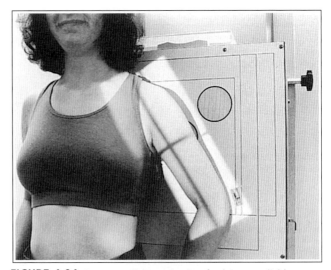

FIGURE 4-94 Proper patient projection for lateromedial humerus image.

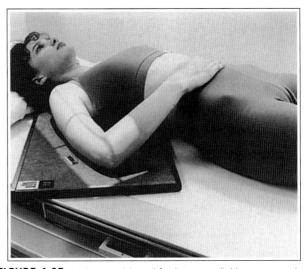

FIGURE 4-95 Patient positioned for lateromedial humerus projection with poor distal humerus alignment.

patient's body in an upright PA projection, with the elbow flexed 90 degrees and the forearm and humerus internally rotated until an imaginary line connecting the humeral epicondyles is perpendicular to the IR; this is termed a *mediolateral projection* (Figure 4-93). Have the patient rotate the humerus internally while the body maintains a PA projection. Do not allow the patient to rotate the body toward the affected humerus instead. Such body obliquity would cause a decrease in density of the proximal humerus compared with the distal humerus (see Image 103), because the shoulder tissue would be superimposed over the proximal humerus. If body rotation cannot be avoided, an increase in exposure (mAs) is required to demonstrate the upper humerus adequately.

• The second method positions the patient's body in an AP projection. The hand is positioned against the patient's side, the elbow is slightly flexed, and the forearm and humerus are internally rotated until an imaginary line connecting the humeral epicondyles is perpendicular to the IR; this is termed a *lateromedial projection* (Figure 4-94). If the patient's forearm is positioned across the body in an attempt to flex the elbow 90 degrees and the distal humerus is not brought away from the IR enough to position the humeral epicondyles perpendicular to the IR (Figure 4-95), the image demonstrates the capitulum posterior to the medial trochlea, a distorted proximal forearm, and the lesser tubercle in partial profile (see Image 104). The difference in the anatomic relationship of the distal humerus between the mediolateral and lateromedial projections is a result of x-ray beam divergence. For a lateral humerus projection, the central ray is centered to the midhumeral shaft, which is located approximately 5 inches (13 cm) from the elbow joint. Because the elbow joint is

placed so far away from the central ray, diverged x-ray beams are used to image the elbow joint. This causes the anatomic structures positioned farthest from the IR to be diverged more distally than the anatomic structures positioned closest to the IR. In the mediolateral projection, the medial trochlea is placed farther from the IR than the capitulum. Consequently, x-ray beam divergence will project the medial trochlea distal to the capitulum. In the lateromedial projection the capitulum is situated farther from the IR; therefore, the x-ray beam divergence will project it distally to the medial trochlea.

• ***Positioning for a humeral fracture.*** When a fracture of the humerus is suspected or a follow-up image is being taken to assess healing of a fracture, the patient's forearm or humerus should not be rotated to obtain a lateral position. Rotation of

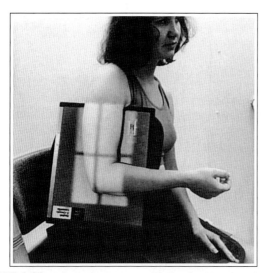

FIGURE 4-96 Proper patient positioning for distal humerus fracture.

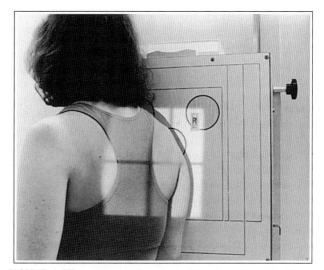

FIGURE 4-97 Proper positioning of a PA oblique (scapular Y) projection for a proximal humerus fracture.

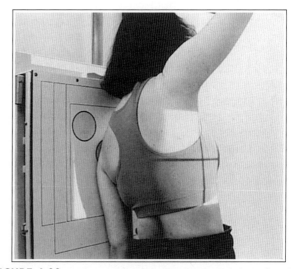

FIGURE 4-98 Proper positioning of a transthoracic lateral projection for a proximal humerus fracture.

the forearm and humerus would increase the risk of radial nerve damage and displacement of the fracture fragments. Because the forearm should not be rotated for a trauma examination, a lateral image of the proximal and distal humerus must be obtained by positioning the patient differently.

- *Distal humeral fracture.* Obtain a lateral distal humerus projection by gently sliding an IR between the patient and the distal humerus. Adjust the IR until the epicondyles are positioned perpendicularly to the IR. Place a flat contact protecting shield between the patient and the IR to absorb any radiation that would penetrate the IR and expose the patient. Finally, center the central ray perpendicularly to the IR and distal humerus (Figure 4-96). This positioning should demonstrate a true lateral projection of the distal humerus with superimposition of the epicondyles and of the radial head and coronoid process (see Image 105).
- *Proximal humeral fracture.* A lateral projection can be achieved by positioning the patient in one of two ways. The first method is best done with the patient in an upright position, a position known as the scapular Y, PA axial projection. Begin by placing the patient in a PA upright projection with the humerus positioned as is, and then rotate the patient toward the affected humerus (approximately 45 degrees) until the scapular body is in a lateral position (Figure 4-97; see Image 106). Precise positioning and evaluating points for this image can be studied by referring to the discussion of the PA oblique (scapular Y) projection (see page 270).

The second method of obtaining a lateral projection of the proximal humerus can be accomplished with an upright or recumbent position. It is known as the transthoracic lateral position (Figure 4-98). The patient's body is placed in a lateral projection with the affected

humerus resting against the grid IR, and the unaffected arm is raised above the patient's head. To prevent superimposition of the shoulders on the image, either (1) elevate the unaffected shoulder by tilting the upper midsagittal plane toward the IR and using a horizontal central ray, or (2) position the shoulders on the same transverse plane and angle the central ray 10 to 15 degrees cephalically.

For both projections, direct the central ray to the midthorax at the level of the affected shoulder. Use breathing technique to blur the vascular lung markings and axillary ribs. With this technique, a long exposure time (3 seconds) is used while the patient breathes shallowly (costal breathing) during the exposure. A transthoracic projection with accurate positioning should sharply demonstrate the affected proximal humerus halfway between the sternum and the thoracic verte-brae, without superimposition of the unaffected shoulder (see Image 107).

The long axis of the humerus is aligned with the long axis of the collimated field.

- If the patient's humerus can remain aligned with the long axis of the IR while the elbow and shoulder joints are included on the IR, align the long axis of the collimated light field with the long axis of the humerus to allow for tight transverse collimation. For many adult humeral images, it may be necessary to position the humerus diagonally on the IR to include the elbow and shoulder joint. If using screen-film or digital radiography (DR) systems for this positioning, the collimator head or tube column should be turned or rotated to align the long axis of the collimated light field with the long axis of the humerus. If a grid is used, do not rotate the tube column or grid cutoff will result. This is not recommended with CR systems. If the collimator head or tube column cannot be adjusted for diagonal positioning, leave the transversely collimated field open enough to include the elbow and shoulder joint. With this setup the collimated field includes a large portion of the patient's thorax. Therefore the thorax is exposed to unnecessary radiation but can be protected by laying a flat contact shield across it. Remember to leave at least 3 inches (7.5 cm) of space between the humeral head and the shield to allow for magnification, so that the shoulder joint is not obscured by the shield.

The humeral midpoint is at the center of the exposure field. The shoulder and elbow joints, the proximal humerus and forearm, and the lateral humeral soft tissue are included within the collimated field.

- To place the humeral midpoint in the center of the image, palpate (1) the acromion angle (Figure 4-99) for a mediolateral projection or (2) the coracoid process for a lateromedial projection and the medial epicondyle. Position the central ray with the humeral midpoint at a level halfway between the two palpable landmarks. To include the elbow and shoulder joints on the image, the degree of radiation beam divergence used when imaging a long body part needs to be considered.

- *IR length and positioning.* Choose an IR that is long enough to allow at least 1 inch (2.5 cm) of IR to extend beyond each joint space; a 14- × 17-inch (35- × 44-cm) screen-film or computed radiography IR placed lengthwise should be adequate. On a patient with a long humerus, it may be necessary to position the humerus somewhat diagonally on the IR to obtain the needed IR length. For the CR system, it is not advisable to

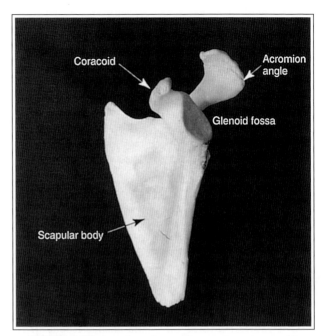

FIGURE 4-99 Location of acromion angle and coracoid.

position the part diagonally unless the system is set to handle this alignment. Palpate the joints to ensure that the IR extends beyond them. The elbow is located approximately 0.75 inch (2 cm) distal to the medial epicondyles. The shoulder joint is located at the same level as the palpable coracoid and acromion angle.

- *Central ray centering and collimation.* Once the humerus is accurately positioned with the IR and the central ray is centered to the humeral midpoint, open the longitudinal collimated field until it extends 1 inch (2.5 cm) beyond the elbow and shoulder joint. If the collimation does not extend beyond both joints, adjust the centering point of the central ray until both the elbow and shoulder joint are included within the collimated field without demonstrating an excessive light field beyond them. Transverse collimation should be within 0.5 inch (1.25 cm) of the skin line laterally and to (1) the lateral scapular border for the mediolateral projection or (2) the coracoid for the lateromedial projection.

Lateral Humeral Projection Analysis

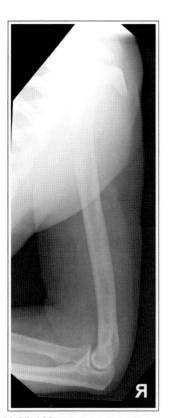

IMAGE 103 Mediolateral projection.

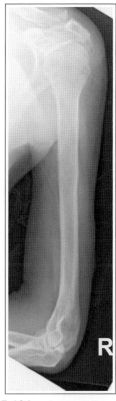

IMAGE 104 Lateromedial projection.

Analysis. The density is lighter at the proximal humerus than at the distal humerus. The torso was not in a PA projection but was rotated toward the humerus, increasing the tissue thickness at the proximal humerus.

Correction. Rotate the torso away from the proximal humerus into a PA projection.

Analysis. The humerus is not in a lateral projection. The epicondyles are not superimposed, the capitulum is posterior to the medial trochlea, and the proximal forearm is distorted. The forearm was positioned across the patient's body and the distal humerus was not drawn away from the table to place the epicondyles perpendicular to the IR, as shown in Figure 4-95.

Correction. Position the patient as shown in Figure 4-94, with the distal humerus positioned adjacent to the IR, aligning the humeral epicondyles perpendicularly to the IR.

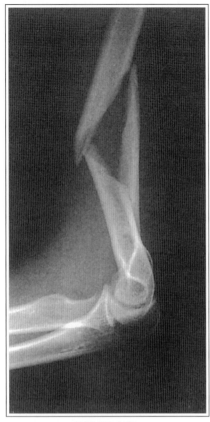

IMAGE 105

Analysis. This is a lateral distal humeral projection demonstrating a fractured distal humerus. The patient was accurately positioned.

Correction. No correction movement is required.

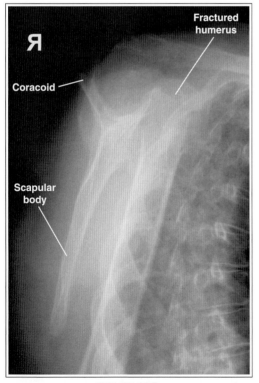

IMAGE 106

Analysis. This is an AP oblique (scapular Y) shoulder projection demonstrating a fractured proximal humerus. The image demonstrates accurate positioning. The scapular body is in a true lateral position. The scapular body, acromion, and coracoid form a Y, with the scapular body as the leg and the acromion and coracoid as the arms.

Correction. No correction movement is required.

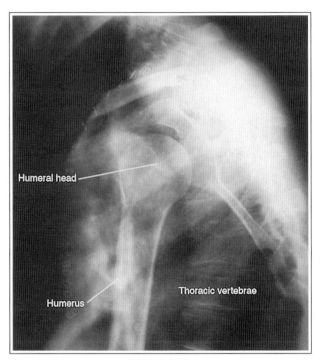

IMAGE 107

Analysis. This is a transthoracic lateral projection of the proximal humerus. The image demonstrates accurate positioning. The unaffected shoulder is superior to the affected shoulder, and the humerus is clearly demonstrated halfway between the thoracic vertebrae and the sternum.

Correction. No correction movement is required.

REFERENCE

1. Epner RA, Bowers WH, Guilford WB: Ulnar variance—the effect of wrist positioning and roentgen filming techniques, *J Hand Surg* 7:298–305, 1982.

Shoulder

OBJECTIVES

After completion of this chapter, you should be able to do the following:

- Identify the required anatomy on shoulder, clavicular, acromioclavicular (AC) joint, and scapular images.
- Describe how to properly position the patient, image receptor (IR), and central ray for shoulder, clavicular, AC joint, and scapular projections.
- State how to properly mark and display shoulder, clavicular, AC joint, and scapular projections.
- List the image analysis requirements for shoulder, clavicular, AC joint, and scapular projections with accurate positioning.
- State how to properly reposition the patient and/or central ray when shoulder, clavicular, AC joint, and scapular projections show poor positioning.
- State the kilovoltage routinely used for shoulder, clavicular, AC joint, and scapular projections and describe which anatomic structures are visible when the correct technique factors are used.
- Discuss why a compensating filter is needed on anteroposterior (AP) shoulder and clavicular projections.
- State where the humerus might be positioned if a shoulder dislocation is demonstrated on AP and

posteroanterior (PA) oblique (scapular Y) shoulder projections.
- Discuss how the visualization of the proximal humerus changes as the humeral epicondyles are placed at different angles to the IR.
- Explain how the scapula is affected when the humerus is abducted.
- State how the central ray angulation can be adjusted to offset longitudinal scapular foreshortening on a kyphotic patient.
- List the anatomic structures that form the Y on a PA oblique (scapular Y) shoulder projection.
- Discuss why non–weight-bearing and weight-bearing images are required for the AP AC joint projection.
- Describe how the shoulder is retracted to obtain an AP projection of the scapula.
- Describe the effect of humeral abduction on the degree of patient obliquity needed to position the scapula in a lateral projection.
- State which long axis of the scapular body is placed parallel with the IR as the humerus is abducted.

KEY TERMS

abduct
adduct
anterior shoulder dislocation
articulation
axilla
bilateral

Hill-Sachs defect
kyphosis
longitudinal foreshortening
palpate
posterior shoulder dislocation
protract

recumbent
retract
supraspinatus outlet
transverse foreshortening
unilateral
weight-bearing

IMAGE ANALYSIS CRITERIA

The following image analysis criteria are used for all adult and pediatric shoulder images and should be considered when completing the analysis for each shoulder projection presented in this chapter (Box 5-1).

An optimal kilovoltage peak (kVp) technique, as shown in Table 5-1, sufficiently penetrates the shoulder structures and provides the contrast scale necessary to visualize the shoulder details. If the AP or inferosuperior shoulder thickness measurement is over 4 inches (10 cm), a grid should be used to absorb the scatter radiation produced by the shoulder, increasing detail visibility. To obtain optimal density, set a manual milliampere-seconds (mAs) level based on the patient's shoulder thickness or choose the appropriate automatic exposure control (AEC) chamber when recommended (see Table 5-1).

BOX 5-1 | Shoulder Imaging Analysis Criteria

- The facility's identification requirements are visible.
- A right or left marker identifying the correct side of the patient is present on the image and is not superimposed over the anatomy of interest.
- Good radiation protection practices are evident.
- Bony trabecular patterns and cortical outlines of the anatomic structures are sharply defined.
- Contrast and density are uniform and adequate to demonstrate the surrounding soft-tissue and bony structures.
- Penetration is sufficient to visualize the bony trabecular patterns and cortical outlines of the shoulder and proximal humerus.
- No evidence of removable artifacts is present.

COMPENSATING FILTER

For AP projections of the shoulder, clavicle, and acromioclavicular (AC) joints, uniform density throughout the shoulder is obtained through the use of a compensating filter. When an exposure (mAs) is set or the AEC is accurately positioned over the glenohumeral joint to provide adequate shoulder density, often the laterally located acromion process and clavicular end are overexposed because of the difference in AP body thickness between these two regions. A compensating filter placed over or under the lateral clavicle region can be used to obtain uniform density across the entire shoulder (Figure 5-1). The filter should be positioned as described in Chapter 1.

TABLE 5-1 | Shoulder Technical Data

Projection	kVp	Grid/Nongrid	AEC Chamber(s)	SID
AP, shoulder	65-75	Grid	Center	40-48 inches (100-120 cm)
Inferosuperior axial, shoulder	65-75			40-48 inches (100-120 cm)
AP oblique (Grashey method), glenoid cavity	65-75	Grid	Center	40-48 inches (100-120 cm)
PA oblique (scapular Y), shoulder	65-75	Grid		40-48 inches (100-120 cm)
AP axial (Stryker "Notch" method), proximal humerus	65-75	Grid		40-48 inches (100-120 cm)
Tangential, supraspinatus outlet	65-75	Grid		40-48 inches (100-120 cm)
AP and AP axial, clavicle	65-75	Grid		40-48 inches (100-120 cm)
AP, AC joint	60-70	Nongrid		72 inches (183 cm)
	65-70	Grid		
AP, scapula	65-75	Grid	Center	40-48 inches (100-120 cm)
Lateral, scapula	70-75	Grid		40-48 inches (100-120 cm)

AEC, Automatic exposure control; *SID,* source–image receptor distance.

SHOULDER: ANTEROPOSTERIOR PROJECTION

See Figures 5-1 and 5-2 and Box 5-2.

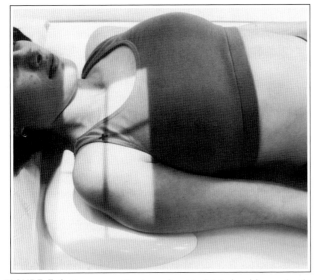

FIGURE 5-1 Proper positioning of neutral AP shoulder projection with compensating filter.

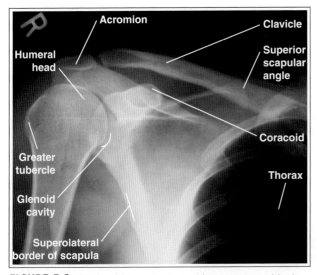

FIGURE 5-2 AP shoulder projection with accurate positioning.

BOX 5-2	Anteroposterior Shoulder Projection Analysis Criteria

- The superolateral border of the scapula is visible without thorax superimposition.
- The clavicle is demonstrated horizontally, with the medial end positioned adjacent to the vertebral column.
- The superior scapular angle is superimposed by midclavicle.
- The humerus is aligned parallel with the body and the glenoid cavity is partially visualized, facing laterally.
- Neutral humerus: the greater tubercle is partially seen in profile laterally and the humeral head is partially seen in profile medially.
- Externally rotated humerus: the greater tubercle is seen in profile laterally and the humeral head in profile medially.
- Internally rotated humerus: the lesser tubercle is seen in profile medially and the humeral head is superimposed by the greater tubercle.
- The glenohumeral joint and coracoid processes are at the center of the exposure field.
- The glenohumeral joint, the lateral two thirds of the clavicle, the proximal third of the humerus, and the superior scapula are included within the collimated field.

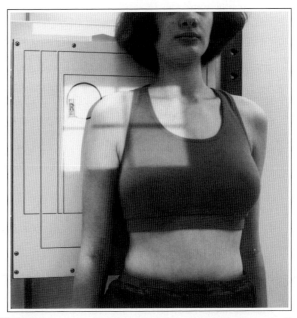

FIGURE 5-3 Proper positioning of neutral AP shoulder projection.

The shoulder girdle is in an AP projection. The scapular body demonstrates transverse foreshortening, showing the glenoid cavity, the superolateral border of the scapula is visible without thorax superimposition, and the clavicle is demonstrated horizontally, with the medial end of the clavicle positioned next to the lateral vertebral column. When the shoulder is not dislocated or the proximal humerus fractured, the posterior portion of the glenoid cavity and the medial margin of the humeral head are superimposed.

- An AP shoulder projection is achieved by placing the patient in a supine or an upright AP projection, with the shoulders positioned at equal distances from the imaging table or upright grid holder (Figure 5-3; also see Figure 5-1). When the patient is positioned in an AP projection, the clavicle should be demonstrated horizontally, with the medial end positioned next to the lateral vertebral column without excessive curvature or longitudinal foreshortening, and the scapular body is at 35 to 45 degrees of obliquity, with the lateral scapula situated more anteriorly than the medial scapula, and the glenoid cavity is visible.

- ***Shoulder retraction.*** The amount of scapular obliquity and glenoid fossa demonstration depends on the degree of shoulder retraction. Retraction or backward movement of the shoulder is a result of the gravitational pull placed on the shoulder when the patient is in a supine position and patient spinal straightening and backward shoulder movement when the patient is in an upright position. It causes the scapular body to be positioned more nearly parallel with the image.

- *Upright positioning for kyphosis.* The kyphotic patient will have less discomfort if in an upright position while the image is taken. If it is not possible to place the kyphotic patient in an upright position, use angled sponges under the shoulders and thorax to place the shoulders at equal distances from the imaging table. An imaging table sponge also helps ease patient discomfort.

- *Detecting rotation.* Rotation on an AP shoulder projection is detected by evaluating the details of the scapular body, glenoid cavity, and clavicle. When the patient is rotated toward the affected shoulder (places affected shoulder closer to IR than unaffected shoulder), the scapular body is positioned closer to or parallel with the IR and appears wider on the image. The thorax is superimposed over the superolateral scapular region, the glenoid cavity and scapular neck are positioned more in profile, and the clavicle is longitudinally foreshortened, with the medial clavicular end shifted away from the vertebral column (see Image 1). When the patient is rotated away from the affected shoulder, the scapular body demonstrates increased transverse foreshortening, the thorax is superimposed over a smaller amount of the scapula, the glenoid cavity is better demonstrated, and the medial clavicular end is superimposed over the vertebral column (see Image 2).

- *Effect of shoulder dislocation.* The AP shoulder projection is taken to detect proximal humerus fractures and shoulder dislocations. When there is no fracture or dislocation, the humeral head is centered to and slightly superimposed over the glenoid cavity. Proximal humerus fractures result in the humeral head being shifted away from this location, often not seeming to be associated with the humerus at all (see Image 3). Shoulder dislocation can result in positioning of the humeral head anteriorly or posteriorly and inferior to the glenoid cavity. Anterior dislocation, which is more common (95%), results in the humeral head being demonstrated anteriorly, beneath the coracoid process (see Image 4). Posterior dislocations, which are uncommon (2% to 4%), result in the humeral head being demonstrated posteriorly, beneath the acromion process or spine of the scapula.

The scapular body is demonstrated without longitudinal foreshortening. The superior scapular angle is superimposed by the midclavicle.

- The tilt of the midcoronal plane determines the degree of longitudinal scapular foreshortening. When the midcoronal plane is vertical and positioned parallel with the IR, the scapula is demonstrated without foreshortening.

- *Detecting scapular foreshortening.* If the upper midcoronal plane is tilted anteriorly (forward) the superior scapular angle will be demonstrated superior to the midclavicle (see Images 5 and 6). If the upper midcoronal plane is tilted posteriorly (backward) the superior scapular angle will be shown inferior to the midclavicle (see Image 7). The severity of foreshortening will increase with an increase in the degree of midcoronal plane tilt.

- *Compensating for kyphosis.* For the kyphotic patient, little can be done to improve patient positioning, but a cephalic central ray angulation can be used to offset the forward angle of the scapula. The central ray should be angled perpendicular to the scapular body.

The humerus is aligned parallel with the body, and the glenoid cavity faces laterally.

- Proper positioning for the AP shoulder projection is accomplished with zero humeral abduction. When the humerus is abducted, it is demonstrated away from the body, the glenoid cavity shifts superiorly, and the scapular body glides around the thorax, moving anteriorly (see Image 8). This scapular movement increases as humeral abduction increases beyond 60 degrees.

The glenohumeral joint space and the coracoid process are at the center of the exposure field. The glenohumeral joint, the lateral two thirds of the clavicle, the proximal third of the humerus, and the superior scapula are included within the collimation field.

- When the central ray is centered 1 inch (2.5 cm) inferior to the palpable coracoid process, the glenohumeral joint is centered within the collimated field. The coracoid process can be palpated 1 inch (2.5 cm) inferior to the midpoint of the lateral half of the clavicle and medial to the humeral head (Figure 5-4). Even on very muscular patients, the concave pocket formed inferior to the lateral half of the clavicle and medial to the humeral head can be used to center the central ray.

- Center the IR to the central ray and open the longitudinal collimation enough to include the top of the shoulder. Transversely collimate to within 0.5 inch (1.25 cm) of lateral humeral skin line.

- An 8- × 10-inch (18- × 25-cm) or 10- × 12-inch (25- × 30-cm) IR placed crosswise should be adequate to include all the required anatomic structures. The IR may be placed lengthwise to demonstrate more of the humerus.

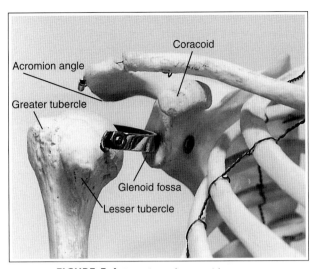

FIGURE 5-4 Location of coracoid process.

HUMERAL HEAD POSITIONING

The position of the humeral epicondyles with respect to the IR determines which anatomic aspect of the humeral head is demonstrated in profile.

- *Positioning for suspected fracture or dislocation.* On a patient with suspected shoulder dislocations or humeral fractures the humerus should not be rotated. Take the exposure with the humerus positioned as it is.

In *neutral rotation,* the greater tubercle is partially demonstrated in profile laterally and the humeral head is partially demonstrated in profile medially (see Figure 5-1).

- Accurate neutral humeral head rotation is accomplished by placing the patient's palm against the thigh, which will align the humeral epicondyles at a 45-degree angle with the IR (see Figure 5-3).

In *external rotation,* the greater tubercle is demonstrated in profile laterally, the humeral head is demonstrated in profile medially, and the vertical cortical outline of the lesser tubercle is visible approximately halfway between the greater tubercle and the medial aspect of the humeral head (see Image 9).

- Accurate external humeral head rotation is obtained by externally rotating the patient's arm until the humeral epicondyles are aligned parallel with the IR (Figure 5-5).
- An arrow or word marker should be used to indicate external humeral rotation. If the arrow is used, it should point laterally.

Locating the Greater and Lesser Tubercles and Humeral Head

- A method of determining where the greater tubercle and humeral head will be positioned on an image is to use the palpable humeral epicondyles. The lateral epicondyle is aligned with the greater tubercle, and the medial epicondyle is aligned with the humeral

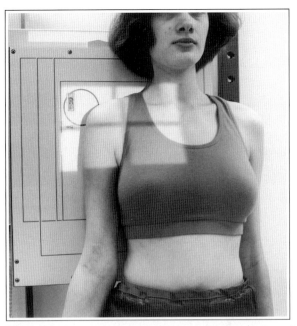

FIGURE 5-5 Proper positioning of AP shoulder projection with external humerus rotation.

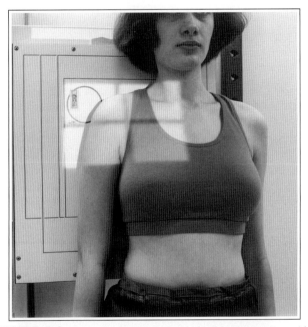

FIGURE 5-6 Proper positioning of AP shoulder projection with neutral humerus.

head. This means that when the humeral epicondyles are in profile, the greater tubercle and humeral head also will be. The lesser tubercle is anteriorly located at a right angle to the greater tubercle.

In *internal rotation,* the lesser tubercle is demonstrated in profile medially and the humeral head is superimposed by the greater tubercle (see Image 10).

- Accurate internal humeral head rotation is obtained by internally rotating the patient's arm until the humeral epicondyles are aligned perpendicular with the IR (Figure 5-6).

- Internal humeral rotation may also cause the scapula to move anteriorly, transversely foreshortening the scapular body, and may cause the humeral head to demonstrate increased glenoid fossa superimposition.
- An arrow or word marker should be used to indicate internal humeral rotation. If the arrow is used, it should point medially.

Anteroposterior Shoulder Projection Analysis

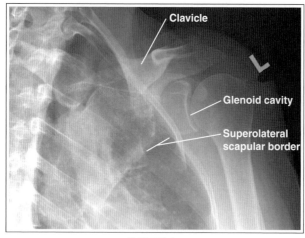

IMAGE 1

Analysis. The glenoid cavity is almost in profile, with only a small amount of the articulating surface demonstrated, the superolateral border of the scapula is superimposed by the thorax, and the clavicle is longitudinally foreshortened. The patient was rotated toward the affected shoulder.

Correction. Rotate the patient away from the affected shoulder into an AP projection, with the shoulders positioned at equal distances from the imaging table.

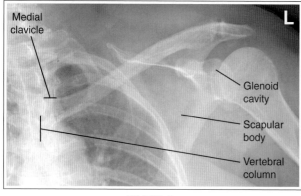

IMAGE 2

Analysis. The scapular body is drawn from beneath the thorax and is foreshortened, the glenoid cavity is demonstrated on end, and the medial clavicular end is superimposed over the vertebral column. The patient was rotated toward the unaffected shoulder.

Correction. Rotate the patient toward the affected shoulder into an AP projection, with the shoulders positioned at equal distances from the imaging table.

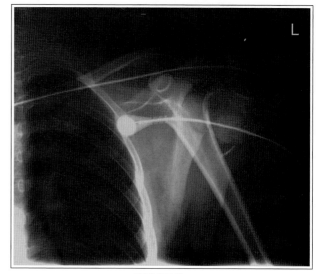

IMAGE 3

Analysis. The humeral head is demonstrated lateral to the glenoid cavity and the humeral head has been broken away from the proximal humerus. There is a proximal humerus fracture.

Correction. No correction movement is needed. When a proximal humerus fracture is suspected, the patient's arm should not be rotated to position the greater and lesser tubercles in the required position for a AP shoulder projection. Take the image with the arm positioned as is.

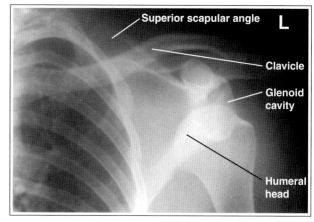

IMAGE 4

Analysis. The humeral head is demonstrated below the coracoid process, and the superior scapular angle is shown superior to the clavicle. The patient's shoulder is dislocated, and the upper midcoronal plane was tilted anteriorly.

Correction. Do not adjust humeral positioning. Tilt the upper midcoronal plane toward the IR.

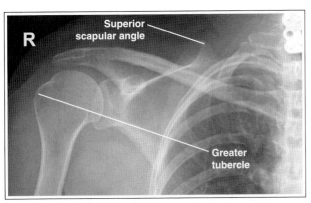

IMAGE 5

Analysis. The superior scapular angle is demonstrated superior to the clavicle. The patient's upper midcoronal plane was tilted anteriorly. The greater tubercle is in profile laterally.

Correction. Tilt the upper midcoronal plane posteriorly until it is parallel with the IR. For a kyphotic patient whose vertebral column cannot be straightened, bring the central ray perpendicular to the scapular body by angling it cephalically. No corrective movement is necessary if the greater tubercle is wanted in profile. If a neutral position is desired, position the humeral epicondyles at a 45-degree angle with the IR (see Figure 5-3). To demonstrate the lesser tubercle in profile, internally rotate the arm until the humeral epicondyles are perpendicular to the IR (see Figure 5-6).

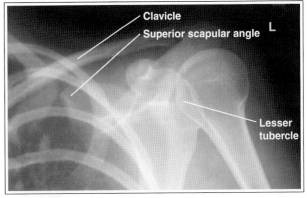

IMAGE 7

Analysis. The superior scapular angle is demonstrated inferior to the clavicle. The patient's upper midcoronal plane was tilted posteriorly. The lesser tubercle is demonstrated in profile medially, and the greater tubercle and humeral head are superimposed. The patient's humerus was internally rotated until the humeral epicondyles were perpendicular to the IR.

Correction. Tilt the upper midcoronal plane anteriorly until it is parallel with the IR. No corrective movement is necessary if the lesser tubercle is wanted in profile. If a neutral position is desired, position the humeral epicondyles at a 45-degree angle to the IR (see Figure 5-3). To demonstrate the greater tubercle in profile, externally rotate the arm until the humeral epicondyles are parallel with the IR (see Figure 5-5).

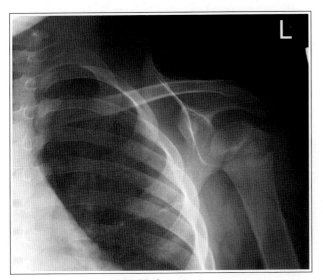

IMAGE 6 Pediatric.

Analysis. The superior scapular angle is demonstrated superior to the clavicle. The patient's upper midcoronal plane was tilted anteriorly.

Correction. Tilt the upper midcoronal plane posteriorly until it is parallel with the IR.

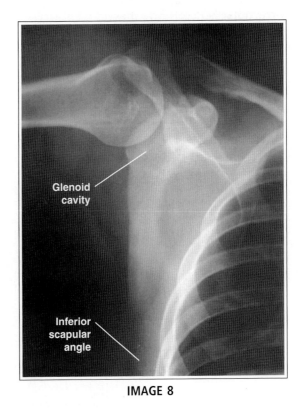

IMAGE 8

Analysis. The humerus is demonstrated at a 90-degree angle with the body, the glenoid cavity faces superiorly, and the lateral scapular body is drawn away from the thorax. The humerus was abducted.

Correction. Position the humerus next to the patient's body.

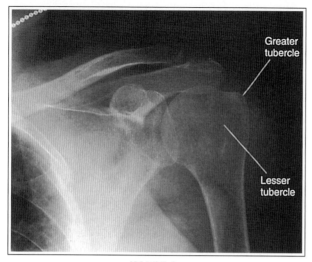

IMAGE 9

Analysis. The greater tubercle is demonstrated in profile laterally, the humeral head is demonstrated medially, and the cortical margin of the lesser tubercle is visible approximately halfway between the greater tubercle and the humeral head. The patient's humerus was externally rotated until the humeral epicondyles were parallel with the IR.

Correction. No corrective movement is necessary if the greater tubercle is wanted in profile. If a neutral position is desired, position the humeral epicondyles at

a 45-degree angle with the IR (see Figure 5-3). To demonstrate the lesser tubercle in profile, internally rotate the arm until the humeral epicondyles are perpendicular to the IR (see Figure 5-6).

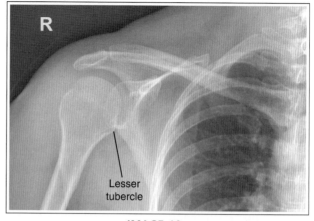

IMAGE 10

Analysis. The lesser tubercle is demonstrated in profile medially, and the greater tubercle and humeral head are superimposed. The patient's humerus was internally rotated until the humeral epicondyles were perpendicular to the IR.

Correction. No corrective movement is necessary if the lesser tubercle is wanted in profile. If a neutral position is desired, position the humeral epicondyles at a 45-degree angle with the IR (see Figure 5-3). To demonstrate the greater tubercle in profile, externally rotate the arm until the humeral epicondyles are parallel with the IR (see Figure 5-5).

SHOULDER: INFEROSUPERIOR AXIAL PROJECTION (LAWRENCE METHOD)

See Figures 5-7, 5-8, and 5-9 and Box 5-3.

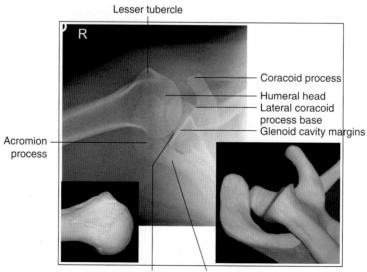

FIGURE 5-7 Inferosuperior axial shoulder projection with accurate positioning obtained with humeral epicondyles positioned parallel with floor.

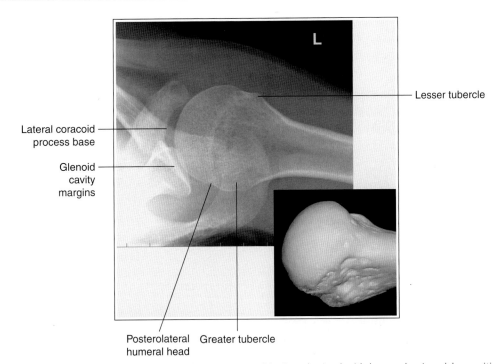

Lateral coracoid process base

Glenoid cavity margins

Lesser tubercle

Posterolateral humeral head   Greater tubercle

FIGURE 5-8 Inferosuperior axial shoulder projection with accurate positioning obtained with humeral epicondyles positioned at 45 degrees with floor.

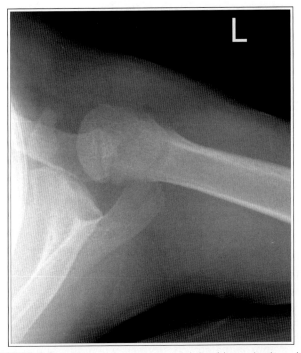

FIGURE 5-9 Pediatric inferosuperior axial shoulder projection with accurate positioning.

The inferior and superior margins of the glenoid cavity are almost superimposed, with only a small amount of humeral head superimposition. The lateral edge of the coracoid process base is aligned with the inferior glenoid cavity margin.

- The inferosuperior axial projection of the shoulder is obtained by placing the patient supine on the imaging table in an AP projection with the affected

BOX 5-3	**Inferosuperior Axial Shoulder Projection (Lawrence Method) Analysis Criteria**

- The inferior and superior margins of the glenoid cavity are almost superimposed, with only a small amount of humeral head superimposition.
- The lateral edge of the coracoid process base is aligned with the inferior glenoid cavity margin.
- The proximal humerus is seen without distortion, and the long axis of the humeral shaft is seen with minimal foreshortening.
- Epicondyles parallel with floor: the lesser tubercle is seen in profile anteriorly.
- Epicondyles at 45-degree angle with floor: the lesser tubercle is seen in partial profile anteriorly and the posterolateral aspect of the humeral head is seen in profile posteriorly.
- The entire coracoid process is demonstrated in profile.
- The humeral head is at the center of the exposure field.
- The glenoid cavity, coracoid process, scapular spine, acromion process, and one third of the proximal humerus are included within the collimated field.

shoulder next to the lateral edge of the imaging table. The patient's arm is then abducted 90 degrees from the body, and a horizontal beam is directed to the axilla, parallel with the glenohumeral joint space (Figure 5-10).

Positioning for suspected fracture or dislocation. On a patient with suspected proximal humeral fractures or shoulder dislocations, the humerus should not be elevated or rotated to avoid farther displacement and nerve damage (see Images 11 and 12). To obtain a lateral projection of the shoulder and

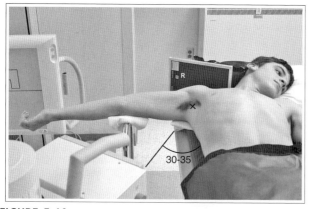

FIGURE 5-10 Proper positioning of inferosuperior axial shoulder projection.

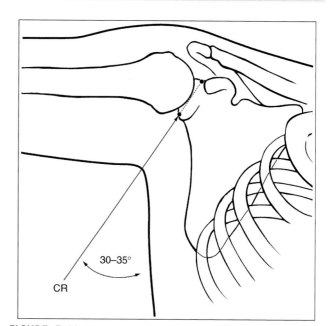

FIGURE 5-11 Placement of glenoid cavity with arm abducted 90 degrees. *CR*, Central ray.

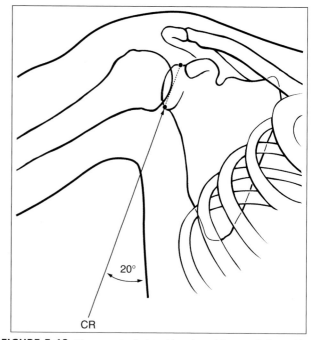

FIGURE 5-12 Placement of glenoid cavity with arm abducted less than 90 degrees. *CR*, Central ray.

proximal humerus when a fracture or dislocation is suspected, perform the PA oblique (scapular Y) projection as described on page 270).

- ***Effect of humeral abduction on central ray alignment.*** Because no palpable structures are present to help align the central ray with the glenohumeral joint, we must rely on our knowledge of scapular movement on humeral abduction to align it. Abduction of the arm is accomplished by combined movements of the glenohumeral joint and the scapula as it glides around the thoracic cavity. The ratio of movement in these two articulations is two parts glenohumeral to one part scapulothoracic, with the initial movement being primarily glenohumeral. If the patient's arm is not abducted, the glenoid cavity is angled approximately 20 degrees with the lateral body surface.

  In a patient who is not experiencing severe pain with the 90-degree humeral abduction, the scapular movement angles the glenoid cavity to approximately 30 to 35 degrees with the lateral body surface (Figure 5-11). Consequently, to align the central ray parallel with the glenohumeral joint on such a patient, the angle between the lateral body surface and central ray should be 30 to 35 degrees. This angle is best accomplished by first determining the 23- and 45-degree angles (see Chapter 1) and then aligning the central ray between these two angles. Thirty-four degrees is halfway between the 23- and 45-degree angles (see Figure 5-10).

  Because the glenoid cavity faces superiorly when the arm is abducted, if a patient is unable to abduct the arm fully, the angle between the lateral body surface and central ray needs to be decreased to align it parallel with the glenohumeral joint (Figure 5-12). Because the first 60 degrees of humeral abduction involves primarily movement of the glenohumeral joint without accompanying scapular movement, the angle between the central ray and lateral body surface should be

approximately 20 degrees when the humerus is abducted up to 60 degrees.

- ***Detecting inaccurate central ray alignment.*** Inaccurate alignment of the central ray with the glenohumeral joint space can be signified on an image by the increased demonstration of the articulating surface of the glenoid cavity and misalignment of the inferior glenoid cavity margin with the lateral edge of the coracoid process base. Whether the angle between the central ray and the lateral body surface should be increased or decreased can be determined by viewing the relationship of the coracoid process base to the inferior glenoid cavity margin. Because the inferior glenoid cavity margin is situated farther from the IR, it will be projected to one side of the coracoid process base instead of being aligned with it if the central ray is aligned inaccurately. If the central ray to lateral body surface angle is too small, the inferior glenoid cavity margin will be projected laterally to the lateral edge of the coracoid process base. (Closely compare the coracoid process base and glenoid cavity relationships in Figure 5-7 and Image 13.) If the angle is too large, the inferior margin will be projected medially to the lateral edge of the coracoid process base (see Image 14).

The proximal humerus is demonstrated without distortion, and the long axis of the humeral shaft is demonstrated with minimal foreshortening.

- Poor alignment of the IR with the central ray and with the humerus results in image distortion. Distortion caused by poor IR and central ray alignment can be eliminated by aligning the central ray with the patient's glenohumeral joint and then positioning the IR vertically at the top of the affected shoulder so it is perpendicular to the central ray. Distortion of the humeral shaft and head can be reduced when the patient's humerus is placed in 90-degree abduction. If the patient is unable to abduct the arm to 90 degrees, the humeral shaft and head demonstrate foreshortening (see Image 15). The severity of the distortion depends on how close to 90 degrees the patient was able to abduct the humerus. The more the humerus is abducted, the less distortion is demonstrated.

The proximal humerus is positioned as indicated by your facility.
When humeral epicondyles are positioned parallel with the floor, the lesser tubercle is demonstrated in profile anteriorly (see Figure 5-7).

- The lesser tubercle is placed in profile when the arm is extended and then externally rotated until an imaginary line connecting the epicondyles is positioned parallel with the floor.

When humeral epicondyles are positioned at a 45-degree angle with the floor, the lesser tubercle is demonstrated in partial profile anteriorly and the posterolateral aspect of the humeral head is in profile posteriorly (see Figure 5-8).

- The lesser tubercle is placed in partial profile, and the posterolateral aspect of the humeral head is positioned in profile when the arm is extended and then externally rotated until an imaginary line connecting the humeral epicondyles is placed at a

45-degree angle with the floor (see Figure 5-10). The lateral epicondyle is positioned closer to the floor. This humerus positioning is especially helpful in identifying a compression fracture of the posterolateral aspect of the humeral head. This compression fracture, a result of an anterior shoulder dislocation, is known as the Hill-Sachs defect.

- If the humeral epicondyles are positioned at an angle greater than 45 degrees with the floor, or if the patient's elbow is flexed so that the hand of the affected arm can be used to hold the IR in place, the lesser tubercle and posterolateral humeral head will not be demonstrated. The greater tubercle will be demonstrated in profile posteriorly and the humeral head anteriorly when the humerus is externally rotated enough to place the humeral epicondyles perpendicular to the floor (see Image 16). For some patients, this degree of external rotation can only be accomplished by involving the vertebral column as described in the next section.

The entire coracoid process is demonstrated in profile.

- The coracoid process is demonstrated in profile when the scapular body is placed parallel with the imaging table because the patient is positioned supine. With excessive external arm rotation, the inferior scapula tilts anteriorly as the vertebral column arches to accomplish this arm rotation. This tilting results in the base of the coracoid process moving beneath the glenoid cavity, decreasing its visibility (see Image 17).

The humeral head is centered within the collimated field. The glenoid cavity, coracoid process, scapular spine, acromion process, and one third of the proximal humerus are included within the collimation field.

- *Including the posterior surface.* To ensure that the scapular spine is included within the image, elevate the patient's shoulder 2 to 3 inches (5 to 7.6 cm) from the imaging table with a sponge or folded washcloth. If the shoulder is not elevated, the posterior portion of the humerus and shoulder may not be included on the image (see Image 18).

- *Including the coracoid.* To include the coracoid process on the image, instruct the patient to turn the face away from the affected shoulder and then laterally flex the neck, tilting the head toward the unaffected shoulder. Place an IR at the top of the patient's shoulder perpendicular to the imaging table and resting snugly against the patient's neck. If the IR is not positioned snugly against the patient's neck, the coracoid process and possibly the glenoid cavity and proximal humerus may not be included on the image (see Image 19).

- *Centering the humeral head.* To align the central ray with the glenohumeral joint, center the central ray horizontally to the midaxillary region at the same level as the coracoid process. (Palpate to locate the coracoid process before humeral abduction.) The humeral head is centered in the collimated field for the axial shoulder, even though the central ray is centered to the glenohumeral joint, because the IR cannot be positioned medially enough to center the joint in the center.

- Open the longitudinal collimation slightly beyond the coracoid process, and transversely collimate to within 0.5 inch (1.25 cm) of the proximal humeral skin line.

- An 8- × 10-inch (18- × 25-cm) IR placed crosswise should be adequate to include all the required anatomic structures.

Inferosuperior Axial Shoulder Projection Analysis

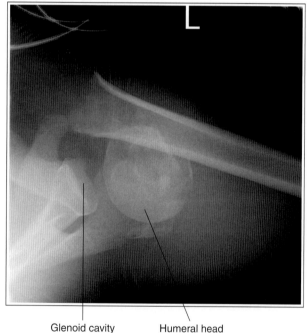

Glenoid cavity   Humeral head
IMAGE 11

Analysis. The humeral head has been broken away from the proximal humerus, demonstrating a displaced proximal humerus fracture.

Correction. No correction movement is needed. When a proximal humerus fracture is suspected, the patient's arm should not be abducted or rotated. Instead, a PA oblique (scapular Y) projection of the proximal humerus should be performed.

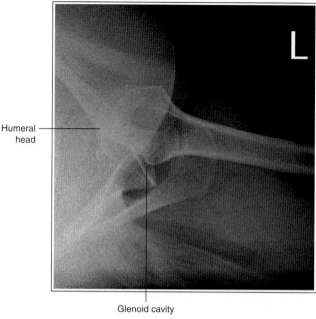

Humeral head

Glenoid cavity

IMAGE 12

Analysis. The humeral head is demonstrated anterior to the glenoid cavity. The patient's shoulder is anteriorly dislocated.

Correction. No correction movement is needed. When a proximal humerus fracture is suspected, the patient's arm should not be abducted or rotated. Instead, a PA oblique (scapular Y) projection of the proximal humerus should be performed.

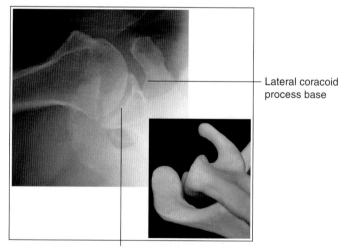

Lateral coracoid process base

Inferior glenoid cavity margin
IMAGE 13

Analysis. The glenohumeral joint is closed, and the inferior glenoid cavity margin is demonstrated lateral to the coracoid process base. The angle formed between the lateral body surface and the central ray was less than required to align the central ray parallel with the glenohumeral joint.

Correction. Increase the angle between the lateral body surface and the central ray to 30 to 35 degrees.

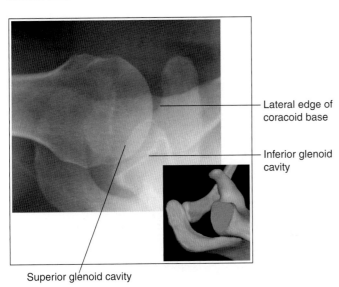

Lateral edge of coracoid base

Inferior glenoid cavity

Superior glenoid cavity

IMAGE 14

Analysis. The glenohumeral joint is closed, and the inferior glenoid cavity margin is demonstrated medially to the lateral edge of the coracoid process base and superior glenoid cavity margin, indicating that the angle between the lateral body surface and the central ray was too large.

Correction. Decrease the angle between the lateral body surface and central ray. If the patient is able to abduct the arm to 90 degrees, the lateral body surface and central ray angle should be 30 to 35 degrees. If the patient is unable to abduct the arm, a smaller angle is required (see Figure 5-12).

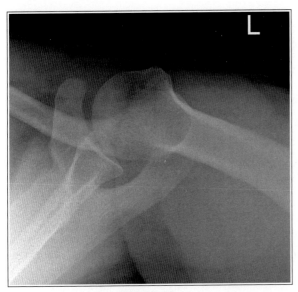

L

IMAGE 15

Analysis. The glenoid cavity and coracoid process are accurately demonstrated, but the humerus is foreshortened and the humeral head is distorted. The arm was not abducted 90 degrees from the body.

Correction. If possible, have the patient abduct the humerus 90 degrees from the body. If the patient cannot abduct the humerus, no corrective movement is necessary.

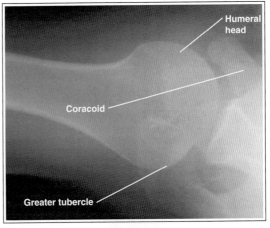

Humeral head

Coracoid

Greater tubercle

IMAGE 16

Analysis. The greater tubercle is in profile posteriorly. The entire coracoid process is not demonstrated in profile. The humerus was externally rotated enough to position the humeral epicondyles perpendicular to the floor.

Correction. Internally rotate the humerus until the epicondyles are at a 45-degree angle with the floor if the posterolateral humeral head is desired in profile or until they are parallel with the floor if the lesser tubercle is desired in profile.

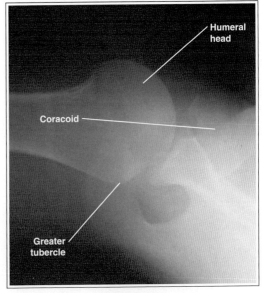

Humeral head

Coracoid

Greater tubercle

IMAGE 17

Analysis. The greater tubercle is in profile posteriorly, and the coracoid process base is partially obscured by the glenoid cavity. The humerus was externally rotated enough to position the humeral epicondyles perpendicular to the floor, and the inferior scapula was tilted anteriorly.

Correction. Internally rotate humerus until the epicondyles are at a 45-degree angle with floor if the posterolateral humeral head is desired in profile and until they are parallel with the floor if the lesser tubercle is desired in profile. This arm movement will also result in the scapula being positioned parallel with the imaging table, increasing coracoid process visibility.

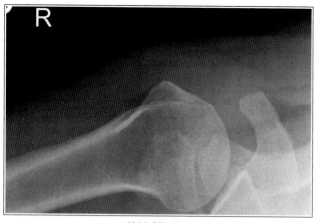

IMAGE 18

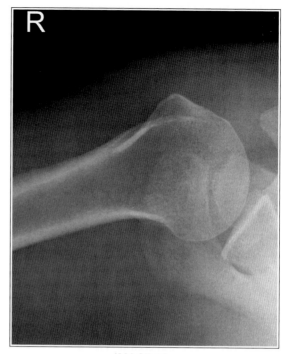

IMAGE 19

Analysis. The posterior aspect of the shoulder is not included on the image. The patient's shoulder was not adequately elevated off the imaging table.

Correction. Elevate the shoulder 2 to 3 inches (5 to 7.6 cm) off the imaging table with a sponge or folded washcloth.

Analysis. The coracoid process is not included on the image. The patient's head was not turned or the neck laterally flexed toward the unaffected shoulder enough to adequately position the IR medially.

Correction. Turn the patient's face, and laterally flex the neck and tilt the head toward the unaffected shoulder. Then snugly position the edge of the IR against the patient's neck.

GLENOID CAVITY: AP OBLIQUE PROJECTION (GRASHEY METHOD)

See Figures 5-13 and 5-14 and Box 5-4.

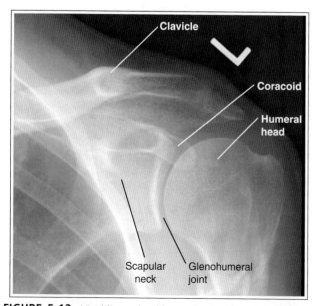

FIGURE 5-13 AP oblique shoulder projection (Grashey Method) with accurate positioning.

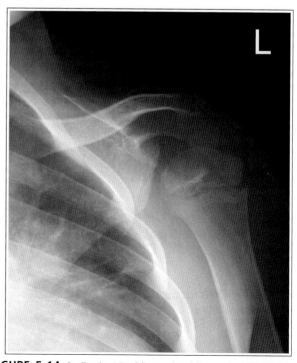

FIGURE 5-14 Pediatric AP oblique shoulder projection (Grashey Method) with accurate positioning.

BOX 5-4	Anteroposterior Oblique Projection (Grashey Method) Analysis Criteria

- The glenoid cavity in profile with open glenohumeral joint space.
- The lateral coracoid process is superimposing the humeral head by about 0.25 inch (0.6 cm).
- The glenohumeral joint is at the center of the exposure field.
- The glenoid cavity, humeral head, coracoid and acromion processes, and distal clavicle are included within the collimated field.

The glenoid cavity is demonstrated in profile, with the glenohumeral joint space open, the lateral coracoid process demonstrates approximately 0.25 inch (0.6 cm) of superimposition of the humeral head, the glenoid cavity is shown without thorax superimposition, and the clavicle is longitudinally foreshortened.

- To obtain an image that demonstrates the glenoid cavity in profile and an open glenohumeral joint space, the patient's scapular body must be positioned parallel with the IR. This is accomplished by placing the patient in an upright AP projection and then rotating the patient's body approximately 35 to 45 degrees toward the affected shoulder (Figure 5-15). A 35- to 45-degree AP oblique projection routinely opens the glenohumeral joint space as long as the patient is upright and the affected shoulder is in a neutral position without protraction.
- *Effect of shoulder protraction on the required degree of patient obliquity.* Protraction or forward movement of the shoulder occurs as a result of pressure that is placed on the affected shoulder when the patient leans against the upright IR holder. The sternoclavicular and AC joints function cooperatively to allow the shoulder to be drawn anteriorly. When the shoulder is drawn anteriorly, the scapula glides around the thorax, moving the lateral portion of the scapula anteriorly. This increase in anterior shoulder positioning places the scapular body at a larger angle with the IR, therefore requiring an increase in patient obliquity to bring the scapular body parallel with the IR for the AP oblique (Grashey method) projection. An image taken with the patient leaning against the IR holder will demonstrate an open glenohumeral joint, but a portion of the thorax will be superimposed over the glenoid cavity (see Image 20). An increase in patient obliquity is also necessary when the examination is performed on a kyphotic or recumbent patient. Because of the vertebral column curvature, the kyphotic patient's shoulders are situated anteriorly, aligning them similarly to protracted shoulders. In this situation, an image can be obtained that demonstrates the glenoid cavity in profile and an open glenohumeral joint space, although the thorax often is superimposed over them. In the recumbent position, the pressure of the body on the shoulder forces the shoulder of interest anteriorly and superiorly when the patient is rotated. Images taken with the patient in this position demonstrate the glenoid cavity situated slightly superiorly and the clavicle aligned more vertically (see Image 21).

- *Recommended method of determining degree of body obliquity.* The most accurate method of determining the amount of patient obliquity necessary for all AP oblique (Grashey) shoulder projections is to palpate the patient's coracoid process and acromion angle and then rotate the patient toward the affected shoulder until the coracoid process is superimposed over the acromion angle, aligning an imaginary line connecting them perpendicular to the IR (Figure 5-16).

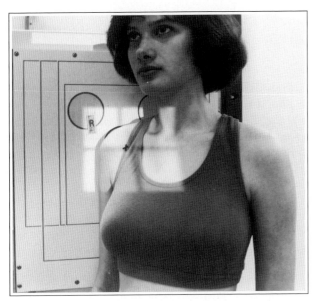

FIGURE 5-15 Proper positioning for AP oblique shoulder projection (Grashey Method).

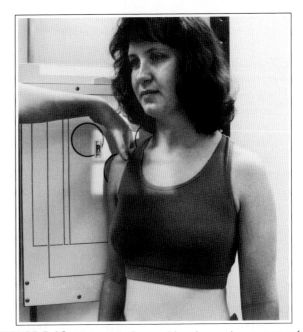

FIGURE 5-16 Alignment of coracoid and acromion processes for AP oblique shoulder projection (Grashey Method).

- *Detecting incorrect obliquity.* Incorrect body obliquity will be identified on an image as a closed glenohumeral joint space. Whether the body has been rotated too much or too little to accomplish this closed joint can be determined by evaluating the relationship of the coracoid process with the humeral head, the degree of thorax superimposition on the glenoid cavity and scapular neck, and the longitudinal clavicle foreshortening. If obliquity was excessive, the glenohumeral joint space is closed, more than 0.25 inch (0.6 cm) of the lateral tip of the coracoid process is superimposed over the humeral head, the thorax demonstrates increased glenoid cavity and scapular neck superimposition, and the clavicle demonstrates excessive longitudinal foreshortening (see Image 22). If obliquity was insufficient, the glenohumeral joint space is closed, the lateral tip of the coracoid process demonstrates less than 0.25 inch (0.6 cm) of humeral head superimposition, the thorax is not superimposed over the scapular neck, and the clavicle demonstrates little foreshortening (see Image 23).
- *Evaluating the recumbent patient's image.* When evaluating an AP oblique (Grashey) shoulder projection on a recumbent patient, you cannot use clavicular foreshortening as a guide to determine repositioning because it is vertically positioned, although you can evaluate its proximity to the scapular neck. If obliquity was excessive, the glenohumeral joint is closed, the lateral tip of the coracoid process is superimposed over more than 0.25 inch (0.6 cm) of the humeral head, and the clavicle is superimposed over the scapular neck (see Image 24). If the obliquity was insufficient, then the glenohumeral joint is closed, the lateral tip of the coracoid process is superimposed over less than 0.25 inch (0.6 cm) of the humeral head, and the clavicle is not superimposed over the scapular neck (see Image 25).
- *Repositioning for inadequate obliquity.* When repositioning for an excessive or insufficient obliquity on an AP oblique (Grashey) projection, remember that the glenohumeral joint space is narrow and that the necessary repositioning movement is only half the distance demonstrated between the anterior and posterior margins of the glenoid cavity. In most cases, you need to move the patient only a few degrees to obtain an open joint space, so it is important to carefully evaluate and make mental notes on how the patient was positioned for the initial examination. If a repeat is necessary, start with the patient position used for the initial examination and then adjust the position from this starting point.

The glenohumeral joint is at the center of the exposure field. The glenoid cavity, humeral head, coracoid and acromion processes, and distal clavicle are included within the collimation field.

- Center a perpendicular central ray at a level 1 inch (2.5 cm) inferior and medial to the palpable coracoid process to place the glenohumeral joint at the center of the exposure field. The coracoid process can be palpated 0.75 inch (2 cm) inferior to the midpoint of the lateral half of the clavicle and medial to the humeral head. Even on very muscular patients, the concave pocket formed inferior to the lateral half of the clavicle and medial to the humeral head can be used to center the central ray.
- Center the IR to the central ray and open the longitudinal collimated field enough to include the shoulder top and transversely collimate to the lateral humeral skin line.
- An 8- × 10-inch (18- × 25-cm) IR placed crosswise should be adequate to include all the required anatomic structures.

Anteroposterior Oblique Projection Shoulder Projection Analysis (Grashey Method)

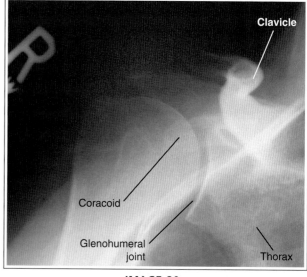

IMAGE 20

Analysis. The glenohumeral joint space is open, and the lateral tip of the coracoid process is superimposed over the humeral head by approximately 0.25 inch (0.6 cm). The clavicle demonstrates excessive longitudinal foreshortening, and the thorax is superimposed over the inferior glenohumeral joint space. The image was taken with the shoulder protracted and the patient rotated more than 45 degrees to obtain an open glenohumeral joint space. Shoulder protraction results when the patient leans against the upright IR holder or is in a supine position. Because the clavicle is not vertical, it can be determined that this examination was conducted with the patient leaning against the upright holder.

Correction. Position the patient's upper midcoronal plane in a vertical position, and place the affected shoulder in a neutral position. Do not allow the patient to lean against the upright IR holder. Less patient obliquity will be required with this new positioning.

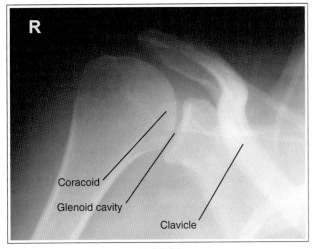

IMAGE 21

Analysis. The glenohumeral joint space is open, the glenoid cavity is situated slightly superiorly, and the clavicle is aligned somewhat vertically. This examination was taken with the patient in a recumbent position.

Correction. No positioning change is required. The goal of the examination is to obtain an image with an open and unobstructed glenohumeral joint space.

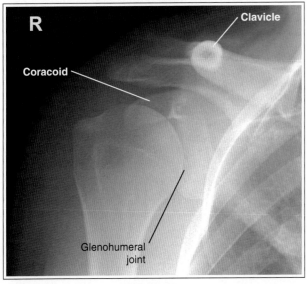

IMAGE 22

Analysis. The glenohumeral joint space is closed, more than 0.25 inch (0.6 cm) of the lateral tip of the coracoid process is superimposed over the humeral head, and the clavicle demonstrates excessive longitudinal foreshortening. Patient obliquity was excessive.

Correction. Decrease the degree of patient obliquity. The amount of decrease required is only half the distance between the anterior and posterior margins of the glenoid cavity.

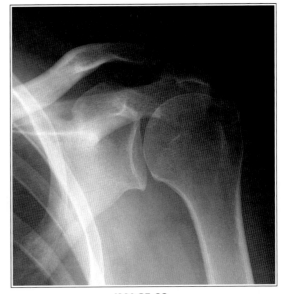

IMAGE 23

Analysis. The glenohumeral joint space is closed, the lateral tip of the coracoid process superimposes less than 0.25 inch (0.6 cm) of the humeral head, and the clavicle demonstrates little foreshortening. Patient obliquity was insufficient.

Correction. Increase the degree of patient obliquity, thereby moving the coracoid process toward the humeral head and shifting the anterior and posterior margins of the glenoid cavity toward each other.

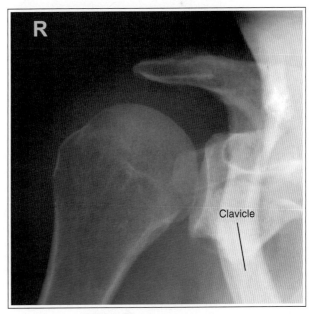

IMAGE 24 Recumbent patient.

Analysis. The glenohumeral joint space is closed, more than 0.25 inch (0.6 cm) of the coracoid process tip is superimposed over the humeral head, and the clavicle is superimposed over the scapular neck. The patient was in a recumbent position. Patient obliquity was excessive.

Correction. Decrease the degree of patient obliquity.

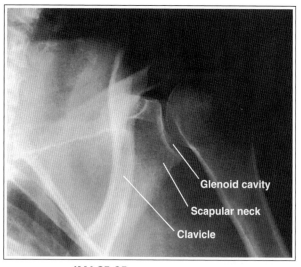

IMAGE 25 Recumbent patient.

Analysis. The glenohumeral joint space is closed, less than 0.25 inch (0.6 cm) of the coracoid process tip is superimposed over the humeral head, and the clavicle is not superimposed over the scapular neck. The patient was in a recumbent position. Patient obliquity was insufficient.

Correction. Increase the degree of patient obliquity.

SCAPULAR Y: POSTEROANTERIOR OBLIQUE PROJECTION

See Figure 5-17 and Box 5-5.

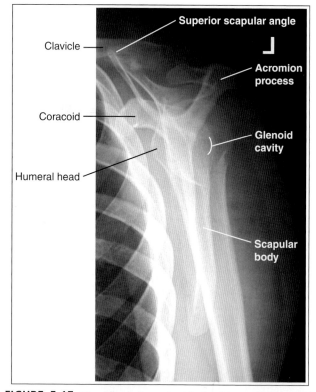

FIGURE 5-17 PA oblique (scapular Y) shoulder projection with accurate positioning.

The scapula demonstrates the least amount of magnification.

- The standing anterior oblique patient position places the scapula closer to the IR, resulting in the least amount of scapular magnification and the greatest scapular detail.

BOX 5-5	**Posteroanterior Oblique (Scapular Y) Shoulder Projection Analysis Criteria**

- The scapula demonstrates the least possible magnification.
- The lateral and vertebral scapular borders are superimposed.
- The scapular body and the acromion and coracoid processes form a Y.
- The relationship between the humeral head and glenoid cavity is demonstrated.
- The superior scapular angle is superimposed over the clavicle.
- The midscapular body is at the center of the exposure field.
- The scapula, including the inferior and superior angles, the coracoid and acromion processes, and the proximal humerus, are included within the collimated field.

The scapular body is in a lateral projection. The lateral and vertebral scapular borders are superimposed, and the scapular body is not superimposed over the thoracic cavity. The scapular body and the acromion and coracoid processes form a Y, with the scapular body as the leg and the acromion and coracoid processes as the arms. The glenoid cavity is demonstrated on end at the converging point of the arms and leg of the Y.

- To place the scapular body in a lateral projection, begin by placing the patient in an upright PA projection, with the affected arm hanging freely. This nonelevated arm position aligns the vertebral border of the scapula parallel with the IR when the scapula is in a lateral projection, allowing the coracoid and acromion processes to be demonstrated in profile. From this PA projection, rotate the patient's body 45 to 60 degrees toward the affected scapula until the lateral and vertebral scapular borders are superimposed (Figure 5-18).

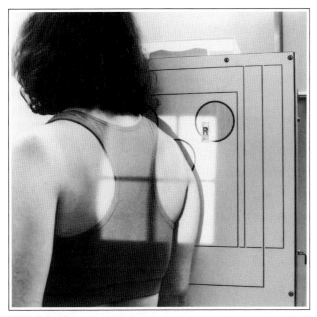

FIGURE 5-18 Proper positioning of PA oblique (scapular Y) shoulder projection.

- *Amount of body obliquity required.* The degree of body obliquity required to superimpose the scapular borders for the PA oblique projection has been questioned. Some textbooks have stated that the midcoronal plane should form a 60-degree angle with the IR. This degree of obliquity originated from the observations made by Rubin and colleagues[2] of the Y shoulder formation while they were evaluating 60-degree oblique chest images. A later study of the PA oblique projection presented by De Smet[1] found that a 45-degree anterior obliquity was the optimal obliquity for this image.

  The controversy between these two observations may lie in the position of the humerus. For a 60-degree PA oblique chest projection, the patient's humerus is abducted and the hand is placed on the patient's crest. When the patient is rotated, the shoulder is retracted (drawn backward). This humerus and shoulder positioning causes the scapula to glide around the thoracic cavity, moving toward the spinal column. When the scapula is in this posterior position, the patient's body needs to be rotated more to bring the scapular body lateral. The 1979 report by De Smet stated that the humerus is to hang freely.[1] Because the humerus and shoulder are not forced backward when the arm hangs freely, the scapula is positioned slightly more anteriorly, therefore needing less obliquity to bring it into a lateral projection.

- *Using scapular palpation to determine accurate degree of body obliquity.* Accurate patient obliquity can be obtained by palpating the coracoid process and the acromion angle and then rotating the patient until an imaginary line drawn between them is aligned parallel with the IR. This positioning sets up the Y formation, with the scapular body positioned between the acromion and coracoid processes. Once the correct obliquity is determined, have the patient step toward the IR until the patient's shoulder just touches the upright grid and IR holder. The exact degree of obliquity varies from patient to patient, depending on shoulder roundness, arm position, and pressure placed on the shoulder when the patient touches the IR holder.

- *AP oblique projection.* For a patient who is supine, the scapular Y image can be obtained by means of an AP oblique projection. Palpate the acromion and coracoid processes and vertebral scapular borders in the same way as described for the standing PA oblique projection, and rotate the patient toward the unaffected shoulder until the vertebral scapular border lies midway between the acromion and coracoid processes. The anatomic relationship of the bony structures of the scapula should be aligned identically on PA and AP oblique projections. The AP oblique projection, however, demonstrates increased magnification of the scapula and humerus (see Image 26).

- *Detecting mispositioning.* If the patient obliquity is not accurate for the PA oblique projection, the Y formation of the scapula is not formed, the medial and lateral borders of the scapular body are not superimposed but are visualized next to each other, and the glenoid cavity is not demonstrated on end.

  To determine whether patient obliquity needs to be increased or decreased to superimpose the medial and lateral borders of scapular body and position the glenoid cavity on end, identify the borders of the scapula. The lateral border is thick, with two cortical outlines that are separated by approximately 0.25 inch (0.6 cm), whereas the cortical outline of the vertebral border demonstrates a single thin line. If the lateral border is demonstrated next to the ribs, and the vertebral border is visualized laterally, patient obliquity was excessive (see Image 27). If the vertebral border is demonstrated next to the ribs and the lateral border is visible laterally, patient obliquity was insufficient to superimpose the borders (see Image 28).

If the shoulder is not dislocated, the humeral head and glenoid cavity and the humeral shaft and scapular body are superimposed. If the shoulder is dislocated, the humeral head and shaft are shown anterior or posterior to the glenoid cavity and scapular body, respectively. If the proximal humerus is fractured, the humeral head and glenoid cavity are superimposed, but the midshaft will be demonstrated anteriorly or posteriorly to the scapular body. Each of these situations should demonstrate the scapular Y formation described previously.

- Two indications for the PA oblique projection are to determine whether a shoulder dislocation or proximal humeral fracture exists. The position of the humeral head and shaft in relation to the glenoid cavity and scapular body should not be a positioning concern to the imaging technologist. As long as the scapula is positioned in a Y formation, proper positioning has been obtained. When the shoulder is being imaged to rule out a dislocation or proximal humeral fracture, the patient's humerus should not be moved.
- *Detecting shoulder dislocation.* The cortical outline of the glenoid cavity is visible as a circular density at the junction of the coracoid and acromion processes and the scapular body. Normally, the humeral head is superimposed over this junction. When the humeral head is not positioned over the glenoid cavity, a shoulder dislocation exists and will result in positioning of the humeral head anterior or posterior and inferior to the glenoid cavity. An anterior dislocation, which is more common (95%), results in the humeral head's being demonstrated anteriorly, beneath the coracoid process (see Image 29). A posterior dislocation, which is uncommon (2% to 4%), results in the humeral head's being demonstrated posteriorly, beneath the acromion process (Figure 5-19).

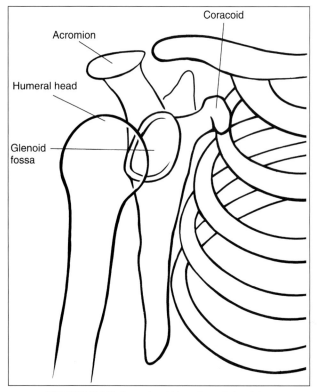

FIGURE 5-19 Posterior dislocation of shoulder.

- *Detecting proximal humeral fracture.* The PA oblique (scapular Y) projection will demonstrate the alignment of the humeral head and shaft in a lateral position without requiring the patient to move the arm. An image taken of a patient with a proximal humeral fracture will demonstrate superimposition of the humeral head and glenoid cavity, but the humeral shaft will be positioned anteriorly or posteriorly to the scapular body (see Image 30). It is important that correct alignment of the scapula be accomplished when a fracture is suspected, because poor alignment may result in misdiagnosis. Images 30 and 31 are from the same patient. Compare the accuracy of the scapular Y formation and the alignment of the humeral head and shaft on these images.

The scapula is demonstrated without longitudinal foreshortening, and the superior scapular angle is superimposed over the clavicle.

- Longitudinal foreshortening of the scapula is prevented when the midcoronal plane remains vertical. Foreshortening is a result of leaning the patient's upper midcoronal plane and shoulder toward the IR. This forward position causes the glenoid cavity and the acromion and coracoid processes to move inferiorly and the superior scapular angle and spine to move superiorly. A longitudinally foreshortened scapula image demonstrates the superior scapular angle above the clavicle (see Image 32).
- *Positioning for kyphosis.* On a patient with spinal kyphosis the scapula is longitudinally foreshortened because of the forward curvature of the vertebral column. To offset this curvature and obtain a scapula without foreshortening, the central ray may be angled perpendicular to the vertebral scapular border. This angulation can be obtained by palpating the vertebral scapular border and aligning the central ray perpendicular to it. For PA oblique projections, the angulation would be caudal and, for AP oblique projections, the angulation would be cephalad.

The midscapular body is at the center of the exposure field. The entire scapula, which includes the inferior and superior angles, the coracoid and acromion processes, and the proximal humerus, is included within the collimation field.

- To place the midscapular body in the center of the exposure field, center a perpendicular central ray to the vertebral border of the scapula halfway between the inferior scapular angle and the acromial angle. Each of these anatomic structures is palpable and should be used to ensure accurate positioning.

- Center the IR to the central ray, and open the longitudinal collimation enough to include the acromion process and inferior scapular angles. Transversely collimate to within the lateral humeral skin line.
- A 10- × 12-inch (25- × 30-cm) IR placed lengthwise should be adequate to include all the required anatomic structures.

Posteroanterior Oblique (Scapular Y) Shoulder Projection Analysis

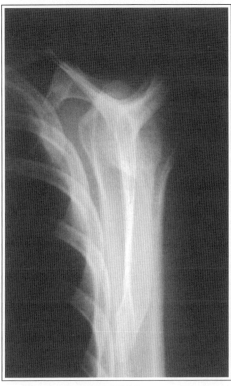

IMAGE 26

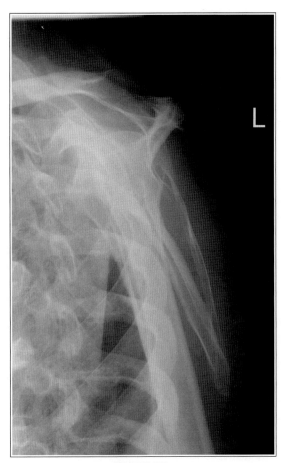

IMAGE 27

Analysis. The vertebral and lateral borders of the scapular body are superimposed, the coracoid and acromion processes form the upper arms of a Y, and the cortical outline of the glenoid cavity is visualized at the Y's arm and leg junction. The patient was accurately positioned. Note the increased amount of magnification of the scapula and humerus compared with the image shown in Figure 5-15. This image was taken with the patient in an AP oblique projection.

Correction. No corrective movement is necessary. If the patient can stand, the PA oblique position would demonstrate less magnification.

Analysis. The lateral and vertebral borders of the scapula are demonstrated without superimposition, and the glenoid cavity is not demonstrated on end but is shown medially. The lateral scapular border is demonstrated next to the ribs, and the vertebral border is visible laterally. The patient was rotated more than necessary to superimpose the borders of the scapular body.

Correction. Decrease the patient obliquity. The amount of decrease is half the distance demonstrated between the vertebral and lateral scapular borders. The measurement should be taken at the midscapular body region.

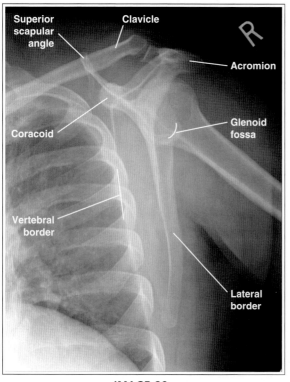

IMAGE 28

Analysis. The lateral and vertebral borders of the scapula are demonstrated without superimposition, and the glenoid cavity is not demonstrated on end but appears laterally. The vertebral scapular border is demonstrated next to the ribs, whereas the lateral border is visible laterally. The patient was not rotated enough to superimpose the borders of the scapular body.

Correction. Increase the patient obliquity.

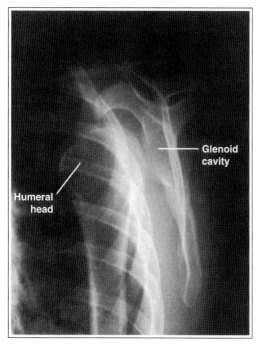

IMAGE 29

Analysis. The scapular body and acromion and coracoid processes are accurately positioned into a Y formation, and the cortical outline of the glenoid cavity is demonstrated at the junction of the arms and leg of the Y. The humeral head and shaft are demonstrated anterior to the glenoid cavity and scapular body, respectively. The shoulder is anteriorly dislocated.

Correction. No corrective movement is required.

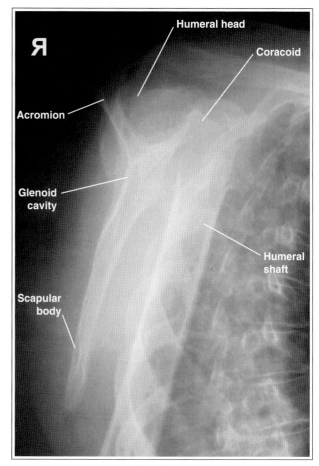

IMAGE 30

Analysis. The scapular body and acromion and coracoid processes are accurately positioned into a Y formation, and the cortical outline of the glenoid cavity is demonstrated at the junction of the arms and leg of the Y. The humeral head and glenoid cavity are superimposed, and the humeral shaft is anterior to the scapular body. The proximal humerus is fractured.

Correction. No corrective movement is required.

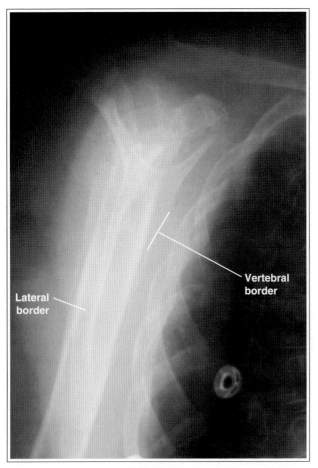

IMAGE 31

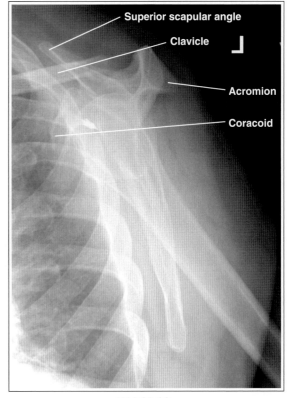

IMAGE 32

Analysis. The lateral and vertebral borders of the scapula are demonstrated without superimposition, and the humeral shaft and scapular body are superimposed. The vertebral scapular border is demonstrated next to the ribs, whereas the lateral border is visible laterally. The patient was not rotated enough to superimpose the borders of the scapular body. The proximal humerus is fractured.

Correction. Increase the patient obliquity.

Analysis. The scapular body, acromion, and coracoid processes are accurately aligned, but the superior scapular angle is demonstrated superior to the clavicle. The scapula is foreshortened. The patient's upper midcoronal plane and shoulder were leaning toward the IR.

Correction. Position the patient with the shoulders on the same transverse plane and tilt the upper midcoronal plane away from the IR until the midcoronal plane is vertical.

PROXIMAL HUMERUS: ANTEROPOSTERIOR AXIAL PROJECTION (STRYKER "NOTCH" METHOD)

See Figure 5-20 and Box 5-6.

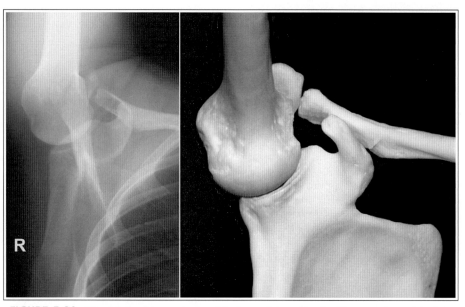

FIGURE 5-20 AP axial shoulder projection (Stryker notch method) with accurate positioning.

BOX 5-6	Anteroposterior Axial Shoulder Projection (Stryker Notch Method) Analysis Criteria

- The coracoid process is situated directly lateral to the conoid tubercle of the clavicle.
- The posterolateral aspect of the humeral head is in profile laterally, and the greater and lesser tubercles are seen in partial profile.
- The coracoid process is superimposed over the lateral clavicle.
- The coracoid process is at the center of the exposure field.
- The humeral head, coracoid process, lateral clavicle, and glenoid cavity are included within the collimated field.

The patient's shoulder is in an AP projection. The coracoid process is situated directly lateral to the conoid tubercle of the clavicle.

- An AP axial (Stryker notch method) projection of the patient's shoulder is obtained by placing the patient in a supine position with the shoulders at equal distances from the imaging table (Figure 5-21).
- *Detecting rotation.* Rotation on an AP axial projection is detected by evaluating the relationship of the coracoid process with the conoid tubercle (an eminence on the inferior surface of the clavicle to which the conoid ligament is attached). The coracoid process is situated just lateral to the conoid tubercle on a nonrotated image. If the patient is rotated away from the affected shoulder, the coracoid process is situated medial to this position and, if the patient is rotated toward the affected

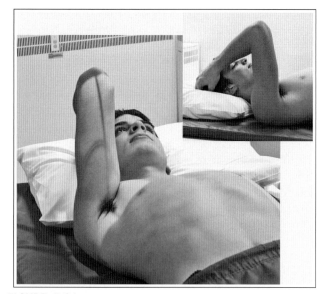

FIGURE 5-21 Proper positioning of AP axial shoulder projection (Stryker notch method).

shoulder, the coracoid process is situated lateral to this position.

The posterolateral aspect of the humeral head is demonstrated in profile laterally, and the greater and lesser tubercles are demonstrated in partial profile. The coracoid process is superimposed over the lateral clavicle.

- The AP axial projection is obtained to diagnose a Hill-Sachs defect of the shoulder. The Hill-Sachs defect is a posterolateral notch defect in the humeral head created by impingement of the articular surface of the humeral head against the anteroinferior rim of the glenoid cavity. The AP axial projection of the shoulder is obtained by placing the patient supine on the imaging table in an AP projection, with the affected arm elevated until the humerus is vertical (90-degree angle with torso). The elbow is then flexed, and the palm of the hand is placed on the top of the patient's head. The central ray is then angled 10 degrees cephalad.

- *Poor humeral positioning and central ray angulation.* Accurate humeral positioning with the 10 degrees of cephalic central ray angulation places the posterolateral aspect of the humeral head in profile laterally and demonstrates the greater and lesser tubercles in partial profile. Poor humeral positioning and central ray angulation result in the posterolateral aspect of the humeral head being obscured. Distinguish poor humeral positioning from poor central ray angulation by evaluating the coracoid process and lateral clavicle relationship. When the central ray is angled 10 degrees cephalad, the coracoid process is superimposed over the lateral clavicle. If less than a 10-degree cephalad angle is used, the coracoid process will be demonstrated inferior to the clavicle and the humeral shaft will demonstrate increased foreshortening (see Image 33). If more than a 10-degree cephalad angle is used, the coracoid process will be demonstrated superior to the clavicle and the humeral shaft will demonstrate decreased foreshortening.

- *Humeral abduction and posterolateral humeral head visualization.* When the central ray is angled accurately but the humerus is inadequately abducted, the coracoid process is superimposed over the lateral clavicle and the posterolateral aspect of the humeral head will be obscured. If the humerus is elevated beyond vertical, the humeral shaft will be demonstrated with decreased foreshortening (see Image 34) and the humeral head will be demonstrated more on end. If the humerus is elevated to a position less than vertical, the humeral shaft will demonstrate increased foreshortening and a decrease in density (see Image 35).

- *Distal humeral tilting and posterolateral humeral head visibility.* Visibility of the posterolateral aspect of the humeral head is also dependent on the degree of medial and lateral tilt of the distal humerus. When the humerus is positioned vertically and parallel with the midsagittal plane, the posterolateral humeral head is demonstrated. If the distal humerus is allowed to tilt laterally, the humerus is rotated, the lesser tubercle appears in profile medially, and the greater tubercle and posterolateral humeral head

are obscured (see Image 34). If the distal humerus is allowed to tilt medially, the lesser tubercle is obscured, and the greater tubercle is demonstrated in profile laterally (see Image 36).

The coracoid process is centered within the collimated field. The humeral head, coracoid process, lateral clavicle, and glenoid cavity are included within the collimation field.

- Center a 10-degree cephalic central ray to the coracoid process to place it at the center of the exposure field. The coracoid process can be palpated 0.75 inch (2 cm) inferior to the midpoint of the lateral half of the clavicle and medial to the humeral head. Even on very muscular patients, the concave pocket formed inferior to the lateral half of the clavicle and medial to the humeral head can be used to center the central ray. The coracoid process should be palpated before the arm is elevated.

- Center the IR to the central ray, open the longitudinal collimated field enough to include the shoulder, and transversely collimate to within 0.5 inch (1.25 cm) of the lateral humeral skin line.

- An 8- × 10-inch (18- × 25-cm) IR placed lengthwise should be adequate to include all the required anatomic structures.

Anteroposterior Axial Shoulder Projection (Stryker Notch Method) Analysis

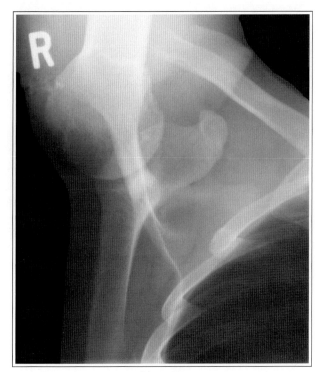

IMAGE 33

Analysis. The coracoid process is inferior to the clavicle, and the humeral shaft demonstrates increased foreshortening. The central ray was angled less than the required 10 degrees cephalad.

Correction. Place a 10-degree cephalic angle on the central ray.

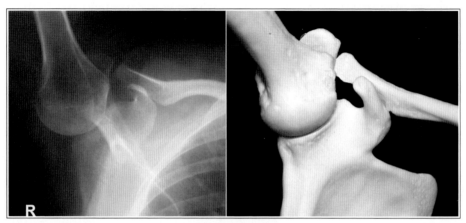

IMAGE 34

Analysis. The coracoid process is superimposed over the lateral clavicle, and the humeral shaft demonstrates decreased foreshortening. The posterolateral humeral head and greater tubercle are obscured, and the lesser tubercle is demonstrated in profile. The humerus was elevated beyond a vertical position, and the distal humerus was tilted laterally.

Correction. Adduct the humerus until it is in a vertical position, and tilt the distal humerus medially until the humerus is aligned parallel with the midsagittal plane.

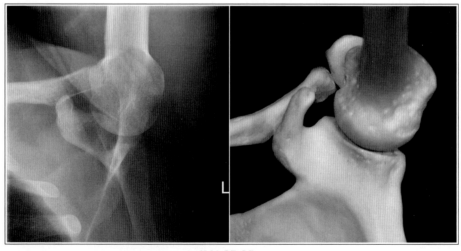

IMAGE 35

Analysis. The posterolateral humeral head is obscured, and the humeral shaft demonstrates increased foreshortening and a decrease in density. The humerus was elevated less than vertically.

Correction. Elevate the humerus until it is placed at a 90-degree position with the patient's torso.

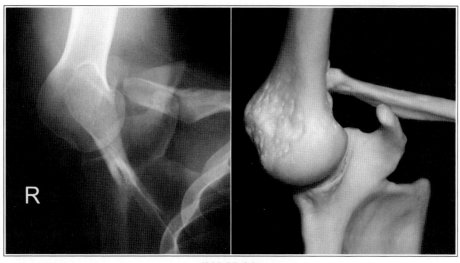

IMAGE 36

Analysis. The posterolateral humeral head and lesser tubercle are obscured. The greater tubercle is in profile laterally. The distal humerus was tilted medially.

Correction. Tilt the distal humerus laterally until it is parallel with the midsagittal plane.

SUPRASPINATUS "OUTLET": TANGENTIAL PROJECTION (NEER METHOD)

See Figure 5-22 and Box 5-7.

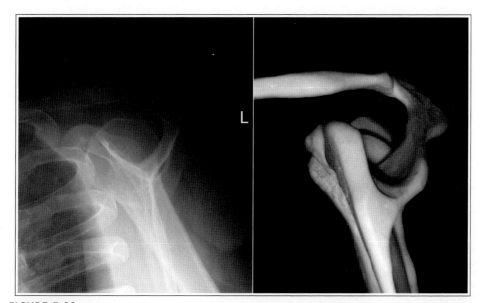

FIGURE 5-22 Tangential supraspinatus outlet projection (Neer method) with accurate positioning.

The lateral and vertebral scapular borders are superimposed, demonstrating a lateral scapula. The scapular body and acromion and coracoid processes form a Y, with the scapular body as the leg and the acromion and coracoid processes as the arms. The glenoid cavity is demonstrated on end at the converging point of the arms and leg of the Y.

- To place the scapular body in a lateral projection, begin by placing the patient in an upright PA projection, with the affected arm abducted slightly or hanging freely. The arm position aligns the vertebral border of the scapula parallel with the IR when the scapula is in a lateral projection, allowing the coracoid and acromion processes to be demonstrated in

BOX 5-7	Tangential Supraspinatus Outlet Projection (Neer Method) Analysis Criteria

- The lateral and vertebral scapular borders are superimposed, demonstrating a lateral scapula.
- The scapular body, acromion, and coracoid form a Y, with the glenoid cavity demonstrated on end.
- The lateral clavicle and acromion process form a smooth continuous arch; the superior scapular angle is at the level of the coracoid process tip and is positioned about 0.5 inch (1.25 cm) inferior to the clavicle.
- The AC joint is at the center of the exposure field.
- The acromion process, lateral clavicle, superior scapular spine, coracoid process, and half of the scapular body are included within the collimated field.

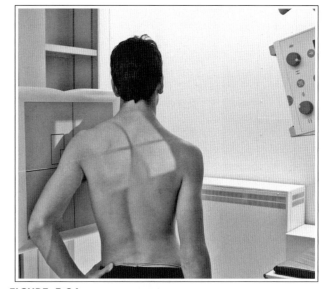

FIGURE 5-24 Proper tangential supraspinatus outlet projection (Neer method) with arm abducted.

profile. From this PA projection, rotate the patient's body toward the affected scapula until the midcoronal plane is approximately 45 degrees for the nonabducted arm position (Figure 5-23) and 60 degrees for the abducted arm position or until the lateral and vertebral scapular borders are superimposed (Figure 5-24). Also see Figure 5-22.

- *Amount of body obliquity required.* The degree of body obliquity required to obtain a lateral scapula varies with the degree of arm abducted. When the tangential projection is obtained with the patient's arm abducted (see Figure 5-24), the shoulder is retracted (drawn backward) as the patient is rotated because the humerus does not rotate with the body. This shoulder retraction causes the scapula to glide around the thoracic cavity, moving toward the spinal column. When the scapula is in this posterior position, the patient's body needs to be rotated more to bring the scapular body lateral. When the patient's arm is allowed to hang freely for the image,

the shoulder is not retracted, resulting in the scapular body being positioned more anteriorly and therefore requiring less obliquity to bring it into a lateral projection (see Figure 5-23).

- *Using scapular palpation to determine accurate degree of body obliquity.* The proper degree of body rotation for any arm position is determined by palpating the lateral and vertebral scapular borders. Because the superior portions of the lateral and vertebral borders are heavily covered with muscles, it is best to palpate them just superior to the inferior scapular angle. Once these anatomic structures are located, rotate the patient's body until the vertebral border of the scapula is superimposed over the lateral border and the inferior scapular angle is positioned in profile.

- *Detecting mispositioning.* If the patient obliquity is not accurate for the tangential projection, the Y formation of the scapula is not attained, the medial and lateral borders of the scapular body are not superimposed but are demonstrated next to each other, and the glenoid cavity is not demonstrated on end. To determine whether patient obliquity needs to be increased or decreased to superimpose the scapular body and position the glenoid cavity on end, identify the borders of the scapula. The lateral border is thick, with two cortical outlines that are separated by approximately 0.25 inch (0.6 cm), whereas the cortical outline of the vertebral border demonstrates a single thin line. If the vertebral border is demonstrated next to the ribs and the lateral border is visible laterally, patient obliquity was insufficient to superimpose the borders (see Image 37). If the lateral border is demonstrated next to the ribs and the vertebral border is visible laterally, patient obliquity was excessive (see Image 38).

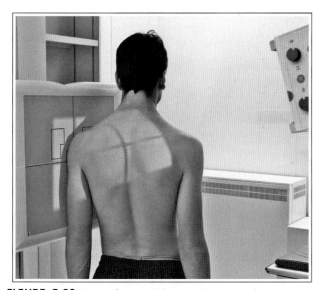

FIGURE 5-23 Proper tangential supraspinatus outlet projection (Neer method) with arm dangling (nonabducted).

The supraspinatus outlet is open and the inferior aspect of the lateral clavicle and acromion is demonstrated in profile. The lateral clavicle and acromion process form a smooth continuous arch and the superior scapular angle is at the level of the coracoid process tip, positioned about 0.5 inch (1.25 cm) inferior to the clavicle.

- The supraspinatus muscle runs along the supraspinatus fossa, beneath the acromion, and attaches to the greater tubercle. Narrowing of the supraspinatus outlet is caused by a variation in the shape or slope of the acromion or acromioclavicular joint because of spur or osteophyte formations. This narrowing is the primary cause of shoulder impingement and rotator cuff tears. The tangential projection is taken to identify spur or osteophyte formations on the inferior surfaces of the lateral clavicle and acromion process angle. For these inferior surfaces to be visualized best, the central ray must transverse the area at a 10- to 15-degree angle. This alignment is accomplished by positioning the midcoronal plane vertically, angling the central ray 10 to 15 degrees caudally, and centering the central ray to the AC joint; it is demonstrated on a tangential outlet image when the superior scapular angle is at the level of the coracoid process tip and visible about 0.5 inch (1.25 cm) inferior to the clavicle.
- *Positional causes of supraspinatus outlet narrowing.* If the tangential projection is taken without the 10- to 15-degree caudal angle, with the patient's upper midcoronal plane tilted anteriorly toward the IR, or with the central ray centered too inferiorly, the supraspinatus outlet narrows and the superior scapular angle is visualized closer than 0.5 inch (1.25 cm) inferior to the clavicle (see Image 39). The supraspinatus outlet will be closed and the superior scapular angle seen superior to the clavicle if the central ray is angled in the wrong direction (see Image 40).

The AC joint is at the center of the exposure field. The acromion process, lateral clavicle, superior scapular spine, coracoid process, and half of the scapular body should be included within the collimation field.

- To place the AC joint in the center of the exposure field, center the central ray to the superior aspect of the humeral head.
- Center the IR to the central ray, and open the longitudinal collimation enough to include the acromion process and lateral clavicle. Transverse collimate to within 0.5 inch (1.25 cm) of the lateral humeral skin line.
- An 8- × 10-inch (18- × 25-cm) IR placed lengthwise should be adequate to include all the required anatomic structures.

Tangential (Supraspinatus Outlet) Projection (Neer Method) Analysis

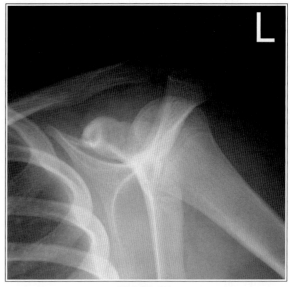

IMAGE 37

Analysis. The lateral and vertebral borders of the scapula are demonstrated without superimposition, and the glenoid cavity is not demonstrated on end but is demonstrated laterally. The vertebral scapular border is demonstrated next to the ribs, whereas the lateral border is demonstrated laterally. The patient was not rotated enough to superimpose the scapular body.

Correction. Increase the patient obliquity.

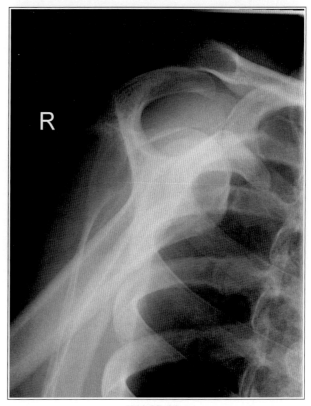

IMAGE 38

Analysis. The lateral and vertebral borders of the scapula are demonstrated without superimposition, and the glenoid cavity is not demonstrated on end but appears medially. The lateral scapular border is demonstrated next to the ribs, and the vertebral border is demonstrated laterally. The patient was rotated more than necessary to superimpose the borders of the scapular body.

Correction. Decrease the patient obliquity.

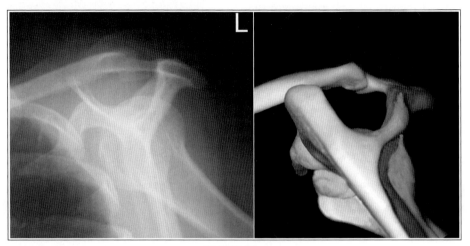

IMAGE 39

Analysis. The supraspinatus outlet is narrowed. The superior scapular angle is superimposing the lateral clavicle and the coracoid is inferior to it. The inferior aspects of the lateral clavicle and acromion are seen on end instead of profile. The upper midcoronal plane was tilted anteriorly toward the IR; the central ray was not angled 10 to 15 degrees caudally nor was it centered to inferior on the patient.

Correction. Position the midcoronal plane vertically, place a 10- to 15-degree caudal angle on the central ray, and center to the AC joint.

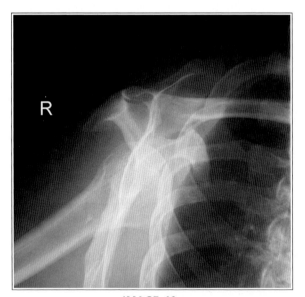

IMAGE 40

Analysis. The supraspinatus outlet is closed and the superior scapular angle is seen superior to the lateral clavicle. The central ray was angled 10 to 15 degrees cephalically.

Correction. Angle the central ray 10 to 15 degrees caudally.

CLAVICLE: ANTEROPOSTERIOR PROJECTION

See Figure 5-25 and Box 5-8.

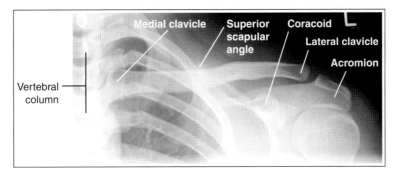

FIGURE 5-25 AP clavicular projection with accurate positioning.

BOX 5-8	Anteroposterior Clavicle Projection Analysis Criteria

- The medial clavicular end lies next to the lateral edge of the vertebral column.
- The midclavicle is superimposed on the superior scapular angle.
- The midclavicle is at the center of the exposure field.
- The clavicle and the acromion process are included within the collimated field.

The clavicle is demonstrated in an AP projection without longitudinal foreshortening. The medial clavicular end lies next to the lateral edge of the vertebral column.

- An AP projection of the clavicle is obtained by placing the patient in a supine or upright position with the shoulders at equal distances from the imaging table or upright IR holder (Figure 5-26).
- *Positioning for kyphosis.* The kyphotic patient will have less discomfort if the image is taken with the patient in an upright position. If it is not possible to place the kyphotic patient in an upright position, use angled sponges under the shoulders and thorax to place the shoulders at equal distances from the imaging table. An imaging table sponge also helps with patient comfort.
- *Detecting clavicular rotation.* Rotation and therefore longitudinal foreshortening on an AP clavicle projection is detected by evaluating the relationships of the medial clavicular end with the vertebral column. If the patient is rotated away from the affected clavicle, the medial end of the clavicle is superimposed over the vertebral column (see Image 41). If the patient is rotated toward the affected clavicle, the medial end of the clavicle draws away from the vertebral column and the clavicle is longitudinally foreshortened (see Image 42).
- *PA versus AP projection.* Although a PA projection would position the clavicle closer to the IR, resulting in less magnification and greater image detail, the AP projection is the more commonly performed because it causes less patient discomfort during positioning and allows the clavicle to be easily palpated.

The clavicle is demonstrated without inferosuperior foreshortening. The midclavicle is superimposed on the superior scapular angle.

- Inferosuperior foreshortening of the clavicle results when the patient's upper midcoronal plane is allowed to tilt anteriorly or posteriorly. This tilting can often be avoided by instructing the patient to arch the upper thorax and shoulders backward, straightening the vertebral column.
- *Detecting inferosuperior foreshortening.* Inferosuperior foreshortening of the clavicle is demonstrated when the superior scapular angle is visible superiorly or inferiorly to the midclavicle. If the upper midcoronal plane is tilted anteriorly (forward), the superior scapular angle will be demonstrated superior to the midclavicle (see Image 43). If the upper midcoronal plane is tilted posteriorly (backward), the superior scapular angle is shown inferior to the midclavicle (see Image 44).

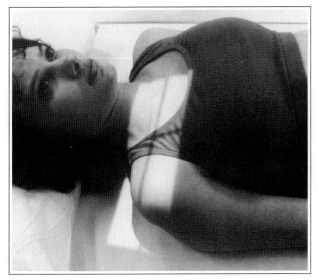

FIGURE 5-26 Proper positioning of AP clavicular projection.

The midclavicle is at the center of the exposure field. The entire clavicle and the acromion process are included within the collimation field.

- The midclavicle is located by palpating the medial and lateral ends of the clavicle and centering the central ray halfway between them.

- Center the IR to the central ray and open the longitudinal and transverse collimation enough to include all aspects of the medial and lateral clavicular ends.
- A 10- × 12-inch (25- × 30-cm) IR placed crosswise should be adequate to include all the required anatomic structures.

Anteroposterior Clavicle Projection Analysis

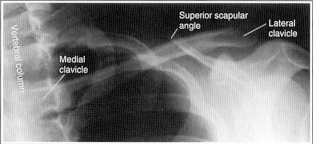

IMAGE 41

Analysis. The medial end of the clavicle is superimposed over the vertebral column. The patient was rotated away from the affected clavicle for this image.

Correction. Place the patient in an AP projection by rotating the patient toward the affected clavicle. The shoulders should be placed at equal distances from the IR.

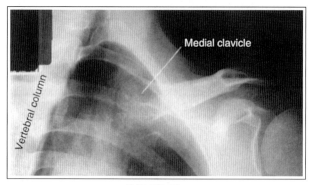

IMAGE 42

Analysis. The medial end of the clavicle is drawn away from the vertebral column, and the clavicle is longitudinally foreshortened. The patient was rotated toward the affected shoulder for this image.

Correction. Place the patient in an AP projection by rotating the patient away from the affected clavicle. The shoulders should be placed at equal distances from the IR.

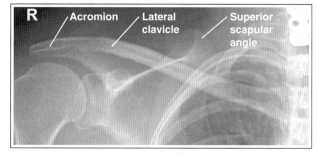

IMAGE 43

Analysis. The superior scapular angle is projected superiorly to the midclavicle. The clavicle has been inferosuperiorly foreshortened. The upper midcoronal plane was tilted anteriorly.

Correction. Instruct the patient to arch the upper thorax and shoulders backward, straightening the upper vertebral column and midcoronal plane.

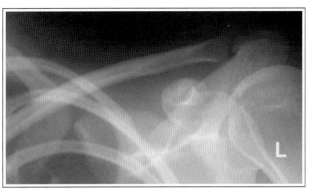

IMAGE 44

Analysis. The superior scapular angle is projected inferiorly to the midclavicle. The clavicle has been transversely foreshortened. The upper midcoronal plane was tilted posteriorly. The medial end of the clavicle is not included on the image. The central ray was positioned too laterally.

Correction. Instruct the patient to arch the upper thorax and shoulders forward, straightening the upper vertebral column and midcoronal plane. Center the central ray approximately 1 inch (2.5 cm) medially, and open collimation enough to include the medial end of the clavicle.

CLAVICLE: ANTEROPOSTERIOR AXIAL PROJECTION (LORDOTIC POSITION)

See Figure 5-27 and Box 5-9.

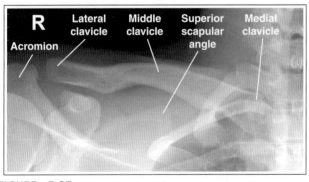

FIGURE 5-27 AP axial clavicular projection with accurate positioning.

BOX 5-9	Anteroposterior Axial Clavicle Projection Analysis Criteria

- The medial end of clavicle lies next to the lateral edge of the vertebral column.
- The medial end of clavicle is superimposed over the first, second, or third rib.
- The middle and lateral thirds of clavicle are seen superior to the acromion process and the clavicle bows upwardly.
- The midclavicle is at the center of the exposure field.
- The clavicle and the acromion process are included within the collimated field.

The clavicle is demonstrated without rotation. The medial end of the clavicle lies next to the lateral edge of the vertebral column.

- An AP axial projection of the clavicle is accomplished by placing the patient in a supine or

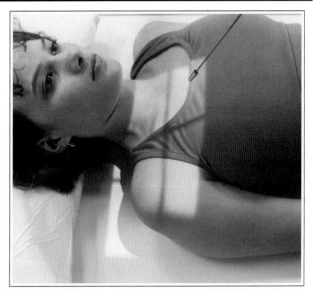

FIGURE 5-28 Proper positioning of AP axial clavicular projection.

upright position with shoulders positioned at equal distances from the imaging table or upright IR holder (Figure 5-28).

- *Detecting clavicular rotation.* Rotation on an AP axial clavicle projection is detected by evaluating the relationships of the medial clavicular end with the vertebral column. If the patient is rotated away from the affected clavicle, the medial end of the clavicle is superimposed over the vertebral column. If the patient is rotated toward the affected clavicle, the medial end of the clavicle is drawn away from the vertebral column and the clavicle is longitudinally foreshortened. (See Images 41 and 42. Rotation on the AP and AP axial clavicle projections are similar, but the clavicle on the AP axial projection would be situated more superiorly on the thorax.)

The medial end of the clavicle is superimposed over the first, second, or third rib, the middle and lateral thirds of the clavicle are demonstrated superior to the acromion process, and the clavicle bows slightly upward.

- A 15- to 30-degree cephalic angle is used on the AP axial projection of the clavicle to project more of the clavicle superior to the thorax region and to demonstrate the degree of fracture displacement, when present. Even though the amount of angulation used may vary among radiology departments, all images result in superior projection of the clavicle. The larger the angle, the more superiorly the clavicle is projected. Ideally, because 80% of clavicle fractures occur at the middle third and 15% at the lateral third, the central ray should be angled enough to project the lateral and middle thirds of the clavicle superior to the thorax and scapula.

    Compare Images 45 and 46, and note how an increase in cephalic angulation has projected the lateral and middle thirds of the clavicle above the scapula. The clavicle fracture demonstrated on these images is obvious, but a subtle nondisplaced fracture could be obscured by the scapular structures if an AP axial projection were not included in the examination.

The midclavicle is at the center of the exposure field. The entire clavicle and the acromion process are included within the collimation field.

- The midclavicle is located by palpating the lateral and medial ends of the clavicle and centering the central ray halfway between the ends.
- Center the IR to the central ray and open the longitudinal and transverse collimation enough to include all aspects of the lateral and medial clavicular ends.
- An 8- × 10-inch (18- × 25-cm) or 10- × 12-inch (25- × 30-cm) IR placed crosswise should be adequate to include all the required anatomic structures.

Anteroposterior Axial Clavicle Projection Analysis

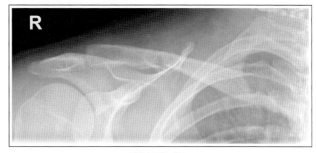

IMAGE 45

Analysis. The lateral and middle thirds of the clavicle are superimposed by the scapula. The cephalic central ray angulation was not adequate to project the lateral and middle thirds of the clavicle superior to the scapula. A midclavicular fracture is present.

Correction. Increase the cephalic central ray angulation enough to project the clavicle above the scapula.

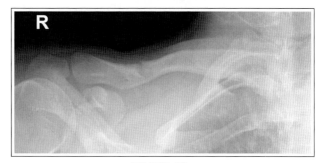

IMAGE 46

Analysis. The lateral and middle thirds of the clavicle are projected above the scapula. A nondisplaced fracture of the middle third of the clavicle is evident.

Correction. No corrective movement is necessary.

ACROMIOCLAVICULAR JOINT: AP PROJECTION

See Figures 5-29 and 5-30 and Box 5-10.

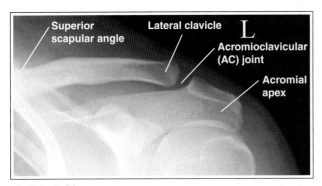

FIGURE 5-29 AP acromioclavicular joint projection (without weights) with accurate positioning.

BOX 5-10	Anteroposterior Acromioclavicular Joint Projection Analysis Criteria

- The weight-bearing image displays a word or arrow marker to indicate that it is the weight-bearing image.
- The lateral clavicle is almost horizontal, and about 0.125 inch (0.3 cm) of space is present between the lateral clavicle and acromial apex.
- The lateral clavicle demonstrates minimal acromion process superimposition, and the midclavicle is superimposed over the scapular spine.
- The AC joint is at the center of the exposure field.
- The lateral clavicle and acromion process are included within the collimated field.

The weight-bearing image displays a word or arrow marker, pointing downward, to indicate that it is the weight-bearing image.

The lateral clavicle and acromion process are demonstrated in an AP projection. The lateral clavicle is almost horizontal, and approximately 0.125 inch (0.3 cm) of space is present between the lateral clavicle and the acromial apex.

- An AP projection of the AC joint is obtained by placing the patient in an upright position with both shoulders positioned at equal distances from the upright IR holder (Figure 5-31).
- *Weight-bearing AC joint images.* To evaluate the AC joint for possible injury to the AC ligament, which extends between the lateral clavicular end and the acromion process, the AP projection should be taken first without weights. Then a second AP projection should be taken with the patient holding 5- to 8-lb weights (Figure 5-32).

If injury to the AC ligament has occurred, the AC joint space is wider on the weight-bearing image than on the image taken without weights. For the weight-bearing image, equal weights should be attached to the arms, regardless of whether the examination is unilateral (one side) or bilateral (both sides), keeping the shoulders on the same transverse plane. Attach the weights to the patient's wrists or slide them onto the patient's forearms after the elbows are flexed to 90 degrees, and instruct the patient to allow the weights to depress the shoulders.

- *Detecting rotation.* Rotation on an AP AC joint projection is detected by evaluating the relationships of the lateral clavicle with the acromion apex and of the scapular body with the thoracic cavity. If the patient was rotated toward the affected AC joint, the lateral end of the clavicle and the acromion apex are rotated out of profile, resulting in a narrowed or closed AC joint. The thoracic cavity also moves toward the scapular body, increasing the amount of scapular body

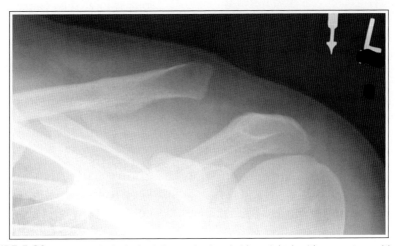

FIGURE 5-30 AP acromioclavicular joint projection (with weights) with accurate positioning.

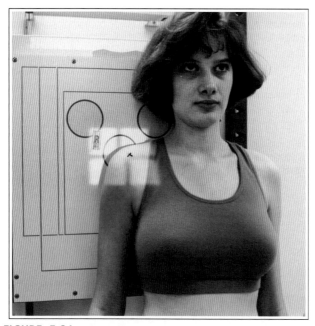

FIGURE 5-31 Proper positioning of AP acromioclavicular joint projection (without weights).

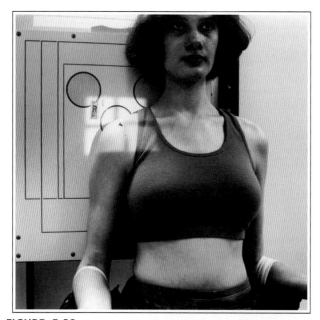

FIGURE 5-32 Proper positioning of AP acromioclavicular joint projection (with weights).

superimposition (see Image 47, right shoulder). If the patient is rotated away from the affected AC joint, the lateral end of the clavicle and the acromion apex demonstrate a slightly greater AC joint space with only a small amount of rotation and may be closed with a greater degree of rotation. The scapular body demonstrates decreased thoracic cavity superimposition (see Image 47, left shoulder).

The lateral clavicle demonstrates minimal acromion process superimposition, and the midclavicle is superimposed over the scapular spine. The lateral clavicle and acromion process are demonstrated without transverse foreshortening.

- Inferosuperior foreshortening of the clavicle and acromion process results when the patient's upper midcoronal plane is allowed to tilt anteriorly or posteriorly. This tilting can often be avoided by instructing the patient to arch the upper thorax and shoulders backward, straightening the vertebral column.
- *Detecting inferosuperior foreshortening.* Inferosuperior foreshortening of the clavicle and acromion process is demonstrated when the lateral clavicle demonstrates greater or less than minimal superimposition of the acromion process and the superior scapular angle appears superiorly or inferiorly to the midclavicle. If the upper midcoronal plane is tilted anteriorly (forward), the lateral clavicle will demonstrate increased acromion process superimposition and the superior scapular angle will be demonstrated superior to the midclavicle (see Image 48). If the upper midcoronal plane is tilted posteriorly (backward), the lateral clavicle will demonstrate decreased acromion process superimposition and the superior scapular angle will be visible inferior to the midclavicle (see Image 49).
- *Positioning for kyphosis.* For the kyphotic patient, little can be done to improve patient positioning, but a cephalic central ray angulation can be used to offset the forward angle of the scapula. The central ray should be angled enough to align it perpendicular to the scapular body.

The AC joint of interest is at the center of the exposure field, and the lateral clavicle and acromion process are included within the collimation field.

- *Unilateral AC joint images.* Center a perpendicular central ray to the AC joint of interest. The AC joint is located by palpating along the clavicle until the most lateral tip is reached, and then moving approximately 0.5 inch (1 cm) inferiorly. Center the IR to the central ray, and open the longitudinally and transversely collimated field to approximately a 5-inch (10-cm) field size. An 8- × 10-inch (18- × 25-cm) IR placed crosswise should be adequate to include all the anatomic structures.
- *Bilateral AC joint image.* Center a perpendicular central ray to the midsagittal plane at a level 1 inch (2.5 cm) superior to the jugular notch. Center the IR to the central ray, and open the longitudinally collimated field to approximately a 5-inch (10-cm) field size. Transverse collimate should be left open the full IR length. A 15- × 17-inch

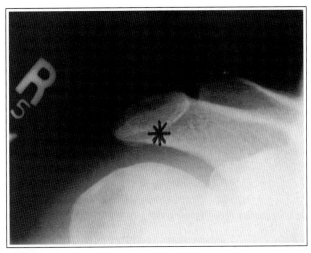

FIGURE 5-33 Acromioclavicular joint projection taken without weights and showing good centering. *Star,* Location of central ray.

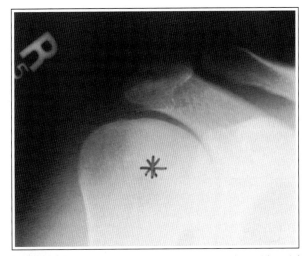

FIGURE 5-34 Acromioclavicular joint projection taken with weights and showing poor centering. Star indicates location of central ray.

(35- × 43-cm) or 7- × 17-inch (15- × 43-cm) IR placed crosswise should be adequate to include both AC joints. This method is not recommended because it unnecessarily exposes the thyroid and uses diverged x-rays to record the AC joints.

- *Alternate central ray.* An AP axial projection of the AC joint is taken with a 15-degree cephalic central ray angle centered at the level of the AC joint. This projection demonstrates the AC joint superior to the acromion process.
- *Ensuring identical central ray alignment with and without weights.* Repalpate for the AC joint to ensure that the same centering is obtained when the patient is given weights. Because the shoulders are depressed when weights are used, the AC joint moves inferiorly. If the central ray is not centered the same for both images, x-ray beam divergence may result in a false reading. Compare Figures 5-33 and 5-34, images of the same patient, taken without weights and with weights, respectively. Because the central ray was not centered in the same location, it is uncertain whether the separation demonstrated on the weight-bearing image is a result of ligament injury or poor central ray centering.

Anteroposterior Acromioclavicular Joint Projection Analysis

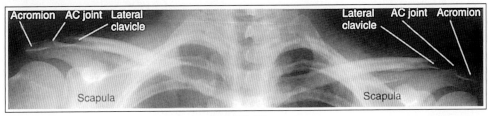

IMAGE 47

Analysis. This image was taken with the central ray centered on the vertebral column to position both AC joints on one receptor. This method is not recommended because it unnecessarily exposes the thyroid and uses diverged x-rays to record the AC joints. When bilateral AC joint images are ordered, each AC joint should be imaged separately, as described earlier. The right AC joint is closed and the right scapular body demonstrates greater thoracic superimposition than the left; the left AC joint is open. The patient was rotated toward the right shoulder.

Correction. Take the image of each AC joint on a separate receptor. Rotate the patient toward the left shoulder until the shoulders are at equal distances from the IR.

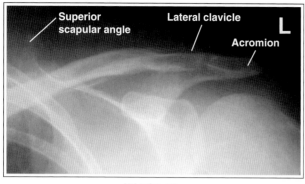

IMAGE 48

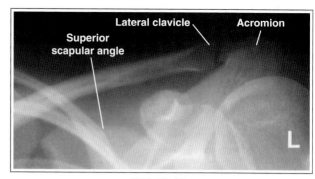

IMAGE 49

Analysis. The lateral end of the clavicle is completely superimposed on the acromion process, and the superior scapular angle appears superior to the midclavicle. The upper midcoronal plane was tilted anteriorly, transversely foreshortening the clavicle and acromion process.

Correction. Instruct the patient to arch the upper thorax and shoulders backward, straightening the upper vertebral column and midcoronal plane.

Analysis. The acromion process is demonstrated without clavicular superimposition, and the superior scapular angle appears inferior to the midclavicle. The upper midcoronal plane was tilted posteriorly, inferosuperiorly foreshortening the clavicle and acromion process.

Correction. Instruct the patient to arch the upper thorax and shoulders forward, straightening the upper vertebral column and midcoronal plane.

SCAPULA: ANTEROPOSTERIOR PROJECTION

See Figure 5-35 and Box 5-11.

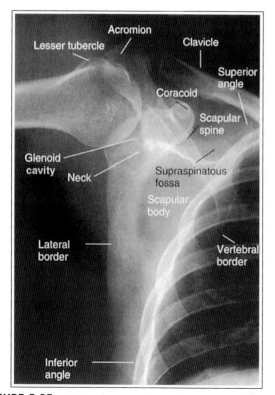

FIGURE 5-35 AP scapular projection with accurate positioning.

BOX 5-11	Anteroposterior Scapula Projection Analysis Criteria

- The anterior and posterior margins of the glenoid cavity are almost superimposed.
- The superior scapular angle is about 0.25 inch (0.6 cm) inferior to the clavicle.
- The lateral border of scapula is seen without thoracic cavity superimposition, and the supraspinatus fossa and superior angle of the scapular are seen without superimposition of the clavicle.
- The thoracic cavity is superimposed over the vertebral border of the scapula.
- The humeral shaft demonstrates 90 degrees of abduction.
- The midscapular body is at the center of the exposure field.
- The entire scapula is included within the collimated field.

Density is uniform across the scapular body.

- *Image density of shoulder girdle and thoracic cavity.* Although the AP thickness is approximately the same across the entire scapula, the overall image density is not uniform. On AP scapular projections, the medial portion of the scapula, which is superimposed by the thoracic cavity, demonstrates darker density (less brightness) than the lateral scapula, which is superimposed by the soft tissue of the shoulder girdle. This image density difference is a result of the difference in atomic density that exists between the thoracic cavity and the shoulder soft tissue.

The thoracic cavity is largely composed of air, which contains very few atoms in a given area, whereas the same area of soft tissue contains many compacted atoms. As the radiation goes through the patient's body, fewer photons are absorbed in the thoracic cavity than in the shoulder girdle, because fewer atoms with which the photons can interact are present in the thoracic cavity. Consequently, more photons penetrate the thoracic cavity to expose the IR than penetrate the shoulder girdle.

- *Respiration and image density.* Taking the exposure on expiration can help decrease the image density of the portion of the scapula that is superimposed by the thoracic cavity by reducing the air and slightly compressing the tissue in this area. If the AP scapular projection is taken on inspiration, the medial scapular body demonstrates increased density (see Image 50).

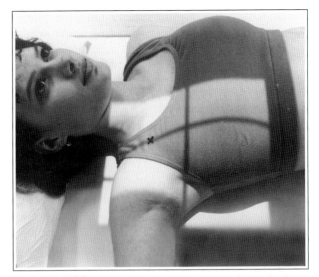

FIGURE 5-36 Proper positioning of AP scapular projection.

The bony trabecular patterns and cortical outlines of the scapula are sharply defined.

- Patient respiration also determines how well the scapular details are demonstrated. Some positioning textbooks suggest that a breathing technique be used to visualize the vertebral border and medial scapular body through the air-filled lungs better. Although visualization of this anatomy would be improved with such a technique, it is difficult to obtain a long enough exposure time (3 seconds) to blur the ribs and vascular lung markings adequately when the overall exposure (mAs) necessary for an AP scapula projection is so small. If an adequate exposure time cannot be set to use breathing technique, the exposure should be taken on expiration.

The scapula is demonstrated in an AP projection without transverse foreshortening. The anterior and posterior margins of the glenoid cavity are nearly superimposed.

- When the patient's body is positioned in an AP projection, with the arms against the sides, the scapular body is placed at a 35- to 45-degree angle with the IR, with the lateral scapula situated more anteriorly than the medial scapula. This positioning results in transverse foreshortening of the scapular body.
- *Positioning for an AP scapular projection.* An AP scapular projection is obtained by abducting the humerus and then supinating the hand and flexing the elbow to rotate the arm externally (Figure 5-36). Each of these arm movements, with the sternoclavicular and AC joints, works to retract the shoulder (force it backward). Humeral abduction causes the scapula to glide around the thoracic surface, moving the scapula laterally, and shoulder retraction reduces transverse scapular

foreshortening as it forces the lateral aspect of the scapula posteriorly. This movement of the scapula places it very close to an AP projection. To take advantage of gravity and obtain maximum shoulder retraction, take the image with the patient in a supine position.

- *Detecting poor shoulder retraction.* Poor retraction of the scapula can be identified by evaluating the image of the scapular body and glenoid cavity. If the patient's arm is not sufficiently externally rotated and abducted, and the shoulder sufficiently retracted, the transverse scapular body is foreshortened and the glenoid cavity is demonstrated somewhat on end (see Image 51).

The scapula is demonstrated in an AP projection without longitudinal foreshortening. The superior scapular angle is approximately 0.25 inch (0.6 cm) inferior to the clavicle.

- *Longitudinal foreshortening.* Longitudinal foreshortening of the scapular body is caused by poor midcoronal plane positioning and could result when the AP scapular projection is taken with the patient in the upright position or when the patient is kyphotic. To prevent such foreshortening, position the patient's midcoronal plane vertically when the patient is upright. A longitudinally foreshortened scapula can be identified on a scapular image that has the arm adequately abducted when the superior scapular angle is more or less than 0.25 inch (0.6 cm) inferior to the clavicle. When the superior scapular angle is demonstrated less than 0.25 inch (0.6 cm) from the clavicle, the upper midcoronal plane was tilted anteriorly. When the superior scapular angle appears more than 0.25 inch (0.6 cm) inferior to the clavicle, the upper midcoronal plane was tilted posteriorly.

- *Angulation for kyphosis.* Longitudinal foreshortening of the scapular body on the kyphotic patient cannot be improved with patient positioning, but a cephalic central ray angulation can be used to offset the forward angle of the scapula. Angle the central ray to align it perpendicular to the scapular body.

The lateral border of the scapula is demonstrated without thoracic cavity superimposition, and the supraspinatus fossa and the superior angle of the scapula are demonstrated without superimposition of the clavicle. The thoracic cavity is superimposed over the vertebral border of the scapula. The humeral shaft demonstrates 90 degrees of abduction.

- Demonstrating the lateral portion of the scapula with adequate density often causes the medial scapula, which is superimposed by the thoracic cavity, to demonstrate excessive density (low brightness). To increase the proportion of scapular body demonstrated without thoracic cavity superimposition, the humerus is abducted.
- *Effect of humeral abduction.* Abduction of the humerus is accomplished by combined movements of the shoulder joint and rotation of the scapula around the thoracic cage. The ratio of movement in these two articulations is two parts glenohumeral to one part scapulothoracic. When the arm is abducted, the lateral scapula is drawn from beneath the thoracic cavity and the glenoid cavity moves superiorly. Because the first 60 degrees of humeral abduction involves primarily movement of the glenohumeral joint without accompanying scapular movement, it takes at least 90 degrees of humeral abduction to demonstrate the lateral border of the scapula without thoracic cavity superimposition, and the supraspinatus fossa and superior angle without clavicle superimposition. The farther the arm is abducted, the more of the lateral scapular body is demonstrated without thoracic cavity superimposition. With 0 to 60 degrees of humeral abduction, the inferolateral border of the scapula is superimposed by the thoracic cavity and the clavicle is superimposed over the supraspinatus fossa and superior scapular angle. Image 50 demonstrates an image taken with 60 degrees of abduction, and Image 52 was taken without humeral abduction.
- *Positioning for trauma.* Trauma patients often experience great pain with arm abduction. Because of this pain, the abduction movement may take place

almost entirely at the glenohumeral articulation, instead of involving the combined movements of the glenohumeral and scapulothoracic articulations. When the scapulothoracic articulation is not involved with the movement of humeral abduction, the inferolateral border and inferior angle of the scapula may remain superimposed by the thoracic cavity, and the supraspinatus fossa and superior border may remain superimposed by the clavicle (see Image 53). In this situation, little can be done to draw the scapula away from the thoracic cavity, although the exposure can be taken on expiration and a technique used that better demonstrates the parts of the scapula superimposed by the thorax. An AP projection of the scapular body can be obtained in a trauma situation by using the AP oblique (Grashey method) shoulder projection, as discussed earlier in this chapter. In this position, the patient is rotated toward the affected shoulder, bringing the scapula AP. The central ray should be centered 2 inches (5 cm) inferior to the coracoid process and the kVp and exposure reduced to prevent the dark density (less brightness) caused by the air-filled lungs.

The midscapular body is at the center of the exposure field. The entire scapula, consisting of the inferior and superior angles, the coracoid and acromion processes, and glenoid cavity, is included within the collimation field.

- To ensure that the entire scapula, from the coracoid process to the inferior angle, is included on the image, center a perpendicular central ray approximately 2 inches (5 cm) inferior to the palpable coracoid process. The coracoid process can be palpated 0.75 inch (2 cm) inferior to the midpoint of the lateral half of the clavicle and medial to the humeral head. Even for very muscular patients the concave pocket formed inferior to the lateral half of the clavicle and the medial humeral head can be used to center the central ray. The coracoid process should be palpated before the arm is abducted. This positioning accurately aligns the longitudinal and transverse aspects of the scapula. If the arm cannot be adequately abducted, the transverse centering should be 0.5 inch (1 cm) more medial.
- Center the IR to the central ray, and open the longitudinal collimation to the top shoulder skin line. Transversely collimate to within 0.5 inch (1.25 cm) of the lateral body skin line.
- A 10- × 12-inch (25- × 30-cm) IR placed lengthwise should be adequate to include all the required anatomic structures.

Anteroposterior Scapular Projection Analysis

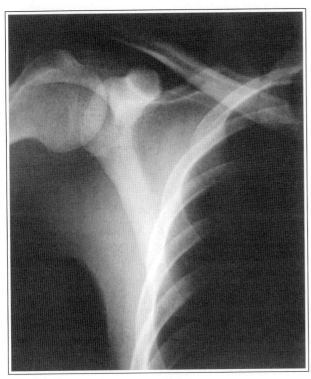

IMAGE 50

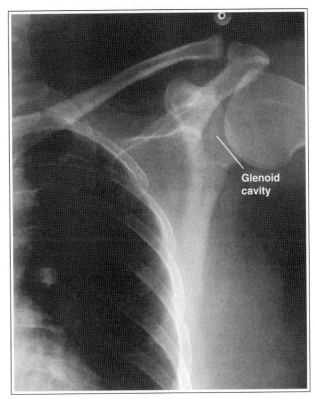

Glenoid cavity

IMAGE 51

Analysis. The portion of the scapula superimposed by the thoracic cavity demonstrates excessive density. The examination was taken on inspiration. The inferolateral border of the scapula is superimposed by the thoracic cavity and the superior angle is superimposed by the clavicle. The humeral shaft is inadequately abducted.

Correction. Take the exposure on expiration or use a breathing technique, and abduct the arm to 90 degrees.

Analysis. The transverse axis of the scapular body is foreshortened, and the articulating surface of the glenoid cavity is demonstrated. This AP scapular projection was taken with the patient in an upright position, resulting in insufficient shoulder retraction.

Correction. Place the patient supine to maximize shoulder retraction, or instruct the patient to retract the shoulder toward the IR.

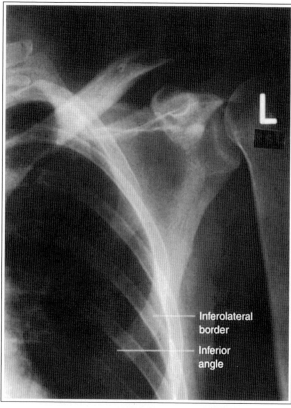

IMAGE 52

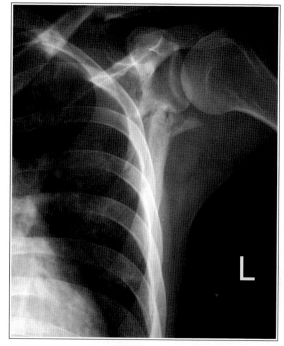

IMAGE 53

Analysis. The inferolateral border of the scapula is superimposed by the thoracic cavity, and the superior angle is superimposed by the clavicle. The humeral shaft is not abducted 90 degrees with the body.

Correction. Abduct the humerus 90 degrees from the body. This adjustment will draw the inferolateral border of the scapula away from the thoracic cavity and shift the superior angle away from the clavicle.

Analysis. The inferolateral border of the scapula is superimposed by the thoracic cavity. The humeral shaft was abducted to about 60 degrees, but a scapular fracture prevented the scapula moving from beneath the thorax.

Correction. No correction movement is needed.

SCAPULA: LATERAL PROJECTION (LATEROMEDIAL OR MEDIOLATERAL)

See Figure 5-37 and Box 5-12.

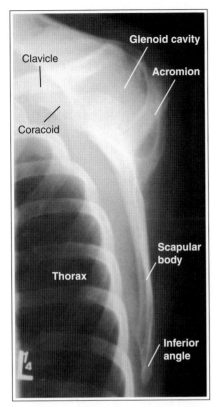

FIGURE 5-37 Lateral scapular projection with accurate positioning.

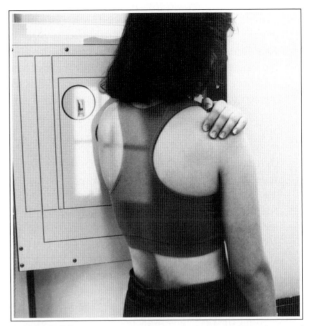

FIGURE 5-38 Proper positioning of standing lateral scapular projection.

BOX 5-12	Lateral Scapula Projection Analysis Criteria

- Lateral and vertebral scapular borders are superimposed.
- Scapular body is seen without superimposing the thoracic cavity.
- Humerus is drawn away from the superior scapular body, and the superior scapular angle is superimposed over the coracoid process base.
- Midscapular body is at the center of the exposure field.
- Entire scapula is included within the collimated field.

The scapular body is in a lateral projection. The lateral and vertebral scapular borders are superimposed, and the scapular body is demonstrated without superimposing the thoracic cavity.

- The scapular body is placed in a lateral projection by first placing the patient in an upright PA projection, with the affected arm drawn across the chest so that the hand can grasp the unaffected shoulder. From this position, rotate the patient's body toward the affected scapula until the lateral and vertebral scapular borders are superimposed (Figure 5-38).

- The degree of body obliquity required to superimpose the scapular borders depends on the degree of humeral elevation. As the humerus is elevated, the inferior angle of the scapula glides around the thoracic cage, moving the scapula more anteriorly. The more the scapula glides around the thorax, the less body obliquity is required to superimpose the vertebral and lateral scapular borders.

- To position the long axis of the scapular body parallel with the IR and demonstrate it with the least amount of foreshortening, elevate the arm to a 90-degree angle with the body.

- The proper degree of body rotation for any arm position is determined by palpating the lateral and vertebral scapular borders. Because the superior portions of the lateral and vertebral borders are heavily covered with muscles, it is best to palpate them just superior to the inferior scapular angle. Adjusting the arm position slightly while palpating can also help in locating the scapular borders and inferior angle. Once these anatomic structures are located, rotate the patient's body until the vertebral border of the scapula is superimposed over the lateral border and the inferior scapular angle is positioned in profile. Because abduction of the humerus shifts the scapula laterally, the amount of rotation is dependent on the amount of humerus elevation. When the humerus is elevated to 90 degrees, approximately 30 degrees of patient obliquity is necessary. If the arm is elevated less than 90 degrees, the amount of obliquity needs to be increased and, if the arm is elevated more than 90 degrees, the amount is decreased.

- *Positioning the supine patient.* For the supine patient a lateral scapula projection is obtained by placing the patient in an AP oblique projection. The lateral and vertebral scapular borders and the inferior scapular angle should be palpated using the same method as described for the standing patient; however, the patient is rotated toward the unaffected shoulder to superimpose the vertebral and lateral scapular borders and place the inferior angle in profile (Figure 5-39).

- *Detecting inaccurate rotation.* If the body was not accurately rotated for a lateral scapular projection, the borders of the scapula are not superimposed but are demonstrated next to each other. When such a projection has been produced, one can determine whether patient obliquity was excessive or insufficient by identifying the scapular borders. The lateral border is thick, being identified by two cortical outlines that are separated by approximately 0.25 inch (0.6 cm), whereas the cortical outline of the vertebral border is a single thin line. If the lateral border is demonstrated next to the ribs and the vertebral border is demonstrated laterally, the patient has been rotated too much (see Image 54). If the vertebral border is demonstrated next to the ribs and the lateral border is demonstrated laterally, the patient was not rotated enough to superimpose the borders (see Image 55).

The humerus is drawn away from the superior scapular body, and the superior scapular angle is superimposed over the coracoid process base.

- Eighty percent of scapular fractures involve the body or neck of the scapula. The neck of the scapula is best visualized on the AP projection, because it is demonstrated on end in the lateral position. If a fracture of the scapular body is present or suspected, the lateral projection should be taken to demonstrate the AP alignment of the fracture.

- *Effect of humeral elevation on scapular visualization.* To demonstrate the scapular body best, position its long axis parallel with the long axis of the IR by elevating the humerus to a 90-degree angle with the patient's body (Figures 5-40 and 5-41).

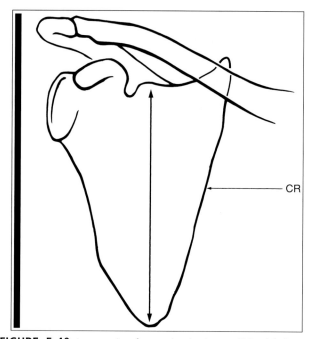

FIGURE 5-40 Long axis of scapular body parallel with image receptor. *CR,* Central ray.

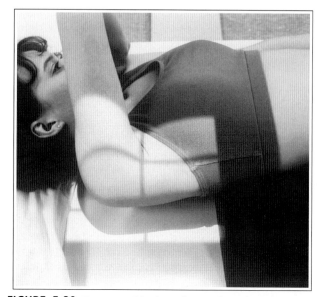

FIGURE 5-39 Proper positioning of recumbent lateral scapular projection.

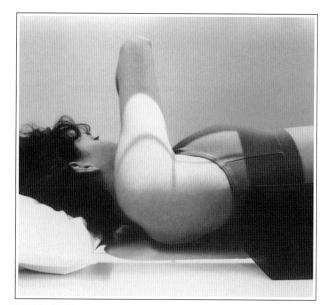

FIGURE 5-41 Proper arm positioning for lateral scapula projection.

This positioning causes the scapula to glide anteriorly around the thoracic cavity and tilts the glenoid fossa slightly upward, placing the long axis of the scapular body parallel with the IR (see Figure 5-35). The humerus is also drawn away from the superior scapular body, allowing it to be visualized without humeral superimposition.

- If humeral elevation is increased above 90 degrees, with the patient still grasping the opposite shoulder, the lateral border of the scapula is placed parallel with the IR (Figures 5-42 and 5-43). This positioning distorts the superior scapular body

and demonstrates the superior scapular angle and scapular spine below the coracoid and acromion processes, respectively (see Image 56). If the humerus is not elevated but rests on the patient's chest, with the patient still grasping the opposite shoulder, the vertebral border of the scapula is positioned parallel with the image (Figures 5-44 and 5-45). This arm positioning produces a shoulder image similar to that obtained for the PA oblique (scapular Y) projection—the superior scapular body is superimposed over the glenoid cavity and the proximal humerus, the coracoid and acromion processes are visible in profile, and the AP relationship of the humeral head and glenoid cavity is demonstrated (see Image 57).

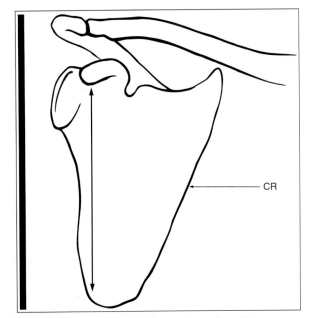

FIGURE 5-42 Lateral border of scapula parallel with image receptor. *CR,* Central ray.

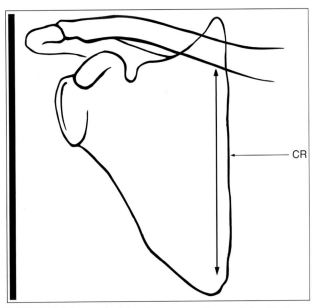

FIGURE 5-44 Vertebral border of scapula parallel with image receptor. *CR,* Central ray.

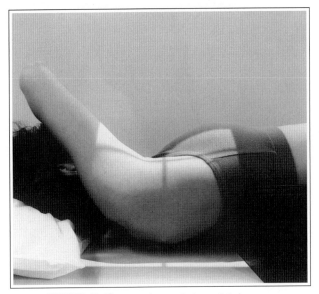

FIGURE 5-43 Arm elevated above 90 degrees.

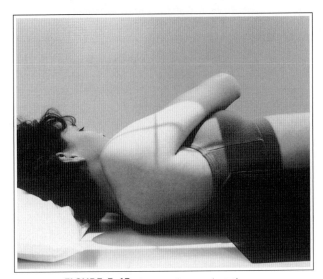

FIGURE 5-45 Arm resting against thorax.

The midscapular body is at the center of the exposure field. The entire scapula, consisting of the inferior angle and the coracoid and acromion processes, is included within the collimation field.

- To place the midscapular body in the center of the exposure field, center a perpendicular central ray to the midscapular body.
- Center the IR to the central ray, and open the longitudinal collimation enough to include both the acromion and inferior scapular angles. Transversely collimate to within 0.5 inch (1.25 cm) of the closest lateral skin line.
- A 10- × 12-inch (25- × 30-cm) IR placed lengthwise should be adequate to include all the required anatomic structures.

Lateral Scapular Projection Analysis

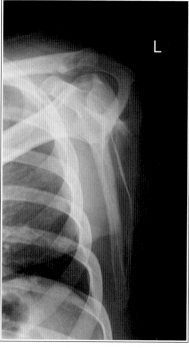

IMAGE 54

Analysis. The lateral and vertebral borders of the scapula are demonstrated without superimposition. The lateral border is next to the ribs, and the vertebral border is demonstrated laterally. The patient was rotated more than required for this image.

Correction. Decrease the patient obliquity. The amount of change required is half of the distance demonstrated between the lateral and vertebral borders. When patient obliquity is decreased, the lateral border moves away from the thoracic cavity and the vertebral border moves closer to the thoracic cavity.

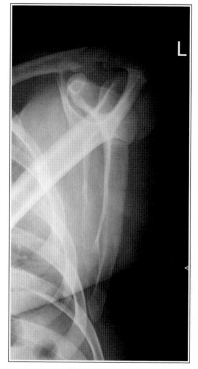

IMAGE 55

Analysis. The lateral and vertebral borders of the scapula are demonstrated without superimposition. The thick lateral border is demonstrated laterally, and the vertebral border is visible next to the ribs. The patient was not rotated enough for this image.

Correction. Increase the patient obliquity. The amount of change necessary is half the distance demonstrated between the lateral and vertebral borders.

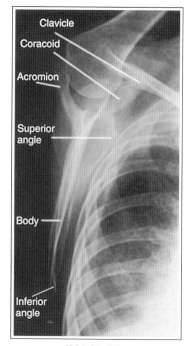

IMAGE 56

Analysis. The lateral and vertebral borders of the scapula are superimposed, indicating that patient obliquity was adequate. Note that the superior angle is demonstrated next to the thoracic cavity, inferior to the coracoid process. The patient's arm was elevated more than 90 degrees, positioning the lateral border of the scapula parallel with the IR (Figures 5-42 and 5-43).

Correction. Depress the arm, positioning it at a 90-degree angle with the body. This depression causes the inferior angle to draw posteriorly around the thoracic cavity. Because of this posterior scapular movement, it is necessary to increase patient obliquity slightly to obtain a lateral scapula. It is suggested that the scapular borders and inferior angle be repalpated to obtain accurate patient obliquity.

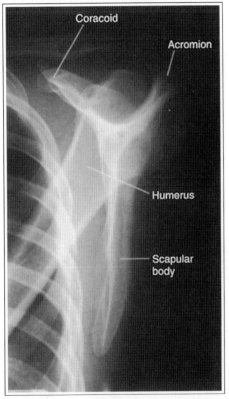

IMAGE 57

Analysis. The superior scapular body is superimposed by the glenoid cavity, the proximal humeral head and the coracoid and acromion processes are clearly demonstrated, and the glenoid cavity is demonstrated "on end." The patient's arm was not elevated but rested on the patient's chest, positioning the vertebral border of the scapula parallel with the IR (see Figures 5-44 and 5-45).

Correction. For the scapular body to be demonstrated best, the arm should be elevated to approximately 90 degrees with the body. If the coracoid and acromion processes or the AP relationship between the glenoid fossa and humeral head is of interest, no corrective movement is necessary.

REFERENCES

1. De Smet AA: Anterior oblique projection in radiography of the traumatized shoulder, *AJR Am J Roentgenol* 134:515–518, 1980.
2. Rubin SA, Gray RL, Green WR: The scapular "Y": A diagnostic aid in shoulder trauma, *Radiology* 110:725–726, 1974.

OBJECTIVES

After completion of this chapter, you should be able to do the following:

- Identify the required anatomy on lower extremity images.
- Describe how to properly position the patient, image receptor (IR), and central ray for lower extremity images.
- State how to properly mark and display lower extremity images.
- List the image analysis criteria used to determine the accuracy of lower extremity images and state how to improve images when the criteria are not met.
- List the image requirements for accurate positioning for lower extremity images.
- Discuss how the degree of central ray angulation is adjusted for an AP axial foot projection and how the degree of obliquity is adjusted for an AP oblique foot projection in patients with high and low longitudinal arches.
- Describe how the central ray angulation is adjusted when a patient is unable to dorsiflex the foot for an axial calcaneal projection.
- Describe what effect the anode heel effect has on lower leg and femoral images and how the leg should be positioned to take advantage of it.
- Explain how the central ray angulation used for AP and AP oblique knee projections is determined by the thickness of the patient's upper thigh and buttocks, and discuss why this adjustment is required.

- State how to determine what central ray angulation to use for an AP knee projection in a patient who cannot fully extend the knee.
- State which anatomic structures are placed in profile on AP oblique knee projections with accurate positioning.
- List the soft tissue structures of interest found on lower extremity images. State where they are located and why their visualization is important.
- State how the patient's knee is positioned for a lateral knee projection if a patella fracture is suspected.
- State the relationship of the medial and lateral femoral condyles, and describe the degree of femoral inclination demonstrated in a patient in an erect and recumbent lateral projection.
- State the femoral length and pelvic width that demonstrate the least amount of femoral inclination.
- Describe how patellar subluxation is demonstrated on a tangential knee projection.
- State the importance of securing the legs and instructing the patient to relax the quadriceps femoris muscles for a tangential knee projection.
- Explain how the positioning setup for a tangential knee projection is adjusted for a patient with large posterior calves.

KEY TERMS

adductor tubercle
dorsal
dorsiflex
dorsoplantar
intermalleolar line

lateral mortise
plantar
plantar-flex
subluxation
talar domes

tarsi sinus
valgus deformity
varus deformity

IMAGE ANALYSIS CRITERIA

The following image analysis criteria are used for all adult and pediatric lower extremity images and should be considered when completing the analysis for each lower extremity projection presented in this chapter (Box 6-1).

BOX 6-1	Lower Extremity Imaging Analysis Criteria

- The facility's identification requirements are visible.
- A right or left marker identifying the correct side of the patient is present on the image and is not superimposed over the anatomy of interest.
- Good radiation protection practices are evident.
- Bony trabecular patterns and cortical outlines of the anatomic structures are sharply defined.
- Contrast and density are uniform and adequate to demonstrate the surrounding soft tissue and bony structures.
- Penetration is sufficient to visualize the bony trabecular patterns and cortical outlines of the lower extremity.
- No evidence of removable artifacts is present.

- *Visibility of lower extremity details.* An optimal kilovoltage peak (kVp) technique, as shown in Table 6-1, sufficiently penetrates the bony and soft tissue structures of the lower extremity and provides a contrast scale necessary to visualize the bony details. To obtain optimal density, set a manual milliampere-seconds (mAs) value based on the part thickness. If the patient's lower extremity thickness measures less than 4 inches (10 cm), a grid is not required. If the patient's lower extremity thickness measures more than 4 inches (10 cm), a grid should be used because this thickness would produce enough scatter radiation to negatively affect image contrast. When a grid is used, increase the kVp to approximately 70 to penetrate the structure and to provide an adequate scale of contrast. Increase the exposure (mAs) by the standard density conversion factor for the grid ratio being used to compensate for the scatter and the primary radiation that the grid will absorb.

TABLE 6-1	Lower Extremity Technical Data		
Projection	**kVp**	**Grid**	**SID**
Toe	55–65		40–48 inches (100–120 cm)
Foot	55–65		40–48 inches (100–120 cm)
Axial (dorsoplantar), calcaneus	60–65		40–48 inches (100–120 cm)
Lateral, calcaneus	55–65		40–48 inches (100–120 cm)
Ankle	55–65		40–48 inches (100–120 cm)
Lower Leg	55–65		40–48 inches (100–120 cm)
AP, knee	Nongrid: 50–60 Grid: 65–75	If measures over 10 cm	40–48 inches (100–120 cm)
Lateral, knee	Nongrid: 50–60 Grid: 65–75	If measures over 10 cm	40–48 inches (100–120 cm)
AP oblique, knee	Nongrid: 50–60 Grid: 65–75	If measures over 10 cm	40–48 inches (100–120 cm)
PA axial (Holmblad method), intercondylar fossa	60–70		40–48 inches (100–120 cm)
AP axial (Béclère method), intercondylar fossa	60–70		40–48 inches (100–120 cm)
Tangential (Merchant method), patella and patellofemoral joint	60–70		48–72 inches (120–180 cm)
Femur	70–80	Grid	40–48 inches (100–120 cm)

SID, Source–image receptor distance.

TOE(S): ANTEROPOSTERIOR AXIAL PROJECTION

See Figures 6-1, 6-2, and 6-3 and Box 6-2.

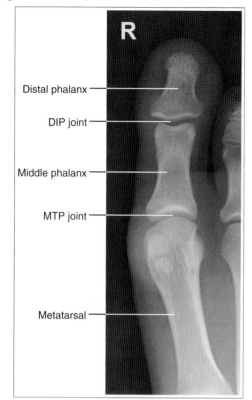

FIGURE 6-1 First AP axial toe projection with accurate positioning. *DIP,* Distal interphalangeal; *MTP,* metatarsophalangeal.

Distal phalanx

DIP joint

Middle phalanx

MTP joint

Metatarsal

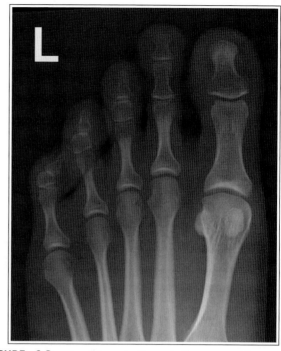

FIGURE 6-3 AP axial projection of the toes with accurate positioning.

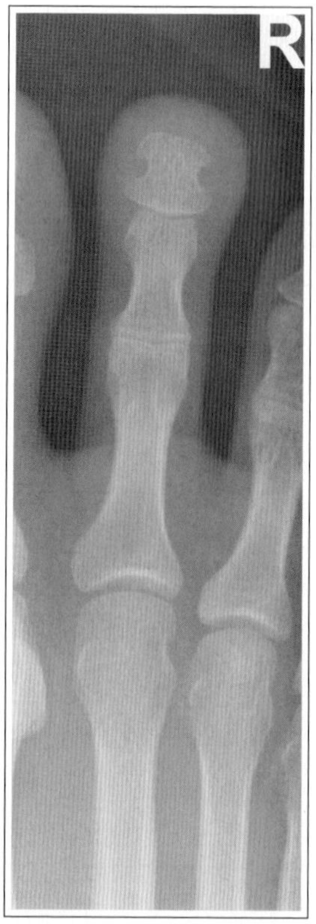

FIGURE 6-2 Second AP axial toe projection with accurate positioning.

BOX 6-2	**Anteroposterior Axial Toe(s) Projection Analysis Criteria**

- Soft tissue width and midshaft concavity are equal on both sides of phalanges.
- The IP and MTP joints are open and the phalanges are seen without foreshortening.
- No soft tissue or bony overlap from adjacent digits is present.
- MTP joint is at the center of the exposure field for a toe image and third MTP joint is at the center when all toes are imaged.
- Phalanges and half of the metatarsal(s) are included within the collimated field.

IP, Interphalangeal; *MTP,* metatarsophalangeal.

The digit demonstrates no rotation. Soft tissue width and midshaft concavity are equal on both sides of the phalanges.

- An AP axial projection of the toe is obtained by flexing the supine patient's knee until the plantar foot surface rests flat against the image receptor (IR). The lower leg, ankle, and foot should remain

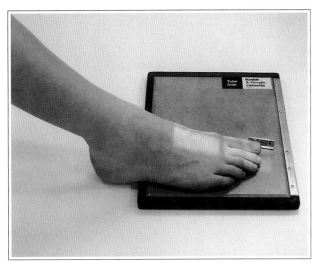

FIGURE 6-4 Proper patient positioning for AP axial toe projection.

aligned, and equal pressure should be applied across the plantar surface (Figure 6-4).

- *Detecting toe rotation.* Toe rotation is controlled by the position of the foot. Take a few minutes to study a toe skeleton and note that in an AP projection, concavity of the midshaft of the proximal phalanx is equal on both sides. Also, note that the posterior (plantar) surface of the proximal phalanx demonstrates more concavity than the anterior (dorsal) surface. As the skeleton is rotated medially or laterally, the amount of concavity increases on the side toward which the posterior surface is rotated, whereas the side toward which the anterior surface is rotated demonstrates less concavity. The same observations can be made about the soft tissue that surrounds the phalanges. More soft tissue thickness is present on the posterior surface than the anterior surface, so the side demonstrating the greatest soft tissue width on an image will be the side toward which the posterior surface is rotated. Look for this midshaft concavity and soft tissue width variation to indicate rotation on an AP axial toe projection. With lateral toe rotation, phalangeal soft tissue width and midshaft concavity are greater on the side positioned away from the lateral foot surface (see Image 1). With medial toe rotation, phalangeal soft tissue width and midshaft concavity are greater on the side positioned away from the medial foot surface (see Image 2). If the patient's toenail is visualized,

which is often the case with the first toe, it can also be used to determine the direction of toe rotation. The nail rotates in the same direction as the foot.

The interphalangeal (IP) and metatarsophalangeal (MTP) joints appear as open spaces, and the phalanges are demonstrated without foreshortening.

- The IP and MTP joint spaces are open and the phalanges are demonstrated without foreshortening when the toe(s) was fully extended and a 10- to 15-degree proximal (toward the calcaneus) central ray was centered to the MTP joint(s). The central ray angulation is required to align the central ray placement closer to parallel with the joint spaces and perpendicular to the phalanges, preventing closed joint spaces and foreshortened phalanges (see Image 3).
- *Central ray angulation for nonextendable toes.* For patients who have extremely flexed toes that will not extend, the toes and forefoot may be elevated on a radiolucent sponge to bring the phalanges parallel with the IR.

No soft tissue or bony overlap from adjacent digits is present.

- Spreading the toes slightly prevents soft tissue and bone from overlapping from adjacent toes. It is difficult to evaluate the soft tissue of an affected toe when it is superimposed by other soft tissue.

The MTP joint is at the center of the exposure field for an AP toe projection and the third MTP joint is at the center when all the toes are imaged. The phalanges and half of the metatarsal(s) are included within the collimated field.

- Centering the central ray to the MTP joint for a toe image or to the third MTP for images of the toes places the joint(s) in the center of the image.
- Open the longitudinal collimation to include the toe(s) and the distal half of the metatarsal(s). To include half of the metatarsal(s), extend the light field 2 inches (5 cm) proximal to the between-toe interconnecting tissue. Transverse collimation should be to within 0.5 inch (1.25 cm) of the toe or foot skin line.
- One third of an 8- × 10-inch (18- × 24-cm) detailed screen-film or computed radiography IR placed crosswise should be adequate to include all the required anatomic structures.

Anteroposterior Axial Toe Projection Analysis

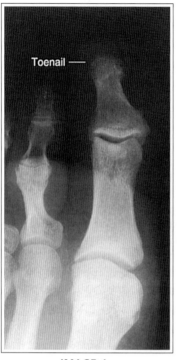

IMAGE 1

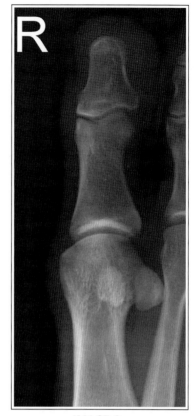

IMAGE 2

Analysis. The phalanges demonstrate greater soft tissue width and midshaft concavity on the medial surface. The toe was laterally rotated.

Correction. Medially rotate the foot and toe until they are flat against the IR.

Analysis. The phalanges demonstrate greater soft tissue width and midshaft concavity on the lateral surface. The toe and foot were medially rotated.

Correction. Laterally rotate the foot until the toe(s) of interest is flat against the IR.

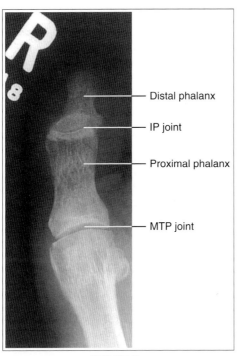

Distal phalanx

IP joint

Proximal phalanx

MTP joint

IMAGE 3

Analysis. The IP and MTP joint spaces are closed, and the phalanges are foreshortened. The patient's toe was flexed, and the central ray was not aligned parallel with the joint spaces or perpendicular to the phalanges.

Correction. If the patient's condition allows, extend the toe, placing it flat against the IR. If the patient is unable to extend the toe, elevate it on a radiolucent sponge until the central ray is aligned parallel with the joint spaces or perpendicular to the phalanges of interest.

TOE(S): ANTEROPOSTERIOR OBLIQUE PROJECTION

See Figures 6-5 and 6-6 and Box 6-3.

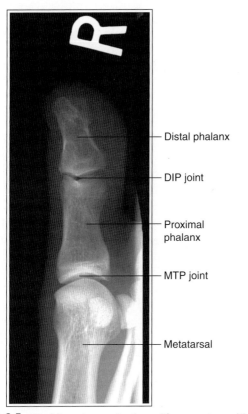

Distal phalanx

DIP joint

Proximal phalanx

MTP joint

Metatarsal

FIGURE 6-5 AP oblique toe projection with accurate positioning. *DIP,* Distal interphalangeal; *MTP,* metatarsophalangeal.

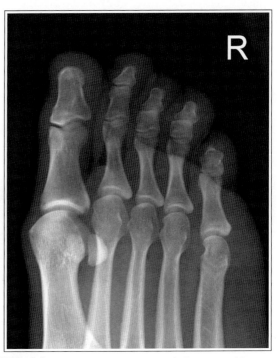

FIGURE 6-6 AP oblique projections of the toes with accurate positioning.

BOX 6-3 | **Anteroposterior Oblique Toe(s) Projection Analysis Criteria**

- Twice as much soft tissue width and more phalangeal and metatarsal concavity are present on the side of the digit rotated away from the IR.
- IP and MTP joint(s) are open and the phalanges are demonstrated without foreshortening.
- No soft tissue or bony overlap from adjacent digits.
- MTP joint is at the center of the exposure field for a toe image and third MTP joint is at the center when all toes are imaged.
- Phalanges and half of the metatarsal(s) are included within the collimated field.

IP, Interphalangeal; *IR*, image receptor; *MTP*, metatarsophalangeal.

The digit(s) is rotated 45 degrees. Twice as much soft tissue width and more phalangeal and metatarsal concavity are present on the side of the digit rotated away from the IR.

- An AP oblique toe(s) projection is obtained by placing the affected foot on the IR and then rotating the foot until the affected toe is rotated 45 degrees from the AP projection (Figure 6-7). When the first through third toes are of interest, the foot should be rotated medially. When the fourth and fifth toes are of interest, the foot should be rotated laterally. The variation in rotation for the different toes is to obtain an AP oblique projection with the least amount of OID.
- *Verifying toe rotation on AP oblique projections.* To verify the accuracy of rotation on an AP oblique toe projection and to determine the proper way to reposition the patient when digit obliquity was insufficient or excessive, study the midshaft concavity of the proximal phalanx and compare the soft tissue width on both sides of the digit. An AP oblique toe projection taken at 45 degrees of obliquity demonstrates more phalangeal midshaft concavity and twice as much soft tissue width on the side positioned farther from the IR. When the midshaft concavity of the proximal phalanx and soft tissue width are closer to equal on both sides of the digit, the toe was not adequately rotated (see Image 4).

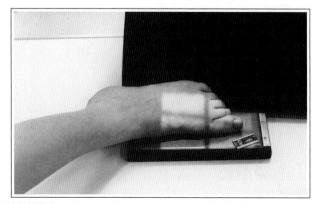

FIGURE 6-7 Proper patient positioning for AP oblique toe projection.

When more than twice the width of soft tissue is present on one side of the digit than on the other and when the posterior aspect of the proximal phalanx's midshaft demonstrates more concavity than the anterior aspect, the toe was rotated more than 45 degrees for the image (see Image 5).

The IP and MTP joints are visible as open spaces, and the phalanges are demonstrated without foreshortening.

- The IP and MTP joint spaces are open and the phalanges are demonstrated without foreshortening when the toe(s) was fully extended and a perpendicular central ray was centered to the MTP joint. This toe positioning and central ray placement align the joint spaces perpendicular to the IR and parallel with the central ray. They also prevent foreshortening of the phalanges, because the long axes of the phalanges are aligned parallel with the IR and perpendicular to the central ray. If the toe was not extended, the resulting image demonstrates closed joint spaces and foreshortened phalanges (see Image 6).
- *Central ray angulation for nonextendable toes.* In patients who are unable to extend their toes, the central ray should be angled proximally (toward the calcaneus) until it is perpendicular to the phalanx of interest or parallel with the joint space of interest or the toes and forefoot may be elevated on a sponge to bring phalanges closer to parallel with the IR.

No soft tissue or bony overlap from adjacent digits is present.

- The adjacent toes should be drawn away from the affected toe to prevent overlapping. It may be necessary to use tape or another immobilization device to maintain the unaffected toe's position. If the unaffected toes are not drawn away, they may be superimposed over the affected toe (see Image 7).

The MTP joint is at the center of the exposure field for an AP toe projection or the third MTP joint is at the center for images of the toes. The phalanges and half of the metatarsal(s) are included within the collimated field.

- Centering the central ray to the MTP joint for a toe or to the third MTP for toes places the joint(s) in the center of the image and aids in opening the joint spaces.
- Open the longitudinal collimation to include the toe(s) and the distal half of the metatarsal(s). To include half of the metatarsal(s), extend the light field 2 inches (5 cm) proximally to the between-toe interconnecting tissue. Transverse collimation should be to within 0.5 inch (1.25 cm) of the toe or foot skin line.
- One third of an 8- × 10-inch (18- × 24-cm) detailed screen-film or computed radiography IR placed crosswise should be adequate to include all the required anatomic structures.

Anteroposterior Oblique Toe Projection Analysis

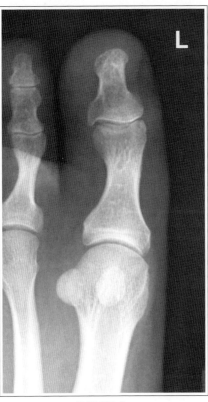

IMAGE 4

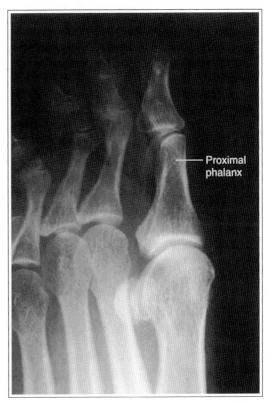

IMAGE 5

Analysis. Soft tissue width and midshaft concavity on both sides of the phalanges are almost equal. The toe was rotated less than 45 degrees.

Correction. Increase toe and foot obliquity until the affected toe is at a 45-degree angle with the IR.

Analysis. The proximal phalanx demonstrates more concavity on the lateral aspect of the toe than the medial aspect. The toe has been rotated close to a lateral position.

Correction. Decrease toe and foot obliquity until the affected toe is at a 45-degree angle with the IR.

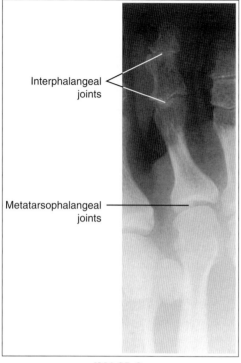

Interphalangeal
joints

Metatarsophalangeal
joints

IMAGE 6

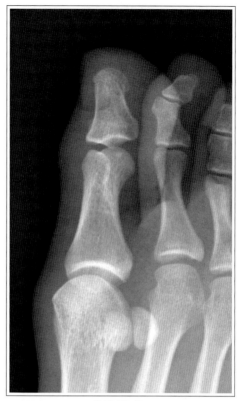

IMAGE 7

Analysis. The IP and MTP joint spaces are obscured, and the phalanges are foreshortened. The patient's toe was flexed, and the central ray was not angled to open these joints or to demonstrate the phalanges without foreshortening.

Correction. If the patient's condition allows, extend the toe, placing it flat against the IR. If the patient's toe cannot be extended, angle the central ray until it is aligned perpendicularly to the phalanx of interest or parallel with the joint space of interest.

Analysis. Soft tissue and bony overlap of the adjacent digit onto the affected digit are present. The toes were not spread apart.

Correction. Draw the unaffected toes away from the affected toe. It may be necessary to use tape or another immobilization device if the patient is unable to maintain the position.

TOE(S): LATERAL PROJECTION (MEDIOLATERAL AND LATEROMEDIAL)

See Figures 6-8 and 6-9 and Box 6-4.

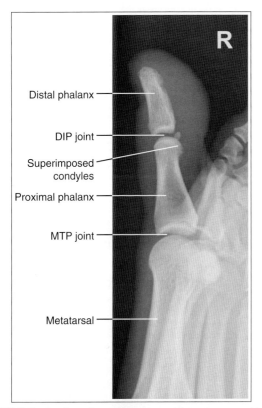

FIGURE 6-8 First lateral toe projection with accurate positioning. *DIP,* Distal interphalangeal; *MTP,* metatarsophalangeal.

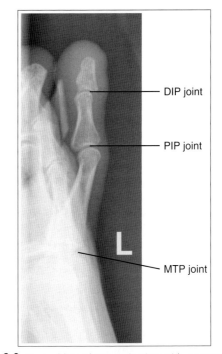

FIGURE 6-9 Second lateral toe projection with accurate positioning. *DIP,* Distal interphalangeal; *MTP,* metatarsophalangeal; *PIP,* proximal interphalangeal.

BOX 6-4	Lateral Toe Projection Analysis Criteria

- Posterior surface of the proximal phalanx demonstrates more concavity than the anterior surface, and the condyles of the proximal phalanx are superimposed.
- There is no soft tissue or bony overlap from adjacent toes.
- The PIP joint is at the center of the exposure field.
- The phalanges and MTP joint space are included within the collimated field.

MTP, Metatarsophalangeal; *PIP,* proximal interphalangeal.

The digit is demonstrated in a lateral projection. The posterior surface of the proximal phalanx demonstrates more concavity than the anterior surface, and the condyles are superimposed. The soft tissue outline of the nail, when shown, is in profile anteriorly.

- A lateral toe projection is obtained by rotating the foot and toe until the affected toe is lateral. Whether the foot is medially or laterally rotated to achieve this goal depends on which toe is being imaged. When the first, second, and third toes are imaged, rotate the foot medially (Figure 6-10). When the fourth and fifth toes are imaged, rotate the foot laterally (Figure 6-11).
- *Inadequate toe rotations.* In a lateral projection, the posterior (plantar) surface of the proximal phalanx demonstrates more concavity than the anterior (dorsal) surface and the condyles are superimposed. Inadequate rotation demonstrates almost equal concavity on the posterior and anterior surfaces of the proximal phalanx and the condyles without superimposition (see Image 8). Evaluate the degree

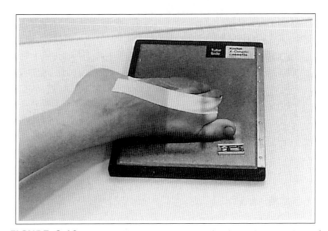

FIGURE 6-10 Proper patient positioning for lateral projection of the first toe.

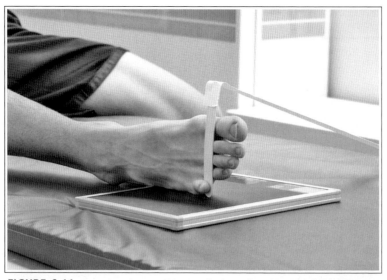

FIGURE 6-11 Proper patient positioning for lateral projection of the fifth toe.

of metatarsal head superimposition to determine whether the toe was rotated too much or not enough when a poor lateral toe projection is produced. Compare Images 8 and 9. In Image 8, the metatarsal heads are shown without superimposition, indicating that the amount of foot and toe rotation should be increased. In Image 9, the metatarsal heads demonstrate slight superimposition, indicating that the amount of foot and toe rotation should be decreased.

No soft tissue or bony overlap from adjacent toes is present.

- The adjacent toes should be drawn away from the affected toe to prevent overlapping. It may be necessary to use tape or another immobilization device to maintain the unaffected toe's position. If the unaffected toes are not drawn away, they may be superimposed over the affected toe (see Image 10).

The proximal interphalangeal (PIP) joint is at the center of the exposure field. The phalanges and MTP joint space are included within the collimated field.

- Centering a perpendicular central ray to the PIP joint places the joint in the center of the image.
- Open the longitudinal collimation to include the distal phalanx and MTP joint space. The MTP joint space is located approximately 1 inch (2.5 cm) proximal to the between-toe interconnecting tissue. Transverse collimation should be to within 0.5 inch (1.25 cm) of the toe skin line.
- One third of an 8- × 10-inch (18- × 24-cm) detailed screen-film or computed radiography IR placed crosswise should be adequate to include all the required anatomic structures.

Lateral Toe Projection Analysis

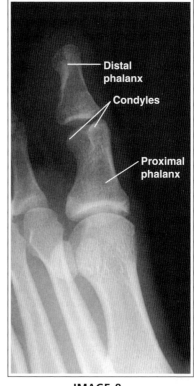

IMAGE 8

Analysis. The proximal phalanx demonstrates almost equal midshaft concavity, the condyles are shown without superimposition, and the metatarsal heads are shown without superimposition. The foot and toe were not rotated enough for the toe to be placed in a lateral position.

Correction. Increase the patient's toe and foot obliquity until the affected toe is in a lateral position. For this patient it may also be necessary to draw the unaffected toes away from the affected toe to prevent superimposition.

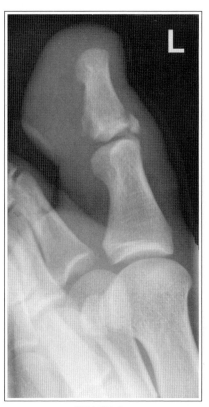

IMAGE 9

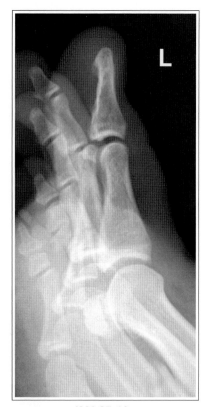

IMAGE 10

Analysis. The proximal phalanx demonstrates almost equal midshaft concavity, the condyles are shown without superimposition, and the metatarsal heads are slightly superimposed. The foot and toe were rotated too much for the toe to be placed in a lateral position.

Correction. Decrease the patient's toe and foot obliquity until the affected toe is in a lateral projection.

Analysis. Soft tissue and bony overlap of digits are present. The adjacent unaffected digits were not drawn away from the affected digit.

Correction. The patient's unaffected toes should be drawn away from the affected toe. It may be necessary to use tape or another immobilization device to help the patient maintain this position.

FOOT: ANTEROPOSTERIOR AXIAL PROJECTION (DORSOPLANTAR)

See Figure 6-12 and Box 6-5.

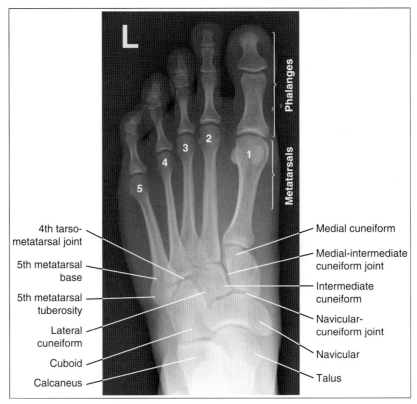

FIGURE 6-12 AP axial foot projection with accurate positioning.

BOX 6-5   Anteroposterior Axial Foot Projection Analysis Criteria

- The foot demonstrates uniform density across the phalanges, metatarsals, and tarsals.
- The joint space between the medial (first) and intermediate (second) cuneiforms is open, about 0.75 inch (2 cm) of the calcaneus is demonstrated without talar superimposition, and concavity on both sides of the first metatarsal midshaft is equal.
- The TMT and navicular-cuneiform joint spaces are open.
- The third metatarsal base is at the center of the exposure field.
- The proximal calcaneus, talar neck, tarsals, metatarsals, phalanges, and foot soft tissue are included within the collimated field.

TMT, Tarsometatarsal.

The foot demonstrates uniform density across the phalanges, metatarsals, and tarsals.

- When an exposure (mAs) is set that will adequately demonstrate the proximal metatarsals and tarsals, the distal metatarsals and phalanges are often overexposed because of the difference in AP foot thickness in these two regions (see Image 11). A wedge-type compensating filter placed over the phalanges and MTP joints can be used to absorb some of the photons that reach these areas, thereby obtaining more uniform foot density (Figure 6-13). Position the thinnest part of the filter 1 inch (2.5 cm) proximally to the between-toe interconnecting tissue and the thickest over the phalanges.

The foot demonstrates an AP projection. The joint space between the medial (first) and intermediate (second) cuneiforms is open, approximately 0.75 inch (2 cm) of the calcaneus is demonstrated without talar superimposition, and concavity on both sides of the first metatarsal midshaft is equal.

- An AP projection of the foot is obtained by flexing the supine patient's knee and placing the plantar foot surface against the IR (Figure 6-14). The lower leg, ankle, and foot should remain aligned, and equal pressure should be applied across the plantar surface.
- *Effect of foot rotation.* If the lower leg, ankle, and foot are not aligned or if more pressure is placed on the medial or lateral plantar surface, foot rotation will result, and the medial and intermediate cuneiform joint space will be closed. When the foot is laterally rotated, the navicular tuberosity, which superimposes itself on an AP projection, is rolled

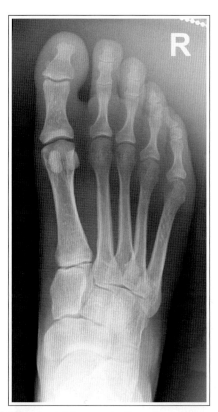

FIGURE 6-13 AP axial foot projection with compensating filter used on the toes.

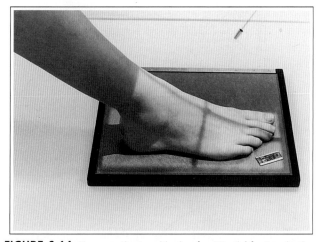

FIGURE 6-14 Proper patient positioning for AP axial foot projection.

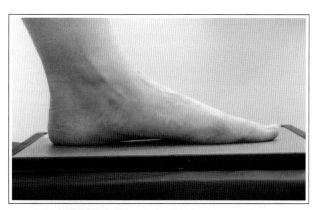

FIGURE 6-15 Low longitudinal foot arch.

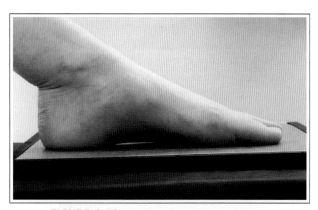

FIGURE 6-16 Average longitudinal foot arch.

standing position. An AP standing foot projection should meet the same evaluating criteria used for a nonstanding AP foot projection.

The tarsometatarsal (TMT) and navicular-cuneiform joint spaces are open.

- The bones of the foot, with their ligamentous and muscular structures, are arranged in a longitudinal arch that is visible on the medial foot surface. This arch places the tarsometatarsal and navicular-cuneiform joint spaces at a set angle with the IR. To demonstrate these joints as open spaces, angle the central ray until it is aligned parallel with them. This is accomplished in most patients by using a 10- to 15-degree proximal (toward the calcaneus) angle or aligning the central ray perpendicularly with the dorsal surface. The exact degree of angulation needed depends on the height of the longitudinal arch. A 10-degree angle should be used when the patient's longitudinal arch is low, as shown in Figure 6-15. A 15-degree angle is needed in a patient with a high arch, as shown in Figure 6-16. Higher arched patients require a slightly higher angle. Omitting or employing an inaccurate central ray angulation results in obstructed TMT and navicular-cuneiform joint spaces (see Image 14).

into profile, and the talus moves over the calcaneus, resulting in less than 0.75 inch (2 cm) of calcaneal demonstration without talar superimposition. An increase in metatarsal base superimposition also occurs (see Images 11 and 12). When the foot is medially rotated, the talus moves away from the calcaneus, resulting in more than 0.75 inch (2 cm) calcaneal visualization without talar superimposition. A decrease in superimposition of the metatarsal bases also occurs (see Image 13).

- **Standing AP projection of the foot.** This image may also be obtained with the patient in a

The third metatarsal base is at the center of the exposure field. The proximal calcaneus, talar neck, tarsals, metatarsals, phalanges, and surrounding foot soft tissue are included within the collimated field.

- To place the third metatarsal base in the center of the image, center the central ray to the midline of the foot at a level 0.5 inch (1.25 cm) distal to the fifth metatarsal tuberosity. The fifth metatarsal tuberosity can be palpated along the lateral foot surface, approximately halfway between the ball of the foot and the calcaneus.
- Open the longitudinal collimation enough to include the phalanges. Transverse collimation should be to within 0.5 inch (1.25 cm) of the foot skin line.
- Half of a 10- × 12-inch (24- × 30-cm) detailed screen-film or computed radiography IR placed lengthwise should be adequate to include all the required anatomic structures.

Anteroposterior Axial Foot Projection Analysis

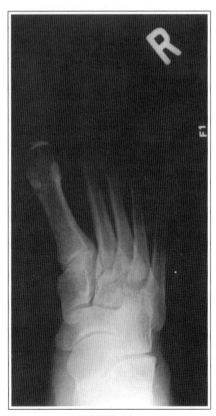

IMAGE 11

Analysis. The phalanges and distal metatarsals are overexposed. A compensating filter was not used on this portion of the foot. The joint space between the medial and intermediate cuneiforms is closed, the navicular tuberosity is demonstrated in profile, and less than 0.75 inch (2 cm) of the calcaneus is demonstrated without talar superimposition. More pressure was placed on the patient's lateral plantar surface than on the medial surface, resulting in lateral foot rotation. The TMT joint spaces are observed. The central ray was not aligned parallel with these joint spaces.

Correction. Position a compensating filter over the phalanges and distal metatarsal. Rotate the foot medially until the pressure over the entire plantar surface is equal. The lower leg, ankle, and foot should be aligned. Direct the central ray 10 to 15 degrees proximally.

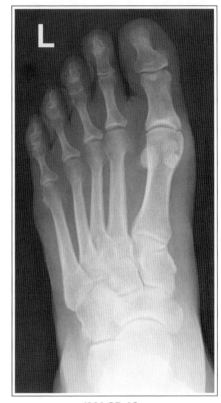

IMAGE 12

Analysis. The joint space between the medial and intermediate cuneiforms is closed, the navicular tuberosity is demonstrated in profile, and less than 0.75 inch (2 cm) of the calcaneus is demonstrated without talar superimposition. The TMT joint spaces are obscured. More pressure was placed on the patient's lateral plantar surface than on the medial surface, resulting in lateral foot rotation, and the central ray was not aligned parallel with these joint spaces.

Correction. Rotate the foot medially until the pressure over the entire plantar surface is equal. The lower leg, ankle, and foot should be aligned. Direct the central ray 10 to 15 degrees proximally (toward the calcaneus), or angle the central ray until it is perpendicular with the dorsal surface.

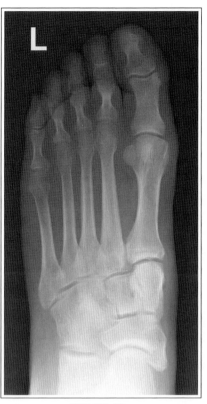

IMAGE 13

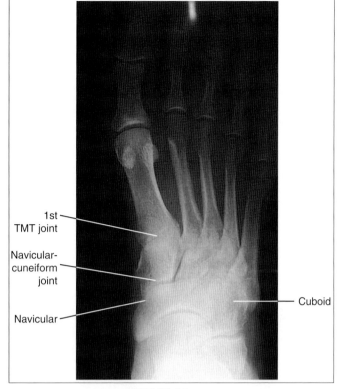

IMAGE 14

Analysis. The joint space between the medial and intermediate cuneiforms is closed, the calcaneus demonstrates no talar superimposition, and the metatarsal bases demonstrate decreased superimposition. More pressure was placed on the patient's medial plantar surface than on the lateral surface, resulting in medial foot rotation.

Correction. Rotate the foot laterally until the pressure over the entire plantar surface is equal. The lower leg, ankle, and foot should be aligned.

Analysis. The TMT and navicular-cuneiform joint spaces are obscured. The central ray was not aligned parallel with these joint spaces.

Correction. Direct the central ray 10 to 15 degrees proximally (toward the calcaneus), or angle the central ray until it is perpendicular with the dorsal surface. Less angulation is needed for patients with low longitudinal arches, whereas more angulation is required for patients with high arches.

FOOT: ANTEROPOSTERIOR OBLIQUE PROJECTION (MEDIAL ROTATION)

See Figures 6-17 and 6-18 and Box 6-6.

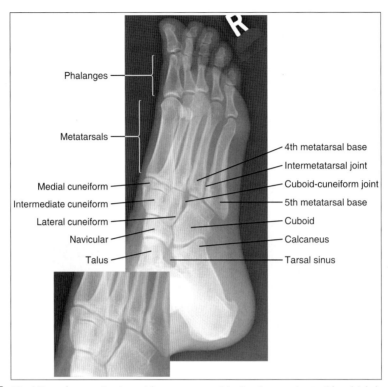

Phalanges

Metatarsals

Medial cuneiform
Intermediate cuneiform
Lateral cuneiform
Navicular
Talus

4th metatarsal base
Intermetatarsal joint
Cuboid-cuneiform joint
5th metatarsal base
Cuboid
Calcaneus
Tarsal sinus

FIGURE 6-17 AP oblique foot projection with accurate positioning in a patient with a high longitudinal arch.

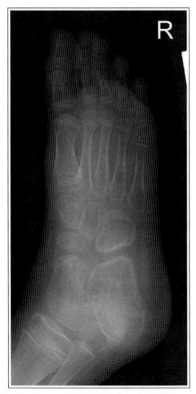

FIGURE 6-18 Pediatric AP oblique foot projection with accurate positioning.

BOX 6-6	Anteroposterior Oblique Foot Projection Analysis Criteria

- The foot demonstrates uniform density across the phalanges, metatarsals, and tarsals.
- The cuboid-cuneiform joint space and second through fifth intermetatarsal joint spaces are open.
- The tarsi sinus and fifth metatarsal tuberosity are visualized.
- The third metatarsal base is at the center of the exposure field.
- The phalanges, metatarsals, tarsals, calcaneus, and foot soft tissue are included within the collimated field.

The foot demonstrates uniform density across the phalanges, metatarsals, and tarsals.

- A wedge-type compensating filter placed over the patient's phalanges and distal metatarsals can be used to obtain uniform foot density. Position the thinnest part of the filter 1 inch (2.5 cm) proximally to the between-toe interconnecting tissue and the thickest over the phalanges.

The foot demonstrates adequate obliquity. The cuboid-cuneiform joint space is open, the first and second intermetatarsal joints are closed, but the second through fifth intermetatarsal joint spaces are open, and the tarsi sinus and fifth metatarsal tuberosity are well demonstrated.

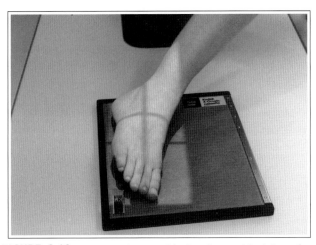

FIGURE 6-19 Proper patient positioning for an AP oblique foot projection.

- To obtain an AP oblique foot projection, begin with the patient in a supine position with the knee flexed until the plantar foot surface rests against the receptor. Medially rotate the patient's leg and foot until the foot forms a 30- to 60-degree angle with the IR (Figure 6-19).
- *Determining required obliquity.* To determine whether a 30- or 60-degree rotation is needed, view the medial aspect of the patient's foot in an AP projection to judge the height of the patient's longitudinal arch. Less obliquity is required in a patient with a low longitudinal arch than in a patient with a high arch. If the patient has a low arch (Figure 6-20; also see Figure 6-15), rotate the patient's foot approximately 30 degrees medially; if the patient's foot has an average arch (Figure 6-21; also see Figure 6-16), rotate the foot approximately 45 degrees medially; and, if the patient's arch is high (Figure 6-22; also see Figure 6-17), rotate the foot approximately 60 degrees. The average arch requires 45 degrees of rotation. As the foot is rotated, keep the lower leg, ankle, and foot aligned to judge the degree of foot obliquity better.
- *Judging the degree of the rotation on AP oblique foot projections.* On lateral foot projections, the height of the longitudinal arches can be compared by evaluating the amount of cuboid demonstrated

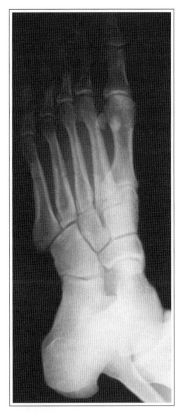

FIGURE 6-21 AP oblique foot projection of a patient with an average longitudinal arch.

posterior to the navicular bone. Note that more cuboid is visible posterior to the navicular bone on the lateral foot projection in Figure 6-22 than in Figure 6-20 and Figure 6-23. A lateral foot projection from a patient with an average longitudinal arch demonstrates approximately 0.5 inch (1.25 cm) of cuboid posterior to the navicular bone, whereas a patient with a high arch will demonstrate approximately 0.75 inch (2 cm) and a patient with a low arch approximately 0.25 inch (0.6 cm). On AP oblique projections, accurate obliquity has been obtained when the cuboid-cuneiform and second through fifth intermetatarsal joint spaces are open. This accuracy is demonstrated on the AP oblique projections in Figures 6-17 and 6-21, even though they were taken with different degrees of obliquity. This can be confirmed

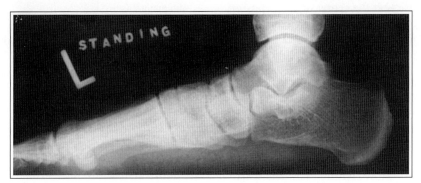

FIGURE 6-20 Lateral foot projection of a patient with a low longitudinal arch.

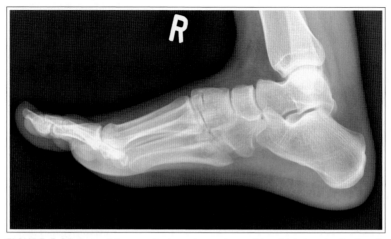

FIGURE 6-22 Lateral foot projection of a patient with a high longitudinal arch.

by studying the amount of first and second metatarsal base superimposition, the amount of space demonstrated between the metatarsal heads, and the demonstration of the sinus tarsi (opening between the calcaneus and talus). When the foot is rotated medially, the first metatarsal base rotates beneath the second metatarsal base, and the second through third metatarsal heads move closer together. The greater the foot obliquity, the greater the superimposition of the metatarsal heads.

- *Underrotation versus overrotation.* If the degree of foot obliquity is inadequate for an AP oblique foot projection, the longitudinally running foot joints (cuneiform-cuboid, navicular-cuboid, and second through fifth intermetatarsal joint spaces) are closed. To determine whether the patient's foot has been underrotated or overrotated, evaluate the intermetatarsal joint spaces between the fourth and fifth metatarsals. If this joint space is closed and the fourth metatarsal base is superimposed over the fifth metatarsal base, the foot was underrotated (see Images 15 and 16). If the fourth-fifth intermetatarsal joint space is closed and the fifth proximal metatarsal is superimposed over the fourth metatarsal tubercle, the foot was overrotated (see Image 17). The fourth metatarsal tubercle is a rounded protruding surface located just distal to the fourth metatarsal base.

The third metatarsal base is at the center of the exposure field. The phalanges, metatarsals, tarsals, calcaneus, and surrounding foot soft tissue are included within the collimated field.

- Centering a perpendicular central ray to the midline of the foot at the level of the fifth metatarsal tuberosity places the base of the proximal third metatarsal in the center of the image.
- Open the longitudinal collimation enough to include the phalanges and calcaneus. Transverse collimation should be to within 0.5 inch (1.25 cm) of the foot skin line.

- Half of a 10- × 12-inch (24- × 30-cm) detailed screen-film or computed radiography IR placed lengthwise should be adequate to include all the required anatomic structures.

Anteroposterior Oblique Foot Projection Analysis

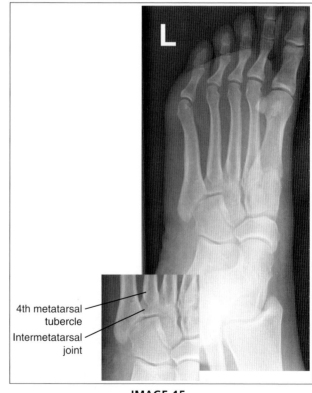

4th metatarsal tubercle

Intermetatarsal joint

IMAGE 15

Analysis. The lateral cuneiform-cuboid, navicular-cuboid, and third through fifth intermetatarsal joint spaces are closed. The fourth metatarsal tubercle is demonstrated without superimposition of the fifth metatarsal. The foot was not medially rotated enough.

Correction. Increase the degree of medial foot rotation. The amount of increase needed is half the amount of fourth and fifth metatarsal base superimposition demonstrated on the image.

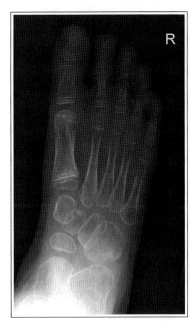

IMAGE 16

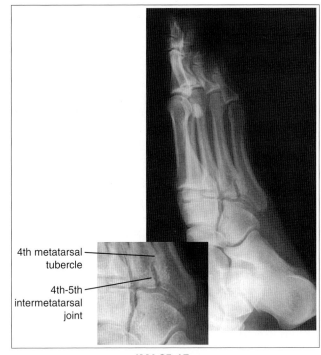

IMAGE 17

Analysis. The lateral cuneiform-cuboid and third through fifth intermetatarsal joint spaces are closed. The foot was not medially rotated enough.

Correction. Increase the degree of medial foot rotation.

Analysis. The lateral cuneiform-cuboid, navicular-cuboid, and intermetatarsal joint spaces are closed, and the fifth proximal metatarsal is superimposed over the fourth metatarsal tubercle. The patient's foot was overrotated.

Correction. Decrease the medial foot rotation.

FOOT: LATERAL PROJECTION (MEDIOLATERAL AND LATEROMEDIAL)

See Figures 6-23 and 6-24 and Box 6-7.

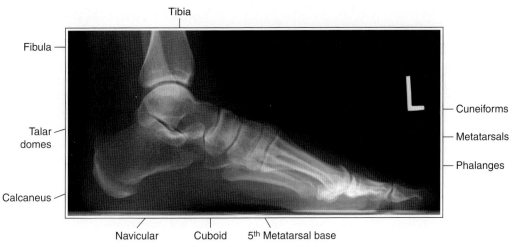

FIGURE 6-23 Mediolateral foot projection with accurate positioning.

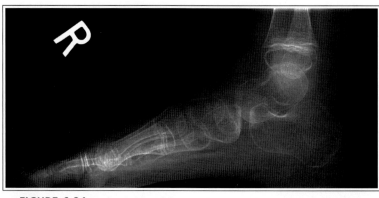

FIGURE 6-24 Pediatric lateral foot projection with accurate positioning.

| BOX 6-7 | **Lateral Foot Projection Analysis Criteria** |

- Contrast and density are adequate to demonstrate the anterior pretalar and posterior pericapsular fat pads.
- The talar domes are superimposed, the tibiotalar joint is open, and the distal fibula is superimposed by the posterior half of the distal tibia.
- The long axis of the foot is positioned at a 90-degree angle with the lower leg.
- The proximal metatarsals are at the center of the exposure field.
- The phalanges, metatarsals, tarsals, talus, calcaneus, 1 inch (2.5 cm) of the distal lower leg, and foot soft tissue are included within the collimated field.

Contrast and density are adequate to demonstrate the anterior pretalar and posterior pericapsular fat pads on the foot and ankle.

- *Fat pads on the foot and ankle.* Two soft tissue structures located around the foot and ankle may indicate joint effusion and injury, the anterior pretalar fat pad and posterior pericapsular fat pad. The anterior pretalar fat pad is visible anterior to the ankle joint and rests next to the neck of the talus (Figure 6-25). Surrounding the ankle joint is a fibrous, synovium-lined capsule attached to the borders of the tibia, fibula, and talus. On injury or disease invasion the synovial membrane secretes synovial fluid, resulting in distention of the fibrous capsule. Anterior fibrous capsule distention results in displacement of the anterior pretalar fat pad. Because neither the fibrous capsule nor the ankle ligaments can be detected on plain radiography, displacement of this fat pad indicates joint effusion and the possibility of underlying injuries.
- The posterior fat pad is positioned within the indentation formed by the articulation of the posterior tibia and talar bones (see Figure 6-25). This fat pad is displaced in the same manner as the anterior pretalar fat pad, although it is less sensitive and requires more fluid evasion to be displaced.

The foot is in a lateral projection. The talar domes are superimposed, the tibiotalar joint is open, and the distal fibula is superimposed by the posterior half of the distal tibia.

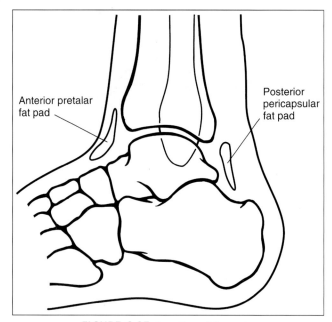

Anterior pretalar fat pad

Posterior pericapsular fat pad

FIGURE 6-25 Location of fat pads.

- To obtain a lateral foot projection, begin with the patient in a supine position with the leg extended and the foot dorsiflexed until its long axis forms a 90-degree angle with the lower leg (Figure 6-26). Rotate the patient toward the affected leg until the lateral foot surface is against the IR, and then adjust the degree of rotation until this surface is aligned parallel with the IR (Figure 6-27). For most patients, this positioning places the lower leg parallel with the imaging table. If this is not the case, as for a patient with a large upper thigh, the foot and IR should be elevated with an immobilization device until the lower leg is brought parallel with the imaging table.
- *Accurate longitudinal arch visualization:* This position may not bring the medial plantar foot surface perpendicular to the IR. If this is so, do not try to adjust the leg in an attempt to position this surface perpendicular to the IR. The true relationship of this surface to the IR and the metatarsals to one another depends on the height of the patient's

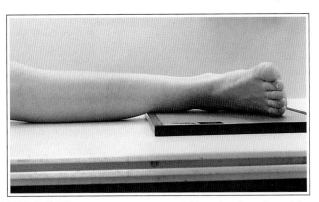

FIGURE 6-26 Accurate positioning of lower leg for a lateral foot projection.

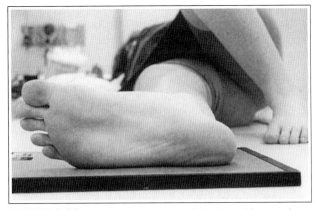

FIGURE 6-27 Accurate positioning of the lateral foot surface.

longitudinal arch and the incline of the calcaneus. Adjusting the patient's plantar surface may result in poor talar dome positioning and an erroneous longitudinal arch height.

The height of the longitudinal arch can be determined by measuring the amount of cuboid demonstrated posterior to the navicular bone. The average lateral foot projection demonstrates approximately 0.5 inch (1.25 cm) of the cuboid, as shown in Figure 6-23. Because the bones that form the foot arch are held in position by ligaments and tendons, weakening of these tissues may result in a decreased or low arch. On a lateral foot projection, this decrease in arch height is demonstrated as a decrease in the amount of cuboid demonstrated posterior to the navicular bone. Figure 6-20 shows a lateral foot projection of a patient with a low longitudinal arch and approximately 0.25 inch (0.6 cm) of cuboid posterior to the navicular bone, whereas Figure 6-22 shows a patient with a high arch and approximately 0.75 inch (2 cm) of cuboid posterior to the navicular bone.

- *Talar domes.* The domes of the talus are formed by the most medial and lateral aspects of the talar's trochlear surface. On a lateral foot projection, they appear as domed structures that articulate with the tibia. On a properly positioned lateral foot

projection, the talar domes should be superimposed and appear as one and the tibiotalar joint should be open. When the lateral foot is mispositioned, the domes are individually demonstrated, and they obscure the tibiotalar joint. Proximal-distal misalignment of the domes results from poor knee and lower leg positioning, and AP misalignment of the domes results from poor foot positioning.

- *Effect of lower leg and knee positioning on proximal-distal talar dome superimposition.* Often, if the knee is not fully extended (Figure 6-28) or if the distal tibia is not elevated to place the lower leg parallel with the IR in patients with large upper thighs, the proximal tibia is positioned farther from the imaging table than the distal tibia. The resulting image demonstrates the lateral talar dome proximal to the medial talar dome, the height of the longitudinal arch appears less than it actually is because the cuboid shifts anteriorly and the navicular bone moves posteriorly in this position, and the talocalcaneal joint will be narrowed (see Image 18). If the distal tibia is positioned farther from the table than the proximal tibia, the medial talar dome is demonstrated proximal to the lateral dome, the height of the longitudinal arch appears higher than it actually is because the cuboid shifts proximally and the navicular bone moves anteriorly in this position, and the talocalcaneal joint will be widened (see Image 19).

When viewing a lateral foot projection that demonstrates one of the talar domes proximal to the other, evaluate the height of the longitudinal arch and the degree of narrowing or widening of the talocalcaneal joint to determine which dome is the proximal dome. If the navicular bone is superimposed over more of the cuboid than expected and the talocalcaneal joint is narrowed, the lateral

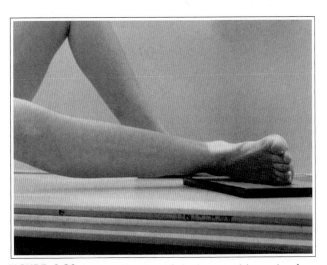

FIGURE 6-28 Poor positioning of the knee and lower leg for a lateral foot projection.

dome is the proximal dome; if the navicular bone is superimposed over less of the cuboid than expected and the talocalcaneal joint is wider, the medial dome is the proximal dome.

- **Effect of foot positioning on AP talar dome superimposition.** To demonstrate accurate AP alignment of the talar domes, position the lateral surface of the foot parallel with the IR. If this surface is not parallel with the IR, one of the talar domes is demonstrated anterior to the other. When the leg is rotated more than needed to place the lateral foot surface parallel with the IR, as shown in Figure 6-29, the medial talar dome is demonstrated anterior to the lateral talar dome (see Image 20). If the leg is not rotated enough to place the lateral foot surface parallel with the IR, as shown in Figure 6-30, the medial talar dome is demonstrated posterior to the lateral talar dome (see Image 21).

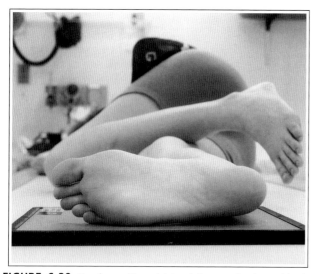

FIGURE 6-29 Poorly positioned lateral foot projection with the calcaneus elevated (leg externally rotated).

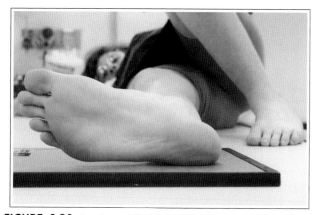

FIGURE 6-30 Poorly positioned lateral foot projection with the calcaneus depressed (leg internally rotated).

When viewing a lateral foot projection that demonstrates one of the talar domes anterior to the other, evaluate the position of the fibula in relation to the tibia to determine how to reposition the patient. On most lateral foot projections with accurate positioning, the fibula is positioned in the posterior half of the tibia. If the fibula is demonstrated more posteriorly than this relationship on a lateral foot projection with poor positioning, the medial talar dome is anterior and the patient was positioned with the forefoot depressed and the heel elevated (leg externally rotated), as shown in Figure 6-29. If the fibula is demonstrated more anteriorly than this relationship, the medial talar dome is posterior and the patient was positioned with the forefoot elevated and the heel depressed (leg internal rotation), as shown in Figure 6-30.

The long axis of the foot is positioned at a 90-degree angle with the lower leg.

- In most cases, when a patient is relaxed, the foot rests in plantar flexion. Plantar flexion results in a forced flattening of the anterior pretalar fat pad, reducing its usefulness in the detection of joint effusion (see Image 22). Consequently, it is best to dorsiflex the foot, placing its long axis at a 90-degree angle with the lower leg. This positioning also places the tibiotalar joint in a neutral position and helps keep the leg and foot from rolling too far anteriorly. Anterior foot rotation elevates the heel and rotates the foot.

The proximal metatarsals are at the center of the exposure field. The phalanges, metatarsals, tarsals, talus, calcaneus, 1 inch (2.5 cm) of the distal lower leg, and surrounding foot soft tissue are included within the collimated field.

- Centering a perpendicular central ray halfway between the distal toes and heel and the AP aspect of the foot places the bases of the metatarsals at the center of the exposure field.
- Open the longitudinal collimation enough to include the patient's toes and heel. Transverse collimation should be to a point 1 inch (2.5 cm) proximal to the medial malleolus (Figure 6-31).
- A diagonally placed 8- × 10-inch (18- × 24-cm) or a 10- × 12-inch (24- × 30-cm) detailed screen-film or computed radiography IR placed crosswise should be adequate to include all the required anatomic structures.

WEIGHT-BEARING LATEROMEDIAL PROJECTION

A standing lateromedial foot projection is accomplished by placing the IR against the medial aspect of the foot and aligning the lateral foot surface parallel with the

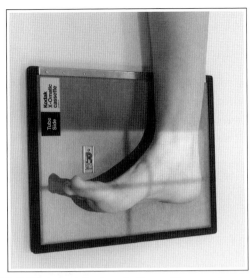

FIGURE 6-31 Lateral foot projection with accurate central ray (*CR*) centering and collimation.

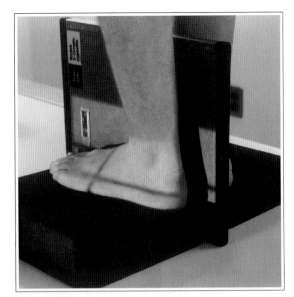

FIGURE 6-33 Poorly positioned lateral (lateromedial) foot projection.

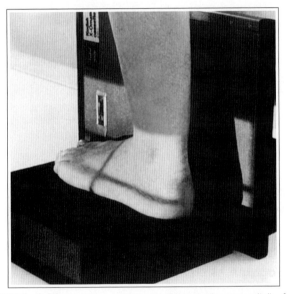

FIGURE 6-32 Properly positioned lateral (lateromedial) foot projection.

Lateral Foot Projection Analysis

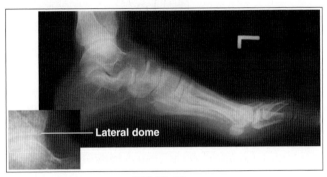

IMAGE 18

IR, as shown in Figure 6-32. Even pressure should be applied to both feet. Notice that the patient's heel is situated slightly away from the IR when the lateral foot surface is parallel with the IR. The resulting image should meet all the analysis requirements listed for the mediolateral projection.

The most common misposition for the standing lateromedial projection of the foot shows the medial talar dome positioned anterior to the lateral talar dome and the distal fibula positioned too posteriorly on the tibia (see Image 20). This misposition is a result of aligning the medial foot surface parallel with the IR, as shown in Figure 6-33, rather than the lateral surface. When such an image is obtained, move the patient's heel away from the IR (leg internally rotated).

Analysis. The tibiotalar joint space is obscured, and one talar dome is demonstrated proximal to the other dome. Because the navicular bone is superimposed over most of the cuboid and the talocalcaneal joint is narrowed, the lateral talar dome is the proximal dome. The proximal tibia was elevated, as shown in Figure 6-29.

Correction. Extend the knee, positioning the lower leg parallel with the IR, as shown in Figure 6-26. If the knee was extended for this image, elevate the lower leg until it is positioned parallel with the IR.

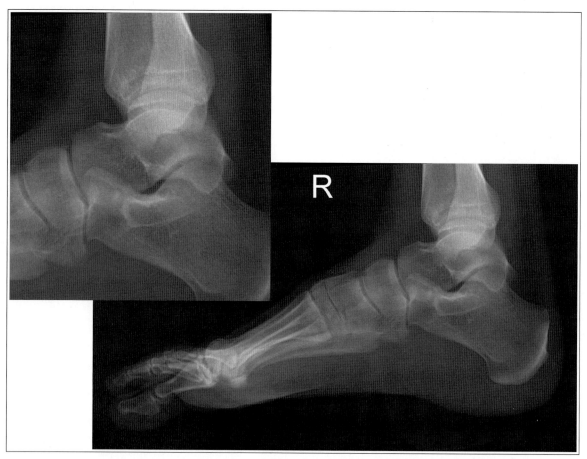

IMAGE 19

Analysis. The tibiotalar joint space is obscured, and one talar dome is demonstrated proximal to the other dome. Because more than 0.5 inch (1.25 cm) of cuboid is visible posterior to the navicular bone and the talocal-caneal joint is widened, the medial dome is the proximal dome. The distal tibia was elevated.

Correction. Position the lower leg parallel with the IR.

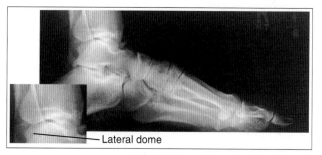

IMAGE 20

Analysis. The medial talar dome is positioned anterior to the lateral dome, as indicated by the posterior position of the fibula on the tibia. The lateral foot surface was not positioned parallel with the IR. If this is a mediolateral projection, the forefoot was depressed and heel was elevated (leg externally rotated), as shown in Figure 6-29. If this is a standing lateromedial projection, the medial surface of the patient's heel was placed next to the IR, as shown in Figure 6-33.

Correction. For a mediolateral projection, elevate the patient's forefoot and depress the patient's heel (internally rotate the leg) until the lateral foot surface is positioned parallel with the IR, as shown in Figure 6-27. For a standing lateromedial projection, draw the patient's heel away from the IR until the lateral foot surface is positioned parallel with the IR, as shown in Figure 6-32.

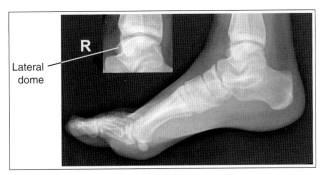

IMAGE 21

Analysis. The medial talar dome is positioned posterior to the lateral dome, as indicated by the anterior position of the distal fibula on the tibia. The lateral foot surface was not positioned parallel with the IR but was positioned with the forefoot elevated and heel depressed (leg internally rotated), as shown in Figure 6-30.

Correction. Depress the patient's forefoot and elevate the heel (externally rotated leg) until the lateral foot surface is positioned parallel with the IR, as shown in Figure 6-27.

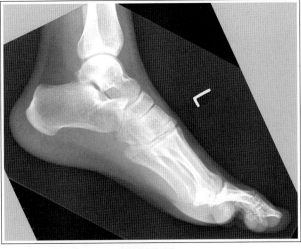

IMAGE 22

Analysis. The lower leg and long axis of the foot do not form a 90-degree angle. The patient's foot was in plantar flexion. A small amount of foot rotation is also present.

Correction. Dorsiflex the foot until the lower leg and long axis of the foot form a 90-degree angle.

CALCANEUS: AXIAL PROJECTION (PLANTODORSAL)

See Figure 6-34 and Box 6-8.

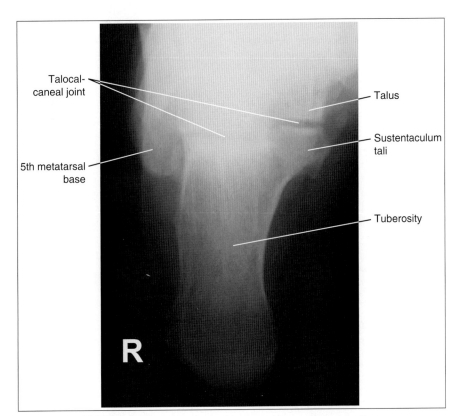

FIGURE 6-34 Axial calcaneal image with accurate projection.

| BOX 6-8 | **Axial Calcaneus Projection Analysis Criteria** |

- The talocalcaneal joint is open and the calcaneal tuberosity is demonstrated without distortion.
- The second through fourth distal metatarsal are not demonstrated on the medial or lateral aspect of the foot, respectively.
- The proximal calcaneal tuberosity is at the center of the exposure field.
- The calcaneal tuberosity and talocalcaneal joint space are included within the collimated field.

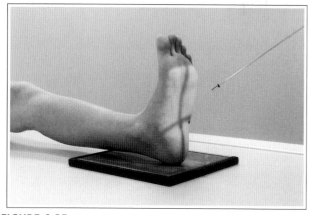

FIGURE 6-35 Properly positioned axial calcaneal image projection.

The talocalcaneal joint is demonstrated as an open space, and the calcaneal tuberosity is demonstrated without distortion.

- The talocalcaneal joint space is demonstrated as an open space, and the calcaneal tuberosity appears without distortion, when the correct central ray angulation and foot position are used. For a patient who has foot mobility, place the foot in a neutral-vertical position and direct a 40-degree central ray angulation toward the plantar foot surface (Figure 6-35). This positioning places the central ray parallel with the talocalcaneal joint space and perpendicular to the calcaneal tuberosity (Figure 6-36).

- *Compensating for plantar-flexed or dorsiflexed foot.* When the patient's foot is dorsiflexed beyond a 90-degree position with the lower leg or is plantar-flexed, the central ray needs to be adjusted to maintain its accurate position with the calcaneal joint space and tuberosity. If the patient's foot is dorsiflexed beyond the vertical position and a 40-degree angulation is used, the calcaneal joint spaces would be obscured and the tuberosity elongated (Figure 6-37; see Image 23). In this situation the central ray angulation should be decreased to maintain accurate central ray alignment. If the patient's foot is plantar-flexed and a 40-degree central ray angulation is used, the calcaneal joint space is obscured and the tuberosity foreshortened (see Image 24 and Figure 6-38). In this situation the central ray angulation should be increased to maintain accurate central ray alignment. The angulation required for each of these situations can be estimated by locating the base of the fifth metatarsal and the distal point of the fibula. The fifth metatarsal base is palpable on the lateral foot surface approximately halfway between the ball of the foot and the heel. Once these structures are located, angle the central ray parallel with an imaginary line drawn between them. When the axial calcaneal projection is taken with the foot in plantar flexion and the central ray is angled as just discussed to demonstrate the talocalcaneal joint space, the

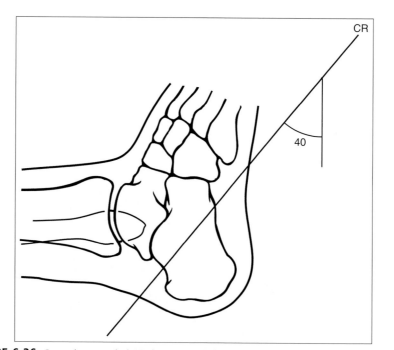

FIGURE 6-36 Central ray angled 40 degrees with foot in 90-degree position. *CR,* Central ray.

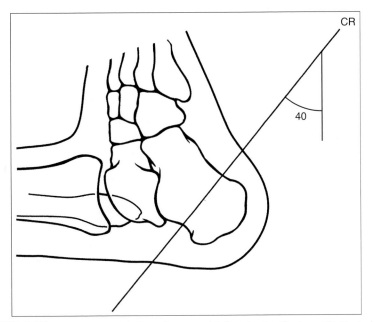

FIGURE 6-37 Central ray angled 40 degrees with foot in dorsiflexion. *CR,* Central ray.

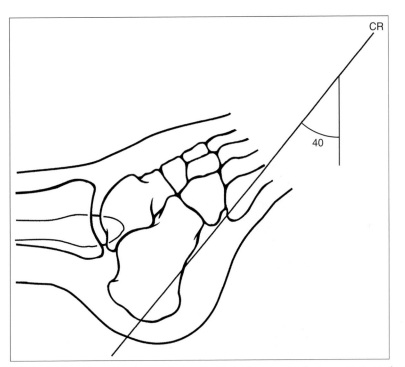

FIGURE 6-38 Central ray angled 40 degrees with foot in plantar flexion. *CR,* Central ray.

calcaneal tuberosity will be elongated because of the acute angle created between the central ray and IR (see Image 25).

The second through fourth distal metatarsals are not demonstrated on the medial or lateral aspect of the foot, respectively.

- To prevent calcaneal tilting, place the patient supine on the imaging table, with the leg fully extended and the foot dorsiflexed until its long

axis is placed in a vertical position, without medial or lateral rotation or foot inversion or eversion. If the ankle is internally rotated or the foot inverted, the first and second metatarsals are demonstrated medially. If the ankle is externally rotated or the foot everted, the fourth and fifth metatarsals are demonstrated laterally (see Images 25 and 26).

The proximal calcaneal tuberosity is at the center of the exposure field. The calcaneal tuberosity and the talocalcaneal joint space are included within the collimated field.

- Centering the central ray to the midline of the foot at the level of the fifth metatarsal base places the proximal tuberosity in the center of the exposure field.
- Open the longitudinal collimation enough to include the patient's entire heel. Transverse collimation should be to within 0.5 inch (1.25 cm) of the heel skin line.
- Half of an 8- × 10-inch (18- × 24-cm) IR detailed screen-film or computed radiography IR placed crosswise should be adequate to include all the required anatomic structures.

Axial Calcaneal Projection Analysis

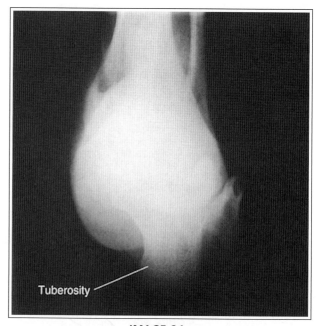

IMAGE 24

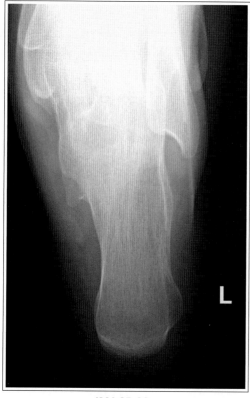

IMAGE 23

Analysis. The talocalcaneal joint space is obscured, and the calcaneal tuberosity is foreshortened. The foot was in plantar flexion, and the standard 40-degree central ray angulation was used.

Correction. If patient condition allows, dorsiflex the foot to a vertical, neutral position. If the patient cannot dorsiflex the foot, increase the central ray angulation, aligning the central ray with the fifth metatarsal base and the distal point of the fibula. Because of the acute angle that will be set up between the central ray and IR with this method, the calcaneal tuberosity will be elongated (see Image 23).

Analysis. The talocalcaneal joint space is obscured, and the calcaneal tuberosity is elongated. The foot was dorsiflexed beyond the vertical position, and a 40-degree central ray angulation was used.

Correction. Plantar-flex the foot to a vertical position and use a 40-degree angulation. If the patient cannot plantar-flex the foot, decrease the degree of central ray angulation, aligning the central ray with the fifth metatarsal base and the distal point of the fibula.

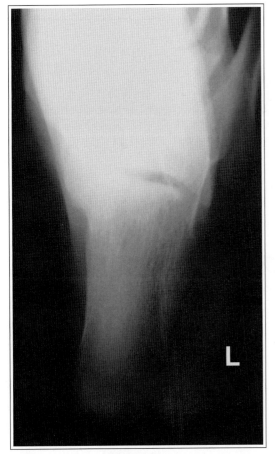

IMAGE 25

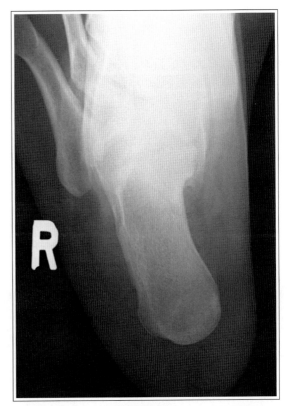

IMAGE 26

Analysis. The talocalcaneal joint space is shown as an open space and the calcaneal tuberosity demonstrates elongation. The foot was in plantar flexion, and the central ray was angled so that it was aligned with an imaginary line that connects the fifth metatarsal tuberosity and the distal point of the fibula. The fourth and fifth metatarsals are demonstrated on the lateral aspect of the foot. The ankle was externally rotated, and/or the foot was everted.

Correction. Elongation is not preventable if the patient's foot cannot be dorsiflexed because of the acute angle created between the central ray and IR. Internally rotate the leg until the ankle is in an AP projection, and/or bring the foot to a neutral position without eversion.

Analysis. The fourth and fifth metatarsals are demonstrated on the lateral aspect of the foot. The ankle was externally rotated, and/or the foot was everted.

Correction. Internally rotate the leg until the ankle is in an AP projection, and/or bring the foot to a neutral position without eversion.

CALCANEUS: LATERAL PROJECTION (MEDIOLATERAL)

See Figure 6-39 and Box 6-9.

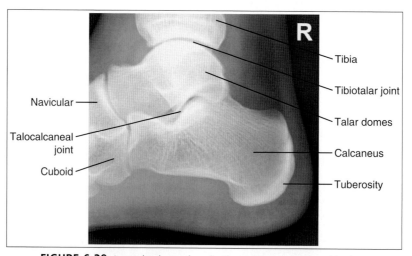

FIGURE 6-39 Lateral calcaneal projection with accurate positioning.

BOX 6-9	**Lateral Calcaneus Projection Analysis Criteria**

- The talar domes are superimposed, the tibiotalar joint space is open, and the distal fibula is superimposed by the posterior half of the distal tibia.
- The long axis of the foot is positioned at a 90-degree angle with the lower leg.
- The midcalcaneus is at the center of the exposure field.
- The tibiotalar joint, talus, calcaneus, and calcaneus-articulating tarsal bones are included within the collimated field.

The calcaneus and distal tibia and fibula are in a lateral projection. The domes of the talus are superimposed, the tibiotalar joint space is open, and the distal fibula is superimposed by the posterior half of the distal tibia.

- To obtain a lateral calcaneal projection, begin with the patient in a supine position, with the leg extended (Figure 6-40) and the foot dorsiflexed until its long axis forms a 90-degree angle with the lower leg. Rotate the patient toward the affected leg until the lateral foot surface is against the IR; then, adjust the degree of rotation until the surface is aligned parallel with the IR (Figure 6-41). For most patients, this positioning places the lower leg parallel with the imaging table. If this is not the case, as with a patient with a large upper thigh, the foot and IR should be elevated to place the lower leg parallel with the imaging table.

- *Talar domes:* The domes of the talus are formed by the most medial and lateral aspects of the talar's trochlear surface. They are visible on a lateral calcaneal projection as domed structures that articulate with the tibia. When a lateral calcaneus projection has been obtained, the talar domes should be superimposed and appear as one, and the tibiotalar joint should be open. If the lateral calcaneus is mispositioned, the domes are individually demonstrated and obscure the tibiotalar joint. Misalignment of the domes will result from poor knee and foot positioning.

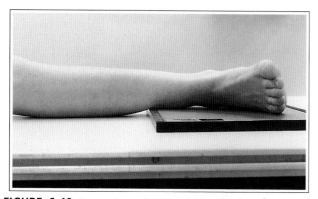

FIGURE 6-40 Proper lower leg positioning for lateral calcaneal projection.

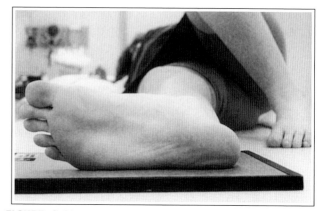

FIGURE 6-41 Proper lateral foot surface positioning for lateral calcaneal projection.

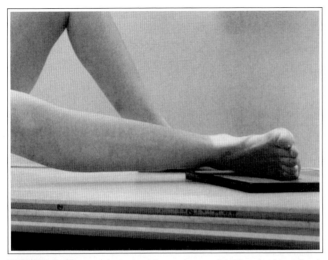

FIGURE 6-42 Poor knee and lower leg positioning for lateral calcaneal projection.

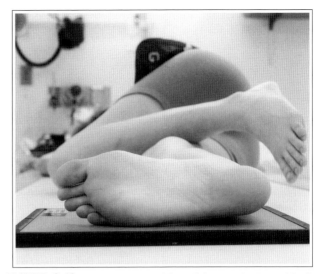

FIGURE 6-43 Poorly positioned lateral foot projection with the calcaneus elevated (leg internally rotated).

- *Effect of lower leg positioning on talar dome superimposition.* Often, if the knee is not fully extended (Figure 6-42) or if the distal tibia is not elevated to place the lower leg parallel with the IR (in a patient with a large upper thigh), the proximal tibia is positioned farther from the imaging table than the distal tibia. The resulting image demonstrates the lateral talar dome proximal to the medial talar dome, and the height of the longitudinal arch appears less than it actually is because the cuboid shifts anteriorly and the navicular bone moves posteriorly in this position; the talocalcaneal joint will be narrowed (see Image 27). If the distal tibia is positioned farther from the imaging table than the proximal tibia, the medial talar dome is demonstrated proximal to the lateral dome, and the height of the longitudinal arch appears higher than it actually is because the cuboid shifts posteriorly, the navicular bone moves anteriorly, and the talocalcaneal joint will be wider (see Image 28).

  When viewing a lateral calcaneal projection that demonstrates one of the talar domes proximal to the other, evaluate the height of the longitudinal arch and the degree of narrowing or widening of the talocalcaneal joint to determine which dome is the proximal dome. If the navicular bone is superimposed over more of the cuboid than expected and the talocalcaneal joint is narrowed, the lateral dome is the proximal dome; if the navicular bone is superimposed over less of the cuboid than expected and the talocalcaneal joint is wider, the medial dome is the proximal dome.

- *Effect of foot positioning on talar dome superimposition.* To demonstrate accurate AP alignment of the talar domes, the lateral surface of the foot should be positioned parallel with the IR. If this surface is not parallel with the IR, the talar domes are demonstrated with one anterior to the other. When the leg is rotated more than needed to place the lateral foot

surface parallel with the IR, as shown in Figure 6-43, the medial talar dome is demonstrated anterior to the lateral talar dome (see Image 29). If the leg is not rotated enough to place the lateral foot surface parallel with the IR, as shown in Figure 6-44, the medial talar dome is demonstrated posterior to the lateral talar dome (see Image 30). When imaging a lateral calcaneus projection that demonstrates one of the talar domes anterior to the other, image the position of the fibula in relation to the tibia to determine how the patient should be repositioned. On most lateral calcaneus projections with accurate positioning, the fibula is positioned in the posterior half of the tibia. On a lateral calcaneus projection with poor positioning, if the fibula is demonstrated more posteriorly, the medial talar dome is anterior and the patient was positioned with the forefoot depressed and the heel elevated (leg externally rotated), as shown in Figure 6-43. If the fibula is demonstrated more anteriorly (leg internally rotated), the medial domes are posterior and the patient was positioned with the forefoot elevated and the heel depressed, as shown in Figure 6-44.

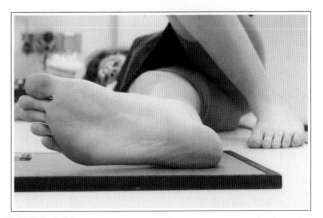

FIGURE 6-44 Poorly positioned foot projection with the calcaneus depressed (leg externally rotated).

The long axis of the foot is positioned at a 90-degree angle with the lower leg.

- In most cases, when a patient is relaxed, the foot rests in plantar flexion, making it difficult for the patient to maintain a lateral position. Often, the patient rotates the foot too far anteriorly, elevating the heel and rotating the foot (see Image 31). Consequently, it is best to dorsiflex the patient's foot, placing its long axis at a 90-degree angle with the lower leg.

The midcalcaneus is at the center of the exposure field. The tibiotalar joint, talus, calcaneus, and calcaneus-articulating tarsal bones are included within the collimated field.

- Center a perpendicular central ray 1 inch (2.5 cm) distal to the medial malleolus to place the calcaneus in the center of the exposure field. Centering to the midcalcaneus better demonstrates the calcaneus and the surrounding calcaneotarsal and talocalcaneal articulations, allowing for accurate calcaneal inclination measurements and for visualization of calcaneal tuberosity displacement.
- Open the longitudinal collimation enough to include the calcaneus and tibiotalar joint, which is located at the level of the palpable medial malleolus. Including the tibiotalar joint on all lateral calcaneal projections provides a method of judging rotation and determining how to reposition when a rotated lateral calcaneal projection has been obtained. Transverse collimation should be to the calcaneal tuberosity and the calcaneotarsal joint spaces. Ensure that the calcaneotarsal joint spaces are included by extending the transverse collimation at least 2 inches (5 cm) anterior to the medial malleolus (Figure 6-45).
- Half of an 8- × 10-inch (18- × 24-cm) detailed screen-film or computed radiography IR placed crosswise should be adequate to include all the required anatomic structures.

Lateral Calcaneal Projection Analysis

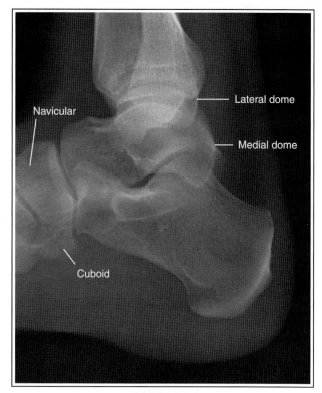

IMAGE 27

Analysis. The tibiotalar joint space is obscured, and one talar dome is demonstrated proximal to the other dome. Because the navicular bone is superimposed over most of the cuboid and the talocalcaneal joint is narrowed, the lateral dome is the proximal dome. The proximal tibia was elevated, as shown in Figure 6-42.

Correction. Extend the knee to position the lower leg parallel with the IR, as shown in Figure 6-40. If the knee was extended for this image, elevate the lower leg until it is positioned parallel with the IR.

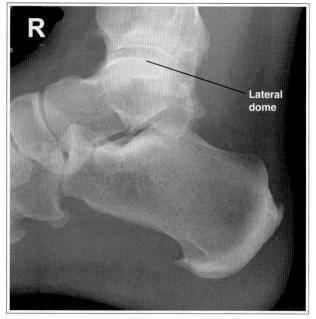

IMAGE 28

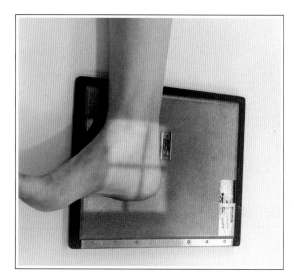

FIGURE 6-45 Accurate lateral calcaneal projection with central ray (*CR*) centering and collimation.

Analysis. The tibiotalar joint space is obscured, and one talar dome is demonstrated proximal to the other dome. Because more than 0.5 inch (1.25 cm) of cuboid is demonstrated posterior to the navicular bone and the talocalcaneal joint is widened, the medial dome is the proximal dome. The distal tibia was elevated.

Correction. Position the lower leg parallel with the IR.

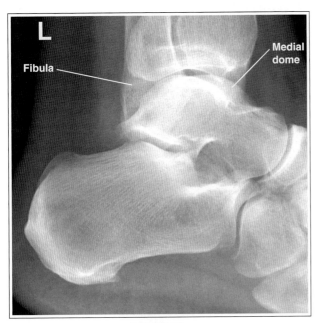

IMAGE 29

Analysis. The medial talar dome is positioned anterior to the lateral talar dome, as indicated by the posterior position of the fibula on the tibia. The lateral foot surface was not positioned parallel with the IR. The patient's forefoot was depressed and the heel was elevated (leg externally rotated), as shown in Figure 6-43.

Correction. Elevate the patient's forefoot and depress the heel (internally rotate the leg) until the lateral foot surface is parallel with the IR, as shown in Figure 6-41.

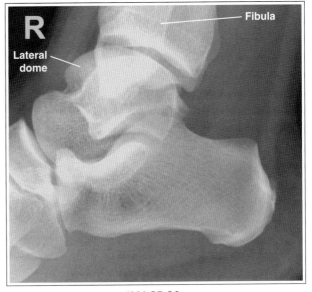

IMAGE 30

Analysis. The medial talar dome is positioned posterior to the lateral dome, as indicated by the anterior position of the distal fibula on the tibia. The lateral foot surface was positioned not parallel with the IR but with the forefoot elevated and the heel depressed, as shown in Figure 6-44.

Correction. Depress the patient's forefoot and elevate the heel until the lateral foot surface is positioned parallel with the IR, as shown in Figure 6-41.

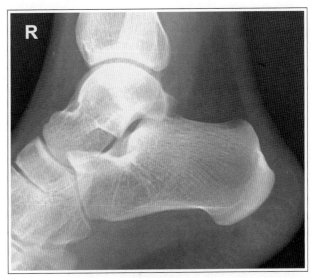

IMAGE 31

Analysis. The lower leg and the long axis of the foot do not form a 90-degree angle. The patient's foot was in plantar flexion.

Correction. Dorsiflex the foot until the lower leg and the long axis of the foot form a 90-degree angle.

ANKLE: ANTEROPOSTERIOR PROJECTION

See Figure 6-46 and Box 6-10.

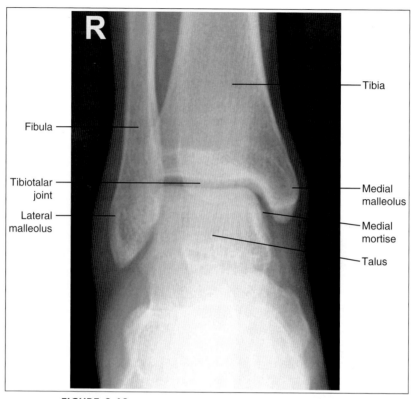

Tibia

Fibula

Tibiotalar joint

Lateral malleolus

Medial malleolus

Medial mortise

Talus

FIGURE 6-46 AP ankle projection with accurate positioning.

| **BOX 6-10** | **Anteroposterior Ankle Projection Analysis Criteria** |

- The medial mortise is open, and the distal tibia and talus are superimposed over the distal fibula by approximately 0.125 inch (0.3 cm), closing the lateral mortise.
- The tibiotalar joint space is open, and the tibia is demonstrated without foreshortening.
- The tibiotalar joint space is at the center of the exposure field.
- The distal fourth of the tibia and fibula, the talus, and surrounding ankle soft tissue are included within the collimated field.

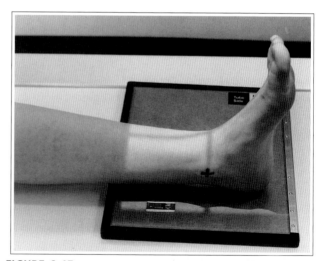

FIGURE 6-47 Proper patient positioning for AP ankle projection.

The ankle is demonstrated in an AP projection. The medial mortise (tibiotalar articulation) is open, and the distal tibia and talus are superimposed over the distal fibula by a small amount (0.125 inch [3 mm]), closing the lateral mortise (fibulotalar articulation).

- An AP projection of the ankle is obtained by positioning the patient supine on the image table, with the leg fully extended and the foot dorsiflexed until its long axis is placed in a vertical position (Figure 6-47). In this position, the intermalleolar line (imaginary line drawn between the medial and lateral malleoli) is at a 15- to 20-degree angle with the IR. The medial malleolus is positioned farther from the IR than the lateral malleolus.

- *Detecting direction of ankle rotation.* If the ankle was not positioned in an AP projection but is rotated laterally or medially, the medial mortise is obscured. When an AP ankle projection demonstrates a closed medial mortise, one can determine which way the patient's leg was rotated by evaluating the amount of tibia and talar superimposition of the fibula and the position of the medial malleolus. In external rotation, the tibia and talus

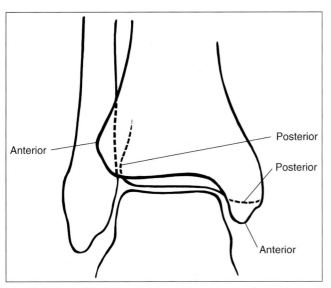

FIGURE 6-48 Anatomy of anterior and posterior ankle.

demonstrate greater superimposition of the fibula and the posterior aspect of the medial malleolus (Figure 6-48) is situated medial to the anterior aspect (see Image 32). In internal rotation, the fibula is demonstrated without talar superimposition (see Image 33).

The tibiotalar joint space is open, and the tibia is demonstrated without foreshortening.

- The tibiotalar joint is open and the tibia is demonstrated without foreshortening if the patient's lower leg was positioned parallel with the IR and the central ray was centered at the level of the tibiotalar joint.
- *Evaluating the openness of the tibiotalar joint.* On an AP ankle projection, determine whether an open joint was obtained and whether the tibia is demonstrated without foreshortening by evaluating the anterior and posterior margins of the distal tibia. On an AP ankle projection with accurate positioning, the anterior margin is demonstrated approximately 0.125 inch (3 mm) proximally to the posterior margin (see Figure 6-48). If the proximal lower leg was elevated or the central ray was centered proximal to the tibiotalar joint, the anterior tibial margin is projected distally, resulting in a narrowed or obscured tibiotalar joint space (see Image 34). If the distal lower leg was elevated or the central ray was centered distal to the tibiotalar joint, the anterior tibial margin is projected more proximally to the posterior margin than on an AP ankle projection, expanding the tibiotalar joint space and demonstrating the tibial articulating surface (see Image 35).
- *Effect of foot positioning on tibiotalar joint visualization.* The position of the foot also determines how well the tibiotalar joint space is demonstrated. The patient's foot should be placed vertically, with its long axis positioned at a 90-degree

angle with the lower leg. When the AP ankle projection is taken with the foot dorsiflexed, the trochlear surface of the talus is wedged into the anterior tibial region, resulting in a narrower appearing joint space. If the foot is plantar-flexed, the calcaneus is moved proximally, beneath the body of the talus, resulting in talocalcaneal superimposition and possibly hindering visualization of the talar trochlear surface.

The tibiotalar joint space is at the center of the exposure field. The distal fourth of the tibia and fibula, the talus, and the surrounding ankle soft tissue are included within the collimated field.

- To place the tibiotalar joint in the center of the image, center a perpendicular central ray to the ankle midway between the malleoli. The medial malleolus is located at the same level as the tibiotalar joint space. Open the longitudinal collimation to include the calcaneus and one fourth of the distal lower leg. Transverse collimation should be to within 0.5 inch (1.25 cm) of the ankle skin line.
- Either half of a 10- × 12-inch (24- × 30-cm) detailed screen-film IR placed crosswise or a single 8- × 10-inch (18- × 24-cm) digital IR placed lengthwise should be adequate to include all the required anatomic structures.

Anteroposterior Ankle Projection Analysis

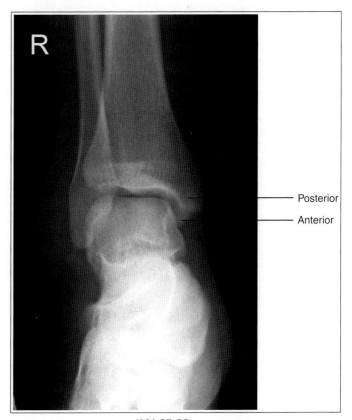

IMAGE 32

Analysis. The ankle was not placed in an AP projection. The medial mortise is obscured, the tibia and talus demonstrate increased superimposition of the fibula, and the posterior aspect of the medial malleolus is situated medial to the anterior aspect. The ankle was externally rotated.

Correction. Rotate the leg internally, placing the long axis of the foot in a vertical position.

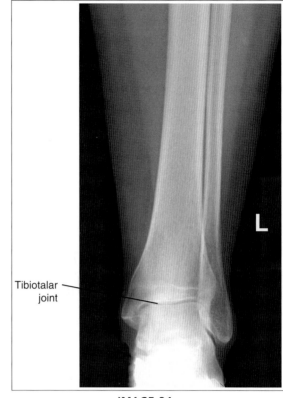

IMAGE 34

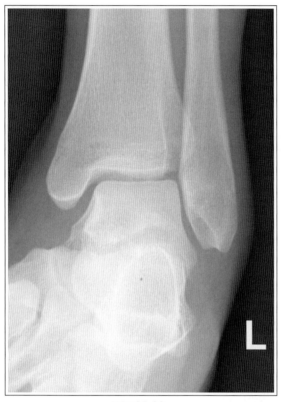

IMAGE 33

Analysis. The ankle was not placed in an AP projection. The fibula is demonstrated without talar superimposition. The ankle was internally rotated.

Correction. Rotate the leg externally, placing the long axis of the foot in a vertical position.

Analysis. The tibiotalar joint is closed. The anterior tibial margin has been projected into the joint space. Either the proximal tibia was elevated because of knee flexion, or the central ray was centered proximal to the tibiotalar joint.

Correction. Extend the knee, lowering the proximal tibia until the lower leg is parallel with the IR, or center the central ray to the tibiotalar joint (located at the level of the medial malleolus).

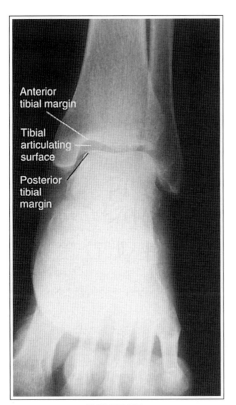

IMAGE 35

Analysis. The tibiotalar joint is distorted. The anterior tibial margin is projected proximal to the posterior margin, and the tibial articulating surface is demonstrated. Either the distal tibia was elevated or the central ray was centered distal to the tibiotalar joint.

Correction. Depress the distal tibia or elevate the proximal tibia until the lower leg is parallel with the IR, or center the central ray to the tibiotalar joint at the level of the medial malleolus.

ANKLE: ANTEROPOSTERIOR OBLIQUE PROJECTION (MEDIAL ROTATION)

See Figures 6-49, 6-50, and 6-51 and Box 6-11.

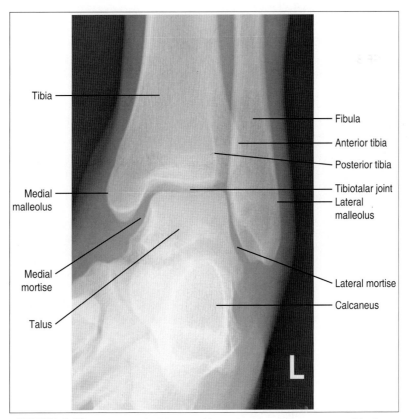

FIGURE 6-49 AP (mortise) oblique ankle projection with accurate positioning.

BOX 6-11	Anteroposterior Oblique Ankle Projection Analysis Criteria

- Mortise (15–20 degree) oblique: The distal fibula is demonstrated without talar superimposition, demonstrating an open lateral mortise, and the lateral and medial malleoli are in profile. The fibula demonstrates slight (0.125 inch [0.3 cm]) tibial superimposition.
- 45-degree oblique: The medial mortise is closed and lateral mortise is partially closed, the fibula is seen without tibial superimposition, and the tarsal sinus is demonstrated.
- The tibiotalar joint space is open and the tibia is seen without foreshortening.
- The calcaneus is visualized distal to the lateral mortise and fibula.
- The tibiotalar joint is at the center of the exposure field.
- The distal fourth of the fibula and tibia, the talus, and the surrounding ankle soft tissue are included within the collimated field.

Mortise (15 to 20 degrees oblique): The ankle demonstrates 15 to 20 degrees of obliquity. The distal fibula is demonstrated without talar superimposition, demonstrating an open lateral mortise (talofibular joint), and the lateral and medial malleoli are in profile. The fibula demonstrates slight (0.125 inch [33 mm]) tibial superimposition.

- To obtain a mortise AP oblique ankle projection with accurate positioning, place the patient in a supine AP projection with the leg extended and the foot positioned vertically (Figure 6-52). The leg and foot are then rotated the desired amount. Make certain that the foot does not invert during rotation. While viewing the plantar surface of the foot, place your index fingers on the most prominent aspects of the lateral and the medial malleoli. Rotate the patient's entire leg internally (medially) 15 to 20 degrees, until your index fingers and the malleoli are positioned at equal distances from the IR (Figure 6-53). An imaginary line drawn between the malleoli (intermalleolar plane) is then aligned parallel with the IR. This rotation moves the fibula away from the talus to demonstrate an open lateral mortise.

- *Identifying poor ankle and leg rotation.* If the ankle and leg are internally rotated less than the needed 15 to 20 degrees, the medial mortise will be open while the lateral mortise will be closed (see Image 36). If the ankle was internally rotated more than 15 to 20 degrees, the image will demonstrate a closed medial mortise and decreased tibial superimposition of the fibula or an open tibiofibular joint, depending on the degree of increased rotation (see Image 37).

45-Degree Oblique:
The ankle demonstrates 45 degrees of obliquity. The lateral mortise is partially closed, the anterior and posterior cortical outlines of the lateral tibia are superimposed, visualizing the fibula without tibial superimposition, and the tarsal sinus is demonstrated. Whether or not there is an open space between the tibia and

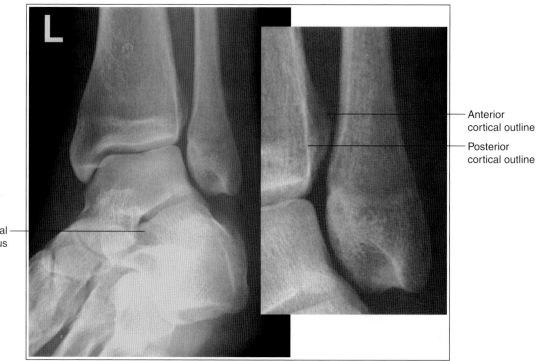

Tarsal sinus

Anterior cortical outline

Posterior cortical outline

FIGURE 6-50 AP (45-degree) oblique ankle projection with accurate positioning.

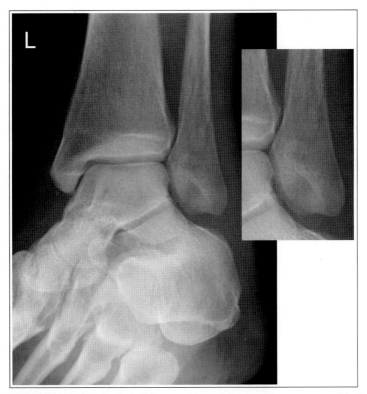

FIGURE 6-51 AP (45-degree) oblique ankle projection with accurate positioning.

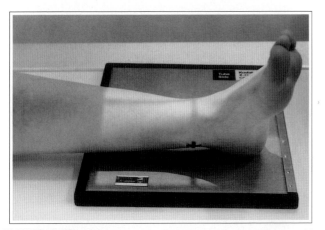

FIGURE 6-52 Proper patient positioning for AP oblique ankle projection.

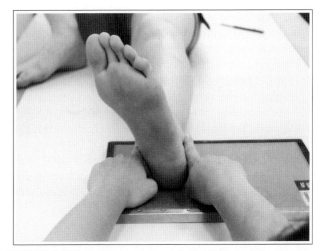

FIGURE 6-53 Aligning the intermalleolar line parallel with IR for AP oblique ankle projection.

fibula on this image will depend on how closely aligned the two structures are with each other (compare the superimposition of the anterior and posterior cortical outlines of the lateral tibia and the openness of the tibiotalar joint spaces in Figures 6-50 and 6-51).

- To obtain a 45-degree AP oblique ankle projection with accurate positioning, place the patient in a supine AP projection, with the leg extended and the foot positioned vertically. The leg and foot are then internally rotated until the long axis of the foot is aligned 45 degrees with the IR (Figure 6-54).

- *Identifying poor ankle and leg rotation.* If the ankle and leg are internally rotated less than 45 degrees, the anterior cortical outline of the lateral tibia will be lateral to the posterior cortical outline of the lateral tibia (see Image 38). If the ankle and leg are internally rotated slightly more than 45 degrees, the anterior cortical outline of the lateral tibia will be medial to the posterior cortical outline of the lateral tibia.

The tibiotalar joint space is open, and the tibia is demonstrated without foreshortening.

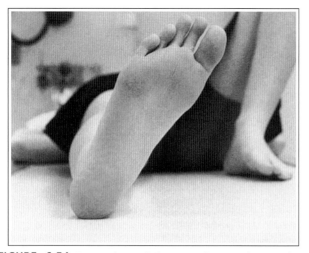

FIGURE 6-54 Proper internal foot rotation: 45-degrees from vertical.

- The tibiotalar joint space is open and the tibia is demonstrated without foreshortening when the patient's lower leg was positioned parallel with the IR and the central ray was centered at the level of the tibiotalar joint (see Figure 6-52).
- *Evaluating the openness of the tibiotalar joint.* On an AP oblique ankle projection, you can determine whether the positioning and central ray alignment goals have been met by evaluating the anterior and posterior margins of the distal tibia. On an AP oblique ankle projection with accurate positioning, the anterior margin should be visualized approximately 0.125 inch (3 mm) proximal to the posterior margin. If the proximal lower leg was elevated or the central ray was centered proximal to the tibiotalar joint, the anterior tibial margin is projected distally, resulting in a narrowed or obscured tibiotalar joint. If the patient's distal lower leg was elevated or the central ray was centered distal to the tibiotalar joint, the anterior tibial margin is projected too far proximal to the posterior margin, expanding the tibiotalar joint space and demonstrating the tibial articulating surface (see Images 39 and 40).

The calcaneus is demonstrated distal to the lateral mortise and fibula.

- To position the calcaneus distal to the lateral mortise and fibula, place the foot in a neutral position by positioning its long axis at a 90-degree angle with the lower leg. If the foot was plantar-flexed for an AP oblique projection, the calcaneus obscures the distal aspect of the lateral mortise and the distal fibula (see Images 41 and 42).

The tibiotalar joint space is at the center of the exposure field. The distal fourth of the fibula and tibia, the talus, and the surrounding ankle soft tissue are included within the collimated field.

- To place the tibiotalar joint in the center of the image, center a perpendicular central ray to the ankle midway between the malleoli. The medial malleolus is located at the same level as the tibiotalar joint space. Open the longitudinal collimation to include the calcaneus and one fourth of the distal lower leg. Transverse collimation should be to within 0.5 inch (1.25 cm) of the ankle skin line.
- Either half of a 10- × 12-inch (24- × 30-cm) detailed screen-film IR placed crosswise or a single 8- × 10-inch (18- × 24-cm) digital IR placed lengthwise should be adequate to include all the required anatomic structures.

Anteroposterior Oblique Ankle Projection Analysis

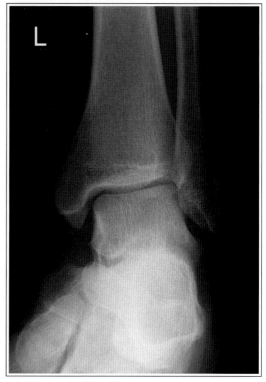

IMAGE 36 Mortise oblique.

Analysis. The lateral mortise (talofibular joint) is closed, and the medial mortise is partially open. The tarsal sinus is not visible. The patient's leg and ankle were not internally rotated enough.

Correction. Rotate the entire leg internally until the most prominent aspects of the lateral and medial malleoli are positioned at equal distances from the IR, as shown in Figure 6-53.

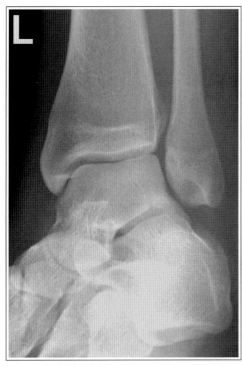

IMAGE 37 Mortise oblique.

Analysis. The medial mortise is closed and there is no tibial superimposition of the fibula. The image was obtained with more than 15 to 20 degrees of leg and ankle obliquity.

Correction. Externally rotate the leg and ankle until the medial and lateral malleoli are positioned at equal distances from the IR.

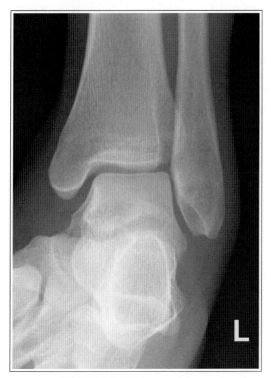

IMAGE 38 45-degree oblique.

Analysis. The lateral and medial mortises are open and the tibia superimposes a portion of the fibula. The tarsi sinus is not demonstrated. The patient's leg and ankle were rotated less than 45 degrees.

Correction. Rotate the leg and foot internally until the long axis of the foot is at a 45-degree angle with the IR.

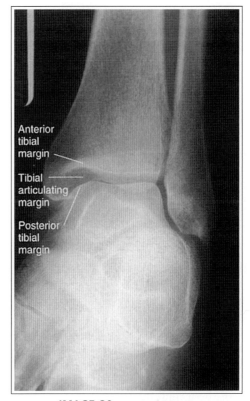

IMAGE 39 Mortise oblique.

Analysis. The tibiotalar joint space is expanded. The anterior tibial margin has been projected proximal to the posterior margin, and the tibial articulating surface is demonstrated. Either the distal tibia was elevated or the central ray was centered distal to the tibiotalar joint.

Correction. Depress the distal tibia or elevate the proximal tibia until the lower leg is placed parallel with the IR, or center the central ray to the tibiotalar joint at the level of the medial malleolus.

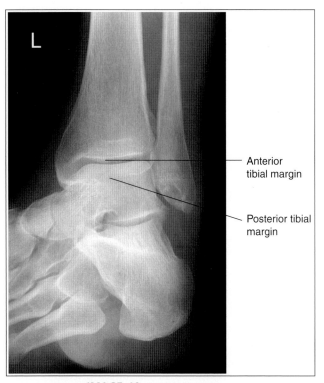

IMAGE 40 45-degree oblique.

Analysis. The tibiotalar joint space is expanded. The anterior tibial margin has been projected proximal to the posterior margin, and the tibial articulating surface is demonstrated. Either the distal tibia was elevated or the central ray was centered distal to the tibiotalar joint.

Correction. Depress the distal tibia or elevate the proximal tibia until the lower leg is placed parallel with the IR, or center the central ray to the tibiotalar joint at the level of the medial malleolus.

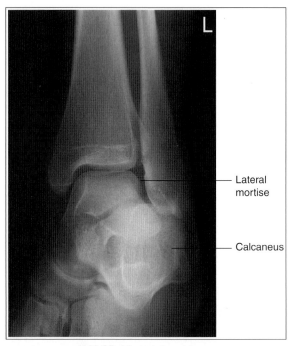

IMAGE 41 Mortise oblique.

Analysis. The calcaneus is obscuring the distal aspect of the lateral mortise and distal fibula. The foot was in plantar flexion when the image was taken.

Correction. Dorsiflex the foot until its long axis forms a 90-degree angle with the lower leg.

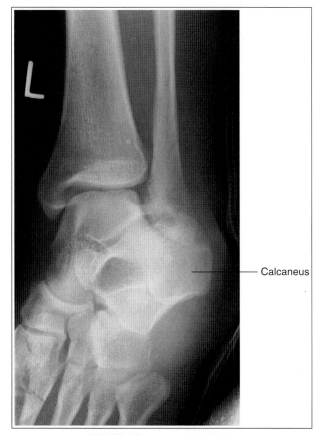

IMAGE 42 45-degree oblique.

Analysis. The calcaneus is obscuring the distal aspect of the lateral mortise and distal fibula. The foot was in plantar flexion when the image was taken.

Correction. Dorsiflex the foot until its long axis forms a 90-degree angle with the lower leg.

ANKLE: LATERAL PROJECTION (MEDIOLATERAL)

See Figure 6-55 and Box 6-12.

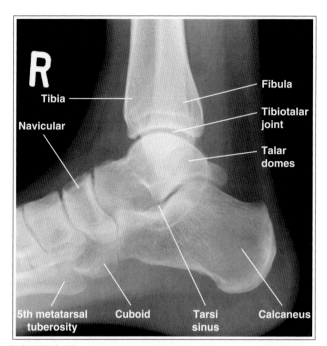

FIGURE 6-55 Lateral ankle projection with accurate positioning.

BOX 6-12	Lateral Ankle Projection Analysis Criteria

- Contrast and density are adequate to demonstrate the anterior pretalar and posterior pericapsular fat pads.
- The talar domes are superimposed, the tibiotalar joint is open, and the distal fibula is superimposed by the posterior half of the distal tibia.
- The long axis of the foot is positioned at a 90-degree angle with the lower leg.
- The tibiotalar joint is at the center of the exposure field.
- The talus, 1 inch (2.5 cm) of the fifth metatarsal base, surrounding ankle soft tissue, and the distal fourth of the fibula and tibia are included within the collimated field.

Contrast and density are adequate to demonstrate the anterior pretalar and posterior pericapsular fat pads on the foot and ankle.

- *Fat pads on the ankle.* Two soft tissue structures located around the ankle may indicate joint effusion and injury—the anterior pretalar fat pad and the posterior pericapsular fat pad. The anterior pretalar fat pad is demonstrated anterior to the ankle joint and rests next to the neck of the talus (Figure 6-56). The posterior fat pad, positioned within the indentation formed by the articulation of the posterior tibia and talar bones (see Figure 6-56), is displaced in the same manner as the anterior

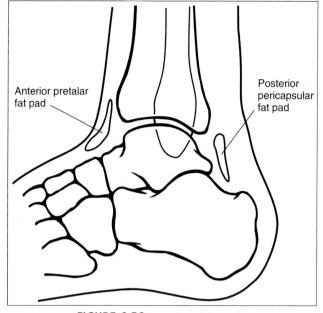

FIGURE 6-56 Location of fat pads.

pretalar fat pad, although it is less sensitive and requires more fluid evasion to be displaced.

The ankle is in a lateral projection. The domes of the talus are superimposed, the tibiotalar joint is open, and the distal fibula is superimposed by the posterior half of the distal tibia.

- To obtain a lateral ankle projection, begin with the patient in a supine position, with the leg extended (Figure 6-57) and the foot dorsiflexed until its long axis forms a 90-degree angle with the lower leg. Rotate the patient and affected leg until the lateral foot surface is against the IR, and then adjust the degree of rotation until the surface is aligned parallel with the IR (Figure 6-58). For most patients, this positioning places the lower leg parallel with the imaging table. If this is not the case, as with a patient with a large upper thigh, the foot and IR should be elevated until the lower leg is parallel with the imaging table.

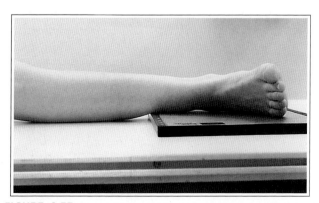

FIGURE 6-57 Proper knee and lower leg positioning for lateral ankle projection.

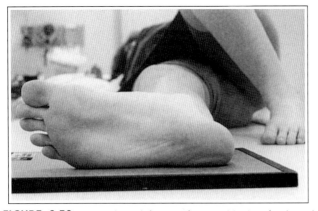

FIGURE 6-58 Proper lateral foot surface positioning for lateral ankle projection.

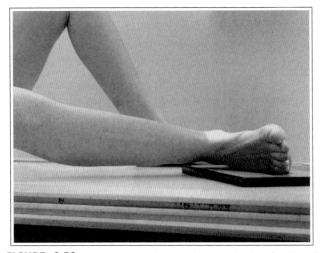

FIGURE 6-59 Poor knee and lower leg positioning for lateral ankle projection.

- *Effect of lower leg positioning on talar dome superimposition.* Often, if the knee is not fully extended (Figure 6-59) or if the distal tibia is not elevated to place the lower leg parallel with the IR in a patient with large upper thighs, the proximal tibia is positioned farther from the imaging table than the distal tibia. The resulting image demonstrates the lateral talar dome proximal to the medial talar dome and the height of the longitudinal arch appears less than it actually is because the cuboid shifts anteriorly and the navicular bone moves posteriorly in this position and the talocalcaneal joint will be narrowed (see Image 43). If the distal tibia is positioned farther from the table than the proximal tibia, the medial talar dome is demonstrated proximal to the lateral dome, and the height of the longitudinal arch appears greater than it actually is because the cuboid shifts posteriorly and the navicular bone moves anteriorly in this position and the talocalcaneal joint will be

widened (see Image 44). When viewing a lateral ankle projection that demonstrates one of the talar domes proximal to the other, evaluate the height of the longitudinal arch and the degree of talocalcaneal joint visualization to determine which dome is the proximal dome. If the navicular bone is superimposed over more of the cuboid than expected and a narrowed talocalcaneal joint is seen, the lateral dome is the proximal dome. If the navicular bone is superimposed over less of the cuboid than expected and a wider talocalcaneal joint is seen, the medial dome is the proximal dome.

- *Effect of foot positioning on talar dome superimposition.* To demonstrate accurate AP alignment of the talar domes, position the lateral surface of the foot parallel with the IR. If this surface is not parallel with the IR, the talar domes are demonstrated one anterior to the other. When the leg is rotated more than needed to place the lateral foot surface parallel with the IR (leg externally rotated), as shown in Figure 6-60, the medial talar dome is demonstrated anterior to the lateral talar dome (see Image 45). If the leg is not rotated enough to place the lateral foot surface parallel with the IR (leg internally rotated), as shown in Figure 6-61, the medial talar dome is demonstrated posterior to the lateral talar dome (see Image 46). When taking a lateral ankle projection that demonstrates one of the talar domes anterior to the other, observe the position of the fibula in relation to the tibia to determine how the patient should be repositioned. On most lateral ankle projections with accurate positioning, the fibula is positioned in the posterior half of the tibia. On a lateral projection with poor positioning, if the

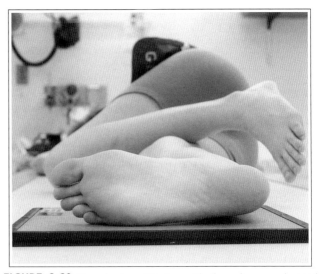

FIGURE 6-60 Poor foot positioning with the calcaneus elevated (leg externally rotated).

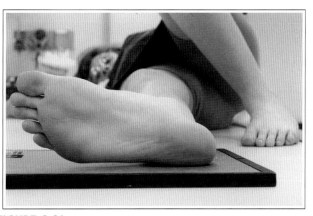

FIGURE 6-61 Poor foot positioning with the calcaneus depressed (leg internally rotated).

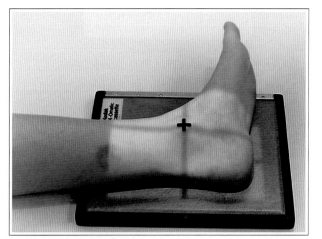

FIGURE 6-62 Lateral ankle projection with proper central ray (*CR*) centering and collimation.

fibula is demonstrated more posteriorly, the medial dome is anterior and the patient was positioned with the forefoot depressed and the heel elevated (leg externally rotated), as shown in Figure 6-60. If the fibula is demonstrated more anteriorly, the medial domes are posterior and the patient was positioned with the forefoot elevated and the heel depressed (leg internally rotated), as shown in Figure 6-61.

The long axis of the foot is positioned at a 90-degree angle with the lower leg.

- In most cases, when the patient is relaxed, the foot rests in plantar flexion. Plantar flexion results in a forced flattening of the anterior pretalar fat pad, reducing its usefulness in the detection of joint effusion (see Image 47). Consequently, it is best to dorsiflex the patient's foot, placing its long axis at a 90-degree angle with the lower leg. This positioning also places the tibiotalar joint in a neutral position and helps prevent the leg from rolling too far anteriorly. Anterior foot rotation elevates the heel and rotates the foot.

The tibiotalar joint is at the center of the exposure field. The talus, 1 inch (2.5 cm) of the fifth metatarsal base, the surrounding ankle soft tissue, and the distal fourth of the fibula and tibia are included within the collimated field.

- Centering a perpendicular central ray to the ankle midline at the level of the palpable medial malleolus places the tibiotalar joint in the center of the collimated field (Figure 6-62).
- Open the longitudinal collimation enough to include the calcaneus and one fourth of the distal tibia and fibula. Transversely collimate to include 3 inches (7.5 cm) of the proximal forefoot, ensuring that approximately 1 inch (2.5 cm) of the fifth metatarsal base is included on the image. An

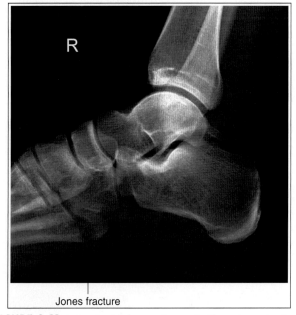

Jones fracture

FIGURE 6-63 Lateral ankle image demonstrating a Jones fracture.

inversion injury of the foot and ankle may result in a fracture of the fifth metatarsal base, known as a Jones fracture (Figure 6-63). Including the fifth metatarsal base on the lateral ankle projection allows it to be evaluated for a Jones fracture.

- Either half of a 10- × 12-inch (24- × 30-cm) detailed screen-film IR placed crosswise or a single 8- × 10-inch (18- × 24-cm) computed radiography IR placed lengthwise should be adequate to include all the required anatomic structures.

Lateral Ankle Projection Analysis

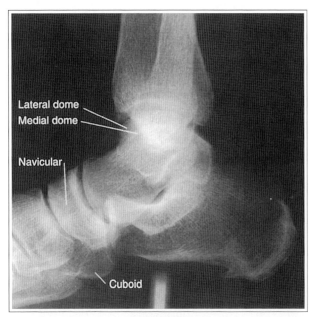

IMAGE 43

Analysis. The tibiotalar joint space is obscured, and one talar dome is demonstrated proximal to the other dome. Because the navicular bone is superimposed over most of the cuboid, and the talocalcaneal joint will be narrowed, the lateral dome is the proximal dome. The proximal tibia was elevated, as shown in Figure 6-59.

Correction. Extend the knee to position the lower leg parallel with the IR, as shown in Figure 6-57. If the knee was extended for this image, elevate the lower leg until it is positioned parallel with the IR.

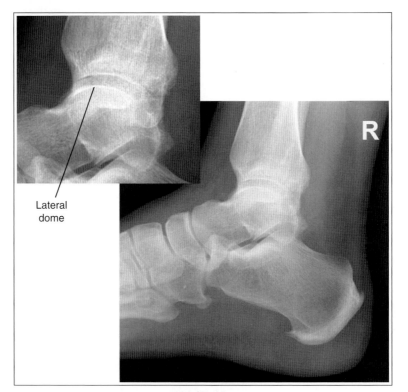

IMAGE 44

Analysis. The tibiotalar joint space is obscured, and one talar dome is demonstrated proximal to the other dome. Because more than 0.5 inch (1.25 cm) of cuboid is visible posterior to the navicular bone and the talocalcaneal joint is widened, the medial dome is the proximal dome. The distal tibia was elevated.

Correction. Depress the distal lower leg until the lower leg is aligned parallel with the IR.

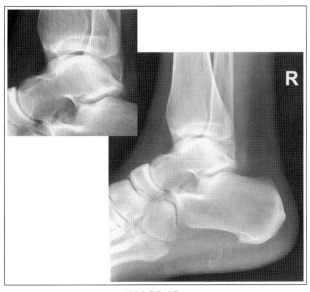

IMAGE 45

Analysis. The medial talar dome is positioned anterior to the lateral talar dome, as indicated by the posterior position of the fibula on the tibia. The lateral foot surface was not positioned parallel with the IR. The patient's forefoot was depressed and the heel elevated (leg externally rotated), as shown in Figure 6-60.

Correction. Elevate the patient's forefoot, and depress the heel (internally rotate the leg) until the lateral foot surface is parallel with the IR, as shown in Figure 6-58.

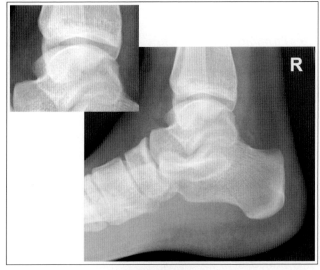

IMAGE 46

Analysis. The medial talar dome is positioned posterior to the lateral dome, as indicated by the anterior position of the distal fibula on the tibia. The lateral foot surface was positioned not parallel with the IR, but with the forefoot elevated and the heel depressed (leg internally rotated), as shown in Figure 6-61.

Correction. Depress the forefoot and elevate the heel (externally rotate the leg) until the lateral foot surface is positioned parallel with the IR, as shown in Figure 6-58.

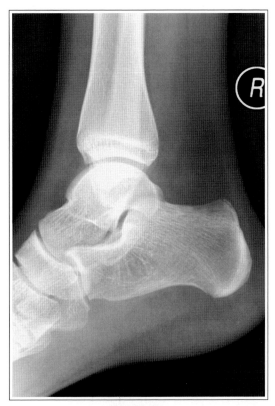

IMAGE 47

Analysis. The lower leg and long axis of the foot do not form a 90-degree angle. The patient's foot was in plantar flexion.

Correction. Dorsiflex the foot until the lower leg and long axis of the foot form a 90-degree angle with the lower leg.

LOWER LEG: ANTEROPOSTERIOR PROJECTION

See Figure 6-64 and Box 6-13.

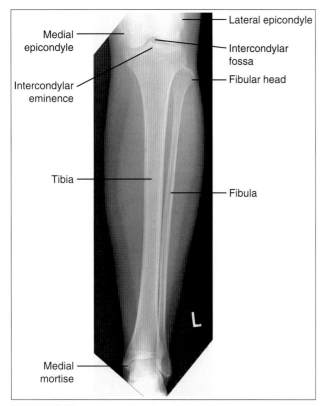

FIGURE 6-64 AP lower leg projection with accurate positioning.

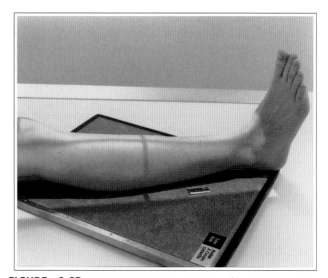

FIGURE 6-65 Proper patient positioning for AP lower leg projection.

BOX 6-13	Anteroposterior Lower Leg Projection Analysis Criteria

- Image density is uniform across the lower leg.
- The tibia demonstrates only minimal superimposition of the proximal and distal fibula, and the fibular midshaft is demonstrated free of tibial superimposition.
- The knee and tibiotalar joint spaces are closed.
- The tibial midshaft is at the center of the exposure field.
- The tibia, fibula, knee and surrounding lower leg soft tissue are included within the collimated field.

Image density is uniform across the lower leg.

- Position the thicker proximal lower leg at the cathode end of the tube and the thinner distal lower leg at the anode end to take advantage of the anode heel effect and obtain more uniform density across the lower leg.

The lower leg demonstrates an AP projection. The tibia demonstrates only minimal superimposition of the proximal and distal fibula, and the fibular midshaft is demonstrated free of tibial superimposition.

- To obtain an AP projection of the lower leg, place the patient in a supine position with the knee fully

extended and the foot placed vertically. Dorsiflex the foot to a 90-degree angle with the lower leg (Figure 6-65).

- **Detecting lower leg rotation.** Rotation of the lower leg can be identified on an AP lower leg projection by evaluating the relationship of the fibula to the tibia. When the patient's leg is externally (laterally) rotated, the fibula shifts toward and eventually beneath the tibia, obscuring the medial mortise (see Image 48). When the patient's leg is internally (medially) rotated, the head of the fibula draws from beneath the tibia (see Image 49).

- **Positioning for fracture.** For a patient with a known or suspected fracture who is unable to position both the ankle and knee into an AP projection simultaneously, position the joint closer to the fracture in the truer position. When the fracture is situated closer to the ankle, the ankle should meet the preceding requirements for a true distal lower leg AP projection (see Image 50). When the fracture is situated closer to the knee, the knee should meet the requirements for accurate positioning for a proximal lower leg AP projection. Depending on the degree of tibial and fibular rotation at the fracture site, the other joint may or may not be accurately positioned for an AP projection.

The knee and tibiotalar joint spaces are closed.

- The proximal tibia slopes distally from the anterior condylar margin to the posterior condylar margin by approximately 5 degrees. When the lower leg is placed parallel with the IR and the central ray is centered to the midshaft of the lower leg, x-rays that diverge in the opposite direction are used to record the image of the proximal tibia (see Figure 6-66). The distal lower leg also slopes distally from the anterior tibial margin to the posterior margin by approximately 3 degrees. Although the x-rays diverge in the same direction as the slope of the distal tibia, they diverge at a greater angle. Because the angle of x-ray divergence is not aligned parallel with either the proximal or distal tibia, the knee and ankle joints are demonstrated as closed spaces on an AP lower leg projection.

The tibial midshaft is at the center of the exposure field. The tibia, fibula, ankle, knee, and surrounding lower leg soft tissue are included within the collimated field.

- A perpendicular central ray is centered to the midpoint of the lower leg to place it in the center of the image.
- To include the ankle and knee joints on the image, you must consider the degree of x-ray beam divergence that occurs when a long body part is imaged (Figure 6-66). A 14- × 17-inch (35- × 43-cm) detailed screen-film or computed radiography IR should be adequate to include both the ankle and knee. When a screen-film system is used, the leg can be positioned diagonally to accommodate the length. For the computed radiography system, it is not advisable to do this unless the system is set to handle this alignment. To ensure that both joints are included, the film should extend 1 to 1.5 inches (2.5 to 4 cm) beyond each joint space. The ankle is located at the level of the medial malleolus, and the knee joint is located 1 inch (2.5 cm) distal to the palpable medial epicondyle.
- Once the lower leg is accurately positioned with the IR, center the central ray to the midpoint of the lower leg and open the longitudinal collimation field until it extends just beyond both the knee and the ankle. For patients with long lower legs, it may be necessary to raise the source–image receptor distance (SID) above the standard to obtain a longitudinally collimated field long enough to include both joints on the same IR. Transverse collimation should be to within 0.5 inch (1.25 cm) of the lower leg skin line.

Anteroposterior Lower Leg Projection Analysis

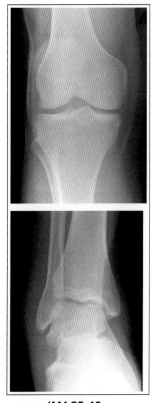

IMAGE 48

Analysis. These are externally rotated AP knee and AP ankle projections that simulate how an externally rotated AP tibial projection would appear.

Correction. Internally (medially) rotate the leg until the foot is vertical.

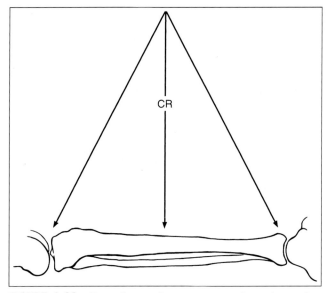

FIGURE 6-66 Effect of x-ray divergence on AP lower leg projection. *CR,* Central ray.

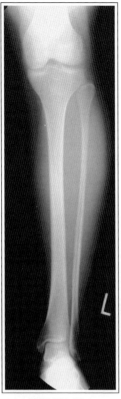

IMAGE 49

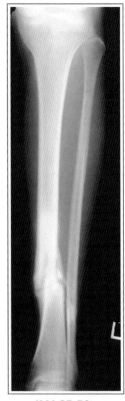

IMAGE 50

Analysis. The proximal and distal fibula demonstrate minimal tibial superimposition. The leg was medially (internally) rotated.

Correction. Laterally (externally) rotate the leg until the foot is vertical.

Analysis. A distal tibial and fibular fracture is present. The ankle joint is positioned in a true AP projection, but the knee joint demonstrates medial rotation. This rotation is caused by rotation at the fracture site.

Correction. No corrective movement is required.

LOWER LEG: LATERAL PROJECTION (MEDIOLATERAL)

See Figures 6-67 and 6-68 and Box 6-14.

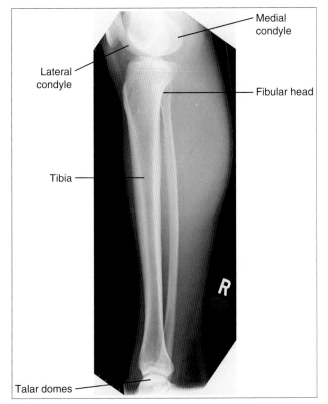

FIGURE 6-67 Lateral lower leg projection with accurate positioning.

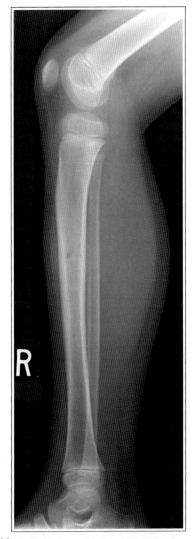

FIGURE 6-68 Pediatric lateral lower leg projection with accurate positioning.

Image density is uniform across the lower leg.

- Position the thicker proximal lower leg at the cathode end of the tube and the thinner distal lower leg at the anode end to take advantage of the anode heel effect and obtain more uniform density across the lower leg.

The lower leg demonstrates a lateral projection. The distal fibula is superimposed by the posterior half of the distal tibia. The fibular midshaft is free of tibial superimposition. The tibia is partially superimposed over the fibular head, and the medial femoral condyle is demonstrated posterior to the lateral condyle if the leg is extended; the condyles are superimposed if the knee is flexed at least 30 degrees (compare Figure 6-67 and Image 51).

- To obtain a lateral lower leg projection, begin by placing the patient in a supine position with the leg extended and the foot dorsiflexed until it forms a 90-degree angle with the lower leg. Next, rotate the leg, positioning the lateral foot surface against the IR and the femoral epicondyles perpendicular to the IR (Figure 6-69).

BOX 6-14	**Lateral Lower Leg Projection Analysis Criteria**

- Image density is uniform across the lower leg.
- The distal fibula is superimposed by the posterior half of the distal tibia.
- The fibular midshaft is free of tibial superimposition.
- The tibia is partially superimposed over the fibular head and the medial femoral condyle is demonstrated posterior to the lateral condyle if the leg is extended or the condyles are superimposed if the knee is flexed to at least 30 degrees.
- The tibial midshaft is at the center of the exposure field.
- The tibia, fibula, ankle, knee, and surrounding lower leg soft tissue are included within the collimated field.

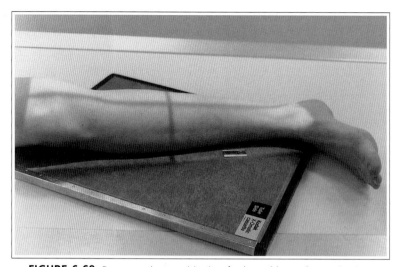

FIGURE 6-69 Proper patient positioning for lateral lower leg projection.

- *Detecting leg rotation.* If the distal lower leg was not placed in a lateral projection, the tibiofibular relationship is altered. If the patient's leg was externally rotated (patella positioned too close to the IR and heel elevated off the IR), the distal fibula is situated too far posterior on the tibia, and the fibular head is demonstrated free of tibial superimposition (see Image 52). If the patient's leg was internally rotated (patella positioned too far away from IR and forefoot elevated off the IR), the distal fibula is situated too far anterior on the tibia and fibular head and neck, and possibly the midshaft is superimposed by the tibia (see Image 53).
- Superimposition of the femoral condyles is not a good indication of rotation on a lateral lower leg projection. The amount of their superimposition depends on the degree of knee flexion and the way in which the diverged x-ray beams are aligned with the medial condyle. See page 364 (lateral knee) for a discussion of central ray alignment and the superimposition of the femoral condyles.
- *Positioning for fracture.* For a patient with a known or suspected fracture who is unable to position both the ankle and knee into a lateral projection simultaneously, position the joint closer to the fracture in the truer position. If the fracture is situated closer to the distal lower leg, the distal lower leg should meet the preceding requirements for a true lateral projection. If the fracture is situated closer to the proximal lower leg, the proximal lower leg should meet the preceding requirements for a lateral projection. Depending on the degree of tibial and fibular rotation at the fracture site, the other end of the lower leg may or may not be in a lateral projection.

The tibial midshaft is at the center of the exposure field. The tibia, fibula, ankle, knee, and surrounding lower leg soft tissue are included within the collimated field.

- A perpendicular central ray is centered to the midpoint of the lower leg to demonstrate the tibial midshaft in the center of the image.
- To include the ankle and knee joints on the image, you must consider the degree of x-ray beam divergence that occurs when a long body part is imaged (see Figure 6-66). A 14- × 17-inch (35- × 43-cm) detailed screen-film or computed radiography IR should be adequate to include both the ankle and knee. When a screen-film system is used, the leg can be positioned diagonally to accommodate the length. For the computed radiography system, it is not advisable to do this unless the system is set to handle this alignment. To ensure that both joints are included, the IR should extend 1 inch (2.5 cm) beyond each joint space. The ankle is located at the level of the medial malleolus, and the knee is located 1 inch (2.5 cm) distal to the palpable medial epicondyle.
- Once the lower leg is accurately positioned with the IR, center the central ray to the midshaft of the tibia, and open the longitudinal collimation until it extends just beyond both the knee and the ankle. For patients with long lower legs that have to be placed diagonally on the IR, it may be necessary to raise the SID above the standard to obtain a longitudinally collimated field long enough to include both joints on the same image. Transverse collimation should be to within 0.5 inch (1.25 cm) of the lower leg skin line.

Lateral Lower Leg Projection Analysis

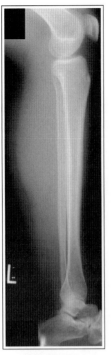

IMAGE 51

Analysis. The distal and proximal ends of the fibula are superimposed by the tibia, whereas the fibular midshaft is free of superimposition. The knee is flexed approximately 45 degrees, and the femoral condyles are superimposed.

Correction. No corrective movement is required, although knee flexion may result in elevation of the proximal lower leg and foreshortening of the tibia and fibula.

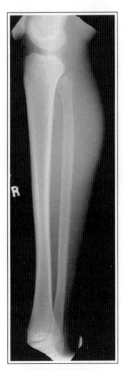

IMAGE 52

Analysis. The distal fibula is situated too far posterior on the tibia, and the fibular head is free of tibial superimposition. The leg was externally rotated.

Correction. Internally rotate the leg until the lateral foot surface is positioned parallel with the IR.

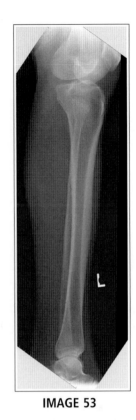

IMAGE 53

Analysis. The distal fibula is situated too far anterior on the tibia and the fibular head and midshaft are superimposed by the tibia. The leg was internally rotated.

Correction. Externally rotate the leg until the lateral foot surface is positioned parallel with the IR.

KNEE: ANTEROPOSTERIOR PROJECTION

See Figure 6-70 and Box 6-15.

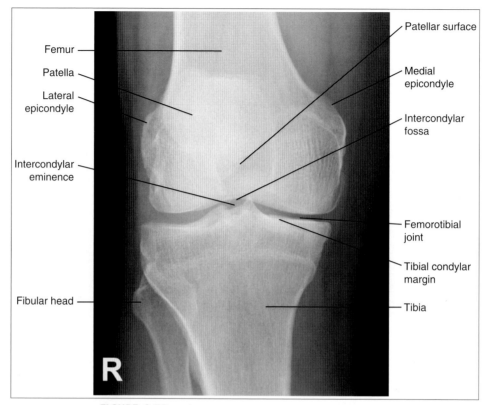

Femur

Patella

Lateral epicondyle

Intercondylar eminence

Fibular head

Patellar surface

Medial epicondyle

Intercondylar fossa

Femorotibial joint

Tibial condylar margin

Tibia

FIGURE 6-70 AP knee projection with accurate positioning.

BOX 6-15	**Anteroposterior Knee Projection Analysis Criteria**

- The medial and lateral femoral epicondyles are in profile, the femoral condyles are symmetrical, the intercondylar eminence is centered within the intercondylar fossa, and the tibia is superimposed over 0.25 inch (0.6 cm) of the fibular head.
- The knee joint space is open, the anterior and posterior condylar margins of the tibia are superimposed, and the fibular head is demonstrated approximately 0.5 inch (1.25 cm) distal to the tibial plateau.
- The patella lies just superior to the patellar surface of the femur and is situated slightly lateral to the knee midline. The intercondylar fossa is partially demonstrated.
- The knee joint is at the center of the exposure field.
- One fourth of the distal femur and proximal lower leg and the surrounding knee soft tissue are included within the collimated field.

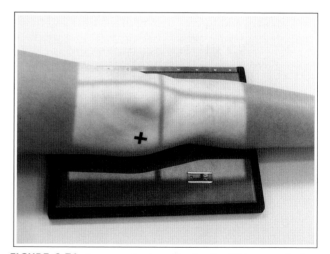

FIGURE 6-71 Proper patient positioning for AP knee projection.

The knee demonstrates an AP projection. The medial and lateral femoral epicondyles are in profile, the femoral condyles are symmetrical, the intercondylar eminence is centered within the intercondylar fossa, and the tibia is superimposed over 0.25 inch (0.6 cm) of the fibular head.

- To obtain an AP knee projection, place the patient in a supine position with the knee fully extended. Internally rotate the leg until an imaginary line drawn between the medial and lateral femoral epicondyles is positioned parallel with the IR (Figure 6-71). This positioning places the medial and lateral femoral epicondyles at equal distances from the IR as well as medially and laterally in profile, respectively. It also centers the intercondylar eminence within the intercondylar fossa and draws the fibular neck and a portion of the fibular head from beneath the tibia.

- *Effect of rotation.* If the femoral epicondyles are not positioned parallel with the IR, an AP projection has not been obtained. If the patient's leg was not internally rotated enough to place the epicondyles at equal distances from the IR, they are not in profile, the medial femoral condyle appears larger than the lateral condyle, and the tibia is superimposed over more than 0.25 inch (0.6 cm) of the fibular head (see Image 54). If the patient's leg was internally rotated more than needed to place the femoral epicondyles at equal distances from the IR, the epicondyles are not demonstrated in profile, the lateral femoral condyle appears larger than the medial condyle, and the tibia is superimposed over less than 0.25 inch (0.6 cm) of the fibular head (see Image 55).

The knee joint space is open, the anterior and posterior condylar margins of the tibia are superimposed, the intercondylar eminence and tubercles are demonstrated in profile, and the fibular head is demonstrated approximately 0.5 inch (1.25 cm) distal to the tibial plateau.

- The anterior and posterior condylar margins of the tibia are superimposed if the correct central ray angulation, as determined by the patient's upper thigh and buttocks thickness, is used. By studying the tibial plateau region, you will see that the tibial plateau slopes distally approximately 5 degrees from the anterior condylar margin to the posterior condylar margin on both the medial and lateral aspects (Figure 6-72). Only if the central ray is aligned parallel with the tibial plateau slope is an open knee joint space obtained.
- *Determining the central ray angulation.* When a patient is placed in a supine position, the degree and direction of the central ray angulation required depend on the thickness of the patient's upper thigh and buttocks. This thickness determines how the lower leg and the tibial plateau align with the IR. Figure 6-73 shows a guideline that can be used to determine the central ray angulation for different body sizes; it illustrates the relationship of the tibial plateau to the imaging table as the patient's upper thigh thickness increases. Note that a decrease occurs in femoral decline, and a shift occurs in the direction of the tibial plateau slope as the thickness of the thigh decreases. Because of this plateau shift, the central ray angulation must also be adjusted to keep it parallel with the plateau and to achieve an open knee joint. For optimal AP knee projections, measure from the patient's anterior superior iliac spine (ASIS) to the imaging table on either side to determine the central ray angulation to use for each knee examination. When measuring this distance, do not include the patient's abdominal tissue. Keep the calipers situated laterally next to the ASIS. If the measurement is less than 18 cm, a 5-degree caudal angle should be used. If the measurement is 19 to

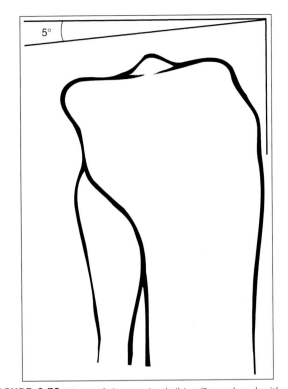

FIGURE 6-72 Slope of the proximal tibia. *(Reproduced with permission from Martensen K: Alternative AP knee method assures open joint space,* Radiol Technol *64:19–23, 1992. Courtesy* Radiologic Technology, *published by the American Society of Radiologic Technologists.)*

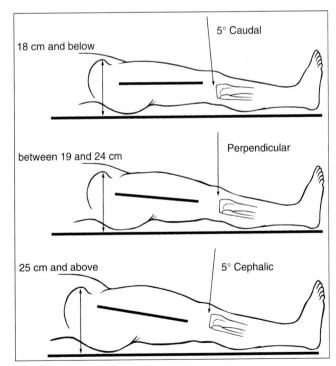

FIGURE 6-73 Determining central ray *(CR)* angle from the patient's thigh thickness. *(Reproduced with permission from Martensen K: Alternative AP knee method assures open joint space,* Radiol Technol *64:19–23, 1992. Courtesy* Radiologic Technology, *published by the American Society of Radiologic Technologists.)*

24 cm, a perpendicular beam should be used. If the measurement is greater than 24 cm, a 5-degree cephalad angle should be used. Using the correct central ray angulation not only results in an open knee joint space but also provides optimal demonstration of the intercondylar eminence and tubercles without foreshortening.

- *Analysis of joint space narrowing.* On an AP knee projection with adequate positioning, joint space narrowing is evaluated by measuring the medial and lateral aspects of the knee joint, which are also referred to as compartments. The measurement of each of these compartments is obtained by determining the distance between the most distal femoral condylar surface and the posterior condylar margin of the tibia on each side. Comparison of these measurements with each other, with measurements from previous images, or with measurements of the other knee determines joint space narrowing or a valgus or varus deformity. In a valgus deformity the lateral compartment is narrower than the medial compartment; in a varus deformity the medial compartment is narrower (see Images 56 and 57). Precise measurements of the compartments are necessary to ensure early detection of joint space narrowing and are best obtained when the knee joint space is completely open. If an inaccurate central ray angulation was used for an AP knee projection, the knee joint is narrowed or obscured, the intercondylar eminence and tubercles are foreshortened, and the tibial plateau is demonstrated.

- *Effect of poor central ray angulation.* When examining an AP knee projection for which an inaccurate central ray angulation was used, you can determine how to adjust the angulation by judging the shape of the fibular head and its proximity to the tibial plateau. If the fibular head is foreshortened and demonstrated more than 0.5 inch (1.25 cm) distal to the tibial plateau, the cephalad angle was too great (see Image 58). If the fibular head is elongated and demonstrated less than 0.5 inch (1.25 cm) distal to the tibial plateau, the caudad angle was too great (see Image 59).

- *Compensating for the nonextendable knee*: If the patient is unable to extend the knee fully, an open knee joint can be obtained by doing the following:

  1. Aligning the central ray perpendicular with the anterior lower leg surface
  2. Decreasing the angulation 5 degrees—placing the central ray parallel with the tibial plateau. For example, if the central ray is perpendicular to the anterior lower leg surface when a 15-degree cephalic angulation is used, the angle should be decreased to 10 degrees if the knee cannot be extended (see Image 60). This setup demonstrates an open knee joint space, a foreshortened distal femur and proximal lower leg, and an elongated intercondylar fossa.

The patella lies just superior to the patellar surface of the femur and is situated slightly lateral to the knee midline. The intercondylar fossa is partially demonstrated.

- The position of the patella and the degree of intercondylar fossa demonstration are determined by the amount of knee flexion. To visualize the patella and fossa as required, the leg must be in full extension. As the knee is flexed, the patella shifts distally and medially onto the patellar surface of the femur and then laterally into the intercondylar fossa, duplicating a C-shaped path that is open laterally (Figure 6-74). Thus, the patella is demonstrated at different locations, depending on the degree of knee flexion. Generally, when the knee is flexed 20 degrees, the patella is demonstrated on the patellar surface. With 30 to 70 degrees of knee flexion, the patella is demonstrated between the patellar surface and the intercondylar fossa. At 90 degrees to full knee flexion, the patella is demonstrated within the intercondylar fossa.

- *Intercondylar fossa visualization with knee flexion.* The extent of intercondylar fossa demonstration also changes with knee flexion. In full extension, only a slight indentation between the distal medial and lateral femoral condyles indicates the location of the intercondylar fossa. As the knee is flexed, the amount of intercondylar fossa that is demonstrated increases. When the knee is flexed to between 50 and 60 degrees, the intercondylar fossa is shown in profile (see Image 60). When the knee is flexed less than 50 degrees or more than 60 degrees, demonstration of the fossa will decrease.

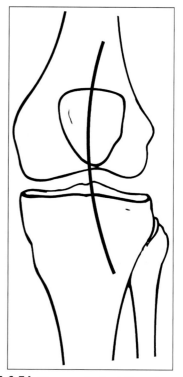

FIGURE 6-74 Movement of patella on knee flexion.

- *Patellar subluxation.* With patellar subluxation (partial patellar dislocation), the patella may be situated more laterally than normal on an AP knee projection (see Image 61). When an image demonstrates a laterally situated patella, evaluate the symmetry of the femoral condyles and the relationship of the tibia and fibular head to rule out external rotation before assuming that the patella is subluxed. External rotation also results in a laterally located patella.

The knee joint is at the center of the exposure field. One fourth of the distal femur and proximal lower leg and the surrounding knee soft tissue are included within the collimated field.

- Center the central ray to the midline of the knee at a level 1 inch (2.5 cm) distal to the palpable medial epicondyle to place the knee joint in the center of the exposure field. (As long as the knee remains extended, an alternative central ray placement is 0.5 inch (1.25 cm) distal to the patellar apex.) Open the longitudinal collimation enough to include one fourth of the distal femur and proximal lower leg. Transverse collimation should be to within 0.5 inch (1.25 cm) of the knee skin line.
- An 8- × 10-inch (18- × 24-cm) or 10- × 12-inch (24- × 30-cm) screen-film or computed radiography IR placed lengthwise should be adequate to include all the required anatomic structures.

Anteroposterior Knee Projection Analysis

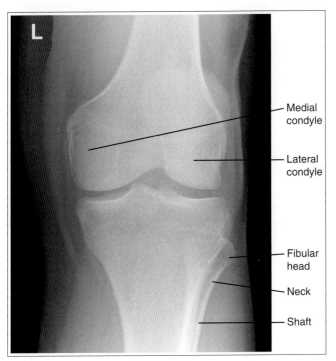

IMAGE 54

Analysis. The femoral epicondyles are not in profile, the medial femoral condyle appears larger than the lateral condyle, and the fibular head demonstrates more than 0.25 inch (0.6 cm) of tibial superimposition. The leg was externally rotated.

Correction. Internally rotate the leg until the femoral epicondyles are at equal distances from the IR.

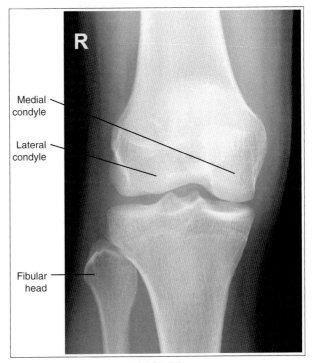

IMAGE 55

Analysis. The femoral epicondyles are not in profile, the lateral femoral condyle appears larger than the medial condyle, and the fibular head demonstrates less than 0.25 inch (0.6 cm) of tibial superimposition. The leg was internally rotated.

Correction. Externally rotate the leg until the femoral epicondyles are at equal distances from the film.

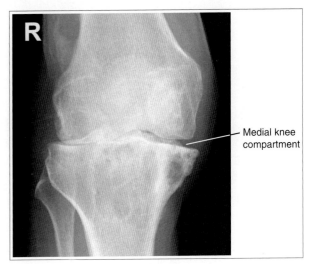

IMAGE 56

Analysis. The lateral knee compartment is narrower than the medial knee compartment. The patient's knee demonstrates a valgus deformity.

Correction. No corrective movement is required.

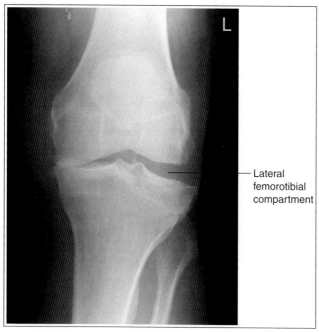

Lateral femorotibial compartment

IMAGE 57

Analysis. The medial knee compartment is narrower than the lateral knee compartment. The patient's knee demonstrates a varus deformity.

Correction. No corrective movement is required.

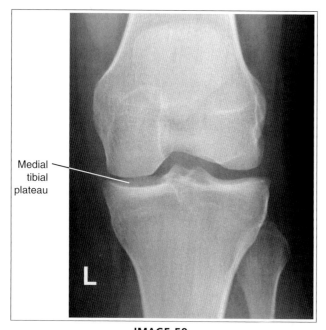

Medial tibial plateau

IMAGE 58

Analysis. The knee joint space is obscured, the medial tibial plateau is demonstrated, the fibular head is foreshortened and demonstrated more than 0.5 inch (1.25 cm) distal to the tibial plateau. Excessive cephalad angulation is indicated.

Correction. Angle the central ray caudally approximately 5 degrees for every 0.25 inch (0.6 cm) of tibial plateau demonstrated. For this image, approximately 0.5 inch (1.25 cm) of the tibial plateau is demonstrated between the anterior and posterior tibial margins. The central ray should be adjusted approximately 10 degrees, because a 5-degree cephalad angle was used. When the image is retaken, a 5-degree caudal angle should be used.

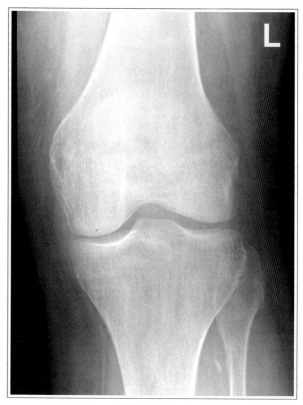

IMAGE 59

Analysis. The medial knee joint space is closed, and the fibular head is elongated and demonstrated less than 0.5 inch (1.25 cm) distal to the tibial plateau. Excessive caudal angulation is indicated.

Correction. If an open medial knee joint space is desired, the central ray should be adjusted cephalically.

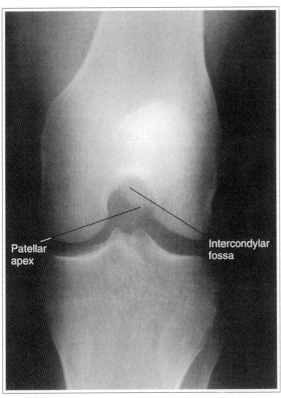

IMAGE 60

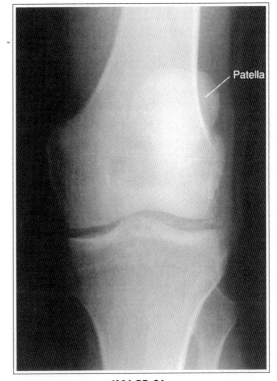

IMAGE 61

Analysis. This is an AP knee projection taken with the knee flexed approximately 50 to 60 degrees and the central ray aligned parallel with the tibial plateau. The knee joint space is open, the intercondylar fossa is demonstrated in profile, and the patellar apex is superimposed over the intercondylar fossa. Because of the acute angle of the lower leg and femur with the IR, the distal femur and proximal lower leg are foreshortened and the intercondylar fossa is slightly elongated.

Correction. If the patient's condition allows, fully extend the knee. If the patient is unable to extend the knee, no corrective movement is required.

Analysis. The knee demonstrates no signs of rotation, even though the patella is superimposed over the lateral aspect of the knee. The patient has a subluxed patella.

Correction. No corrective movement is required.

KNEE: ANTEROPOSTERIOR OBLIQUE PROJECTION (MEDIAL AND LATERAL ROTATION)

See Figures 6-75 and 6-76 and Box 6-16.

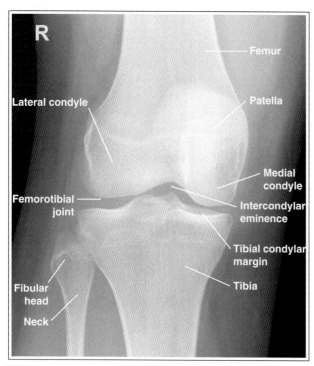

FIGURE 6-75 AP (internal) oblique knee projection with accurate positioning.

BOX 6-16	Anteroposterior Oblique Knee Projection Analysis Criteria

- The knee joint space is open, the anterior and posterior condylar margins of the tibia are superimposed, and the fibular head is approximately 0.5 inch (1.25 cm) distal to the tibial plateau.
- Medial oblique: The fibular head is seen free of tibial superimposition and the lateral femoral condyle is in profile without superimposing the medial condyle.
- Lateral oblique: The fibular head, neck, and shaft are aligned with the anterior edge of the tibia and the medial femoral condyle is in profile without superimposing the lateral condyle.
- The knee joint is at the center of the exposure field.
- One fourth of the distal femur and proximal lower leg and the surrounding knee soft tissue are included within the collimated field.

The knee joint space is open. The anterior and posterior condylar margins of the tibia are superimposed, and the fibular head is approximately 0.5 inch (1.25 cm) distal to the tibial plateau.

- The anterior and posterior condylar margins of the tibia are superimposed by the use of the correct central ray angulation, as determined by the patient's upper thigh and buttocks thickness. By studying the tibial plateau region, you will see that the tibial plateau slopes distally approximately

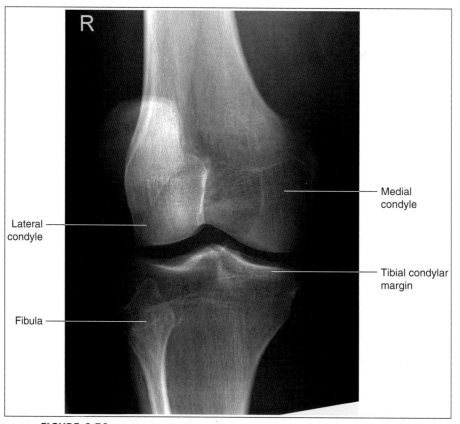

FIGURE 6-76 AP (external) oblique knee projection with accurate positioning.

5 degrees from the anterior condylar margin to the posterior condylar margin on both the medial and lateral aspects. Only if the central ray is aligned parallel with this slope is a truly open joint space obtained.

- *Determining the central ray angulation.* When a patient is placed in a supine position, the degree and direction of the central ray angulation required depend on the thickness of the patient's upper thigh and buttocks, because it is this thickness that will determine the central ray angulation that should be used for different body sizes. Figure 6-77 demonstrates how the relationship of the tibial plateau varies as the patient's upper thigh thickness changes. For optimal AP oblique knee projections, measure each patient from the ASIS to the imaging table, after the patient has been accurately positioned, to determine the correct central ray angulation to use for each examination. When measuring this distance, do not include the patient's abdominal tissue in the measurement. Keep the calipers situated laterally, next to the ASIS. If the measurement is 18 cm or below, a 5-degree caudal angle should be used. If the measurement is 19 to 24 cm, a perpendicular beam should be used. If the measurement is above 24 cm, a 5-degree cephalad angle should be used. It is not uncommon to require a cephalic angle for the AP medial oblique knee projection because

the patient's hip is often elevated to accomplish the needed degree of internal obliquity or to need a caudal angle for the lateral oblique knee image because the patient's hip is placed closer to the imaging table to obtain the needed external obliquity.

- *Effect of poor central ray angulation.* If an inaccurate central ray angulation was used for an AP oblique knee projection, the knee joint space is narrowed or obscured and the anterior and posterior margins of the tibial plateau are not superimposed. When evaluating an AP oblique knee projection for which an inaccurate central ray angulation was used, you can determine how to adjust the angulation by judging the shape of the fibular head and its proximity to the tibial plateau. If the fibular head is foreshortened and demonstrated more than 0.5 inch (1.25 cm) distal to the tibial plateau (see Image 62), the cephalad angle was too great and if the fibular head is elongated and demonstrated less than 0.5 inch (1.25 cm) distal to the tibial plateau, the caudad angle was too great (see Image 63).

The knee joint is at the center of the exposure field. One fourth of the distal femur and proximal lower leg and the surrounding knee soft tissue are included within the collimated field.

- The central ray should be centered to the midline of the knee at the level of the knee joint, which is located 1 inch (2.5 cm) distal to the palpable medial femoral epicondyle, to place the knee joint in the center of the exposure field. Open the longitudinal collimation to include one fourth of the distal femur and the proximal lower leg. Transverse collimation should be within 0.5 inch (1.25 cm) of the knee skin line.
- An 8- × 10-inch (18- × 24-cm) or 10- × 12-inch (24- × 30-cm) screen-film or computed radiography IR placed lengthwise should be adequate to include all the required anatomic structures.

KNEE: MEDIALLY (INTERNALLY) ROTATED ANTEROPOSTERIOR OBLIQUE POSITION

The knee has been rotated 45 degrees internally. The fibular head is demonstrated free of tibial superimposition, and the lateral femoral condyle is in profile, without medial condyle superimposition.

- A medially rotated AP oblique knee projection with accurate positioning is obtained by placing the patient in an AP knee projection, and then internally rotating the leg until an imaginary line drawn between the medial and lateral femoral epicondyles is positioned at a 45-degree angle with the IR

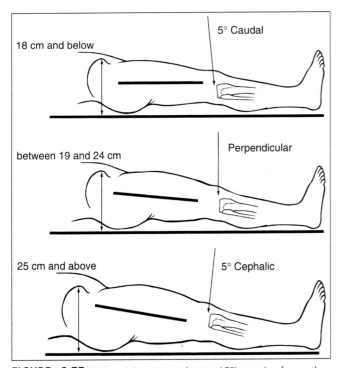

FIGURE 6-77 Determining central ray (*CR*) angle from the patient's thigh thickness. *(Reproduced with permission from Martensen K: Alternative AP knee method assures open joint space, Radiol Technol 64:19–23, 1992. Courtesy Radiologic Technology, published by the American Society of Radiologic Technologists.)*

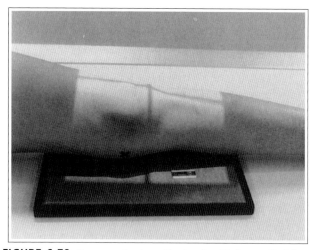

FIGURE 6-78 Proper patient positioning for AP (internal) oblique knee projection.

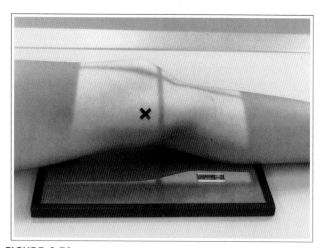

FIGURE 6-79 Proper patient positioning for AP (external) oblique knee projection. X indicates medial femoral epicondyle.

(Figure 6-78). This position places the lateral condyle in profile and rotates the fibular head from beneath the tibia, opening the proximal tibiofibular articulation. If the femoral epicondyles are rotated less than 45 degrees with the IR, the tibia is partially superimposed over the fibular head (see Image 63). If the femoral epicondyles are rotated more than 45 degrees with the IR, the femoral condyles are almost superimposed (see Image 64).

LATERALLY (EXTERNALLY) ROTATED ANTEROPOSTERIOR OBLIQUE PROJECTION

The knee has been rotated 45 degrees externally. The fibular head, neck, and shaft are superimposed by the tibia, and the fibular head is aligned with the anterior edge of the tibia. The medial femoral condyle is in profile, without lateral condyle superimposition.

- A laterally rotated AP oblique knee projection with accurate positioning is obtained by placing the patient in an AP knee projection, and then externally rotating the leg until an imaginary line drawn between the medial and lateral femoral epicondyles is positioned at a 45-degree angle with the IR (Figure 6-79). This position places the medial condyle in profile and rotates the tibia onto the fibula, demonstrating superimposition of the tibia and fibula on the image. If the femoral epicondyles are rotated less than 45 degrees with the IR, the fibular head demonstrates decreased tibial superimposition or will be positioned more toward the center of the tibia (see Image 65). If the femoral epicondyles are rotated more than 45 degrees with the IR, the fibular head is not aligned with the anterior edge of the tibia but is posterior to the placement. The more posteriorly situated is the fibula, the farther away from 45 degrees the patient was positioned (see Image 66).

Anteroposterior Oblique Knee Projection Analysis

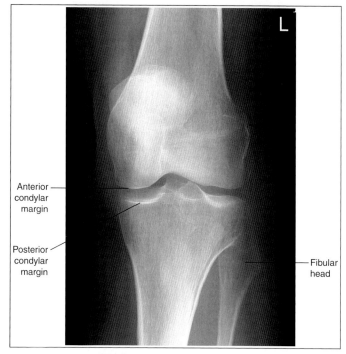

IMAGE 62 Internal oblique.

Analysis. The fibular head is demonstrated without tibial superimposition and the lateral femoral condyle is demonstrated in profile, indicating accurate obliquity. The knee joint space is obscured, and the fibular head is foreshortened and demonstrated more than 0.5 inch (1.25 cm) distal to the tibial plateau. The central ray angulation was too cephalad.

Correction. Decrease the degree of central ray angulation approximately 5 degrees for every 0.25 inch (0.6 cm) of tibial plateau demonstrated. For this image, approximately 0.25 inch of the tibial plateau is demonstrated between the anterior and posterior tibial margins; therefore, the central ray should be adjusted approximately 5 degrees.

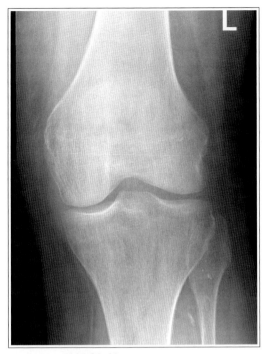

IMAGE 63 Internal oblique.

Analysis. The tibia is partially superimposed over the fibular head. The patient's knee was rotated less than 45 degrees. The joint space is closed, and the fibular head is elongated and demonstrated less than 0.5 inch (1.25 cm) from the tibial plateau. The central ray angulation was too caudal.

Correction. Increase the medial knee obliquity until the femoral epicondyles are aligned at a 45-degree angle with the IR. Increase the degree of central ray angulation approximately 5 degrees for every 0.25 inch (0.6 cm) of tibial plateau demonstrated.

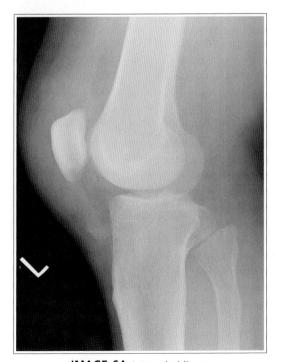

IMAGE 64 Internal oblique.

Analysis. The medial femoral condyle is superimposed over most of the lateral condyle. The patient's knee was rotated more than 45 degrees.

Correction. Decrease the medial knee obliquity until the femoral epicondyles are aligned at a 45-degree angle with the IR.

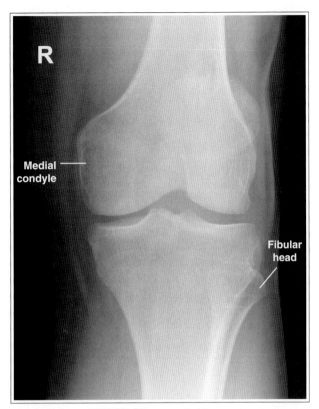

IMAGE 65 External oblique.

Analysis. The fibular head, neck, and shaft are not superimposed by the tibia. The patient's knee was rotated less than 45 degrees.

Correction. Increase the lateral knee obliquity until the femoral epicondyles are aligned at a 45-degree angle with the IR.

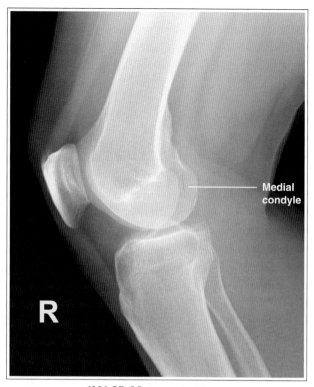

IMAGE 66 External oblique.

Analysis. The fibular head is not aligned with the anterior edge of the tibia but is demonstrated posterior to this placement, and the femoral condyles and the medial condyle are almost superimposed; the medial condyle is posterior. The patient's knee was rotated more than 45 degrees.

Correction. Decrease the lateral knee obliquity until the femoral epicondyles are aligned at a 45-degree angle with the IR.

KNEE: LATERAL PROJECTION (MEDIOLATERAL)

See Figures 6-80 and 6-81 and Box 6-17.

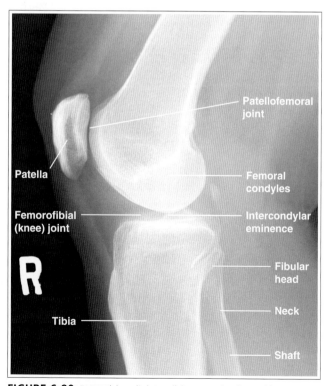

FIGURE 6-80 Lateral (mediolateral) knee projection with accurate positioning.

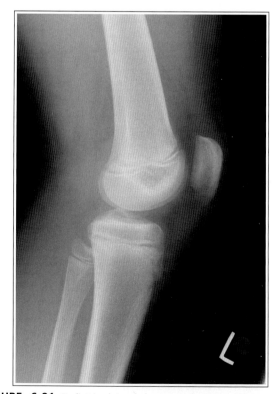

FIGURE 6-81 Pediatric lateral knee projection with accurate positioning.

BOX 6-17	Lateral Knee Projection Analysis Criteria

- Contrast and density are adequate to demonstrate the suprapatellar fat pad.
- The patella is situated proximal to the patellar surface of the femur and the patellofemoral joint is open.
- The distal articulating surfaces of the medial and lateral femoral condyles are superimposed, and the knee joint space is open.
- The anterior and posterior surfaces of the medial and lateral femoral condyles are superimposed, and the tibia is partially superimposed over the fibular head.
- The knee joint is at the center of the exposure field.
- One fourth of the distal femur and proximal lower leg and the surrounding knee soft tissue are included within the collimated field.

Contrast and density are adequate to demonstrate the suprapatellar fat pads.

- *Suprapatellar fat pads.* Two soft tissue structures of interest at the knee are used to diagnose joint effusion and knee injury. They are the posterior and anterior suprapatellar fat pads. Both are located anterior to the patellar surface of the distal femur and are separated by the suprapatellar bursa (Figure 6-82). Fluid that collects in the suprapatellar bursa causes the anterior and posterior suprapatellar fat pads to separate. It is a widening of this space that indicates a diagnosis of joint effusion.

The patella is situated proximal to the patellar surface of the femur, and the patellofemoral joint is open.

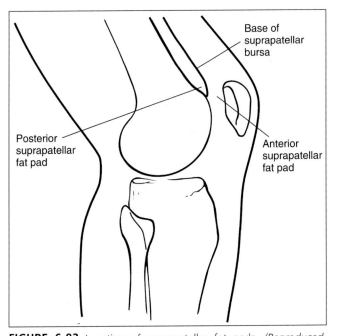

FIGURE 6-82 Location of suprapatellar fat pads. *(Reproduced with permission from Martensen K: The knee, In-Service Reviews in Radiologic Technology, vol 14, no 7, Birmingham, Ala, 1991, In-Service Reviews.)*

- The knee should be flexed 10 to 15 degrees. With less than 20 degrees of knee flexion, the patella is situated proximal to the patellar surface of the femur, the quadriceps are relaxed, and the patella is fairly mobile. In this patellar position the anterior and posterior suprapatellar fat pads can be easily used to evaluate knee joint effusion. Conversely, when the knee is flexed 20 degrees or more, a tightening of the surrounding knee muscles and tendons is present, the patella comes into contact with the patellar surface of the femur, and the anterior and posterior suprapatellar fat pads are obscured, eliminating their usefulness in diagnosing joint effusion (see Image 67). Some authors indicate that 20 to 30 degrees of knee flexion should be used on a lateral knee projection. Facility routines dictate the actual number of degrees that should be used.
- *Positioning for fracture.* If a patellar or other knee fracture is suspected, the knee should remain extended to prevent displacement of bony fragments or vascular injury (Figure 6-83).

The distal articulating surfaces of the medial and lateral femoral condyles are superimposed, and the knee joint space is open.

- Take a few minutes to study a femoral bone. Place it upright with the distal femoral condylar surfaces resting against a flat surface. Note how the femoral shaft inclines medially approximately 10 to 15 degrees. When a patient is in an erect position, this is how the femurs are positioned. This femoral incline gives the body stability (Figure 6-84). The amount of inclination a person displays depends on pelvic width and femoral shaft length. The wider the pelvis and the shorter the femoral shaft length, the more medially the femurs incline.
- When the patient is placed in a recumbent projection for a lateral knee image (Figure 6-85), some of the medial femoral inclination is reduced, resulting in projection of the medial condyle distal to the lateral condyle and into the knee joint space (Figure 6-86). This can be demonstrated by laying the femoral bone on its lateral side. Note how the distal condylar surfaces are no longer on the same plane. The medial condyle is situated distal to the lateral condyle. The amount of distance demonstrated between these two condyles depends on the amount of medial femoral incline the femur displayed in the upright position, the length of the femur, and the width of the pelvis from which the femur originated. If the medial condyle remains in this distal position, it obscures the knee joint space on the image. This is why a cephalic angle is needed for most lateral knee projections.
- *Determining central ray angulation.* Because the degree of femoral inclination varies among patients,

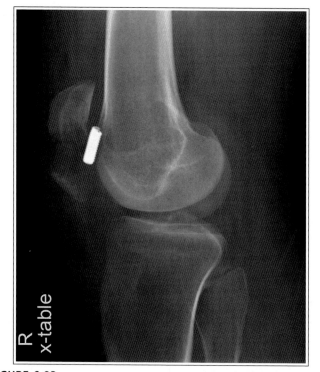

FIGURE 6-83 Cross-table lateral knee projection with fractured patella.

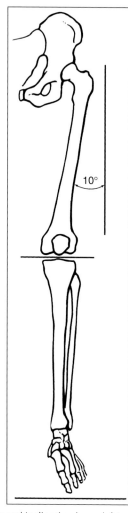

FIGURE 6-84 Femoral inclination in upright position. *(Reproduced with permission from Martensen K: The knee, In-Service Reviews in Radiologic Technology, vol 14, no 7, Birmingham, Ala, 1991, In-Service Reviews.)*

so must the degree of central ray angulation. For a patient with a wide pelvis and short femora, a 5- to 7-degree cephalad angle is the most reliable angulation to use. For a patient with a narrow pelvis and long femora, very little, if any, angulation is required. Although females commonly demonstrate greater pelvic width and femoral inclination and males demonstrate narrower pelvic width and femoral inclination, variations occur in both sexes. Each patient's pelvic width and femoral length should be evaluated to determine the degree of angulation to use.

- *Effect of central ray angulation on femoral condylar superimposition.* If an inaccurate central ray angulation is used on a lateral knee projection, the distal articulating surfaces of the femoral condyles are not superimposed on the image. Whenever this occurs, the knee joint space is narrowed or closed. If a patient required a cephalic angulation to project the medial condyle proximally, but no angle was used, the image demonstrates the distal articulating surface of the medial condyle distal to the distal articulating surface of the lateral condyle (see Image 68). If a patient did not require a cephalic angulation but one was used, or if the cephalad angle was too great, the distal surface of the medial condyle is projected proximal to the distal surface of the lateral condyle (see Image 69). It should also be noted that the tibiofibular joint is better visualized on this image because the proximal tibia is moved proximally, somewhat off the fibular head.

- *Distinguishing lateral and medial condyles.* The first step you should take when evaluating an image on which the distal condylar surfaces are

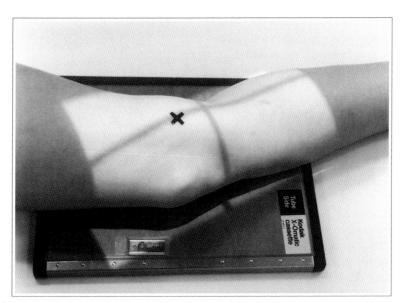

FIGURE 6-85 Proper patient positioning for lateral knee projection. X indicates medial femoral epicondyle.

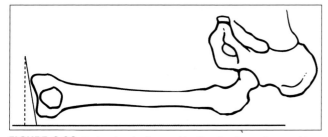

FIGURE 6-86 Reduction in femoral inclination in supine position.

not aligned is to determine which condyle is the lateral and which is the medial. The most reliable method for identifying the medial condyle is to locate the rounded bony tubercle known as the adductor tubercle. It is located posteriorly on the medial aspect of the femur, just superior to the medial condyle. The size and shape of the tubercle are not identical on every patient, although this surface is considerably different from the same surface on the lateral condyle, which is smooth. Once the adductor tubercle is located, the medial condyle is also identified. Another difference between the medial and lateral condyles is evident on their distal articulating surfaces. The distal surface of the medial condyle is convex, and the distal surface of the lateral condyle is flat.

• *Supine (cross-table) lateromedial knee projection.* When a lateral knee projection is taken using a lateromedial projection, with a horizontal central ray, the cephalad central ray angulation described above is not required, as long as the patient's femoral inclination is not reduced or increased by the distal femur being shifted too laterally or medially, respectively. Images 70 and 71 are cross-table lateral knee projections that demonstrate a femoral

condyle within the knee joint space because of poor femoral positioning. Image 70 demonstrates the lateral condyle in the joint space and image 71 demonstrates the medial condyle. When such images are produced, view how far the fibular head is positioned from the tibial plateau. When the distal surfaces of the femoral condyles are accurately superimposed, the fibular head will be positioned about 0.5 inch (1.25 cm) from the tibial plateau. If the central ray (CR) is rotated distally or the leg adducted (moved too medially) for a lateromedial projection of the knee, the lateral condyle will be projected distal to the medial condyle and the fibular head will move farther than 0.5 inch (1.25 cm) from the tibial plateau (see Image 70). If the CR is rotated proximally or the leg abducted (moved too laterally) for a lateromedial projection of the knee, the lateral condyle will be projected proximal to the medial condyle and the fibular head will move closer than 0.5 inch (1.25 cm) from the tibial plateau (see Image 71).

The anterior and posterior surfaces of the medial and lateral femoral condyles are superimposed, and the tibia is partially superimposed over the fibular head.

• How the central ray is aligned with the femur determines the relationship between the tibia and fibula, especially when a cephalic angulation is used. Study a femoral bone that is positioned in a mediolateral projection with the femoral epicondyles placed directly on top of each other. Note that in this position, the medial condyle is situated not only distal but also posterior to the lateral condyle, indicating that the medial condyle must be projected proximally and anteriorly for it to be superimposed over the lateral condyle.

- *Positioning to superimpose the anterior and posterior aspects of the femoral condyles.* Two positioning methods can be used to accomplish this goal. For the first (easier) method, position the femoral epicondyles directly on top of each other, so that an imaginary line drawn between them is perpendicular to the IR. Then, direct the central ray across the femur, as indicated in Figure 6-87. With this method, the central ray projects the medial condyle anteriorly and proximally. This method also demonstrates the fibular head partially superimposed by the tibia, which is an accurate lateral tibiofibular relationship (see Figure 6-80).

- For the second method, align the femoral epicondyles perpendicular to the IR, and then roll the patient's patella toward the IR approximately 0.25 inch (0.6 cm) to move the medial condyle anteriorly onto the lateral condyle. Finally, align the central ray with the femur, as shown in Figure 6-88, projecting the medial condyle proximally. This method produces an image on which the condyles are superimposed but the fibular head is demonstrated without tibial superimposition (see Image 72). Regardless of the method your facility prefers, a true lateral knee projection has not been obtained unless the condyles are superimposed.

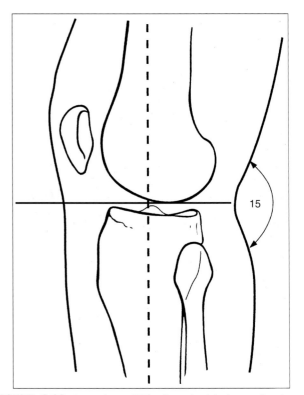

FIGURE 6-88 Central ray (CR) aligned with femur for lateral knee projection. *(Reproduced with permission from Martensen K: The knee, In-Service Reviews in Radiologic Technology, vol 14, no 7, Birmingham, Ala, 1991, In-Service Reviews.)*

- *Effect of knee rotation on femoral condylar superimposition.* When an image is obtained that demonstrates one femoral condyle anterior to the other, the patella must be rolled closer to (leg externally rotated) or farther away from (leg internally rotated) the IR for superimposed condyles to be obtained. The first step in determining which way to roll the knee is to distinguish one condyle from the other. As noted, the most reliable method is to locate the adductor tubercle of the medial condyle. When a lateral knee projection is obtained that demonstrates the adductor tubercle and medial condyle posterior to the lateral condyle, the patella was situated too far from the IR (leg internally rotated) (Figure 6-89; see Image 73). When a lateral

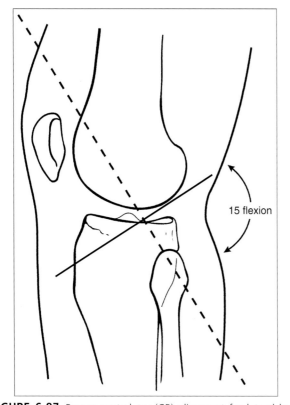

FIGURE 6-87 Proper central ray (CR) alignment for lateral knee projection. *(Reproduced with permission from Martensen K: The knee, In-Service Reviews in Radiologic Technology, vol 14, no 7, Birmingham, Ala, 1991, In-Service Reviews.)*

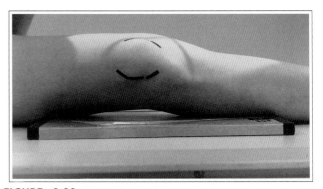

FIGURE 6-89 Poorly positioned lateral knee projection with patella too far from image receptor (leg internally rotated).

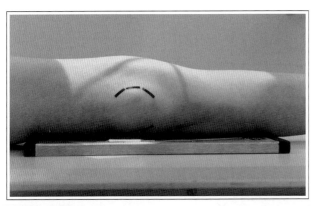

FIGURE 6-90 Poorly positioned lateral knee projection with patella too close to image receptor (leg externally rotated).

knee projection is obtained that demonstrates the medial condyle anterior to the lateral condyle, the patella was situated too close to the IR (leg externally rotated) (Figure 6-90; see Image 74).

Another method used to determine knee rotation is to view the tibiofibular relationship to determine how to reposition for poorly superimposed condyles. If the tibia is superimposed over the fibular head, the patella was positioned too far from the IR. If the fibular head is free of tibial superimposition, the patella was positioned too close to the IR. Although this relationship is reliable for most patients, the alignment of the central ray affects the results. Image 75 demonstrates such a case. If you use the adductor tubercle and medial condyle to determine how this patient should be repositioned, roll the patient's patella toward the IR (externally rotated leg). If you use the tibiofibular relationship, roll the patient's patella away from the IR (internally rotated leg). The adductor tubercle method is more reliable. This patient's patella needed to be rolled toward the IR to superimpose the condyles. It should also be noted that the tibiofibular relationship should not be used when the patient's knee is flexed approximately 90 degrees (see Image 76). When the patient's knee is flexed to this degree, it is femoral elevation and depression that determine the tibiofibular relationship, not leg rotation. To understand this change best, view the skeletal leg in a lateral position with 90 degrees of leg flexion. Observe how the tibiofibular relationship results in increased tibial superimposition of the fibula when the proximal femur is elevated and a decreased tibial superimposition of the fibula as the proximal femur is depressed.

The knee joint is at the center of the exposure field. One fourth of the distal femur and proximal lower leg and the surrounding knee soft tissue are included within the collimated field.

- Center the central ray to the midline of the knee at the level of the knee joint space, which is located 1 inch (2.5 cm) distal to the palpable medial epicondyle, to center the knee joint in the collimated field. Open the longitudinal collimation enough to include one fourth of the distal femur and proximal lower leg. Transverse collimation should be to within 0.5 inch (1.25 cm) of the knee skin line.
- An 8- × 10-inch (18- × 24-cm) or 10- × 12-inch (24- × 30-cm) screen-film or computed radiography IR placed lengthwise should be adequate to include all the required anatomic structures.

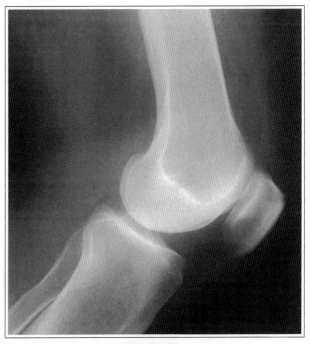

IMAGE 67

Lateral Knee Projection Analysis

Analysis. The patient's knee is overflexed, the patella is in contact with the patellar surface of the femur, and the suprapatellar fat pads are obscured.

Correction. Decrease the amount of knee flexion.

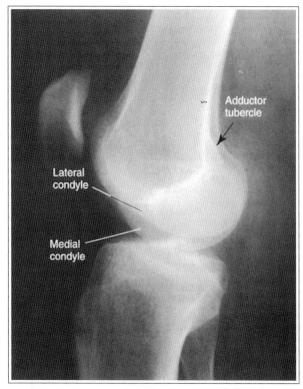

IMAGE 68

Analysis. The distal articulating surfaces of the femoral condyles are not superimposed. The medial condyle is distal to the lateral condyle.

Correction. A cephalic angulation should be used to project the medial condyle proximally. Adjust the angle approximately 5 degrees for every 0.25 inch (0.6 cm) of distance demonstrated between the medial and lateral distal surfaces.

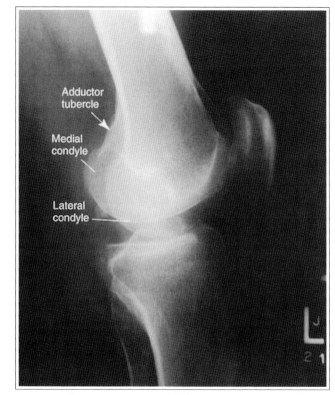

IMAGE 69

Analysis. The distal articulating surfaces of the femoral condyles are not superimposed. The medial condyle has been projected proximally to the lateral condyle. An excessively cephalad angle was used.

Correction. Decrease the central ray angulation approximately 5 degrees for every 0.25 inch (0.6 cm) of distance demonstrated between the medial and lateral distal surfaces.

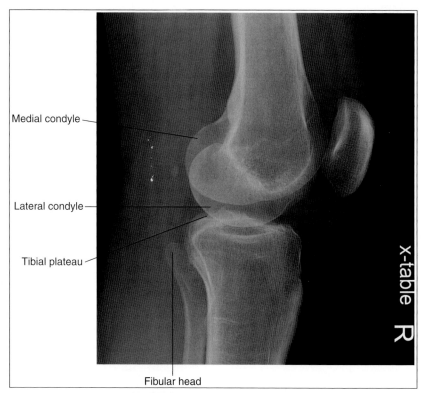

IMAGE 70 Lateromedial projection.

Analysis. The lateral condyle is distal to the medial and the fibular head is more than 0.5 inch (1.25 cm) from the tibial plateau. The CR was rotated distally or the leg adducted (moved too medially).

Correction. Rotate the CR proximally the needed amount or abduct the leg half the distance demonstrated between the two distal condylar surfaces.

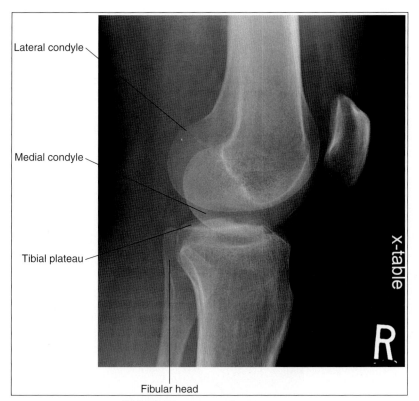

IMAGE 71 Lateromedial projection.

Analysis. The lateral condyle is proximal to the medial and the fibular head is less than 0.5 inch (1.25 cm) from the tibial plateau. The CR was rotated proximally or the leg abducted (moved too laterally).

Correction. Rotate the CR distally the needed amount or adduct the leg half the distance demonstrated between the two distal condylar surfaces.

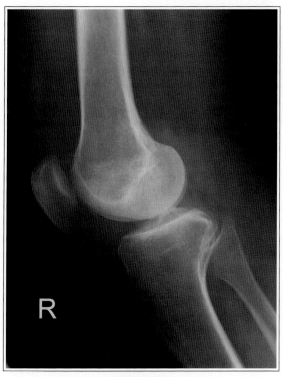

IMAGE 72

Analysis. The femoral condyles are superimposed and the tibiofibular articulation is demonstrated. The image was taken with the femoral epicondyles aligned perpendicular to the IR, and then rolled toward the IR approximately 0.25 inch (0.6 cm) to move the medial condyle anteriorly onto the lateral condyle. The central ray was then aligned with the femur, as shown in Figure 6-88.

Correction. For a more accurate demonstration of the tibia and fibula relationship, position the femoral epicondyles perpendicular to the IR and align the central ray across the femur, as shown in Figure 6-87.

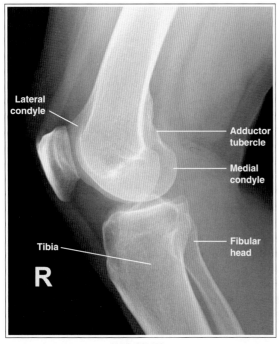

IMAGE 73

Analysis. The anterior and the posterior aspects of the femoral condyles are not superimposed. The medial condyle is situated posteriorly. The patient's patella was positioned too far from the IR (leg internally rotated).

Correction. Roll the patella closer to the IR (externally rotate the leg). Because both condyles will move simultaneously, the amount of adjustment required is only half the distance demonstrated between the posterior surfaces.

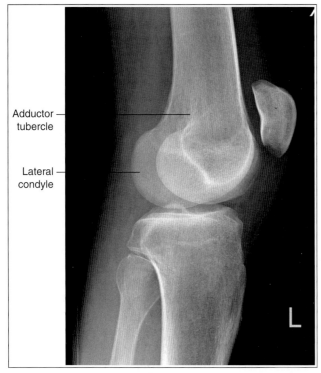

IMAGE 74

Analysis. The anterior and posterior aspects of the femoral condyles are not superimposed. The medial condyle is situated anteriorly. The patella was positioned too close to the IR (leg externally rotated).

Correction. Roll the patella farther away from the IR (internally rotate the leg). Because both condyles will move simultaneously, the amount of adjustment required is only half the distance demonstrated between the posterior surfaces.

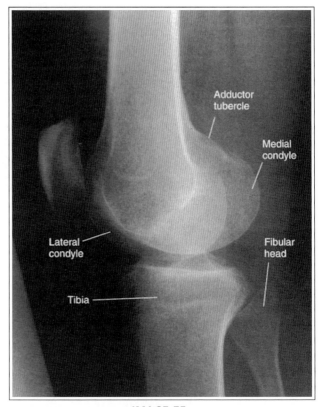

IMAGE 75

Analysis. The AP aspects of the femoral condyles are not superimposed. The medial condyle is situated posteriorly. The patella was positioned too far from the IR (leg internally rotated).

Correction. Roll the patella closer to the IR (externally rotate the leg). Because both condyles move simultaneously, the amount of adjustment required is only half the distance demonstrated between the posterior surfaces.

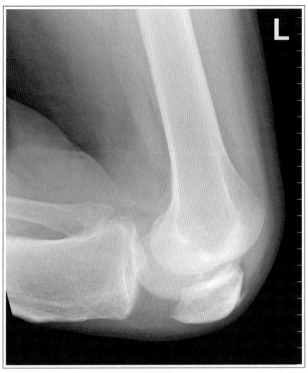

IMAGE 76

Analysis. The knee is flexed 90 degrees, and the medial condyle is demonstrated distal and posterior to the lateral condyle. The fibula is demonstrated without tibial superimposition. The proximal femur was elevated because the patient had a thick proximal thigh, and the patella was positioned too far from the IR.

Correction. Unflex the knee to 10 to 15 degrees of flexion, elevate the distal femur or adjust the central ray angulation cephalically, and rotate the patella closer to the IR.

INTERCONDYLAR FOSSA: POSTEROANTERIOR AXIAL PROJECTION (HOLMBLAD METHOD)

See Figure 6-91 and Box 6-18.

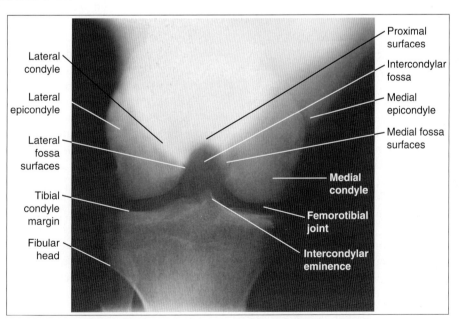

FIGURE 6-91 PA axial knee projection (Holmblad method) with accurate positioning.

The medial and the lateral surfaces of the intercondylar fossa and the femoral epicondyles are in profile, and the fibular head is partially superimposed over the proximal tibia.

- The PA axial projection (Holmblad method) is performed by positioning the patient on hands and knees on the imaging table and then requesting the patient to lean forward until the femur and central

BOX 6-18 | Posteroanterior Axial Knee Projection (Holmblad Method) Analysis Criteria

- The medial and lateral surfaces of the intercondylar fossa and the femoral epicondyles are in profile, and the fibular head is partially superimposed over the proximal tibia.
- The proximal surfaces of the intercondylar fossa are superimposed, and the patellar apex is demonstrated proximal to the intercondylar fossa.
- The knee joint space is open and the tibial plateau and intercondylar eminence and the tubercles are in profile. The fibular head is demonstrated approximately 0.5 inch (1.25 cm) distal to the tibial plateau.
- The intercondylar fossa is at the center of the exposure field.
- The distal femur, proximal tibia, and intercondylar fossa eminence and tubercles are included within the collimated field.

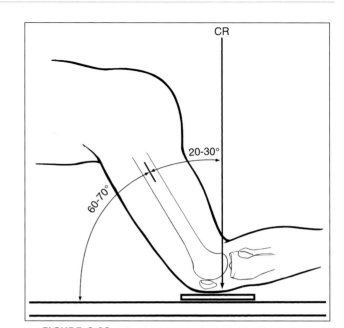

FIGURE 6-93 PA axial knee projection. CR, Central ray.

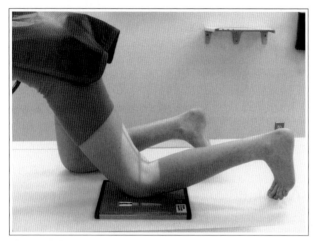

FIGURE 6-92 Proper patient positioning for PA axial knee projection (Holmblad Method).

ray form a 20- to 30-degree angle (femur–imaging table angle is 60 to 70 degrees; Figures 6-92 and 6-93). The IR is positioned under the affected knee.

- *Mechanics of PA axial projection.* To understand how the femur is positioned for this image, study a femoral skeletal bone. Place the femoral bone upright with the distal femoral condylar surfaces resting against a flat surface. While imaging the posterior femoral surface, lean the femur anteriorly until the intercondylar fossa is positioned in profile. In this PA axial projection, note how the femoral shaft inclines medially approximately 10 to 15 degrees. The amount of inclination the femoral bone displays depends on the length of the femoral shaft and the width of the pelvis from which the femur originated. The longer the femur and the wider the pelvis, the more femoral inclination is demonstrated. To obtain an image of the intercondylar fossa with superimposed medial and superimposed lateral surfaces, this inclination should not be offset. If the inclination is offset by shifting the distal femur laterally or the proximal femur medially and positioning the femur

vertically, the medial and lateral aspects of the intercondylar fossa are not superimposed and the patella is situated laterally (see Image 77). This can be demonstrated by placing the femoral skeleton bone vertically and imaging the change in the demonstration of the intercondylar fossa.

- *Effect of foot mispositioning.* Mispositioning of the patient's foot may also result in rotation of the femur and may demonstrate the medial and the lateral aspects of the intercondylar fossa without superimposition. The long axis of the patient's foot should be positioned perpendicular to the imaging table. If the heel was allowed to rotate medially (internally), the medial and lateral aspects of the intercondylar fossa are not superimposed, and the patella is rotated laterally (see Image 77). If the heel was rotated laterally (externally), the medial and lateral aspects of the intercondylar fossa are not superimposed, the patella is demonstrated medially, and the tibia is demonstrated without fibular head superimposition (see Image 78).

The proximal surfaces of the intercondylar fossa are superimposed, and the patellar apex is demonstrated proximal to the intercondylar fossa.

- The proximal surfaces of the intercondylar fossa are superimposed when the femoral shaft is placed at a 60- to 70-degree angle with the imaging table (see Figure 6-92). To study this relationship better, place a femoral skeleton bone in the PA axial projection. While viewing the posterior intercondylar fossa, move the proximal femur closer to and farther away from the imaging table. Note how the proximal surfaces of the fossa are in profile and superimposed only when the femur is at a 60- to 70-degree angle with the imaging table. The position of the femur with respect to the imaging table also determines the position of the patella (see earlier AP knee projection discussion and Figure 6-74). As the knee is flexed (the proximal femur is brought away from the imaging table), the patella moves distally onto the patellar surface of the femur and into the intercondylar fossa. The degree of knee flexion used for the PA axial projection situates the patella just proximal to the fossa.

- *Effect of femur positioning.* If a PA axial projection is obtained that demonstrates the proximal intercondylar fossa's surfaces without superimposition, view the patella's position to determine whether the patient's proximal femur was positioned too close to or too far from the imaging table. If the patellar apex is demonstrated within the fossa, the knee was overflexed (proximal femur positioned too far away from the imaging table; see Image 79). If the patella is demonstrated laterally and proximal to the fossa, the knee was underflexed (proximal femur position too close to the table; see Image 80).

The knee joint space is open and the tibial plateau and intercondylar eminence and tubercles are in profile. The fibular head is demonstrated approximately 0.5 inch (1.25 cm) distal to the tibial plateau.

- To obtain an open knee joint space and demonstrate the tibial plateau and intercondylar eminence and tubercles in profile, dorsiflex the patient's foot and rest the foot on the toes. Because the tibial plateau slopes downward from the anterior tibial margin to the posterior margin, this positioning is necessary to elevate the distal tibia and align the anterior and posterior tibial margins perpendicular to the IR. If the foot is not dorsiflexed and resting on the toes, the knee joint space is narrowed or closed and the tibial plateau is demonstrated (see Images 78 and 80).
- *Determining repositioning for closed knee joint.* If a PA axial knee projection is obtained that demonstrates a closed or narrowed knee joint space and the tibial plateau surface, evaluate the proximity of the fibular head to the tibial plateau to determine the needed adjustment. If the fibular is head is less than 0.5 inch (1.25 cm) from the tibial plateau (see Image 78), the distal lower leg needs to be depressed. If the fibular head is more than 0.5 inch (1.25 cm) from the tibial plateau (see Image 80), the distal lower leg needs to be elevated. The amount of lower leg adjustment required would be half the distance needed to bring the fibular head to within 0.5 inch (1.25 cm) of the tibial plateau. The small amount of lower leg adjustment that would be needed can be accomplished by varying the degree of foot dorsiflexion or plantar flexion.

The intercondylar fossa is at the center of the exposure field. The distal femur, proximal tibia, and intercondylar fossa eminence and tubercles are included within the collimated field.

- Center a perpendicular central ray to the midline of the knee, at a level 1 inch (2.5 cm) distal to the palpable medial femoral epicondyle, to place the intercondylar fossa in the center of the exposure field. Open the longitudinal collimation enough to include the femoral epicondyles. Transverse collimation should be to within 0.5 inch (1.25 cm) of the knee skin line.
- An 8- × 10-inch (18- × 24-cm) screen-film or computed radiography IR placed lengthwise should be adequate to include all the required anatomic structures.

Posteroanterior Axial Knee Projection Analysis

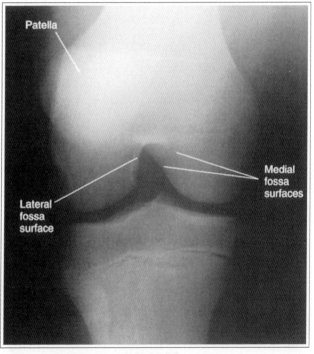

IMAGE 77

Analysis. The medial and the lateral aspects of the intercondylar fossa are not superimposed, and the patella is situated laterally. Either the proximal femur was too medially situated, causing the femur to be too vertical or the heel was rotated medially.

Correction. Position the proximal femur laterally allowing the femur to incline medially, and align the long axis of the patient's foot perpendicular to the imaging table.

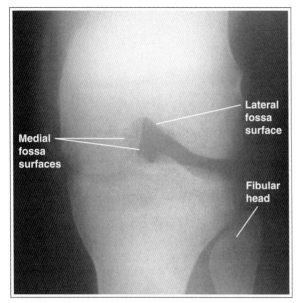

IMAGE 78

Analysis. The medial and lateral aspects of the intercondylar fossa are not superimposed, the patella is situated medially, and the tibia is demonstrated without fibular head superimposition. The heel was laterally rotated. The knee joint is obscured, the tibial plateau is demonstrated, and the fibula is positioned closer than 0.5 inch (1.25 cm) to the tibial plateau.

Correction. Rotate the heel medially until the foot's long axis is aligned perpendicular to the imaging table and depress the distal lower leg by decreasing the amount of foot dorsiflexion.

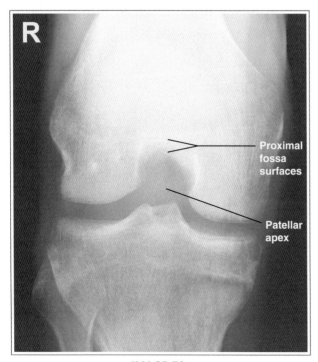

IMAGE 79

Analysis. The proximal surfaces of the intercondylar fossa are demonstrated without superimposition, and the patella is positioned within the intercondylar fossa. The knee was overflexed (femur positioned too far away from the imaging table).

Correction. Extend the knee (position the proximal femur closer to the imaging table). The amount of movement needed is half the distance demonstrated between the anterior and posterior proximal intercondylar fossa's surfaces.

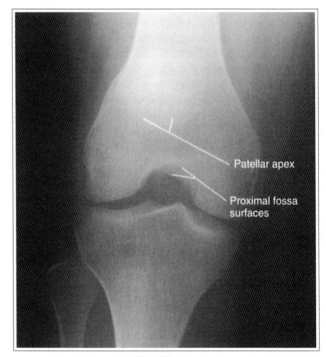

IMAGE 80

Analysis. The proximal intercondylar fossa's surfaces are demonstrated without superimposition, and the patella is positioned too far proximal to the fossa. The knee was underflexed (femur positioned too close to the imaging table). The knee joint is obscured, the tibial plateau is demonstrated, and the fibular head is shown more than 0.5 inch (1.25 cm) from the tibial plateau.

Correction. Flex the knee (position the femur farther away from the imaging table) and elevate the distal lower leg by increasing the amount of foot dorsiflexion.

INTERCONDYLAR FOSSA: ANTEROPOSTERIOR AXIAL PROJECTION (BÉCLÈRE METHOD)

See Figure 6-94 and Box 6-19.

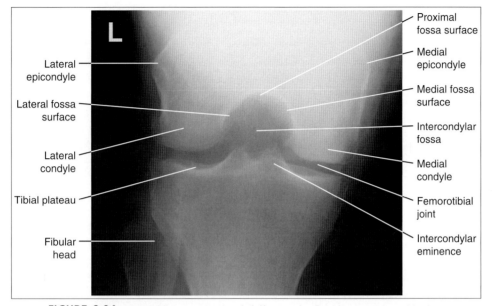

Lateral epicondyle

Lateral fossa surface

Lateral condyle

Tibial plateau

Fibular head

Proximal fossa surface

Medial epicondyle

Medial fossa surface

Intercondylar fossa

Medial condyle

Femorotibial joint

Intercondylar eminence

FIGURE 6-94 AP axial knee projection (Béclère method) with accurate positioning.

BOX 6-19 | **Anteroposterior Axial Intercondylar Fossa Projection (Béclère Method) Analysis Criteria**

- The intercondylar fossa is shown in its entirety, the medial and lateral surfaces of the intercondylar fossa and the femoral epicondyles are in profile, and the tibia is partially superimposed over the fibular head.
- The proximal surface of the intercondylar fossa is in profile and the patellar apex is demonstrated proximal to the fossa.
- The knee joint space is open, the anterior and posterior condylar margins of the tibia are superimposed, the intercondylar eminence and tubercles are in profile, and the fibular head is demonstrated approximately 0.5 inch (1.25 cm) distal to the tibial plateau.
- The intercondylar fossa is at the center of the exposure field.
- The distal femur, proximal tibia, and intercondylar fossa eminence and tubercles are included within the collimated field.

The intercondylar fossa is shown in its entirety, the medial and lateral surfaces of the intercondylar fossa and the femoral epicondyles are in profile, and the tibia is partially superimposed over the fibular head.

- The AP axial projection (Béclère method) is performed by placing the patient on the imaging table in a supine position, with the affected hip and knee in an AP projection and flexed until the long axis of the femur is at a 60-degree angle with the imaging table. Then, adjust the lower leg until the knee is flexed approximately 45 degrees (Figure 6-95). A curved or regular IR is positioned under the knee and is elevated on an immobilization device until it is as close to the posterior knee as possible

and the central ray is aligned parallel with the tibial plateau.

- To demonstrate the intercondylar fossa in its entirety, with superimposed medial and lateral surfaces, the patient's knee needs to be in an AP projection. This is accomplished by internally rotating the leg until an imaginary line connecting the medial and lateral femoral epicondyles is positioned parallel with the imaging table.
- *Effect of rotation.* If the femoral epicondyles are not positioned parallel with the IR, the medial and lateral surfaces of the intercondylar fossa will not be superimposed and in profile, and the intercondylar fossa will not be fully demonstrated. The direction of poor knee rotation can be detected by evaluating the degree of tibial and fibular superimposition and the difference in femoral condylar width. It the patient's leg is not internally rotated enough, the medial femoral condyle appears larger than the lateral condyle and the tibia demonstrates increased fibular superimposition (see Image 81). If the patient's leg is internally rotated more than the amount needed to align the femoral epicondyles parallel with the IR, the lateral femoral condyle will appear larger than the medial condyle, and the tibia will demonstrate decreased superimposition (see Image 82).

The proximal surface of the intercondylar fossa is in profile, and the patellar apex is demonstrated superior to the fossa.

- The proximal surface of the intercondylar fossa is in profile when the central ray is aligned parallel

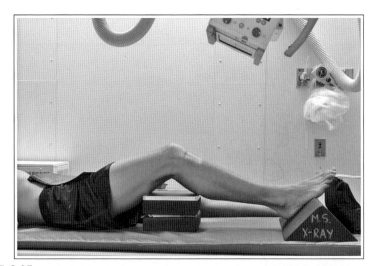

FIGURE 6-95 Proper patient positioning for AP axial projection (Béclère method) knee image.

with it. This is accomplished when the long axis of the femur is flexed at a 60-degree angle with the imaging table.

- *Adjusting for poor proximal intercondylar fossa visualization.* With a set central ray, poor alignment of the proximal surface occurs when the femur is aligned more or less than 60 degrees with the imaging table. If an AP axial projection is achieved and the proximal intercondylar fossa surfaces are demonstrated without superimposition, view the patella apex's position to determine how femoral flexion would need to be adjusted to obtain accurate positioning and demonstrate the entire intercondylar fossa. As the knee is flexed, the patella shifts distally onto the patellar surface of the femur and then into the intercondylar fossa. Therefore, if the long axis of the femur is aligned more than 60 degrees with the imaging table, resulting in increased knee flexion, the patellar apex will be demonstrated within the intercondylar fossa (see Image 83). If the long axis of the femur is aligned less than 60 degrees with the imaging table, resulting in less knee flexion, the proximal intercondylar fossa surfaces will not be aligned and the patellar apex will be shown above the intercondylar fossa (see Image 84).

The knee joint space is open, the anterior and posterior condylar margins of the tibia are superimposed, the intercondylar eminence and tubercles are in profile, and the fibular head is demonstrated approximately 0.5 inch (1.25 cm) distal to the tibial plateau.

- To obtain an open knee joint space and demonstrate the intercondylar eminence and tubercles in profile, the central ray must be aligned parallel with the tibial plateau. This alignment is obtained by first positioning the central ray perpendicular with the anterior lower leg surface and then decreasing the obtained angulation by 5 degrees. The 5-degree decrease is needed because the tibial plateau slopes distally by 5 degrees from the anterior condylar margin to the posterior condylar margin.

- *Effect of poor lower leg positioning.* If an AP axial projection demonstrates a closed or narrowed knee joint space, evaluate the proximity of the fibular head to the tibial plateau. If the fibular head is demonstrated more than 0.5 inch (1.25 cm) distal to the tibial plateau, the distal lower leg was elevated too high or the central ray was too cephalically angled (see Image 85). If the fibular head is demonstrated less than 0.5 inch (1.25 cm) distal to the tibial plateau, the distal lower leg was too depressed or the central ray was too caudally angled (see Image 86).

The intercondylar fossa is at the center of the exposure field. The distal femur, proximal tibia, and intercondylar fossa eminence and tubercles are included within the collimated field.

- Center the central ray to the midline of the knee, at a level 1 inch (2.5 cm) distal to the palpable medial femoral epicondyle, to place the intercondylar fossa in the center of the exposure field. Open the longitudinal collimation enough to include the femoral epicondyles. Transverse collimation should be to within 0.5 inch (1.25 cm) of the knee skin line.

- An 8- × 10-inch (18- × 24-cm) IR placed crosswise or a curved IR should be adequate to include all the required anatomic structures. A curved IR that is built up on an immobilization device enough to place the IR adjacent to the affected knee will demonstrate the least amount of magnification and distortion of the image. If a curved IR is unavailable, an 8- × 10-inch (18- × 24-cm) screen-film or computed radiography IR should be positioned crosswise and built up on an immobilization device, bringing it as close as possible to the affected knee.

Anteroposterior Axial Intercondylar Fossa Projection Analysis

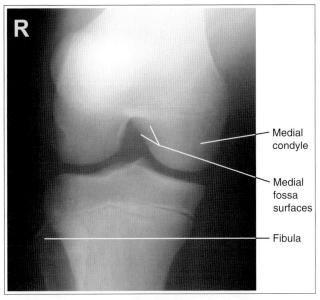

IMAGE 81

Analysis. The medial and the lateral aspects of the intercondylar fossa are not superimposed, the medial femoral condyle is larger than the lateral condyle, and the fibular head demonstrates increased tibial superimposition. The patient's leg was externally rotated.

Correction. Internally rotate the leg until an imaginary line connecting the femoral epicondyles is aligned parallel with the imaging table.

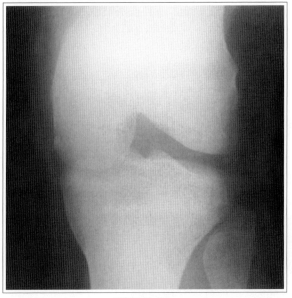

IMAGE 82

Analysis. The medial and lateral aspects of the intercondylar fossa are not superimposed, the lateral femoral condyle is larger than the medial condyle, and the fibular head demonstrates no tibial superimposition. The patient's leg was internally rotated. The knee joint space

is closed, and the fibular head is shown more than 0.5 inch (1.25 cm) distal to the tibial plateau. The distal lower leg was elevated too high, or the central ray was angled too cephalically.

Correction. Externally rotate the leg until an imaginary line connecting the femoral epicondyles is aligned parallel with the imaging table, and depress the distal lower leg until the knee is flexed 45 degrees or adjust the central ray angle caudally.

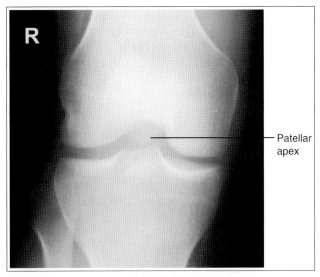

IMAGE 83

Analysis. The proximal surfaces of the intercondylar fossa are not superimposed and the patellar apex is demonstrated within the intercondylar fossa. The long axis of the femur was aligned at more than a 60-degree angle with the imaging table.

Correction. Decrease the degree of hip and knee flexion until the long axis of the femur is aligned 60 degrees with the imaging table.

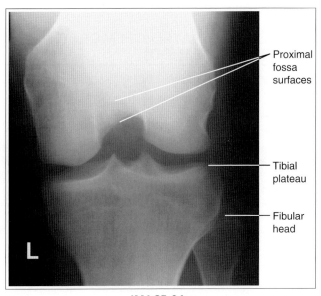

IMAGE 84

Analysis. The proximal surfaces of the intercondylar fossa are not superimposed, and the patellar apex is demonstrated proximal to the intercondylar fossa. The long axis of the femur was aligned at less than a 60-degree angle with the imaging table. The knee joint is closed, and the fibular head is demonstrated more than 0.5 inch (1.25 cm) distal to the tibial plateau. The distal lower leg was elevated too high, or the central ray was angled too cephalically.

Correction. Increase the degree of hip and knee flexion until the long axis of the femur is aligned 60 degrees with the imaging table. Depress the distal lower leg until the knee is flexed 45 degrees, or adjust the central ray caudally.

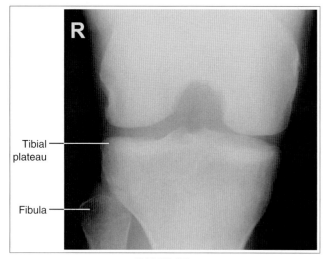

IMAGE 85

Analysis. The knee joint is closed, and the fibular head is demonstrated more than 0.5 inch (1.25 cm) distal to the tibial plateau. The distal lower leg was elevated too high, or the central ray was angled too cephalically.

Correction. Depress the distal lower leg until the knee is flexed 45 degrees, or adjust the central ray caudally.

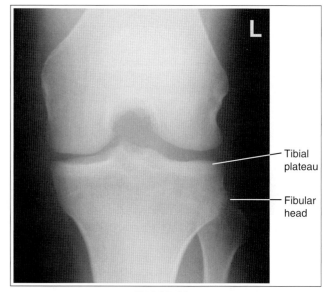

IMAGE 86

Analysis. The knee joint is closed, and the fibular head is demonstrated less than 0.5 inch (1.25 cm) distal to the tibial plateau. The distal lower leg was depressed, or the central ray was angled too caudally.

Correction. Elevate the distal lower leg until the knee is flexed 45 degrees, or adjust the central ray cephalically.

PATELLA AND PATELLOFEMORAL JOINT: TANGENTIAL PROJECTION (MERCHANT METHOD)

See Figure 6-96 and Box 6-20.

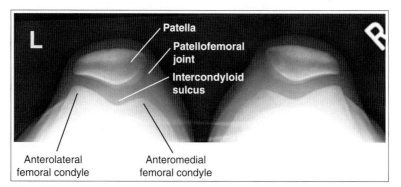

FIGURE 6-96 Tangential knee projection (Merchant method) with accurate positioning.

BOX 6-20	Tangential Patella and Patellofemoral Joint Projection (Merchant Method) Projection Analysis Criteria

- The patellae, anterior femoral condyles, and intercondylar sulci are seen superiorly, and the lateral femoral condyle demonstrates slightly more height than the medial condyle.
- The patellofemoral joint spaces are open with no superimposition of the upper anterior thigh soft tissue, patellae, or tibial tuberosities.
- A point midway between the patellofemoral joint spaces is at the center of the exposure field.
- The patellae, anterior femoral condyles, and intercondylar sulci are included within the collimated field.

Scatter radiation is controlled.

- An optimal 60- to 70-kVp technique sufficiently penetrates the bony and soft tissue structures of the knee and provides high image contrast. If it is necessary to increase the kilovoltage above 70 to penetrate a thicker knee, a grid is not needed, as described earlier for this examination, because of the long object–image receptor distance (OID). When a long OID is used, scatter radiation that would expose the IR when a short OID is used is scattered at a direction away from the IR. Because scatter radiation is not being directed toward the IR, a grid is not needed to absorb the scatter. This is also referred to as the air-gap technique.

The knee demonstrates no rotation. The patellae, anterior femoral condyles, and intercondylar sulci are demonstrated superiorly, and the lateral femoral condyle demonstrates slightly more height than the medial condyle.

- The tangential projection (Merchant method) uses an axial viewer knee-supporting device, as shown in Figure 6-97. This freestanding device maintains the knees at a set degree of flexion, provides straps that restrain the patient's legs, and contains an IR holder that keeps the receptor at the proper angle with the central ray. To obtain a tangential projection of the patellae, place the patient supine on the imaging table with the legs dangling off the end of the table. Set the axial viewer at a standard 45-degree angle, and position it at the end of the imaging table beneath the patient's knees and calves. Situate the patient's ankles between the viewer's receptor holder, and place the receptor on the ankles so that it rests against the viewer's receptor holder (see Figure 6-97).

To demonstrate the knees without rotation and to position the patellae, anterior femoral condyles, and intercondylar sulci superiorly, internally rotate the patient's legs until the palpable femoral epicondyles are aligned parallel with the imaging table. Then, secure the legs in this position by wrapping the axial viewer's Velcro straps around the patient's calves. This positioning places the distal femurs in an AP projection with the imaging table. Because the lateral condyles are situated anterior to the medial condyles, the lateral condyles demonstrate more height on a tangential projection if the legs are adequately rotated. If the legs are not sufficiently rotated, the patellae are situated laterally, and either the anterior femoral condyles demonstrate equal height or the medial condyles demonstrate greater height than the lateral condyles (see Image 87). Both knees may not be rotated equally; often, only one knee is rotated.

- *Patellar position on a tangential projection.* Because this image is taken to demonstrate subluxation (partial dislocation) of the patella, the position of the patellae above the intercondylar sulci on a tangential (axial) projection may vary.

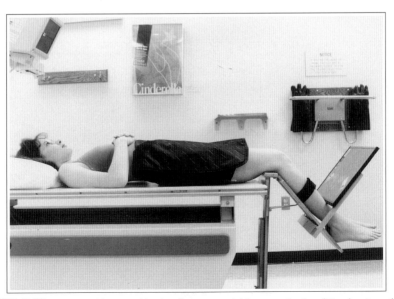

FIGURE 6-97 Proper patient positioning for tangential knee projection (Merchant method).

In a normal knee, the patella is directly above the intercondylar sulcus on a tangential projection, as shown in Figure 6-96. With patellar subluxation, the patella is lateral to the intercondylar sulcus, as shown in Image 88. Do not mistake a subluxed patella for knee rotation. Although both conditions result in a laterally positioned patella, the rotated knee demonstrates the femoral condyles at the same height, whereas with a subluxed patella the lateral condyle is higher than the medial condyle.

- *Positioning to demonstrate patellar subluxation.* To demonstrate patellar subluxation, the quadriceps femoris (four muscles that surround the femoral bone) must be in a relaxed position. This is accomplished by instructing the patient to relax the leg muscles, allowing the calf straps to maintain the internal leg rotation. If the patient does not relax the quadriceps muscles, a patella that would be subluxed on relaxation of the muscles will appear normal.

The patellofemoral joint spaces are open, with no superimposition of the upper anterior thigh soft tissue, patellae, or tibial tuberosities.

- The position of the patient's legs on the axial viewer must be precise for an open patellofemoral joint space to be obtained. The height of the axial viewer is adjustable. It should be set to a height that positions the long axis of the patient's femurs parallel with the table. If the distal femurs are positioned closer to the table than the proximal femurs, the angled central ray traverses the anterior thigh soft tissue, projecting it into the patellofemoral joint space (Figure 6-98 and Image 89). Although the patellofemoral joint space remains open on such an image, the space is underexposed.
- *Knee relationship to axial viewer.* The relationship of the patient's posterior knee curves to the bend of the axial viewer determines whether the central ray will be parallel with the patellofemoral joint spaces. To demonstrate open patellofemoral joint spaces, position the posterior curves of the knees directly above the bend in the axial viewer, as shown in Figure 6-99. If the posterior curves of the knees are situated at or below the bend of the axial viewer (causing the knees to be flexed more than the degree that is set on the axial viewer), the central ray is not parallel with the patellofemoral joint space, and the patellae are resting against the intercondylar sulci (Figure 6-100; see Image 90). If the posterior curves of the knees are situated too far above the bend of the axial viewer (causing the knees to be extended more than the degree set on the axial viewer), the tibial tuberosities are demonstrated within the patellofemoral joint space (Figure 6-101; see Image 91).
- *Positioning and central ray angulation for large calves.* The tibial tuberosities may also be demonstrated within the patellofemoral joint spaces in a patient with large posterior calves, even when the posterior knee curves have been accurately positioned to the bend of the axial viewer. The knees of a patient with large calves are not flexed as much as the axial viewer degree is set. For such patients, the central ray angulation should be increased (5 to 10 degrees) or the axial viewer's angulation should be decreased until the knees are flexed 45 degrees.
- *Determining central ray angulation.* The angle of the central ray and angle placed on the axial viewer also determine how well the patellofemoral joint space is demonstrated. Although 45 degrees is the standard angle, the reviewer is capable of supporting the leg at 30-, 60-, or 75-degree angles as well. Each of these angles requires a predetermined central ray angulation if an open patellofemoral joint is to be obtained.

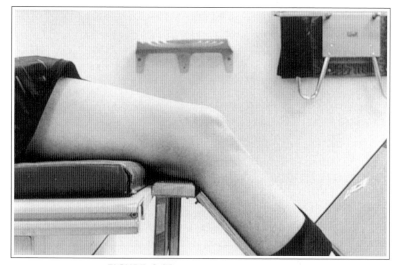

FIGURE 6-98 Poor femur positioning.

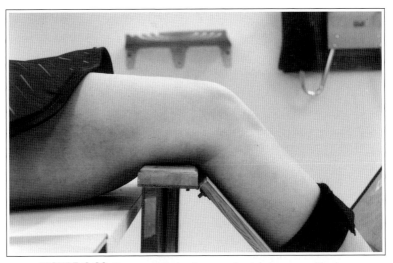

FIGURE 6-99 Proper posterior knee and axial viewer positioning.

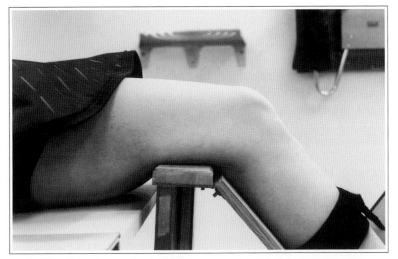

FIGURE 6-100 Posterior knee curve situated below bend in axial viewer.

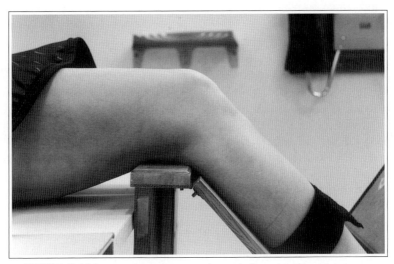

FIGURE 6-101 Posterior knee curve situated above bend in axial viewer.

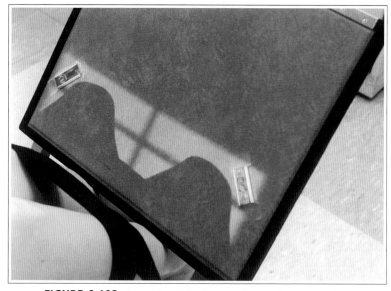

FIGURE 6-102 Proper knee shadows and central ray centering.

The easiest way to determine the central ray angle to use for the different axial viewer angles is to know that the sum of the central ray angle and the axial viewer's angle must equal 105 degrees. For example, if the axial viewer is set at 30 degrees, the central ray angulation must be set at 75 degrees (30 + 75 = 105).

- *Using light field shadow to evaluate positioning.* Evaluate the shadow of the knees that is created on the receptor when the centering light is on before exposing the IR. When the patient has been accurately positioned, these shadows will display oval silhouettes with indentations on each side that outline the patellae (Figure 6-102).

A point midway between the patellofemoral joint spaces is at the center of the exposure field. The patellae, anterior femoral condyles, and intercondylar sulci are included within the collimated field.

- A standard 60-degree caudally angled central ray is centered between the knees at the level of the patellofemoral joint spaces to place the patellofemoral joint spaces in the center of the collimated field (see Figure 6-102). An SID of 72 inches (183 cm) is generally used to offset the magnification caused by the long OID.
- Open the longitudinal collimated field to include the patellae and the distal femurs. Transverse collimation should be to within 0.5 inch (1.25 cm) of the lateral knee skin line.
- A 10- × 12-inch (24- × 30-cm) or 11- × 14-inch (28- × 35-cm) screen-film or computed radiography IR placed crosswise should be adequate to include all the required anatomic structures.

Tangential Patella Projection (Merchant Method) Analysis

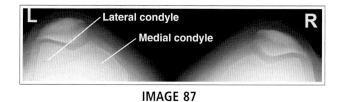

IMAGE 87

Analysis. The patellae are demonstrated directly above the intercondylar sulci and are rotated laterally. The medial femoral condyles demonstrate more height than the lateral condyles. The legs were externally rotated.

Correction. Internally rotate the patient's legs until the patellae are situated superiorly, and then restrain the legs by wrapping the axial viewer's Velcro straps around the calves.

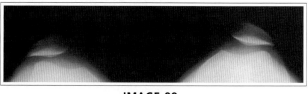

IMAGE 88

Analysis. The femoral condyles are visible superiorly, with the lateral femoral condyles demonstrating more height than the medial condyles. The patellae appear lateral to the intercondylar sulci and demonstrate subluxation.

Correction. No positioning movement is needed.

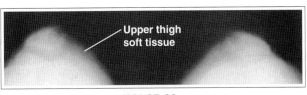

IMAGE 89

Analysis. Soft tissue from the patient's anterior thighs has been projected onto the patellae and patellofemoral joint spaces. The height of the axial viewer was not set high enough to position the femurs parallel with the table. The distal femurs were positioned closer to the table than the proximal femurs, as shown in Figure 6-98.

Correction. Increase the height of the axial viewer until the long axes of the femurs are positioned parallel with the table, as shown in Figure 6-97.

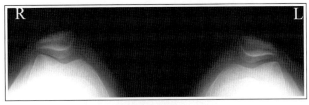

IMAGE 90

Analysis. The patellae are resting against the intercondylar sulci, obscuring the patellofemoral joint spaces. The patient's posterior knee curve was positioned at or below the bend on the axial viewer, as shown in Figure 6-100.

Correction. Slide the patient's knees away from the axial viewer until the patient's posterior knee curvature is just superior to the bend of the reviewer, as shown in Figure 6-99.

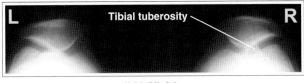

IMAGE 91

Analysis. The tibial tuberosities are demonstrated within the patellofemoral joint spaces. Either the posterior knee curve was positioned too far above the axial viewer's bend, as shown in Figure 6-101, or the patient has large posterior calves.

Correction. Slide the knees toward the axial viewer until the posterior knee curvature is just superior to the bend on the viewer, as shown in Figure 6-99. If the patient was accurately positioned but the calves are large, increase (by 5 to 10 degrees) the central ray angulation or decrease the axial viewer's angulation until the knees are flexed 45 degrees. The total sum of the axial viewer's angle and the central ray angulation will be less than 105 degrees.

FEMUR: ANTEROPOSTERIOR PROJECTION

See Figures 6-103 and 6-104 and Boxes 6-21 and 6-22.

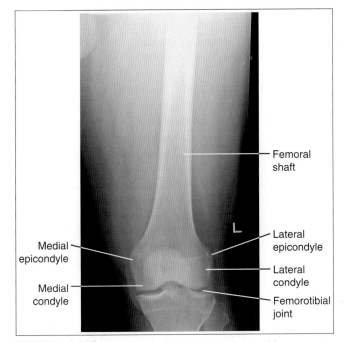

FIGURE 6-103 AP distal femur projection with accurate positioning.

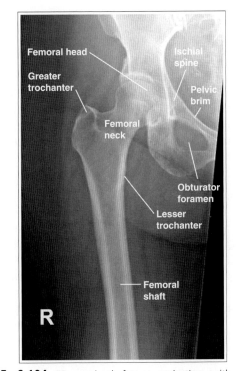

FIGURE 6-104 AP proximal femur projection with accurate positioning.

BOX 6-21	**Anteroposterior Distal Femur Projection Analysis Criteria**

- Image density is uniform across the femur.
- The medial and lateral epicondyles are in profile, the femoral condyles are symmetrical in shape, and the tibia is superimposed over 0.25 inch (0.6 cm) of the fibular head.
- The knee joint space is open but narrowed, and the anterior and posterior margins of the proximal tibia are superimposed.
- The distal femoral shaft is at the center of the exposure field.
- The distal femoral shaft and surrounding femoral soft tissue, the knee joint, and 1 inch (2.5 cm) of the lower leg are included within the collimated field. Any orthopedic apparatus located at the knee is included in its entirety.

BOX 6-22	**Anteroposterior Proximal Femur Projection Analysis Criteria**

- Image density is uniform across the femur.
- The ischial spine is aligned with the pelvic brim, and the obturator foramen is open.
- The femoral neck is demonstrated without foreshortening, the greater trochanter is in profile laterally, and the lesser trochanter is completely superimposed by the proximal femur.
- The proximal femoral shaft is at the center of the exposure field.
- The proximal femoral shaft, hip, and surrounding femoral soft tissue are included within the collimated field. Any orthopedic apparatus located at the hip is included in its entirety.

Image density is uniform across the femur.

- Position the thicker proximal femur at the cathode end of the tube and the thinner distal femur at the anode end to take advantage of the anode heel effect and obtain more uniform density across the femur.

Distal Femur

The distal femur demonstrates an AP projection. The medial and lateral femoral epicondyles are in profile, the femoral condyles are symmetrical in shape, and the tibia is superimposed over 0.25 inch (0.6 cm) of the fibular head.

- To obtain an AP distal femoral projection, place the patient in a supine position with the knee fully extended. Internally rotate the leg until the foot is rotated to a 15- to 20-degree angle and an imaginary line drawn between the medial and lateral femoral epicondyles is positioned parallel with the IR (Figures 6-105 and 6-106). This positioning places the medial and lateral femoral epicondyles at equal distances from the IR, as well as medially and laterally in profile, respectively. It also centers the intercondylar eminence within the intercondylar fossa.

- *Effect of leg rotation.* If the femoral epicondyles are not positioned parallel with the IR, an AP projection has not been obtained. If the leg was not

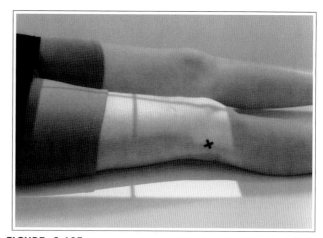

FIGURE 6-105 Proper patient positioning for AP distal femur projection. X indicates lateral femoral epicondyle.

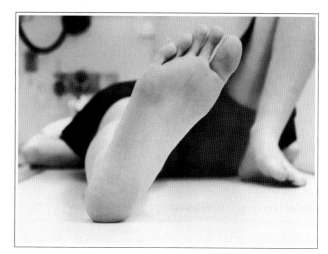

FIGURE 6-106 Proper foot rotation.

externally (laterally) rotated enough to place the epicondyles at equal distances from the IR, the epicondyles are not in profile, the medial femoral condyle is larger than the lateral condyle, and the tibia is superimposed over more than 0.25 inch (0.6 cm) of the fibular head (see Image 92). If the leg was internally (medially) rotated more than needed to place the femoral epicondyles at equal distances from the IR, the epicondyles are not demonstrated in profile, the lateral femoral condyle is larger than the medial condyle, and the tibia is superimposed over less than 0.25 inch (0.6 cm) of the fibular head (see Image 93).

- *Positioning for femoral fracture.* When a patient has a fractured femur, the leg should not be internally rotated, but left as is. Forced internal rotation of a fractured femur may injure the blood vessels and nerves that surround the injured area. Because the leg is not internally rotated when a fracture is in question, the distal femur demonstrates external rotation.

The knee joint space is open but narrowed, and the anterior and posterior margins of the proximal tibia are superimposed.

- An open knee joint space is obtained when the anterior and posterior margins of the proximal tibia are superimposed. Because these margins slope distally from the anterior condylar margin to the posterior condylar margin, and the central ray is centered proximal to the knee joint, x-rays that diverge toward the proximal tibia are aligned close enough to parallel with the slope of the tibia to result in an open joint space. The joint space is narrower because the diverged x-rays project the distal femur partially into the joint space.

The distal femoral shaft is at the center of the exposure field. The distal femoral shaft and surrounding femoral soft tissue, the knee joint, and 1 inch (2.5 cm) of the lower leg are included within the collimated field. Any orthopedic apparatus located at the knee is included in its entirety.

- A perpendicular central ray is centered to the distal femoral shaft to place the shaft in the center of the image. This is accomplished by positioning the lower edge of the receptor approximately 2 inches (5 cm) below the knee joint; the knee joint is located 1 inch (2.5 cm) distal to the medial epicondyle. This lower positioning is needed to prevent the diverged x-ray beams from projecting the knee joint off the IR.
- The longitudinal collimation should be left open the full length of the IR used. Transverse collimation should be to within 0.5 inch (1.25 cm) of the lateral femoral skin line.
- A 14- × 17-inch (35- × 43-cm) screen-film or computed radiography IR placed lengthwise should be adequate to include all the required anatomic structures.
- *Examination of the entire femur.* If the entire femur is of interest and images are taken of the distal and proximal ends of the femur, the images should demonstrate at least 2 inches (5 cm) of femoral shaft overlap. Any orthopedic appliance, such as an intramedullary rod, should be included in its entirety.

Proximal Femur

The pelvis demonstrates an AP projection. The ischial spine is aligned with the pelvic brim, and the obturator foramen is open.

- An AP projection of the pelvis is obtained by placing the patient supine on the imaging table with the legs extended (Figure 6-107). To ensure that the pelvis is not rotated, judge the distance from the ASIS to the imaging table on both sides of the patient. The distances should be equal.
- *Detecting pelvic rotation.* Rotation of the pelvis on an AP femur projection is detected by evaluating the

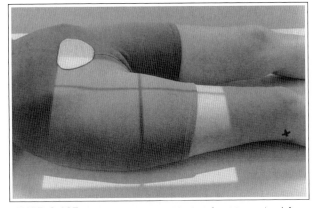

FIGURE 6-107 Proper patient positioning for AP proximal femur projection.

relationship of the ischial spine and the pelvic brim and visualization of the obturator foramen. When the pelvis has been rotated toward the affected femur, the ischial spine is demonstrated without pelvic brim superimposition and visualization of the obturator foramen is decreased (see Chapter 7, Image 1). When the pelvis has been rotated away from the affected femur, the ischial spine is not aligned with the pelvic brim but is demonstrated closer to the acetabulum, and demonstration of the obturator foramen is increased (see Chapter 7, Image 2).

The femoral neck is demonstrated without foreshortening, the greater trochanter is in profile laterally, and the lesser trochanter is completely superimposed by the proximal femur.

- The positions of the patient's foot and femoral epicondyle with respect to the imaging table determine how the femoral neck and trochanters appear on an AP femoral projection.
- *Effect of leg and foot rotation.* Generally, when a patient is relaxed, the legs and feet are externally (laterally) rotated. On external rotation, the femoral neck inclines posteriorly (toward the imaging table) and is foreshortened on an AP femoral projection. Increased external rotation increases the degree of posterior decline and foreshortening of the femoral neck on the image. If the patient's leg was externally (laterally) rotated enough to position the foot at a 45-degree angle and an imaginary line connecting the femoral epicondyles at a 60- to 65-degree angle with the imaging table, the femoral neck is demonstrated on end and the lesser trochanter is demonstrated in profile (Figure 6-108). If the patient's leg is positioned with the foot placed vertically and an imaginary line connecting the femoral epicondyles at approximately a 15- to 20-degree angle with the imaging table, the lesser trochanter is demonstrated in partial profile and the femoral neck is only partially foreshortened (see Image 94).

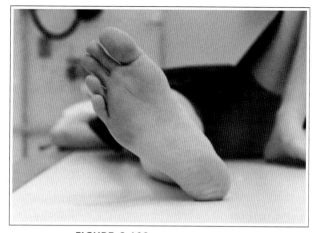

FIGURE 6-108 Poor foot rotation.

For a proximal AP femur projection, which shows the femoral neck without foreshortening and the greater trochanter in profile, the patient's leg should be internally rotated until the foot is tilted 15 to 20 degrees from vertical and the femoral epicondyles are positioned parallel with the imaging table (see Figures 6-106 and 6-107).

- *Positioning for fracture.* When a patient has a fractured proximal femur, the leg should not be internally rotated, but left as is. Forced internal rotation of a fractured proximal femur may injure the blood vessels and nerves that surround the injured area. Because the patient's leg is not internally rotated when a fracture is in question, such an AP femoral projection demonstrates the femoral neck with some degree of foreshortening and the lesser trochanter without femoral shaft superimposition (see Image 95).

The proximal femoral shaft is at the center of the exposure field. The proximal femoral shaft, hip, and surrounding femoral soft tissue are included within the collimated field. Any orthopedic apparatus located at the hip is included in its entirety.

- A perpendicular central ray is centered to the proximal femoral shaft to place it in the center of the image. This is accomplished by positioning the upper edge of the receptor at the level of the ASIS. If the collimated head can be moved, turn it until one of its axes is aligned with the long axis of the femur.
- The longitudinal collimation should be left open the full length of the IR. Transverse collimation should be to within 0.5 inch (1.25 cm) of the lateral femoral skin line. The surrounding femoral soft tissue should be included to allow detection of subcutaneous air or hematomas.
- A 14- × 17-inch (35- × 43-cm) screen-film or computed radiography IR placed lengthwise should be adequate to include all the required anatomic structures.

Anteroposterior Femur Projection Analysis

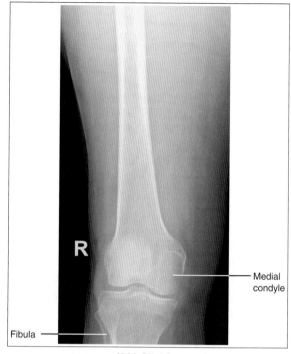

IMAGE 92

Analysis. The femoral epicondyles are not in profile, the medial femoral condyle appears larger than the lateral condyle, and the intercondylar eminence is not centered within the intercondylar fossa. The leg was externally rotated.

Correction. Internally rotate the leg until the femoral epicondyles are at equal distances from the IR.

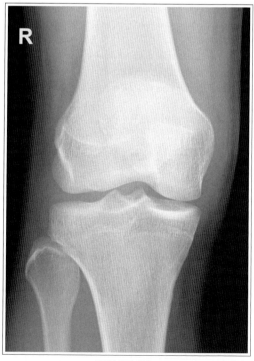

IMAGE 93

Analysis. This is a knee image but it can be evaluated as if it were a distal femur. The femoral epicondyles are not in profile, the lateral femoral condyle appears larger than the medial condyle, and the tibia is superimposed over less than 0.25 inch (0.6 cm) of the fibular head. The leg was internally rotated.

Correction. Externally rotate the leg until the femoral epicondyles are at equal distances from the IR.

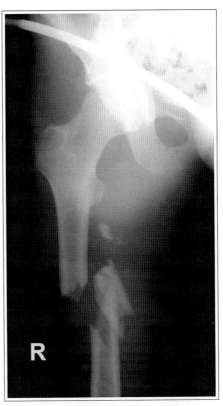

IMAGE 95

Analysis. The femoral neck is partially foreshortened, the lesser trochanter is demonstrated in profile, and the proximal femur demonstrates a fracture. The patient's leg was in external rotation.

Correction. Do not attempt to adjust the patient's leg position if a fracture of the proximal femur is suspected. No corrective movement is needed.

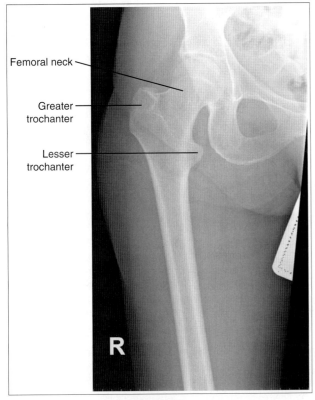

Femoral neck

Greater trochanter

Lesser trochanter

IMAGE 94

Analysis. The femoral neck is partially foreshortened, and the lesser trochanter is demonstrated in profile. The leg was in external rotation, with the femoral epicondyles positioned at approximately a 30-degree angle with the imaging table.

Correction. Internally rotate the patient's entire leg until the foot is tilted 15 to 20 degrees from vertical and the femoral epicondyles are positioned parallel with the imaging table, as shown in Figures 6-98 and 6-99.

FEMUR: LATERAL PROJECTION (MEDIOLATERAL)

See Figures 6-109, 6-110, and 6-111 and Boxes 6-23 and 6-24.

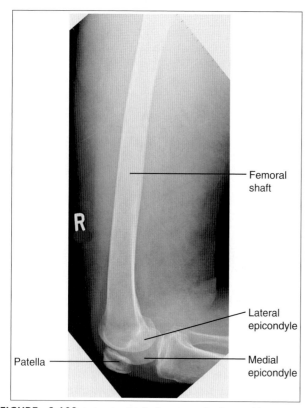

FIGURE 6-109 Lateral distal femur projection with accurate positioning.

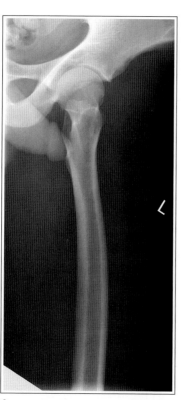

FIGURE 6-110 Lateral proximal femur projection with accurate positioning.

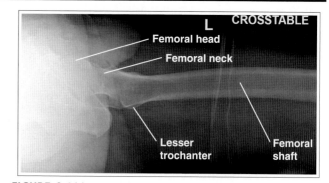

FIGURE 6-111 Cross-table lateral proximal femur projection with accurate positioning.

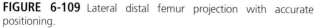

BOX 6-23	**Lateral Distal Femur Projection Analysis Criteria**

- Image density is uniform across the femur.
- The anterior and posterior margins of the medial and lateral femoral condyles are aligned and the tibia is partially superimposed by the fibular head.
- The medial femoral condyle is projected distal to the lateral femoral condyle, closing the knee joint space.
- The distal femoral shaft is at the center of the exposure field.
- The distal femoral shaft, surrounding femoral soft tissue, knee joint, and 1 inch (2.5 cm) of the lower leg are included within the collimated field. Any orthopedic apparatus located at the knee is included in its entirety.

BOX 6-24	**Proximal Distal Femur Projection Analysis Criteria**

- Image density is uniform across the femur.
- The lesser trochanter is in profile medially, and the femoral neck and head are superimposed over the greater trochanter.
- The femoral shaft is seen without foreshortening, the femoral neck is demonstrated on end, and the greater trochanter is demonstrated at the same transverse level as the femoral head.
- The long axis of the femoral shaft is aligned with the long axis of the collimated field.
- The proximal femoral shaft is at the center of the exposure field.
- The proximal femoral shaft, hip joint, and surrounding femoral soft tissue are included within the collimated field. Any orthopedic apparatus located at the hip is included in its entirety.

Image density is uniform across the femur.

- Position the thicker proximal femur at the cathode end of the tube and the thinner distal femur at the anode end to take advantage of the anode heel effect and obtain more uniform density across the femur.

Distal Femur

The anterior and posterior margins of the medial and lateral femoral condyles are aligned, and the tibia is partially superimposed over the fibular head.

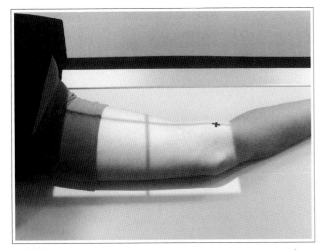

FIGURE 6-112 Proper patient positioning for lateral distal femur projection. X indicates medial femoral epicondyle.

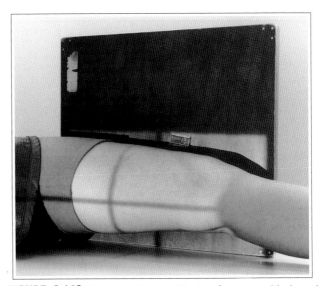

FIGURE 6-113 Proper patient positioning for cross-table lateral distal femur projection.

- To obtain a lateral distal femur projection, place the patient in a supine position with the leg extended. Then rotate the patient onto the lateral aspect of the affected femur until the femoral epicondyles are aligned perpendicular to the IR, and flex affected knee approximately 45 degrees (Figure 6-112). The unaffected leg can be drawn posteriorly and supported or flexed and drawn anteriorly across the proximal femur of the affected leg and supported at hip level. This positioning aligns the anterior and posterior margins of the medial and lateral femoral condyles and places a portion of the fibular head beneath the tibia.
- *Effect of mispositioning.* If the femoral epicondyles are not positioned perpendicular to the IR, the image demonstrates one femoral condyle anterior to the other condyle. The patient's patella must be rolled closer to or farther from the IR by adjusting patient rotation to align the condylar margins. The first step in determining which way to roll the patient's knee is to distinguish one condyle from the other. Because the central ray is centered proximal to the knee joint for a lateral femoral projection, x-ray divergence will cause the medial condyle to project distally to the lateral condyle. Consequently, the distal condyle will be the medial condyle. If a lateral distal femur projection is obtained that demonstrates the medial condyle posterior to the lateral condyle, the patient's patella was situated too far away from the IR (leg internally rotated; see Image 96). If a lateral distal knee projection is obtained that demonstrates the medial condyle anterior to the lateral condyle, the patient's patella was situated too close to the IR (leg externally rotated; see Image 97).
- *Supine femur image.* In patients with a suspected or known fracture, rolling onto the side may cause further soft tissue and bony injury. Consequently, a cross-table lateral distal femur projection should

be taken (Figure 6-113). For this projection, the patient remains in a supine position, the IR is placed against the medial aspect of the femur, and a horizontal beam is directed perpendicular to the IR.

The medial femoral condyle is projected distal to the lateral femoral condyle, closing the knee joint space.

- This image appearance is a result of central ray placement and x-ray divergence. Because the central ray is centered proximal to the femoral condyles, the x-rays used to record the images of the femoral condyles are diverged just as if a caudal angle were used. The divergence projects the medial condyle more distally than the lateral condyle because the medial condyle is situated farther from the IR.

The distal femoral shaft is at the center of the exposure field. The distal femoral shaft, the surrounding femoral soft tissue, the knee joint, and 1 inch (2.5 cm) of the lower leg are included within the collimated field. Any orthopedic apparatus located at the knee is included in its entirety.

- A perpendicular central ray is centered to the distal femoral shaft to place it in the center of the image. This is accomplished by positioning the lower edge of the receptor approximately 2 inches (5 cm) below the knee joint; the knee joint is located 1 inch (2.5 cm) distal to the medial epicondyle. The lower positioning is needed to prevent the diverged x-ray beams from projecting the knee joint off the IR.
- The longitudinal collimation should be left open the full length of the IR. Transverse collimation should be to within 0.5 inch (1.25 cm) of the lateral femoral skin line.

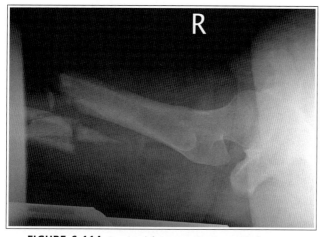

FIGURE 6-114 Proximal femur projection with fracture.

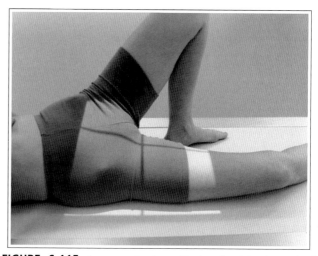

FIGURE 6-115 Proper patient positioning for lateral proximal femur projection.

- A 14- × 17-inch (35- × 43-cm) screen-film or computed radiography IR placed lengthwise should be adequate to include all the required anatomic structures.
- *Examination of the entire femur.* If the entire femur is of interest and images are taken of the distal and proximal ends of the femur, the images should demonstrate at least 2 inches (5 cm) of femoral shaft overlap. If possible, the fracture site should not be located at the overlap between the two images (Figure 6-114). Any orthopedic appliance, such as an intramedullary rod, should be included in its entirety.

Proximal Femur

The lesser trochanter is in profile medially, and the femoral neck and head are superimposed over the greater trochanter.

- To accomplish a lateral proximal femur position, begin by placing the patient supine on the imaging table. Roll the patient's pelvis toward the affected leg until the femur rests against the imaging table and the femoral epicondyles are aligned perpendicular to the imaging table (Figure 6-115). Adjust the pelvis so that it is rolled posteriorly just enough to prevent superimposition; 15 degrees from lateral position is sufficient. This femoral position accurately places the greater trochanter beneath the femoral neck and puts the lesser trochanter in profile medially.
- *Effect of poor pelvis and leg rotation.* If the pelvis is not rotated enough to place the femoral epicondyles perpendicular, the greater trochanter is demonstrated laterally (see Image 98). If the pelvis and leg are rotated too much, positioning the medial epicondyles anterior to the lateral, the greater trochanter is demonstrated medially (see Image 99).

The femoral shaft is demonstrated without foreshortening, the femoral neck is demonstrated on end, and the greater trochanter is demonstrated at the same transverse level as the femoral head.

- The femoral shaft is demonstrated without foreshortening and the femoral neck is demonstrated on end when the femur is positioned flat against the imaging table.
- *Effect of femur abduction.* To understand the relationship between the femoral shaft and neck, study a femoral skeletal bone placed in a lateral projection. Note that when the proximal femur rests against a flat surface in a lateral projection, the femoral neck is on end. With this position, the femoral neck is completely foreshortened. Because of this foreshortening, the femoral neck cannot be evaluated on an image taken in this manner. If the femur is not positioned flat against the imaging table, the femoral neck is shown with decreased foreshortening and the femoral shaft with increased foreshortening (see Image 100).
- *Positioning for fracture.* For a patient with a suspected or known fracture, flexing or abducting the affected leg or rolling the patient onto the affected side may cause further soft tissue and bony injury. Therefore, an axiolateral projection of the proximal femur should be used (Figure 6-116; see Figure 6-111). Consult page 406 for positioning instructions and evaluating criteria for this position.

The long axis of the femoral shaft is aligned with the long axis of the collimated field.

- Aligning the long axis of the femoral shaft with the long axis of the collimated field allows tight collimation without clipping any portion of the femur or surrounding soft tissue.

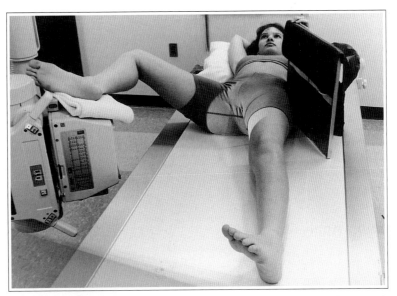

FIGURE 6-116 Proper patient positioning for cross-table lateral proximal femur projection.

- Because the femoral shaft lies across the table when it is abducted, the patient must be rotated on the imaging table until the femur is placed as close to the long axis of the collimation field as possible.

The proximal femoral shaft is at the center of the exposure field. The proximal femoral shaft, hip joint, and surrounding femoral soft tissue are included within the collimated field. Any orthopedic apparatus located at the hip is included in its entirety.

- A perpendicular central ray is centered to the proximal femoral shaft to place it in the center of the image. This is accomplished by positioning the upper edge of the receptor at the level of the ASIS (Figure 6-117). If the collimator head can

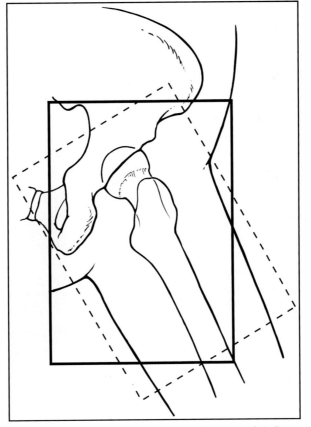

FIGURE 6-117 Central ray centering for lateral proximal femur projection. Dotted line rectangle indicates area covered if collimator head is turned.

be moved, turn it until one of its axes is aligned with the long axis of the femur.

- Leave the longitudinal collimation open the full length of the IR. Transverse collimation should be to within 0.5 inch (1.25 cm) of the lateral femoral skin line. The surrounding femoral soft tissue should be included to detect subcutaneous air or hematomas.

- A 14- × 17-inch (35- × 43-cm) screen-film or computed radiography IR placed lengthwise should be adequate to include all the required anatomic structures.

Lateral Femur Projection Analysis

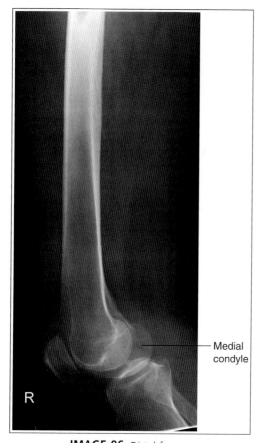

IMAGE 96 Distal femur.

Analysis. The anterior and posterior margins of the medial and lateral femoral condyles are not aligned. The medial condyle is posterior to the lateral condyle. The patella was too far from the IR (leg internally rotated).

Correction. Roll the patient anteriorly, positioning the patella closer to the IR (externally rotate the leg) and the femoral epicondyles perpendicular to the IR. The amount of movement needed is half the distance demonstrated between the anterior and posterior surfaces of the femoral condyles.

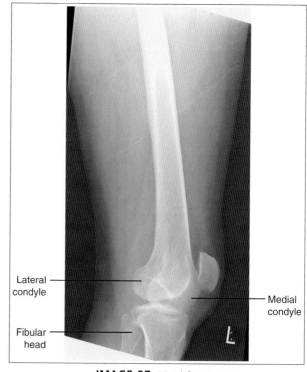

IMAGE 97 Distal femur.

Analysis. The anterior and posterior margins of the medial and lateral femoral condyles are not aligned. The medial condyle is positioned anterior to the lateral condyle. The patella was too close to the IR (leg externally rotated).

Correction. Roll the patient posteriorly, positioning the patella farther from the IR (internally rotate the leg) and the femoral epicondyles perpendicular to the IR. The amount of movement needed is half the distance demonstrated between the anterior or posterior surfaces of the femoral condyles.

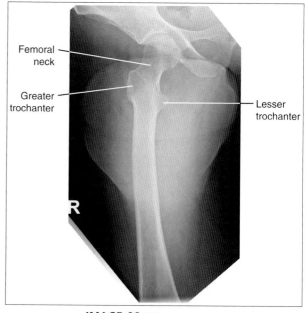

IMAGE 98 Proximal femur.

Analysis. The greater trochanter is positioned laterally. The patient's leg was not rotated enough to position the femoral epicondyles perpendicular to the IR.

Correction. Increase the degree of external leg rotation until the femoral epicondyles are aligned perpendicular to the IR.

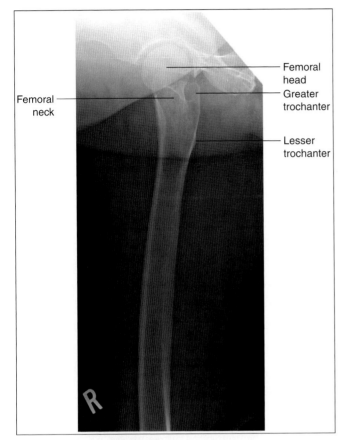

IMAGE 99 Proximal femur.

Analysis. The greater trochanter is demonstrated medially next to the ischial tuberosity and the lesser trochanter is not demonstrated in profile. The leg was rotated more than needed to position the femoral epicondyles perpendicular to the IR.

Correction. Decrease the amount of external leg rotation until the femoral epicondyles are aligned perpendicular to the IR.

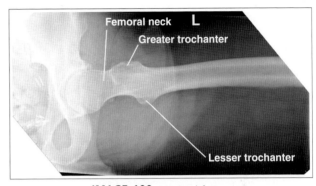

IMAGE 100 Proximal femur.

Analysis. The femoral neck is demonstrated with decreased foreshortening and the femoral shaft with increased foreshortening. The patient's femur was placed at a 45-degree angle with the imaging table.

Correction. The patient's pelvis should be rotated and the leg abducted as needed to place the femur against the imaging table.

OUTLINE

OBJECTIVES

After completion of this chapter, you should be able to do the following:

- Identify the required anatomy on hip, pelvis, and sacroiliac joint projections.
- Describe how to properly position the patient, image receptor (IR), and central ray for hip, pelvic, and sacroiliac joint projections.
- State how to mark and display hip, pelvic, and sacroiliac joint images properly.
- List the requirements for accurate positioning for hip, pelvic, and sacroiliac joint projections and state how to properly reposition the patient when less than optimal projections are produced.
- List the soft tissue fat planes demonstrated on AP hip and pelvis projections, describe their locations, and discuss the importance of using a technique that adequately demonstrates them.
- Explain how leg rotation affects which anatomic structures of the proximal femur are demonstrated on AP hip and pelvis projections.

- Discuss why the leg of a patient with a proximal femoral fracture should never be rotated to obtain AP and lateral projections, and state how these projections should be taken.
- Define the differences demonstrated between the pelvic bones of female and those of male patients.
- Describe how the anatomic structures of the proximal femur are demonstrated differently for AP oblique hip and pelvis projections when the distal femur is elevated at different angles to the imaging table.
- Describe how the anatomic structures of the proximal femur are demonstrated differently for AP oblique hip and pelvis projections when the distal femur is abducted at different angles to the imaging table.
- Describe how to localize the femoral neck for an axiolateral hip projection.
- State which sacroiliac joint is of interest when the patient is rotated for AP oblique sacroiliac joint projections.

KEY TERMS

gluteal fat plane
iliopsoas fat plane

Lauenstein method
obturator internus fat plane

pericapsular fat plane

IMAGE ANALYSIS CRITERIA

The following image analysis criteria are used for all adult and pediatric hip and pelvis images and should be considered when completing the analysis for each hip and pelvis projection presented in this chapter (Box 7-1).

- *Visibility of hip and pelvis details.* An optimal kVp technique, as shown in Table 7-1, sufficiently penetrates the proximal femur, hip, and pelvic structures and provides a contrast scale necessary to visualize the pelvic and femoral details. Use a grid to absorb the scatter radiation produced by the proximal femur, hip, and pelvis, providing a higher contrast image. To obtain optimal density, set a manual milliampere-seconds (mAs) level based on the patient's part thickness or choose the appropriate automatic exposure control (AEC) chamber when recommended. AEC is contraindicated if the patient has hip or pelvic hardware or orthopedic apparatus.

BOX 7-1	Hip and Pelvis Imaging Analysis Criteria

- The facility's identification requirements are visible.
- A right or left marker identifying the correct side of the patient is present on the image and is not superimposed over the anatomy of interest.
- Good radiation protection practices are evident.
- Bony trabecular patterns and cortical outlines of the anatomic structures are sharply defined.
- Contrast and density are uniform and adequate to demonstrate the soft tissue and bony structures.
- Penetration is sufficient to visualize the bony trabecular patterns and cortical outlines of the hip and pelvis.
- No evidence of removable artifacts is present.

HIP: ANTEROPOSTERIOR PROJECTION

See Figure 7-1 and Box 7-2.

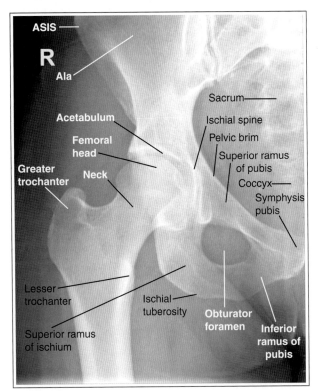

FIGURE 7-1 AP hip projection with accurate positioning.

Contrast and density are adequate to demonstrate the pericapsular gluteal, iliopsoas, and obturator fat planes.

- *Fat planes on AP hip and pelvic projections.* When evaluating AP hip and pelvis projections, the reviewer not only analyzes the bony structures but also studies the placement of the soft tissue fat planes. Four fat planes are of interest on AP hip projections, and their visualization aids in the detection of intraarticular and periarticular disease: obturator internus fat plane, which lies within the pelvic inlet next to the medial brim; the iliopsoas fat plane, which lies medial to the lesser trochanter; the pericapsular fat plane, which is found superior to the femoral neck; and the gluteal fat plane, which lies superior to the pericapsular fat plane (Figure 7-2).

TABLE 7-1	Hip and Pelvis Technical Data			
Projection	kVp	Grid	AEC Chamber(s)	SID
AP, hip	70–85	Grid	Center	40–48 inches (100–120 cm)
AP oblique, hip	70–85	Grid	Center	40–48 inches (100–120 cm)
Axiolateral (inferosuperior), hip	75–85	Grid		40–48 inches (100–120 cm)
AP, pelvis	65–85	Grid	Both outside	40–48 inches (100–120 cm)
AP oblique, pelvis	65–85	Grid	Both outside	40–48 inches (100–120 cm)
AP axial, sacroiliac joints	80–85	Grid	Center	40–48 inches (100–120 cm)
AP oblique, sacroiliac joints	75–85	Grid	Center	40–48 inches (100–120 cm)

AEC, Automatic exposure control; *kVp,* kilovoltage peak; *SID,* source–image receptor distance.

BOX 7-2 | **Hip and Pelvic Projection Analysis Criteria**

- Contrast and density are adequate to demonstrate the pericapsular gluteal, iliopsoas, and obturator fat planes.
- The ischial spine is aligned with the pelvic brim, the sacrum and coccyx are aligned with the symphysis pubis, and the obturator foramen is open.
- The femoral neck is demonstrated without foreshortening, the greater trochanter is in profile laterally, and the lesser trochanter is superimposed by the femoral neck.
- The femoral head or neck are at the center of the exposure field.
- The acetabulum, greater and lesser trochanters, femoral head and neck, and half of the sacrum, coccyx, and symphysis pubis are included within the collimated field.
- Any orthopedic apparatus located at the hip are included in their entirety.

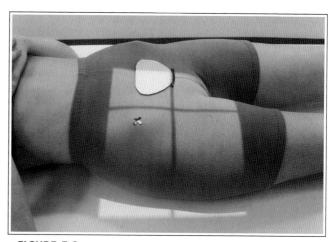

FIGURE 7-3 Proper patient positioning for AP hip projection.

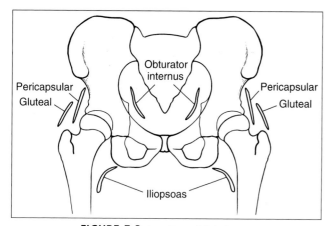

FIGURE 7-2 Location of fat planes.

The pelvis demonstrates an AP projection. The ischial spine is aligned with the pelvic brim, the sacrum and coccyx are aligned with the symphysis pubis, and the obturator foramen is open.

- An AP projection of the hip is obtained by placing the patient supine on the imaging table with the legs extended (Figure 7-3). To ensure that the pelvis is not rotated, judge the distances from the anterior superior iliac spines (ASISs) to the imaging table. The distances on each side should be equal.
- *Detecting pelvis rotation.* Rotation on an AP hip projection is initially detected by evaluating the relationship of the ischial spine and the pelvic brim, the alignment of the sacrum and coccyx with the symphysis pubis, and the degree of obturator foramen demonstration. If the patient was rotated toward the affected hip, the ischial spine is demonstrated without pelvic brim superimposition, the sacrum and coccyx are not aligned with the symphysis pubis but are rotated away from the affected hip, and the obturator foramen is narrowed (see Image 1). If the patient has been rotated away from the affected hip, the ischial spine is not aligned with

the pelvic brim but is demonstrated closer to the acetabulum, the sacrum and coccyx are not aligned with the symphysis pubis, but are rotated toward the affected hip, and the obturator foramen is widened (see Image 2).

The femoral neck is demonstrated without foreshortening, the greater trochanter is in profile laterally, and the lesser trochanter is superimposed by the femoral neck.

- *Accurate leg positioning.* To demonstrate an AP hip projection with the femoral neck shown without foreshortening and the greater trochanter in profile, the patient's leg should be internally rotated until the foot is angled 15 to 20 degrees from vertical and the femoral epicondyles are positioned parallel with the imaging table (Figure 7-4; see Figure 7-1). A sandbag or tape may be needed to help the patient maintain this internal leg rotation.
- *Poor leg positioning.* The relationship of the patient's leg to the imaging table determines how the femoral neck and trochanters are shown on an

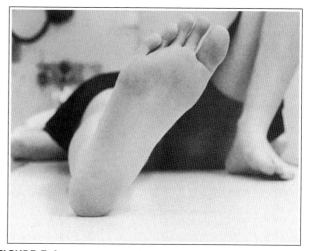

FIGURE 7-4 Proper internal foot rotation, 15 to 20 degrees from vertical.

AP hip projection. In general, when patients are relaxed, their legs and feet are externally (laterally) rotated. On external rotation, the femoral neck declines posteriorly (toward the table) and is foreshortened on an AP hip projection. Increased external rotation increases the degree of posterior decline and foreshortening of the femoral neck on the image. If the patient's leg is externally (laterally) rotated enough to position the foot at a 45-degree angle and an imaginary line connecting the femoral epicondyles at a 60- to 65-degree angle with the imaging table, the femoral neck is demonstrated on end and the lesser trochanter is demonstrated in profile (Figure 7-5; see Image 3). If the patient's leg is positioned with the foot placed vertically and an imaginary line connecting the femoral epicondyles at approximately a 15- to 20-degree angle with the imaging table, the lesser trochanter is demonstrated in partial profile and the femoral neck is only partially foreshortened (see Image 4).

- *Positioning for a fractured or dislocated proximal femur.* When a patient has a dislocated or fractured proximal femur, the leg should not be internally rotated but left as is. Forced internal rotation of a dislocated or fractured proximal femur may injure the blood supply and nerves that surround the injured area. Because the patient's leg is not internally rotated when a fracture is suspected, the resulting AP hip projection may demonstrate the femoral neck with some degree of foreshortening and the lesser trochanter without femoral shaft superimposition (see Image 5).

The femoral head or neck is at the center of the exposure field. The acetabulum, greater and lesser trochanters, femoral head and neck, and half of the sacrum, coccyx, and symphysis pubis are included within the collimated field. Any orthopedic apparatus located at the hip are included in their entirety.

- A perpendicular central ray is centered 1.5 inches (4 cm) distal to the midpoint of a line connecting the ASIS and superior symphysis pubis, to center the hip joint in the center of the exposure field, and a perpendicular central ray is centered 2.5 inches (6.25 cm) distal to the midpoint of a line connecting the ASIS and superior symphysis pubis to place the femoral neck in the center of the exposure field (Figure 7-6). Center the IR to the central ray and open the longitudinal collimation enough to include the ASIS and any hip orthopedic apparatus. Transversely collimate to the patient's midsagittal plane and within 0.5 inch (1.25 cm) of the lateral hip skin line. Including half of the sacrum, coccyx, and symphysis pubis within the exposure field provides a way to evaluate pelvic rotation.

- A 10- × 12-inch (24- × 30-cm) IR placed lengthwise should be adequate to include all the required anatomic structures. A larger IR and lower centering point may be necessary to include hip orthopedic apparatus (Figure 7-7).

- *Gonadal shielding.* Use gonadal shielding on all male patients. Female patients should be shielded, although it is important that no pelvic anatomy be covered by the shield. It is not uncommon for patients with hip fractures to have an associated pelvic fracture. Remember that a shield placed on top of the patient will be greatly magnified.

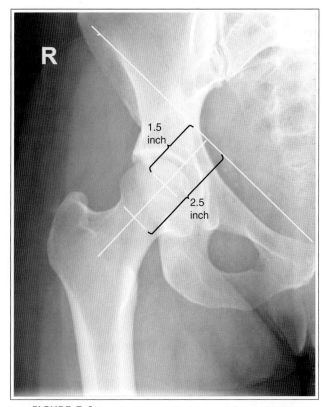

FIGURE 7-6 Localization of hip joint and femoral neck.

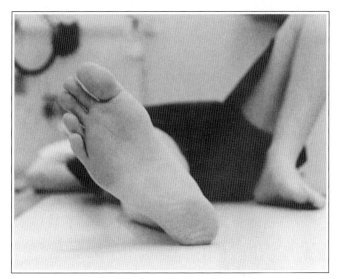

FIGURE 7-5 Poor foot rotation.

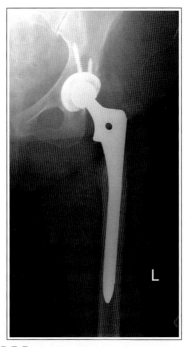

FIGURE 7-7 AP hip projection with metal apparatus.

Anteroposterior Hip Projection Analysis

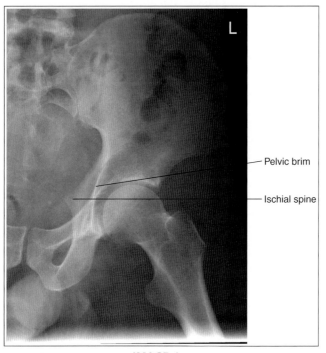

— Pelvic brim

— Ischial spine

IMAGE 1

Analysis. The ischial spine is demonstrated without pelvic brim superimposition, the sacrum and coccyx are not aligned with the symphysis pubis but are rotated away from the affected hip, and the obturator foramen is narrowed. The patient was rotated toward the affected hip. The femoral neck is foreshortened, and the lesser trochanter is demonstrated in profile. The patient's leg was externally rotated.

Correction. Rotate the patient away from the affected hip until the ASISs are positioned at equal distances from the imaging table. Internally rotate the patient's leg until the foot is angled 15 to 20 degrees from vertical and the femoral epicondyles are positioned parallel with the imaging table, as shown in Figure 7-4.

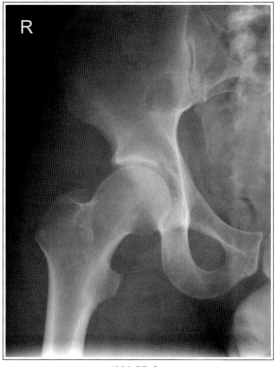

IMAGE 2

Analysis. The ischial spine is not aligned with the pelvic brim but is demonstrated closer to the acetabulum, the sacrum and coccyx are not aligned with the symphysis pubis but are rotated toward the affected hip, and the obturator foramen is clearly demonstrated. The patient was rotated away from the affected hip (left posterior oblique [LPO] position).

Correction. Rotate the patient toward the affected hip until the ASISs are positioned at equal distances from the imaging table.

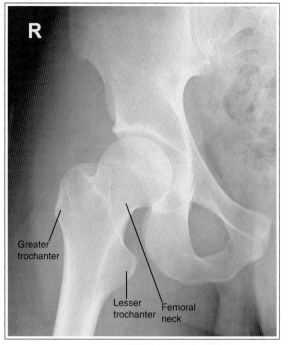

IMAGE 3

Analysis. The femoral neck is completely foreshortened, and the lesser trochanter is demonstrated in profile. The patient's leg was in external rotation with the foot positioned at a 45-degree angle and the femoral epicondyles at a 25- to 30-degree angle with the imaging table, as shown in Figure 7-5.

Correction. Internally rotate the patient's leg until the foot is angled 15 to 20 degrees from vertical and the femoral epicondyles are positioned parallel with the imaging table, as shown in Figure 7-4.

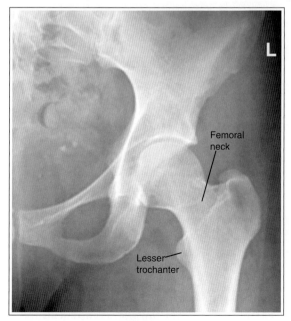

IMAGE 4

Analysis. The femoral neck is partially foreshortened, and the lesser trochanter is demonstrated in profile. The patient's leg was externally rotated, bringing the foot vertical and the femoral epicondyles to approximately a 15- to 20-degree angle with the imaging table.

Correction. Internally rotate the patient's leg until the foot is angled 15 to 20 degrees from vertical and the femoral epicondyles are positioned parallel with the imaging table, as shown in Figure 7-4.

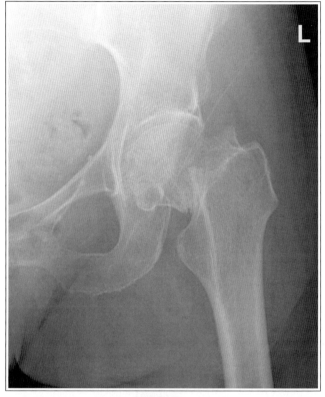

IMAGE 5

Analysis. The femoral neck is partially foreshortened and demonstrates a fracture. The lesser trochanter is demonstrated in profile. The patient's leg was in external rotation.

Correction. Do not attempt to adjust the patient's leg position if a fracture of the proximal femur is suspected. No corrective movement is needed.

HIP: ANTEROPOSTERIOR OBLIQUE PROJECTION (MODIFIED CLEAVES METHOD)

See Figure 7-8 and Box 7-3.

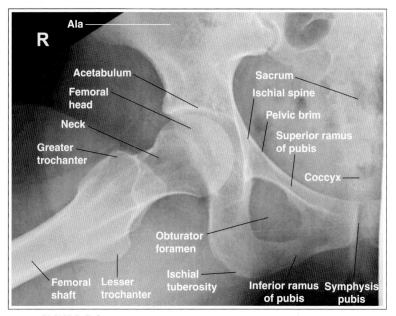

FIGURE 7-8 AP oblique hip projection with accurate positioning.

BOX 7-3	Anteroposterior Oblique Hip Projection Analysis Criteria

- The ischial spine is aligned with the pelvic brim, the sacrum and coccyx are aligned with the symphysis pubis and the obturator foramen is open.
- The lesser trochanter is in profile medially, and the femoral neck is superimposed over the greater trochanter.
- The femoral neck is partially foreshortened, and the proximal greater trochanter is demonstrated at a transverse level halfway between the femoral head and the lesser trochanter.
- The femoral neck is at the center of the exposure field.
- The acetabulum, greater and lesser trochanters, femoral head and neck, and half of the sacrum, coccyx, and symphysis pubis are included within the collimated field.

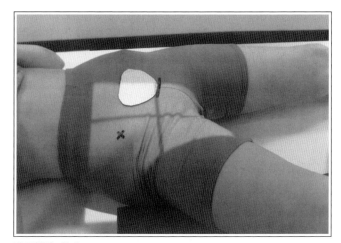

FIGURE 7-9 Proper patient positioning for AP oblique hip projection.

The pelvis demonstrates an AP projection. The ischial spine is aligned with the pelvic brim, the sacrum and coccyx are aligned with the symphysis pubis, and the obturator foramen is open.

- An AP oblique projection of the hip is obtained by placing the patient supine on the imaging table, with the unaffected leg extended and the affected leg flexed and abducted (Figure 7-9). To ensure that the pelvis is not rotated, judge the distances from the ASISs to the imaging table. The distance on each side should be equal.
- *Detecting pelvis rotation.* Rotation of the pelvis on an AP oblique projection is detected by evaluating the relationship of the ischial spine and the pelvic brim, the alignment of the sacrum and coccyx with the symphysis pubis, and the demonstration of the obturator foramen. If the patient was rotated toward the affected hip, the ischial spine is demonstrated without pelvic brim superimposition, the sacrum and coccyx are not aligned with the symphysis pubis but are rotated away from the affected hip, and demonstration of the obturator foramen is decreased (see Image 6). If the patient was rotated away from the affected hip, the ischial spine is not aligned with the pelvic brim but is demonstrated closer to the acetabulum, the sacrum and coccyx are not aligned with the symphysis pubis but are rotated toward the affected hip, and demonstration of the obturator foramen is increased (see Image 7).

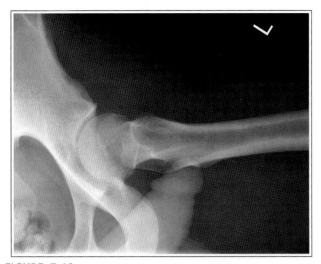

FIGURE 7-10 Lateral hip image obtained using the Lauenstein and Hickey methods.

- *Lauenstein and Hickey methods, lateral hip.* The Lauenstein and Hickey methods are modifications of the AP oblique hip projection. For these methods, the patient is positioned as described for the AP oblique hip projection with the femur flexed and abducted, except that the pelvis is rotated toward the affected hip as needed to position the femur against the imaging table (Figure 7-10).

The lesser trochanter is in profile medially, and the femoral neck is superimposed over the greater trochanter.

- *Accurate femur positioning.* To position the greater trochanter accurately beneath the proximal femur and position the lesser trochanter in profile, flex the patient's knee and hip until the femur is angled at 60 to 70 degrees with the imaging table (20 to 30 degrees from vertical) (Figure 7-11).
- *Effect of distal femur elevation on proximal femur visualization.* For an AP oblique hip projection, the medial and lateral placement of the

greater and lesser trochanters are determined when the patient flexes the knee and hip. Use a femoral skeletal bone for a better understanding of how the relationship of the greater and lesser trochanters to the proximal femur changes as the distal femur is elevated with knee and hip flexion. Begin by placing the femoral bone on a flat surface in an AP position. While slowly elevating the distal femur, observe how the greater trochanter rotates around the proximal femur. First, the greater trochanter moves beneath the proximal femur; then, as elevation of the distal femur continues, it moves from beneath the proximal femur and is demonstrated on the medial side of the femur.

- *Poor distal femur elevation .* If the knee and hip are not flexed enough to place the femur at this angle with the imaging table, the greater trochanter is demonstrated laterally, as it is on an AP projection (see Images 7 and 8). If the knee and hip are flexed too much, placing the femur at an angle greater than 60 to 70 degrees with the imaging table, the greater trochanter is demonstrated medially (see Image 9). The greater trochanter is also demonstrated medially, as shown in Image 9, when the foot and ankle of the affected leg are elevated and placed on top of the unaffected leg. This positioning causes the femur to rotate externally. The foot of the affected leg should remain resting on the imaging table.

The femoral neck is partially foreshortened, and the proximal aspect of the greater trochanter is demonstrated at a transverse level halfway between the femoral head and the lesser trochanter.

- *Accurate leg positioning.* To demonstrate the femoral neck and proximal femur with only partial foreshortening and the proximal greater trochanter at a transverse level halfway between the femoral head and lesser trochanter on an AP oblique hip projection, abduct the femoral shaft to a 45-degree angle from vertical (Figure 7-12).

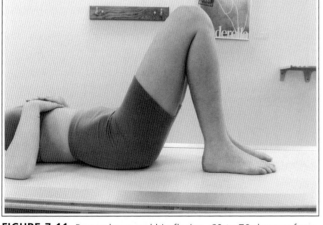

FIGURE 7-11 Proper knee and hip flexion, 60 to 70 degrees from imaging table.

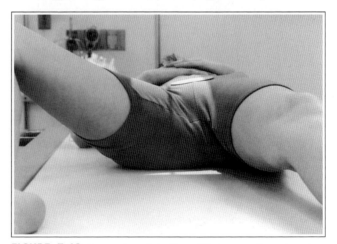

FIGURE 7-12 Proper leg abduction, 45 degrees from imaging table.

- *Effect of leg abduction* . The degree of femoral abduction determines the amount of femoral neck foreshortening and the transverse level at which the proximal greater trochanter is demonstrated between the femoral head and lesser trochanter.

  Use a femoral skeleton bone to understand how leg abduction determines the visualization of the femoral neck and the position of the greater trochanter. Place the femoral bone on a flat surface in an AP position, with the distal femur elevated until the greater trochanter is positioned beneath the proximal femur and the lesser trochanter is in profile (20 to 30 degrees from vertical or 60 to 70 degrees from flat surface). From this position, abduct the femoral bone (move the lateral surface of the femoral bone toward the flat surface). As the bone moves toward the flat surface, observe how the femoral neck is positioned more on end and the greater trochanter moves proximally (toward the femoral head).

- *Poor leg abduction.* If the femoral shaft is abducted 20 to 30 degrees from vertical (60 to 70 degree angle with the imaging table; Figure 7-13) the femoral neck is demonstrated without foreshortening and the proximal greater trochanter is at the same transverse level as the lesser trochanter (see Image 10). If the femoral shaft is abducted to the imaging table (Figure 7-14), the proximal femoral shaft is demonstrated without foreshortening, the proximal greater trochanter is at the same transverse level as the femoral head, and the femoral neck is demonstrated on end (see Image 11).

The femoral neck is at the center of the exposure field. The acetabulum, greater and lesser trochanters, and femoral head and neck, as well as half of the sacrum, coccyx, and symphysis pubis, are included within the collimated field.

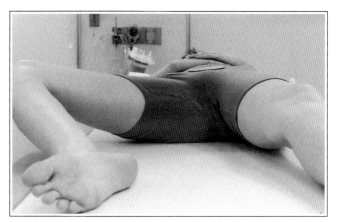

FIGURE 7-14 Femur in maximum abduction, 20 degrees from imaging table.

- Center a perpendicular central ray 2.5 inches (6.25 cm) distal to the midpoint of a line connecting the ASIS and superior symphysis pubis to center the femoral neck in the center of the exposure field. Center the IR to the central ray and open longitudinal collimation to include the ASIS. Transversely collimate to the patient's midsagittal plane and transversely collimate to within 0.5 inch (1.25 cm) of the lateral hip skin line.
- Including half of the sacrum, coccyx, and symphysis pubis within the exposure field provides a way to evaluate pelvic rotation.
- A 10- × 12-inch (24- × 30-cm) IR placed lengthwise should be adequate to include all the required anatomic structures.

AP Oblique Hip Projection Analysis

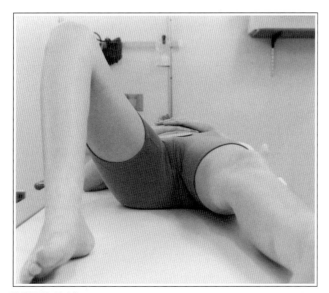

FIGURE 7-13 Femur in only slight abduction, 20 degrees from vertical (70 degrees from imaging table).

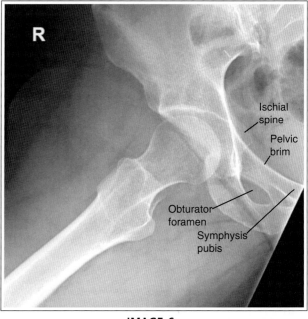

IMAGE 6

Analysis. The ischial spine is demonstrated without pelvic brim superimposition, the sacrum and coccyx are not aligned with the symphysis pubis but are rotated away from the affected hip, and the obturator foramen is not well demonstrated. The patient was rotated toward the affected hip.

Correction. Rotate the patient away from the affected hip until the ASISs are positioned at equal distances from the imaging table.

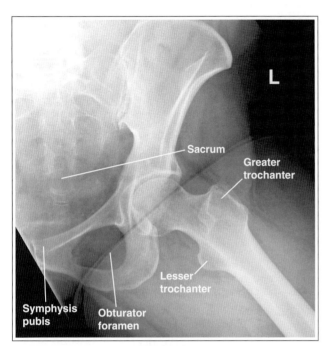

IMAGE 7

Analysis. The ischial spine is not aligned with the pelvic brim but is demonstrated closer to the acetabulum, the sacrum and coccyx are not aligned with the symphysis pubis but are rotated toward the affected hip, and the obturator foramen is well demonstrated. The greater trochanter is partially demonstrated laterally, indicating that the leg was flexed less than the needed 60 to 70 degrees from the imaging table. The patient was rotated away from the affected hip and the leg was not flexed enough.

Correction. Rotate the patient toward the affected hip until the ASISs are positioned at equal distances from the imaging table and increase the degree of knee and hip flexion until the femur is positioned at a 60- to 70-degree angle with the imaging table (see Figure 7-11).

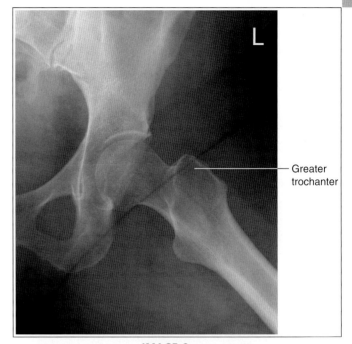

IMAGE 8

Analysis. The greater trochanter is positioned laterally. The patient's knee was not flexed enough to align the femur at a 60- to 70-degree angle with the imaging table (20 to 30 degrees from vertical). The proximal greater trochanter is visible at about the same transverse level as the femoral head, indicating too much femur abduction.

Correction. Decrease the knee flexion until the femur is aligned at a 60- to 70-degree angle with the imaging table, as shown in Figure 7-11.

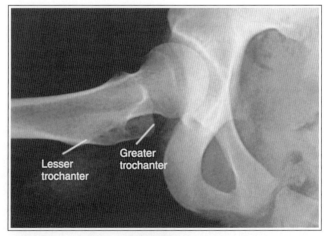

IMAGE 9

Analysis. The greater trochanter is positioned medially. The patient's knee was flexed more than needed, positioning the femur at an angle greater than 60 to 70 degrees with the imaging table (20 to 30 degrees from vertical).

Correction. Decrease the knee flexion until the femur is aligned at a 60- to 70-degree angle with the imaging table, as shown in Figure 7-11.

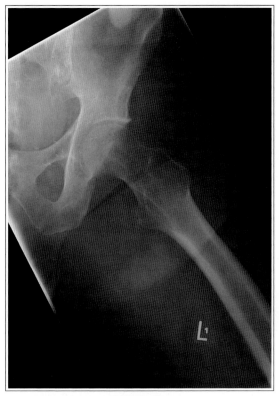

IMAGE 10

Analysis. The femoral neck is demonstrated without foreshortening, and the proximal greater trochanter and the lesser trochanters are demonstrated at approximately the same transverse level. The femur was in only slight abduction, at approximately a 70-degree angle with the imaging table (20 degrees from vertical), as shown in Figure 7-13.

Correction. If the proximal femoral shaft demonstrates too much foreshortening for your facility's standards, have the patient abduct the femur to a 45-degree angle with the imaging table.

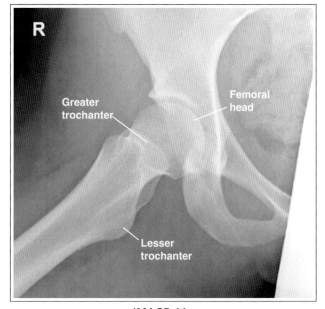

IMAGE 11

Analysis. The femoral neck is demonstrated on end and is entirely foreshortened. The proximal greater trochanter is demonstrated on the same transverse level as the femoral head. The femur was abducted until it was positioned next to the imaging table, as shown in Figure 7-14.

Correction. Decrease the degree of femoral abduction until the femur is at a 45-degree angle with the imaging table, as shown in Figure 7-12.

HIP: AXIOLATERAL (INFEROSUPERIOR) PROJECTION (DANELIUS-MILLER METHOD)

See Figure 7-15 and Box 7-4.

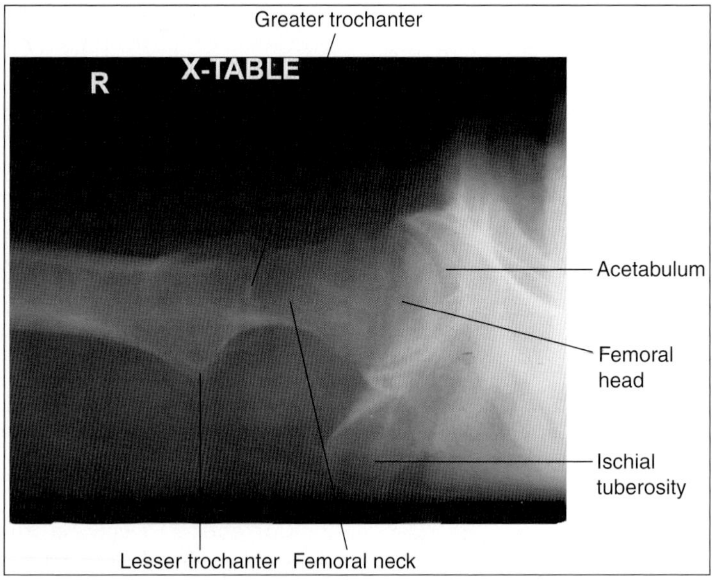

FIGURE 7-15 Axiolateral (inferosuperior) hip projection with accurate positioning.

BOX 7-4 | **Axiolateral Hip Projection Analysis Criteria**

- The proximal femur demonstrates uniform density across it.
- The femoral neck is demonstrated without foreshortening. The proximal greater trochanter and lesser trochanter are demonstrated at approximately the same level.
- The lesser trochanter is in profile posteriorly, and the greater trochanter is superimposed by the femoral shaft.
- The femoral neck is at the center of the exposure field.
- The acetabulum, greater and lesser trochanters, femoral head and neck, and ischial tuberosity are included within the collimated field.
- Any orthopedic apparatus located at the hip are included in their entirety.

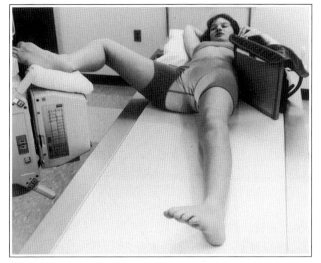

FIGURE 7-16 Proper patient positioning for axiolateral hip projection.

Scatter radiation is controlled. The proximal femur demonstrates uniform density across it.

- Tight collimation and placement of a flat lead contact strip or the straight edge of a lead apron over the top, unused half of the IR, as shown in Figure 7-16, also prevent scatter radiation from reaching the IR.
- *Compensating filter.* Frequently, when an exposure (mAs) is set that adequately demonstrates the hip joint, the proximal femur is overexposed because of the difference in body thickness in these two regions. A wedge-type compensating filter attached to the x-ray tube can be used to obtain uniform image density of the hip joint and proximal femur. Align the thin end of the filter with the femoral neck and the thicker end with the proximal femur.

The femoral neck is demonstrated without foreshortening. The proximal aspects of the greater and lesser trochanters are demonstrated at approximately the same transverse level.

- An axiolateral projection of the hip is obtained by placing the patient on the imaging table in an AP projection, with the unaffected hip positioned next to the lateral edge of the table. Flex the patient's unaffected leg until the femur is as close to a vertical position as the patient can tolerate, and then abduct the leg as far as the patient will allow. Support this leg position by using a specially designed leg holder or suitable support. Flexion and abduction of the unaffected leg move its bony and soft tissue structures away from the affected hip. Inadequate flexion or abduction of the unaffected leg results in superimposition of soft tissue onto the affected hip, preventing visualization of the affected hip (see Image 12).
- *IR placement.* Once the patient's unaffected leg has been positioned, place the grid IR against the patient's affected side at the level of the iliac crest (Figure 7-16). To demonstrate the affected femoral

neck without foreshortening, align the x-ray tube horizontally with the central ray perpendicular to the femoral neck and adjust the distal end of the IR until the receptor's long axis is perpendicular to the central ray and parallel with the femoral neck.

- *Localizing the femoral neck for central ray alignment.* To localize the affected femoral neck, first find the center of an imaginary line drawn between the superior symphysis pubis and the ASIS. Then, bisect that line by drawing a perpendicular line distally (Figure 7-17). This imaginary line parallels the long axis of the femoral neck as long as the leg is not abducted. Once the long axis of the femoral neck has been located, align the central ray perpendicular to it and the IR parallel with it.
- *Effect of central ray and femoral neck misalignment.* Misalignment of the central ray with the femoral neck results in femoral neck foreshortening and a shift in the transverse level at which the greater trochanter is located. If the angle formed between the femur and the central ray is too large, the proximal greater trochanter is demonstrated proximal to the transverse level of the lesser trochanter and is superimposed by a portion of the femoral neck (see Image 13). If the angle between the femur and the central ray is too small, the proximal greater trochanter is demonstrated distal to the transverse level of the lesser trochanter. This mispositioning seldom occurs, because the imaging table and tube position prevent such a small angle.

The lesser trochanter is in profile posteriorly, and the greater trochanter is superimposed by the femoral shaft.

- Rotation of the patient's affected leg determines the relationship of the lesser and greater trochanter to

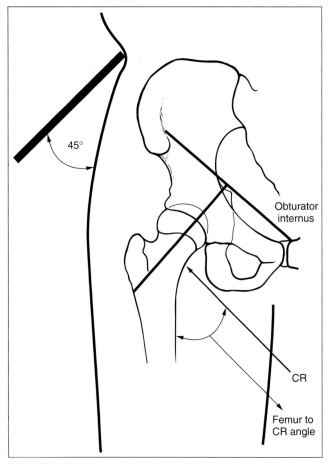

FIGURE 7-17 Locating the femoral neck and proper image receptor placement for small and average patients.

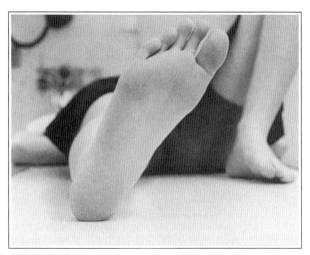

FIGURE 7-18 Proper foot position, 15 to 20 degrees from vertical.

the proximal femur on an axiolateral hip projection. In general, when a patient is placed on the imaging table and the affected leg is allowed to rotate freely, it is laterally (externally) rotated.

- *Effect of leg rotation on proximal femur visualization.* To position the proximal femur in a lateral projection (90 degrees from the AP projection), demonstrating the lesser trochanter in profile posteriorly and superimposing the greater trochanter by the femoral shaft, the affected leg must be internally rotated until an imaginary line drawn between the femoral epicondyles is positioned parallel with the imaging table. The patient's foot is angled internally 15 to 20 degrees from a vertical position (Figure 7-18). If the affected leg is not rotated internally, the greater trochanter is demonstrated posteriorly and the lesser trochanter is superimposed over the femoral shaft (see Image 14). How much greater trochanter is demonstrated without femoral shaft superimposition depends on the degree of external rotation. Greater external rotation increases the amount of greater trochanter shown.

- *Positioning for a proximal femoral fracture or dislocation .* When a patient has a dislocated hip or a suspected or known proximal femoral fracture, the leg should not be internally rotated, but left as is. Forced internal rotation of a dislocated hip or fractured proximal femur may injure the blood supply and nerves that surround the injured area. Because the patient's leg is not internally rotated in such cases, it is acceptable for the greater trochanter to be demonstrated posteriorly and the lesser trochanter to be superimposed over the femoral shaft (see Image 15).

The femoral neck is at the center of the exposure field. The acetabulum, femoral head and neck, greater and lesser trochanters, and ischial tuberosity are included within the collimated field. Any orthopedic apparatus should be included in its entirety.

- Center a perpendicular central ray to the patient's midthigh, at the level of the femoral neck, to place it in the center of the exposure field. The center of the femoral neck is located at a level 2.5 inches (6.25 cm) distal to the midpoint of a line connecting the ASIS and superior symphysis pubis. Open the longitudinal collimation the full length of the IR. Transversely collimate to within 0.5 inch (1.25 cm) of the proximal femoral skin line.

- A 10- × 12-inch (24- × 30-cm) IR placed lengthwise should be adequate to include all the required anatomic structures. A larger IR and lower centering point may be necessary to include hip orthopedic apparatus (Figure 7-19).

- *IR placement alternative.* The level at which the IR is placed along the patient's lateral body surface determines whether the acetabulum and femoral head are included on the IR. For patients with minimal lateral soft tissue thickness, the upper IR edge should be firmly placed in the crease

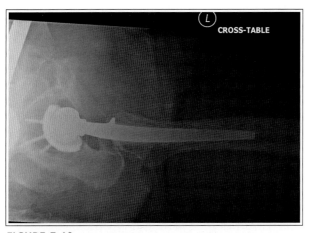

FIGURE 7-19 Axiolateral hip projection with metal apparatus.

formed at the patient's waist, just superior to the iliac crest (see Figure 7-17). For patients with ample lateral soft tissue thickness, the upper IR edge needs to be positioned superior to the iliac crest (Figure 7-20). This superior positioning will result in magnification because of the increase in the object–image receptor distance (OID) but is necessary if the acetabulum and femoral head are to be included on the axiolateral hip projection.

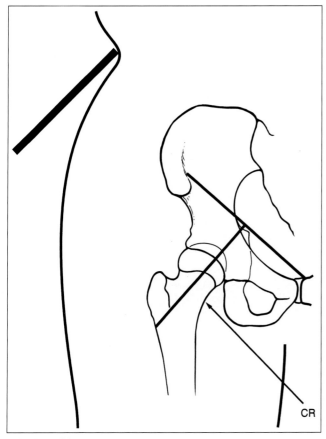

FIGURE 7-20 Proper image receptor placement for large patients.

Axiolateral Hip Projection Analysis

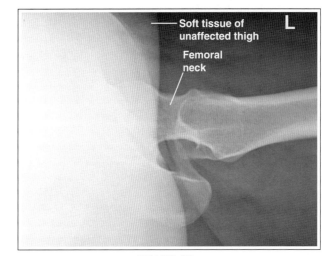

IMAGE 12

Analysis. Soft tissue from the unaffected thigh is superimposing the acetabulum and femoral head of the affected hip. The unaffected leg was not adequately flexed or abducted.

Correction. Flex and abduct the unaffected leg, drawing it away from the affected acetabulum and femoral head. If the patient is unable to adjust the unaffected leg further, the kVp and mAs can be increased to demonstrate this area. A wedge-type compensating filter may also be added to prevent overpenetration of the femoral neck and shaft.

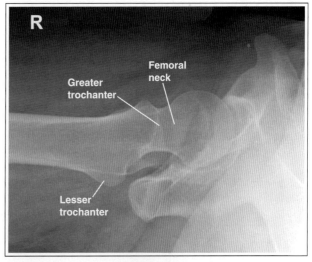

IMAGE 13

Analysis. The proximal greater trochanter is demonstrated at a transverse level proximal to the lesser trochanter, and the femoral neck is partially foreshortened. The angle between the central ray and femur was too large.

Correction. Localize the femoral neck. Position the IR parallel with the femoral neck and the central ray perpendicular to the IR and femoral neck, as shown in Figure 7-17.

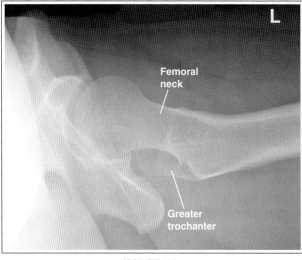

IMAGE 14

IMAGE 15

Analysis. The greater trochanter is demonstrated posteriorly, and the lesser trochanter is superimposed over the femoral shaft. The patient's affected leg was in external rotation.

Correction. Internally rotate the patient's leg until the femoral epicondyles are aligned parallel with the imaging table and the foot is angled internally 15 to 20 degrees from vertical, as shown in Figure 7-18.

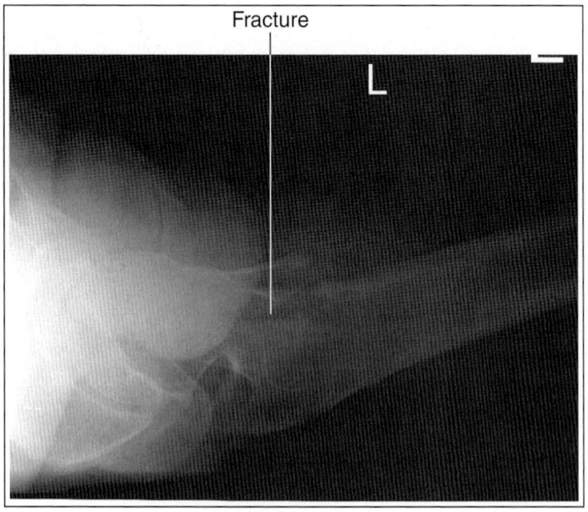

Analysis. A fracture of the femoral neck is present. The greater trochanter is demonstrated posteriorly, and the lesser trochanter is superimposed over the femoral shaft. The patient's leg was in external rotation.

Correction. Do not attempt to adjust the patient's leg position if a fracture of the proximal femur is suspected. No corrective movement is needed.

PELVIS: ANTEROPOSTERIOR PROJECTION

See Figures 7-21 and 7-22 and Box 7-5.

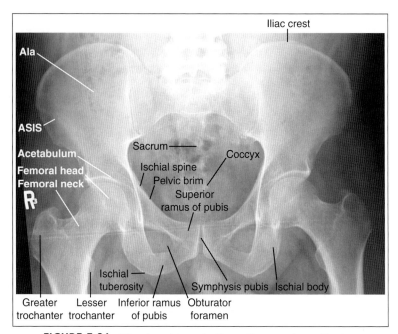

FIGURE 7-21 AP male pelvis projection with accurate positioning.

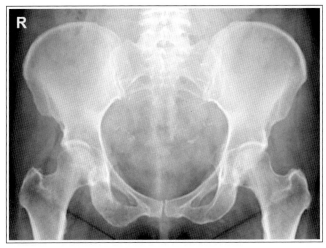

FIGURE 7-22 AP female pelvis projection with accurate positioning.

- *Regarding the male and female pelves*. Be aware of the bony architectural differences that exist between the male and female pelves (Table 7-2). These differences are the result of the need for the female pelvis to accommodate fetal growth during pregnancy and fetal passage during delivery.

Contrast and density are adequate to demonstrate the pericapsular gluteal, iliopsoas, and obturator fat planes of the pelvis.

- Refer to Figure 7-2 for an illustration of each fat plane location.

TABLE 7-2	Male and Female Pelvic Differences	
Parameter	Male	Female
Overall Shape	Bulkier, deeper, narrower	Smaller, shallower, and wider
Ala	Narrower, nonflared	Wider, flared
Pubic arch angle	Acute angle	Obtuse angle
Inlet shape	Smaller, heart shaped	Larger, rounded shape
Obturator foramen	Larger	Smaller

BOX 7-5	Anteroposterior Pelvis Projection Analysis Criteria

- Contrast and density are adequate to demonstrate the pericapsular gluteal, iliopsoas, and obturator fat planes.
- The ischial spines are aligned with the pelvic brim, the sacrum and coccyx are aligned with the symphysis pubis, and the obturator foramina are open and uniform in size and shape.
- The femoral necks are demonstrated without foreshortening, the greater trochanters are in profile laterally, and the lesser trochanters are superimposed by the femoral necks.
- The inferior sacrum is at the center of the exposure field.
- The ilia, symphysis pubis, ischia, acetabula, femoral necks and heads, and greater and lesser trochanters are included within the collimated field.
- Any orthopedic apparatus located at the hip(s) is included in their entirety.

The pelvis demonstrates an AP projection. The ischial spines are aligned with the pelvic brim, the sacrum and coccyx are aligned with the symphysis pubis, and the ilia and obturator foramina are open and uniform in size and shape.

- An AP projection of the pelvis is accomplished by placing the patient supine on the imaging table, with the legs extended and the arms drawn away from the pelvic area (Figure 7-23). To ensure that the pelvis is not rotated, judge the distance from the ASIS to the imaging table on each side. The distances should be equal.
- *Pelvic rotation.* A nonrotated AP pelvis projection demonstrates symmetrical ilia and obturator foramina. Rotation is initially detected by evaluating the relationships of the ischial spines with the pelvic brim and of the sacrum and coccyx with the symphysis pubis. The ischial spines should be aligned with the pelvic brim, and the sacrum and coccyx should be in alignment with the symphysis pubis on a nonrotated pelvis. If the pelvis is rotated into a LPO position, the left ilium is wider than the right, the left obturator foramen is narrower than the right, the left ischial spine is demonstrated without pelvic brim superimposition, and the sacrum and coccyx are not aligned with the symphysis pubis but are rotated toward the right hip (see Image 16).
- If the patient was rotated into a right posterior oblique (RPO) position, the opposite is true. The right ilium is wider than the left, the right obturator foramen is narrower than the left, the right ischial spine is demonstrated without pelvic brim superimposition, and the sacrum and coccyx are rotated toward the left hip.

The femoral necks are demonstrated without foreshortening and the greater trochanters are in profile laterally,

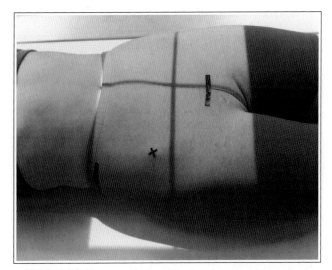

FIGURE 7-23 Proper patient positioning for AP pelvis projection.

whereas the lesser trochanters are superimposed by the femoral necks.

- *Accurate leg positioning.* To demonstrate the femoral necks without foreshortening and the greater trochanters in profile on an AP pelvis projection, the patient's leg should be internally rotated until the feet are angled 15 to 20 degrees from vertical and the femoral epicondyles are positioned parallel with the imaging table (Figure 7-24; see Figure 7-21). Sandbags or tape may be needed to help maintain this internal leg rotation. An AP pelvis projection may not demonstrate the proximal femurs with exactly the same degree of internal rotation. How each proximal femur appears will depend on the degree of internal rotation placed on that leg.

- *Poor leg positioning.* The relationship of the patient's entire leg to the imaging table determines how the femoral necks and trochanters are shown on an AP pelvis projection. In general, when patients are relaxed, their legs and feet are externally (laterally) rotated. On external rotation, the femoral necks decline posteriorly (toward the table) and are foreshortened on an AP pelvis projection. Greater external rotation increases the posterior decline and foreshortening of the femoral necks. If the patient's legs are externally (laterally) rotated enough to position the feet at a 45-degree angle and an imaginary line connecting the femoral epicondyles at a 60- to 65-degree angle with the imaging table, the femoral necks are demonstrated on end and the lesser trochanters are demonstrated in profile (Figure 7-25; see Image 17). If the patient's legs are positioned with the feet placed vertically and an imaginary line connecting the femoral epicondyles at approximately a 15- to 20-degree angle with the imaging table, the lesser trochanter is demonstrated in partial profile and the femoral neck is only partially foreshortened (see Image 18).

- *Positioning for a proximal femoral fracture.* Often, when a fracture of a proximal femur is

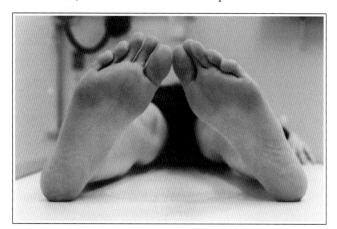

FIGURE 7-24 Proper internal foot positioning, 15 to 20 degrees from vertical.

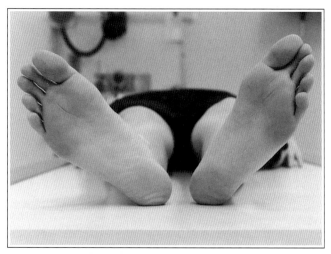

FIGURE 7-25 Poor foot positioning.

suspected, an AP pelvis projection is ordered instead of an AP hip projection because pelvic fractures are frequently associated with proximal femur fractures. If a patient has a suspected fracture or a fractured proximal femur, the leg should not be internally rotated but should be left as is. Forced internal rotation of a fractured proximal femur may injure the blood supply and nerves that surround the injured area. Because the patient's leg is not internally rotated when a fracture is in question, such an AP pelvis projection demonstrates the affected femoral neck with some degree of foreshortening and the lesser trochanter without femoral shaft superimposition.

The inferior sacrum is at the center of the exposure field. The ilia, symphysis pubis, ischia, acetabula, femoral necks and heads, and greater and lesser trochanters are included within the collimated field.

- Center a perpendicular central ray to the midsagittal plane at a level halfway between the symphysis pubis and the midpoint of an imaginary line connecting the ASIS to place the inferior sacrum in the center of the exposure field. Center the IR to the central ray and open the longitudinal collimation the full 14-inch (35-cm) IR length for most adult patients. Transversely collimate to within 0.5 inch (1.25 cm) of the lateral skin line.

- A 14- × 17-inch (35- × 43-cm) IR placed crosswise should be adequate to include all the required anatomic structures.

- *Central ray centering for analysis of hip joint mobility.* When an AP pelvis projection is being taken specifically to evaluate hip joint mobility, the central ray should be centered to the midsagittal plane at a level 1 inch (2.5 cm) superior to the symphysis pubis. Such positioning centers the hip joints on the image but may result in clipping of the superior ilia.

Anteroposterior Pelvis Projection Analysis

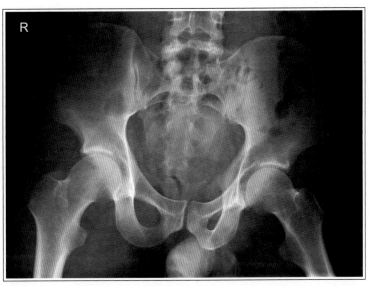

IMAGE 16

Analysis. The left obturator foramen is narrower than the right foramen, the left ischial spine is demonstrated without pelvic brim superimposition, and the sacrum and coccyx are rotated toward the right hip. The lesser trochanters are demonstrated medially and the femoral neck is foreshortened. The pelvis was rotated onto the left hip (LPO) and the legs were externally rotated.

Correction. Rotate the patient toward the right hip until the ASISs are positioned at equal distances from the imaging table and internally rotate the patient's legs until the feet are angled 15 to 20 degrees from vertical and the femoral epicondyles are positioned parallel with the imaging table, as shown in Figure 7-24.

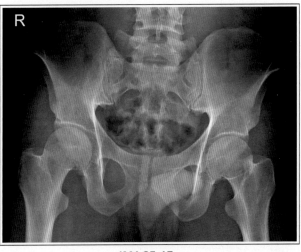

IMAGE 17

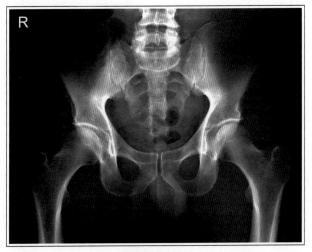

IMAGE 18

Analysis. The femoral necks are completely foreshortened and the lesser trochanters are demonstrated in profile. The patient's legs were externally rotated, with the patient's feet at a 45-degree angle and the femoral epicondyles positioned at a 25- to 30-degree angle with the imaging table, as shown in Figure 7-25.

Correction. Internally rotate the patient's legs until the feet are angled 15 to 20 degrees from vertical and the femoral epicondyles are positioned parallel with the imaging table, as shown in Figure 7-24.

Analysis. The femoral necks are partially foreshortened, and the lesser trochanters are demonstrated in profile. The patient's legs were externally rotated, with the feet vertical and the femoral epicondyles at approximately a 15- to 20-degree angle with the imaging table.

Correction. Internally rotate the patient's legs until the feet are angled 15 to 20 degrees from vertical and the femoral epicondyles are positioned parallel with the imaging table, as shown in Figure 7-24.

PELVIS: ANTEROPOSTERIOR OBLIQUE PROJECTION (MODIFIED CLEAVES METHOD)

See Figure 7-26 and Box 7-6.

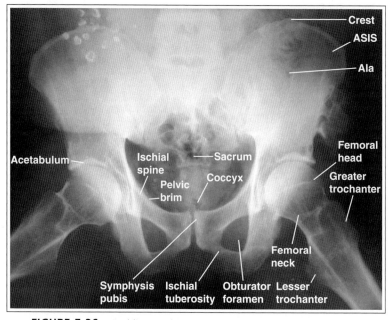

FIGURE 7-26 AP oblique pelvis projection with accurate positioning.

BOX 7-6 | Anteroposterior Oblique Pelvis Projection Analysis Criteria

- Contrast and density are adequate to demonstrate the pericapsular gluteal, iliopsoas, and obturator fat planes.
- The ischial spines are aligned with the pelvic brim, the sacrum and coccyx are aligned with the symphysis pubis, and the obturator foramina are open and uniform in size and shape.
- The lesser trochanters are in profile medially, and the femoral necks are superimposed over the adjacent greater trochanters.
- The femoral necks are partially foreshortened. The proximal greater trochanters are demonstrated at the same transverse level halfway between the femoral heads and lesser trochanters.
- The inferior sacrum is at the center of the exposure field.
- The ilia, symphysis pubis, ischia, acetabula, femoral necks and heads, and greater and lesser trochanters are included within the collimated field.

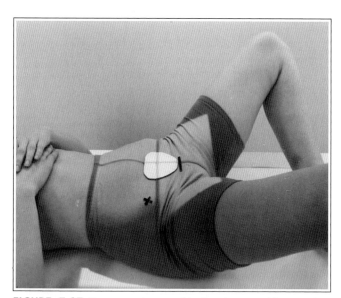

FIGURE 7-27 Proper patient positioning for AP oblique pelvis projection.

The pelvis demonstrates an AP projection. The ischial spines are aligned with the pelvic brim, the sacrum and coccyx are aligned with the symphysis pubis, and the ilia and obturator foramina are open and uniform in size and shape.

- An AP projection of the pelvis is accomplished by placing the patient on the imaging table with the legs flexed and abducted (Figure 7-27). To ensure that the pelvis is not rotated, judge the distance from the ASIS to the imaging table on each side. The distances should be equal.
- *Detecting pelvic rotation.* A nonrotated AP oblique pelvis projection will demonstrate symmetrical ilia

and obturator foramina. Rotation can be detected by evaluating the relationships of the ischial spines with the pelvic brim and of the sacrum and coccyx with the symphysis pubis. The ischial spines should be aligned with the pelvic brim and the sacrum and coccyx should align with the symphysis pubis on a nonrotated pelvis. If the pelvis is rotated into an LPO position, the left ilium is wider than the right, the left obturator foramen is narrower than the right, the left ischial spine is demonstrated without pelvic brim superimposition, and the sacrum and coccyx are not aligned with the symphysis pubis but are rotated toward the right hip (see Image 19). If the patient is rotated into an RPO position, the opposite is true. The right ilium is wider than the left, the right obturator foramen is narrower than the left, the right ischial spine is demonstrated without pelvic brim superimposition, and the sacrum and coccyx are rotated toward the left hip.

The lesser trochanters are in profile medially, and the femoral necks are superimposed over the adjacent greater trochanters.

- *Accurate femur positioning.* To position the greater trochanters beneath the proximal femurs accurately and position the lesser trochanters in profile, flex the patient's knees and hips until the femurs are angled 60 to 70 degrees with the imaging table (20 to 30 degrees from vertical; Figure 7-28).
- *Poor distal femur elevation.* For an AP oblique pelvis projection, the relationship of the greater and lesser trochanters with the proximal femurs is determined when the patient flexes the knees and hips. If the knees and hips are not flexed enough to place the femur at a 60- to 70-degree angle with the imaging table, the greater trochanters are demonstrated laterally, as with an AP projection (see Image 20). If the knees and hips are flexed too much, placing the femurs at an angle greater than 60 to 70 degrees with the imaging table, the greater trochanters are demonstrated medially Image 9).

The femoral necks are partially foreshortened. The proximal aspects of the greater trochanters are demonstrated at a transverse level halfway between the femoral heads and lesser trochanters.

- *Accurate leg positioning.* To demonstrate the femoral necks and proximal femora with only partial

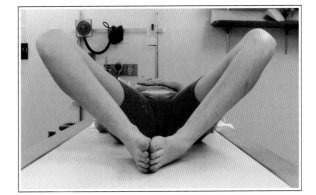

FIGURE 7-29 Proper femoral abduction, 45 degrees from imaging table.

foreshortening and the greater trochanters at a transverse level halfway between the femoral heads and lesser trochanters on an AP oblique pelvis projection, abduct the femoral shafts to a 45-degree angle from vertical (Figures 7-26 and 7-29).
- *Effect of leg abduction.* The degree of femoral abduction determines the amount of femoral neck foreshortening and the transverse level at which the greater trochanters are demonstrated between the femoral heads and lesser trochanters.
- *Poor leg abduction.* If the femoral shafts are abducted to 20 to 30 degrees from vertical (60- to 70-degree angle from the imaging table; Figure 7-30), the femoral necks are demonstrated without foreshortening and the proximal greater trochanters are at the same transverse level as the lesser trochanters on an AP oblique pelvis projection (see Image 21). If the femoral shafts are abducted until they are placed next to the imaging table (Figure 7-31), the proximal femoral shafts are demonstrated without foreshortening, the proximal greater trochanters are at the same transverse level as the femoral heads, and the femoral necks are demonstrated on end on an AP oblique pelvis projection (see Image 22).

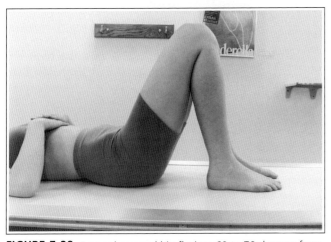

FIGURE 7-28 Proper knee and hip flexion: 60 to 70 degrees from imaging table.

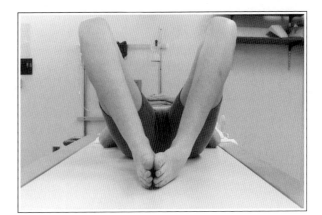

FIGURE 7-30 Femurs in only slight abduction, 20 degrees from vertical.

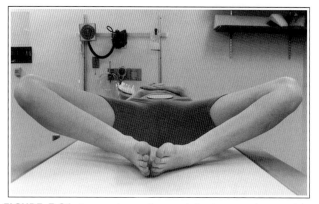

FIGURE 7-31 Femurs in maximum abduction, 20 degrees from imaging table.

- *Importance of symmetrical femoral abduction.* An AP oblique pelvis projection may not demonstrate the proximal femurs with exactly the same degree of femoral abduction. How each proximal femur appears depends on the degree of femoral abduction placed on that leg. As a standard, unless

the AP oblique pelvis projection is ordered to evaluate hip mobility, both femurs should be abducted equally for the image. This symmetrical abduction helps prevent pelvic rotation. It may be necessary to position an angled sponge beneath the patient's femurs to maintain the desired femoral abduction.

The inferior sacrum is at the center of the exposure field. The ilia, symphysis pubis, ischia, acetabula, femoral necks and heads, and greater and lesser trochanters are included within the collimated field.

- Center a perpendicular central ray to the midsagittal plane at a level 1 inch (2.5 cm) superior to the symphysis pubis. Center the IR to the central ray and open the longitudinal collimation the full 14-inch (35-cm) length for most adult patients. Transversely collimate to within 0.5 inch (1.25 cm) of the lateral skin line.
- A 14- × 17-inch (35- x 43-cm) IR placed crosswise should be adequate to include all the required anatomic structures.

Anteroposterior Oblique Pelvis Projection Analysis

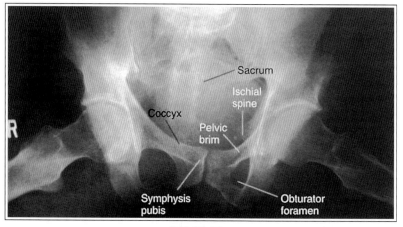

IMAGE 19

Analysis. The left obturator foramen is narrower than the right foramen, the left ischial spine is demonstrated without pelvic brim superimposition, and the sacrum and coccyx are rotated toward the right hip. The patient was rotated onto the left hip (LPO).

Correction. Rotate the patient toward the right hip until the ASISs are positioned at equal distances from the imaging table.

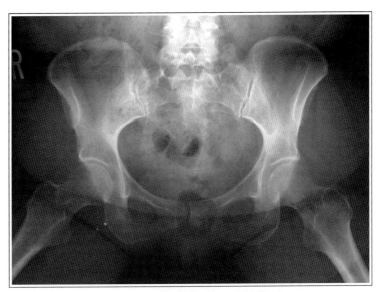

IMAGE 20

Analysis. The greater trochanters are partially demonstrated laterally, indicating that the leg was flexed less than the needed 60 to 70 degrees from the imaging table.

Correction. Increase the degree of knee and hip flexion until the femurs are positioned at a 60- to 70-degree angle with the imaging table.

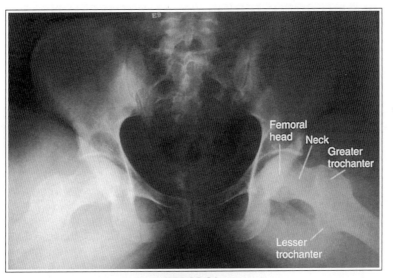

Femoral head
Neck
Greater trochanter
Lesser trochanter

IMAGE 21

Analysis. The femoral necks are demonstrated without foreshortening, and the proximal greater trochanter and lesser trochanter are demonstrated at approximately the same transverse level. The patient's femurs were in only slight abduction, at approximately a 70-degree angle with the imaging table (20 degrees from vertical), as shown in Figure 7-30.

Correction. Consult with reviewers in your facility to determine whether this is an acceptable image. If the proximal femoral shafts demonstrate too much foreshortening, have the patient abduct the femurs to a 45-degree angle with the imaging table.

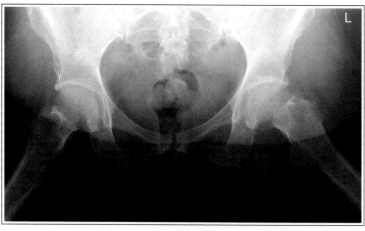

IMAGE 22

Analysis. The femoral necks are demonstrated on end. The proximal greater trochanters are demonstrated on the same transverse level as the femoral heads. The patient's femurs were positioned next to the imaging table, as shown in Figure 7-31.

Correction. Consult with reviewers in your facility to determine whether this is an acceptable image. Because the femoral necks cannot be evaluated because of foreshortening, it may be necessary to have the patient position the femurs at a 45-degree angle with the imaging table.

SACROILIAC JOINTS: ANTEROPOSTERIOR AXIAL PROJECTION

See Figure 7-32 and Box 7-7.

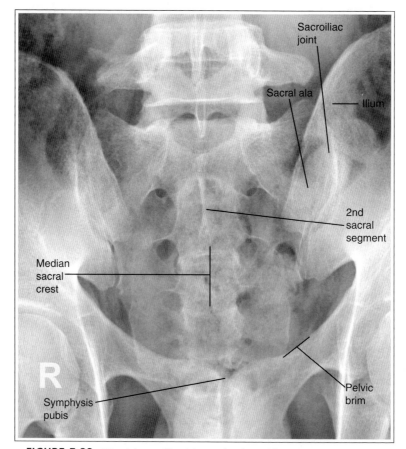

FIGURE 7-32 AP axial sacroiliac joint projection with accurate positioning.

BOX 7-7	**Anteroposterior Axial Sacroiliac Joints Projection Analysis Criteria**

- The median sacral crest is aligned with the symphysis pubis and the sacrum is at equal distance from the lateral wall of the pelvic brim on both sides.
- The sacroiliac joints are demonstrated without foreshortening and the sacrum is elongated, with the symphysis pubis superimposed over the inferior sacral segments.
- The long axis of the median sacral crest is aligned with the long axis of the collimated field.
- The second sacral segment is at the center of the exposure field.
- The sacroiliac joints and the first through fourth sacral segments are included within the collimated field.

The sacroiliac joints are demonstrated in an AP axial projection. The median sacral crest is aligned with the symphysis pubis and the sacrum is at an equal distance from the lateral wall of the pelvic brim on both sides.

- An AP axial projection of the sacroiliac joints is obtained by positioning the patient supine on the imaging table with the legs extended. Position the patient's shoulders and ASISs at equal distances from the imaging table to prevent rotation (Figure 7-33).
- *Detecting sacroiliac joint rotation.* Rotation is detected on an AP axial sacroiliac joint projection by evaluating the alignment of the long axis of the median sacral crest with the symphysis pubis and the distance from the sacrum to the lateral pelvic brim. When the patient is rotated away from the supine position, the sacrum moves in a direction opposite from the movement of the symphysis pubis and is positioned next to the lateral pelvic brim situated farther from the imaging table. If

the patient is rotated into an LPO position, the sacrum is rotated toward the patient's right pelvic brim. If the patient is rotated into an RPO position, the sacrum rotates toward the patient's left pelvic brim.

The sacroiliac joints are demonstrated without foreshortening and the sacrum is elongated, with the symphysis pubis superimposed over the inferior sacral segments.

- The patient is positioned supine, with the legs extended, and the lumbosacral curve causes the proximal sacrum and sacroiliac joints to be angled 30 to 35 degrees with the imaging table and IR. To demonstrate the sacroiliac joints without foreshortening, a 30-degree cephalic angle should be used for male patients and a 35-degree cephalic angle for female patients. Patients with less or greater lumbosacral curvature will require a decrease or increase, respectively, in cephalic angulation to maintain the 30- to 35-degree alignment of the central ray and sacroiliac joints. If an AP axial sacroiliac joint projection is taken with a perpendicular central ray or without enough cephalad angulation, the sacroiliac joints and the first through third sacral segments are foreshortened (see Image 23). If the AP axial sacroiliac joint projection is taken with too much cephalic angulation, the sacrum and sacroiliac joints demonstrate elongation and the symphysis pubis is superimposed over the inferior aspects of the sacrum and sacroiliac joints (see Image 24).

The long axis of the median sacral crest is aligned with the long axis of the exposure field.

- Aligning the long axis of the median sacral crest with the long axis of the exposure field allows for tight collimation and ensures that the central ray is angled directly into the sacroiliac joints. To obtain proper alignment, find the point halfway between the patient's palpable ASISs and then align this point and the palpable symphysis pubis with the center of the collimator's longitudinal light line.

The second sacral segment is at the center of the exposure field. The sacroiliac joints and the first through fourth sacral segments are included within the collimated field.

- Center the central ray to the patient's midsagittal plane at a level 1.5 inches (3 cm) superior to the symphysis pubis. Center the IR to the central ray, and open the longitudinal exposure field to the symphysis pubis. Transversely collimate to approximately a 9-inch (22-cm) collimated field size.
- A 10- × 12-inch (24- × 30-cm) IR placed lengthwise should be adequate to include all the required anatomic structures.

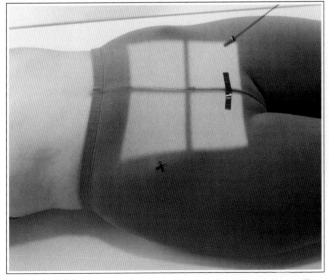

FIGURE 7-33 Proper patient positioning for AP axial sacroiliac joint projection.

Anteroposterior Axial Sacroiliac Joint Projection Analysis

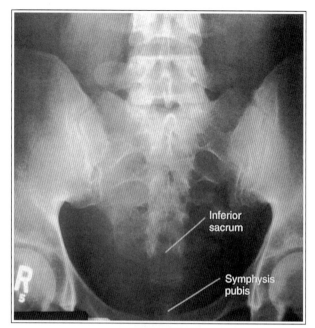

IMAGE 23

Analysis. The sacroiliac joints are foreshortened, and the inferior sacrum is demonstrated without symphysis pubis superimposition. The central ray was inadequately angled.

Correction. Angle the central ray 30 to 35 degrees cephalad.

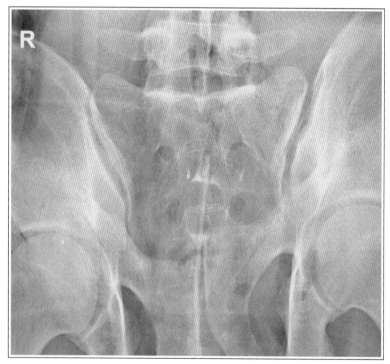

IMAGE 24

Analysis. The sacroiliac joints and sacrum are elongated and the symphysis pubis is superimposed over the inferior aspects of the sacrum and sacroiliac joints. The central ray was angled too cephalically.

Correction. Angle the central ray 30 to 35 degrees cephalad.

SACROILIAC JOINTS: ANTEROPOSTERIOR OBLIQUE PROJECTION (LEFT AND RIGHT POSTERIOR OBLIQUE POSITIONS)

See Figure 7-34 and Box 7-8.

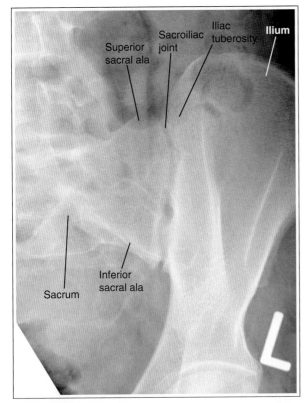

FIGURE 7-34 AP oblique sacroiliac joint projection with accurate positioning.

A right or left marker identifying the sacroiliac joint positioned farther from the IR is present on the image and is not superimposed over the anatomy of interest.

- Because the sacroiliac joint of interest is situated farther from the IR when AP oblique projections are taken, the marker used should identify the sacroiliac joint situated farther from the IR. This differs from the way most oblique projections are marked; routinely, the side marked is the one positioned closer to the IR.

The ilium and sacrum are demonstrated without superimposition, and the sacroiliac joint is open.

- An AP oblique sacroiliac joint projection is obtained by beginning with the patient positioned supine on the imaging table, with the legs extended. From this position, rotate the patient toward the unaffected side until the midcoronal plane is at a 25- to 30-degree angle with the imaging table and IR. The sacral ala and ilium are positioned in profile. Place a radiolucent support beneath the patient's elevated hip and thorax to help maintain the position (Figure 7-35). Both AP oblique projections (RPO and LPO positions) must be obtained to demonstrate the right and left sacroiliac joints. When AP oblique projections are taken, the elevated sacroiliac joint is the joint of interest.

- *Determining accuracy of obliquity.* The accuracy of an AP oblique sacroiliac joint projection can be determined by the lack of ilium and sacral superimposition. The degree of separation or cavity demonstrated between the ilium and sacrum, which represents the sacroiliac joint, varies from patient to patient. The ilia and sacrum fit very snugly together and in older patients the joint spaces between them may be smaller or even nonexistent because of fibrous adhesions or synostosis. If the patient was not rotated enough to place the ilium and sacral ala in profile, the inferior and superior sacral aspects of the ala are demonstrated without ilium superimposition, whereas the lateral sacral ala is superimposed over the iliac tuberosity (see Image 25). The lateral sacrum is also demonstrated without ilium superimposition. If the patient was rotated more than needed to position the ilium and sacral ala in profile, the ilium is superimposed over the lateral sacral ala and the inferior sacrum (see Image 26).

BOX 7-8 | Anteroposterior Oblique Sacroiliac Joints Projection Analysis Criteria

- A right or left marker identifying the sacroiliac joint positioned farther from the IR is present on the image and is not superimposed over the anatomy of interest.
- The ilium and sacrum are demonstrated without superimposition and the sacroiliac joint is open.
- The long axis of the sacroiliac joint is aligned with the long axis of the collimated field.
- The sacroiliac joint of interest is at the center of the exposure field.
- The sacroiliac joint, sacral ala, and ilium are included within the collimated field.

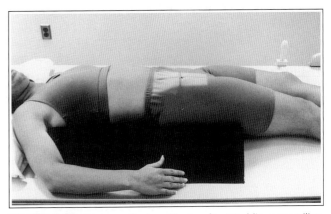

FIGURE 7-35 Proper patient positioning for AP oblique sacroiliac joint projection.

The long axis of the sacroiliac joint is aligned with the long axis of the exposure field.

- Aligning the long axis of the sacroiliac joint with the long axis of the exposure field allows for tight collimation without clipping any portion of the joint.

The sacroiliac joint of interest is at the center of the exposure field. The sacroiliac joint, sacral ala, and ilium are included within the collimated field.

- Center the central ray 1 inch (2.5 cm) medial to the elevated ASIS to position the sacroiliac joint of interest in the center of the exposure field. Center the IR to the central ray and open the longitudinal collimation to the elevated iliac crest. Transverse collimation should be to the elevated ASIS.
- A 10- × 12-inch (24- × 30-cm) IR placed lengthwise should be adequate to include all the required anatomic structures.

Anteroposterior Oblique Sacroiliac Joint Projection Analysis

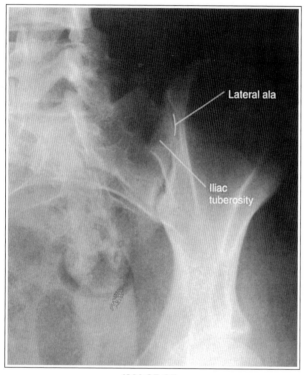

IMAGE 25

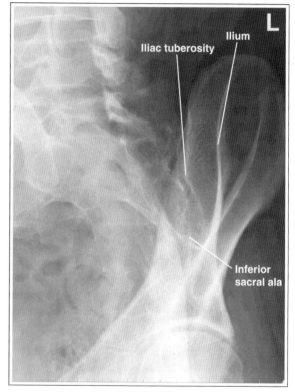

IMAGE 26

Analysis. The sacroiliac joint is closed. The superior and inferior sacral alae are demonstrated without iliac superimposition, and the lateral sacral ala is superimposed over the iliac tuberosity. The patient was not rotated enough.

Correction. Increase the pelvic obliquity. Because both the sacral ala and the ilium move simultaneously, the adjustment made should be only half the amount of superimposition of the sacral ala and iliac tuberosity.

Analysis. The sacroiliac joint is closed. The ilium is superimposed over the inferior sacral ala and the lateral sacrum. Pelvic obliquity was excessive.

Correction. Decrease the pelvic obliquity. Because both the sacral ala and the ilium move simultaneously, the amount of adjustment made should be only half the amount of ilial and sacral superimposition.

Cervical and Thoracic Vertebrae

OBJECTIVES

After completion of this chapter, you should be able to do the following:

- Identify the required anatomy on cervical and thoracic vertebrae projections.
- Describe how to properly position the patient, image receptor (IR), and central ray for cervical and thoracic vertebrae projections.
- State how to properly mark and display each cervical and thoracic vertebrae projections.
- List the image analysis requirements for cervical and thoracic vertebrae projections with accurate positioning and state how to reposition the patient when less than optimal projections are produced.
- Explain how a patient with a suspected subluxation or fracture of the cervical vertebral column is positioned for cervical projections.
- Discuss the curvature of the cervical vertebrae and explain how the intervertebral disk spaces slant and how to obtain open disk spaces on AP projections.

- Describe why a 5-degree cephalic central ray angulation is often required for an AP open-mouth projection of the atlas and axis.
- State how the relationship between the dens and atlas's lateral masses changes when the patient's head is rotated.
- Describe how the prevertebral fat stripe is used as a diagnostic tool.
- Discuss when it is necessary to achieve a lateral cervicothoracic projection of the cervical vertebrae.
- List two methods used to obtain uniform image density on an AP thoracic vertebrae projection.
- Explain the breathing methods used to demonstrate the thoracic vertebrae on a lateral thoracic projection.
- Describe two methods that are used to offset the sagging of the lower thoracic column that results when the patient is in a lateral projection.

KEY TERMS

acanthiomeatal line
costal breathing
external auditory meatus (EAM)

infraorbitomeatal line (IOML)
interpupillary line
occlusal plane

prevertebral fat stripe

IMAGE ANALYSIS CRITERIA

The following image analysis criteria are used for all adult and pediatric cervical and thoracic projections and should be considered when completing the analysis for each projection presented in this chapter (Box 8-1).

- *Visibility of cervical and thoracic vertebral details.* An optimal kilovoltage peak (kVp) technique, as shown in Table 8-1, sufficiently penetrates the cervical and thoracic vertebral structures and provides the contrast scale necessary to visualize the vertebral details. To obtain optimal density, set a manual milliampere-seconds (mAs) level based on the patient's thickness or choose the appropriate automatic exposure control (AEC) chamber. Table 8-1 lists the technical data for the most common projections.

BOX 8-1	Cervical and Thoracic Vertebrae Imaging Analysis Criteria

- The facility's identification requirements are visible.
- A right or left marker identifying the correct side of the patient is present on the image and is not superimposed over the anatomy of interest.
- Good radiation protection practices are evident.
- Bony trabecular patterns and cortical outlines of the anatomic structures are sharply defined.
- Contrast and density are uniform and adequate to demonstrate the soft tissue, air-filled trachea, and bony structures.
- Penetration is sufficient to visualize the bony trabecular patterns and cortical outlines of the vertebral bodies, pedicles, and spinous and transverse processes.
- No evidence of removal artifacts is present.

CERVICAL VERTEBRAE: ANTEROPOSTERIOR AXIAL PROJECTION

See Figure 8-1 and Box 8-2.

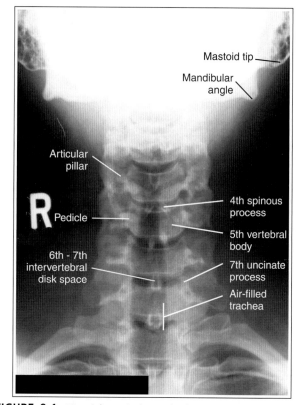

FIGURE 8-1 AP axial cervical vertebral projection with accurate positioning.

The cervical vertebrae demonstrate an AP axial projection. The spinous processes are aligned with the midline of the cervical bodies, the mandibular angles and mastoid tips are at equal distances from the cervical vertebrae, the articular pillars and pedicles are symmetrically demonstrated lateral to the cervical bodies, and the distances from the vertebral column to the medial (sternal) ends of the clavicles are equal.

- An AP axial projection of the cervical vertebrae is obtained by placing the patient supine or upright, with the shoulders positioned at equal distances

TABLE 8-1	Cervical and Thoracic Vertebrae Technical Data				
Projection	**kVp**	**Grid**	**AEC Chamber(s)**	**SID**	
AP axial, cervical vertebrae	70–80	Grid	Center	40–48 inches (100–120 cm)	
AP, open-mouth, C1 and C2	70–80	Grid		40–48 inches (100–120 cm)	
Lateral, cervical vertebrae	70–80	Air-gap technique	Center	72 inches (150–180 cm)	
AP axial oblique, cervical vertebrae	70–80	Air-gap technique	Center	72 inches (150–180 cm)	
Lateral projection (Twining method), cervicothoracic vertebrae	65–85	Grid		40–48 inches (100–120 cm)	
AP, thoracic vertebrae	75–85	Grid	Center	40–48 inches (100–120 cm)	
Lateral, thoracic vertebrae	80–90	Grid	Center	40–48 inches (100–120 cm)	

AEC, Automatic exposure control; *kVp,* kilovoltage peak; *SID,* source–image receptor distance.

BOX 8-2 | **Anteroposterior Axial Cervical Vertebrae Projection Analysis Criteria**

- Spinous processes are aligned with the midline of the cervical bodies, the mandibular angles and mastoid tips are at equal distances from the cervical vertebrae, the articular pillars and pedicles are symmetrically visualized lateral to the cervical bodies, and the distances from the vertebral column to the medial clavicular ends are equal.
- The intervertebral disk spaces are open, the vertebral bodies are demonstrated without distortion, and each vertebra's spinous process is visualized at the level of its inferior intervertebral disk space.
- The third cervical vertebra is demonstrated in its entirety, and the posterior occiput and mandibular mentum are superimposed.
- The long axis of the cervical column is aligned with the long axis of the exposure field.
- The fourth cervical vertebra is at the center of the exposure field.
- The second through seventh cervical vertebrae and the surrounding soft tissue are included within the collimated field.

from the imaging table or upright image receptor (IR; Figure 8-2). The patient's face should be positioned so it is forward, placing the mandibular angles and mastoid tips at equal distances from the imaging table or upright grid holder.

- *Effect of cervical rotation.* When the patient and cervical vertebrae are rotated away from the AP axial projection, the vertebral bodies move toward the side positioned closer to the IR, and the spinous processes move toward the side positioned farther from the IR. The upper (C1 to C4) and lower (C5 to C7) cervical vertebrae can demonstrate rotation independently or simultaneously, depending on which part of the body is rotated. If the head is rotated but the thorax remains in an AP axial projection, the upper cervical vertebrae demonstrate rotation as C1 rotates on C2, and the lower cervical vertebrae remain in an AP

axial projection. If the thorax is rotated but the head remains in a forward position to match, the lower cervical vertebrae demonstrate rotation and the upper cervical vertebrae remain in an AP axial projection. If the patient's head and thorax are rotated simultaneously, the entire cervical column demonstrates rotation (see Image 1).

- *Detecting rotation.* Rotation is present on an AP axial projection in the following situations: (1) if the mandibular angles and mastoid tips are not demonstrated at equal distances from the cervical vertebrae; (2) if the spinous processes are not demonstrated in the midline of the cervical bodies; (3) if the pedicles and articular pillars are not symmetrically demonstrated lateral to the vertebral bodies; and (4) if the medial ends of the clavicles are not demonstrated at equal distances from the vertebral column (see Image 1). The side of the patient positioned closer to the imaging table or upright IR is the side toward which the mandible is rotated and also the side that demonstrates less of the articular pillars and less clavicular and vertebral column superimposition.
- *Positioning for trauma.* When cervical vertebral projections are exposed on a trauma patient with suspected subluxation or fracture, obtain the AP axial projection with the patient positioned as is. Do not attempt to remove the cervical collar or adjust the head or body rotation, mandible position, or cervical column tilting. This might result in greater injury to the vertebrae or spinal cord. Spinal cord injuries may occur from mishandling the patient after the initial injury has taken place.

The intervertebral disk spaces are open, the vertebral bodies are demonstrated without distortion, and each vertebra's spinous process is visualized at the level of its inferior intervertebral disk space.

- The cervical vertebral column demonstrates a lordotic curvature. This curvature and the shape of the vertebral bodies cause the disk-articulating surfaces of the vertebral bodies to slant upward anteriorly to posteriorly.
- *Importance of central ray angulation.* To obtain open intervertebral disk spaces and undistorted vertebral bodies, the central ray must be angled in the same direction as the slope of the vertebral bodies. This can be easily discerned by viewing the lateral cervical projection in Figure 8-3. Studying this lateral cervical projection, you can see that when the correct central ray angulation is used, each vertebra's spinous process is located within its inferior intervertebral disk space. The degree of central ray angulation needed to obtain open intervertebral disk spaces and to align the spinous processes within them accurately depends on the degree of cervical lordotic curvature.
- *Upright versus supine position.* If the AP axial cervical vertebrae projection is performed with the

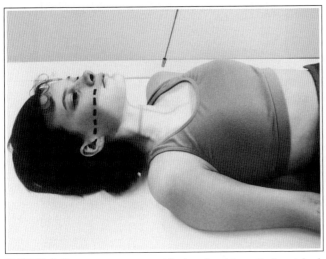

FIGURE 8-2 Proper patient positioning for AP cervical vertebral projection.

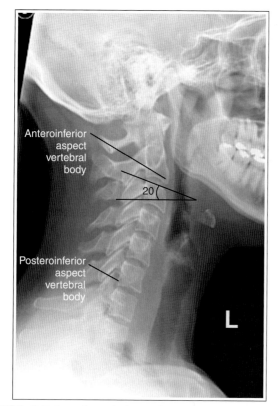

FIGURE 8-3 Lateral cervical vertebrae projection taken with patient upright.

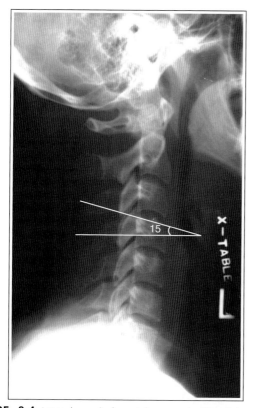

FIGURE 8-4 Lateral cervical vertebrae projection taken with patient supine.

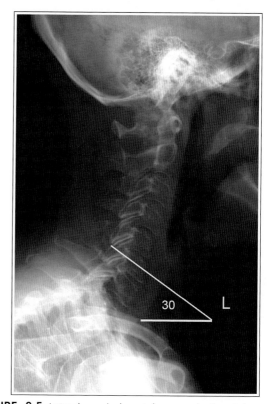

FIGURE 8-5 Lateral cervical vertebrae projection taken on a kyphotic patient.

patient in an upright position, the cervical vertebrae demonstrate more lordotic curvature than if the examination is performed with the patient supine. In a supine position, the gravitational pull placed on the middle cervical vertebrae results in straightening of the cervical curvature. Figure 8-3 demonstrates a lateral cervical projection taken with the patient in an upright position and Figure 8-4 demonstrates a lateral cervical projection taken with the patient supine. Note the difference in lordotic curvature between these two images. Because of this difference, the central ray angulation should be varied when an AP axial cervical vertebrae projection is taken with the patient erect rather than supine. In the erect position, a 20-degree cephalad central ray angulation is needed to align the central ray parallel with the intervertebral disk spaces. In the supine position, a 15-degree cephalad central ray angulation sufficiently aligns the central ray parallel with the intervertebral disk spaces.

- *Kyphotic patient.* The kyphotic patient demonstrates an exaggerated kyphotic curvature of the thoracic vertebrae that will cause excessive lordotic curvature of the cervical vertebrae (Figure 8-5). To demonstrate the upper and lower cervical vertebrae with open intervertebral spaces for an upright AP axial cervical vertebrae projection, it will be necessary to increase the degree of central ray angulation above that routinely needed for a patient without kyphosis. If the AP axial projection is taken with the kyphotic patient in a supine position, a radiolucent sponge should be placed beneath the patient's head to prevent the upper cervical vertebrae from extending toward the imaging table and from superimposing the posterior occiput on the image (see Image 2).

- *Effect of central ray misalignment.* Misalignment of the central ray and intervertebral disk spaces results in closed disk spaces, distorted vertebral bodies, and projection of the spinous processes into the vertebral bodies. If the central ray angulation is not used or is insufficient, the resulting image demonstrates closed intervertebral disk spaces, and each vertebra's spinous process is demonstrated within its vertebral body (see Images 3 and 4). This anatomic relationship also results if the patient's head is tilted toward the x-ray tube for the examination, causing the cervical vertebrae to tilt anteriorly. If the central ray is angled more than needed to align the central ray parallel with the intervertebral disk spaces, or if the patient's cervical vertebral column was extended posteriorly for the examination, the resulting image demonstrates closed intervertebral disk spaces, each vertebra's spinous process is demonstrated within the inferior adjoining vertebral body, and the uncinate processes are elongated (see Image 5).

The third cervical vertebra is demonstrated in its entirety, and the posterior occiput and mandibular mentum are superimposed.

- Accurate positioning of the occiput and mandibular mentum is achieved when an imaginary line connecting the upper occlusal plane (chewing surface of maxillary teeth) and the base of the skull is aligned perpendicular to the imaging table or upright IR. This positioning also aligns the acanthiomeatal line (an imaginary line connecting the point at which the upper lip and nose meet with the external ear opening) perpendicular to the imaging table or upright IR (see Figure 8-2). With this position, you might expect the patient's mandible to be superimposed over the upper cervical vertebrae but this will not be the case because the cephalad central ray angulation used will project the mandible superiorly.
- *Effect of occiput-mentum mispositioning.* Mispositioning of the posterior occiput and the upper occlusal plane results in an obstructed image of the upper cervical vertebrae. If the occlusal plane is positioned superior to the base of the skull (head tilted too far backward), the upper cervical vertebrae are superimposed over the occiput (see Image 6). If the upper occlusal plane is positioned inferior to the base of the skull (chin tucked too far downward), the mandibular mentum is superimposed over the superior cervical vertebrae (see Image 7).

The long axis of the cervical column is aligned with the long axis of the exposure field.

- Aligning the long axis of the cervical column with the long axis of the collimated field ensures that no lateral flexion of the cervical column is present (see Image 8) and allows for tight collimation (see Image 7). This alignment is obtained by aligning the midline of the patient's neck with the collimator's longitudinal light line.

The fourth cervical vertebra is centered within the exposure field. The second through seventh cervical vertebrae and the surrounding soft tissue are included within the collimated field.

- Center the central ray to the patient's midsagittal plane at a level halfway between the external auditory meatus (EAM) and the jugular notch to center C4 to the collimated field.
- Open the longitudinal collimation to the EAM and the jugular notch. Transverse collimation should be to within 0.5 inch (1.25 cm) of the lateral neck skin line.
- An 8- × 10-inch (18- × 24-cm) IR placed lengthwise should be adequate to include all the required anatomic structures.

Anteroposterior Axial Cervical Vertebrae Projection Analysis

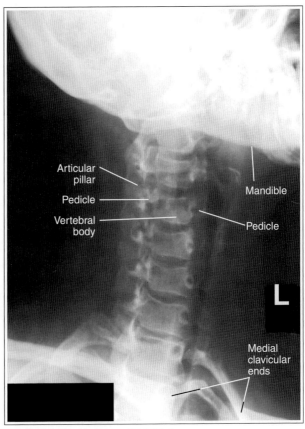

IMAGE 1

Analysis. The spinous processes are not aligned with the midline of the cervical bodies, and the pedicles and articular pillars are not symmetrically demonstrated lateral to the vertebral bodies. The mandible is rotated toward the patient's left side, and the medial end of the left clavicle demonstrates no vertebral column superimposition. The patient was rotated toward the left side (left posterior oblique [LPO] position).

Correction. Rotate the patient toward the right side until the shoulders are at equal distances from the imaging table or upright grid holder, and turn the patient's head toward the right side until the mandibular angles and mastoid tips are at equal distances from the imaging table or upright grid holder.

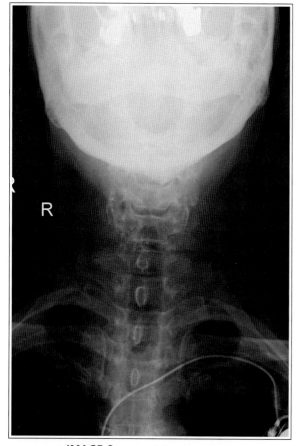

IMAGE 2 Supine kyphotic patient.

Analysis. The intervertebral disk spaces are closed, with the spinous processes of C6 and C7 within their vertebral bodies and the spinous processes of C4 and C5 within the inferior adjoining vertebral bodies. The uncinate processes of C5 and C6 are elongated and C1 through C3 are superimposing the posterior occiput. The central ray angulation was not used or was insufficient to align the central ray parallel with the intervertebral disk spaces of C6 and C7 and too cephalic to align the central ray parallel with the intervertebral disk spaces of C4 and C5, and the upper cervical vertebrae was extended posteriorly to rest the patient's head on the imaging table.

Correction. Increase the degree of cephalic central ray angulation to align it with the C6-C7 intervertebral disk space, tuck the patient's chin toward the chest, and elevate the head on a radiolucent sponge until an imaginary line connecting the upper occlusal plane and base of the skull is aligned perpendicular to the imaging table.

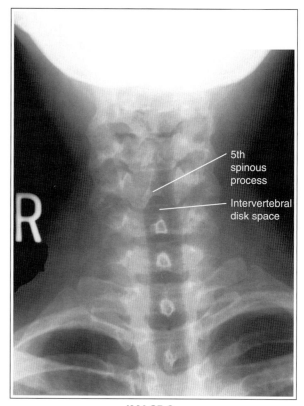

IMAGE 3

Analysis. The anteroinferior aspects of the cervical bodies (see Figure 8-3 for identification) are obscuring the intervertebral disk spaces, and each vertebra's spinous process is demonstrated within its vertebral body. The central ray angulation was not used or was insufficient to align the central ray parallel with the intervertebral disk spaces.

Correction. Increase the degree of cephalic central ray angulation.

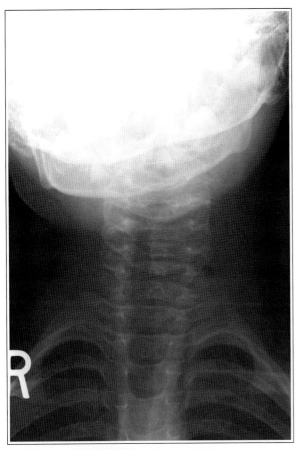

IMAGE 4 Pediatric patient.

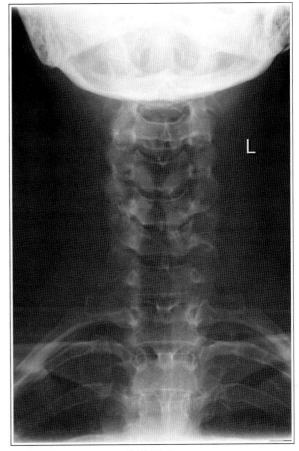

IMAGE 5

Analysis. The anteroinferior aspects of the cervical bodies are obscuring the intervertebral disk spaces, and each vertebra's spinous process is demonstrated within its vertebral body. The central ray angulation was not used or was insufficient to align the central ray parallel with the intervertebral disk spaces.

Correction. Increase the degree of cephalic central ray angulation.

Analysis. The posteroinferior aspects of the cervical bodies (see Figure 8-3 for identification) are obscuring the intervertebral disk spaces, the uncinate processes are elongated, and each vertebra's spinous process is demonstrated within the inferior adjoining vertebral body. The central ray was angled too cephalically to align central ray parallel with the intervertebral disk spaces.

Correction. Decrease the degree of cephalic central ray angulation.

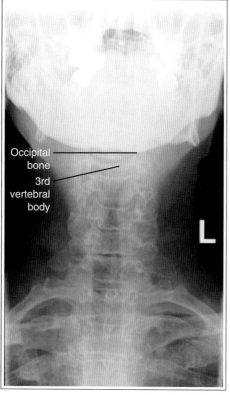

IMAGE 6

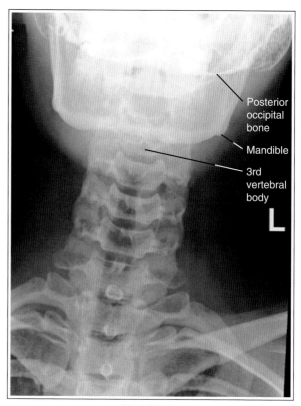

IMAGE 7

Analysis. A portion of the third cervical vertebra is superimposed over the posterior occipital bone, preventing a clear visualization of the third cervical vertebra. The upper occlusal plane was positioned superior to the base of the skull.

Correction. Tuck the chin half the distance demonstrated between the base of the skull and mandibular mentum, or until an imaginary line connecting the upper occlusal plane and the base of the skull is aligned perpendicular to the imaging table or upright grid holder. For this patient, the movement should be approximately 1 inch (2.5 cm).

Analysis. The mandible is superimposed over a portion of the third cervical vertebra. The upper occlusal plane was positioned inferior to the base of the occiput. The long axis of the cervical column is not aligned with the long axis of the collimated field, preventing tight collimation.

Correction. Raise the chin half the distance shown between the base of the skull and mandibular mentum, or until an imaginary line connecting the upper occlusal plane and the inferior base of the posterior occiput is aligned perpendicular to the imaging table or upright grid holder. Align the long axis of the cervical column with the long axis of the collimated field, and increase transverse collimation.

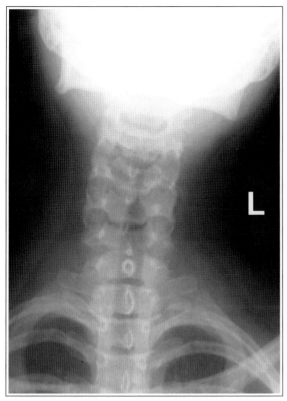

IMAGE 8

Analysis. The head is tilted toward the left side, causing the upper cervical vertebrae to flex laterally. The long axis of the cervical vertebral column was not aligned with the long axis of the collimated field.

Correction. Tilt the head toward the right side until the patient's upper and lower neck midlines are aligned with the collimator's longitudinal light line.

CERVICAL ATLAS AND AXIS: ANTEROPOSTERIOR PROJECTION (OPEN-MOUTH POSITION)

See Figure 8-6 and Box 8-3.

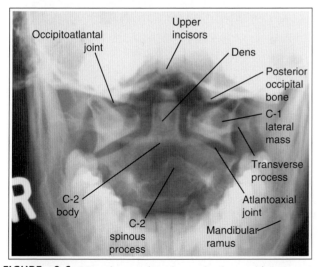

FIGURE 8-6 AP atlas and axis projection with accurate positioning.

The atlas and axis demonstrate an AP projection. The atlas is symmetrically seated on the axis, with the atlas's lateral masses at equal distances from the dens. The

BOX 8-3	Anteroposterior Cervical Atlas and Axis Projection Analysis Criteria

- The atlas is symmetrically seated on the axis, with the atlas's lateral masses at equal distances from the dens.
- The spinous processes of the axis are aligned with the midline of the axis's body, and the mandibular rami are visualized at equal distances from the lateral masses.
- The upper incisors and the base of the skull are seen superior to the dens and the atlantoaxial joint.
- The atlantoaxial joint is open, and the axis's spinous process is demonstrated in the midline and slightly inferior to the dens.
- The dens is at the center of the exposure field.
- The atlantoaxial and occipitoatlantal joints, the atlas's lateral masses and transverse processes, and the axis's dens and body are included within the collimated field.

spinous process of the axis is aligned with the midline of the axis's body, and the mandibular rami are demonstrated at equal distances from the lateral masses.

- An AP projection of the atlas and axis is obtained by placing the patient in a supine or upright position, with the shoulders, mandibular angles, and mastoid tips positioned at equal distances from the imaging table or upright IR (Figure 8-7).

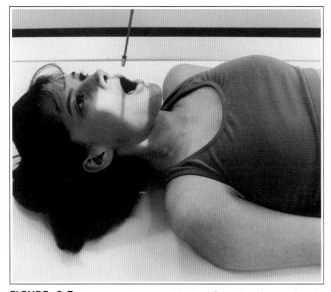

FIGURE 8-7 Proper patient positioning for AP atlas and axis projection.

- *Effect of rotation.* Rotation of the atlas and axis occurs when the head is turned away from an AP projection. On head rotation, the atlas pivots around the dens so that the lateral mass located on the side the face is rotated toward is displaced posteriorly and the mass toe side the face is rotated away from is displaced anteriorly. This displacement causes the space between the lateral mass and dens to narrow on the side the face is rotated away from and to enlarge on the side the face is rotated toward (see Image 9). As the amount of head rotation increases, the axis rotates in the same direction as the atlas, resulting in a shift in the position of its spinous process in the direction opposite that in which the patient's face is turned.
- *Detecting direction of rotation.* To determine how the patient's face was turned, judge the distance between the mandibular rami and lateral masses. The side that demonstrates the greater distance is the side toward which the face was rotated.
- *Positioning for trauma.* When cervical vertebrae projections are taken on a trauma patient with suspected subluxation or fractures, obtain the AP cervical atlas and axis projection with the patient's position left as is. Do not attempt to remove the cervical collar or adjust head or body rotation, mandible position, or cervical vertebral column tilting. To do so might result in increased injury to the vertebrae or spinal cord.

The upper incisors and the base of the skull are demonstrated superior to the dens and the atlantoaxial joint.

- The dens and the atlantoaxial joint are located at the midsagittal plane, at a level 0.5 inch (1.25 cm) inferior to an imaginary line connecting the mastoid tips. To demonstrate them without upper incisor

(front teeth) or posterior occiput superimposition, instruct the patient to open the mouth as widely as possible. Then have the patient tuck the chin until an imaginary line connecting the upper occlusal plane (chewing surface of maxillary teeth) and the base of the skull is aligned perpendicular to the imaging table or upright grid holder. If the patient does not have upper teeth, one should imagine where the occlusal plane would be if the patient had teeth. This positioning also aligns the acanthiomeatal line (an imaginary line drawn between the point where the upper lip and nose meet the external ear opening) perpendicular with the imaging table or upright grid holder. It may be necessary to position a small angled sponge beneath the patient's head to maintain accurate head positioning, especially if the patient's chin has to be tucked so much that it is difficult to open the mouth adequately. The sponge causes the upper occlusal plane and base of the skull to align perpendicularly without requiring as much chin tucking.

- *Relationship of central ray angulation and patient position.* The lateral cervical projection in Figure 8-8 demonstrates how the occlusal plane and the base of the skull should be aligned for an accurate open-mouth AP projection. After studying this image, you might conclude that the atlantoaxial joint will be free of upper incisor or occiput superimposition if the patient maintains this head position and simply drops the jaw.

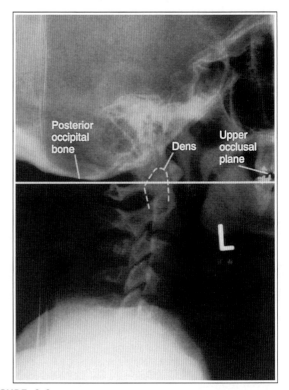

FIGURE 8-8 Lateral cervical vertebral projection demonstrating upper incisor, dens, and posterior occiput relationship.

Because the upper incisors are positioned at a long object–image receptor distance (OID), however, they are greatly magnified, causing them to be projected onto the dens and atlantoaxial joint. In most patients, when the upper occlusal plane and base of the skull are superimposed, magnification causes the upper incisors to be projected approximately 1 inch (2.5 cm) inferior to the base of the skull (see Image 10). For these incisors to be projected superiorly, a 5-degree cephalic angle should be placed on the central ray. The upper incisors will be projected approximately 1 inch (2.5 cm) for every 5 degrees of angulation. This angle adjustment is based on a 40-inch (102-cm) SID; if a longer SID is used, the required angle adjustment would be less, whereas if a shorter SID is used, the angulation adjustment would be greater. If, instead of an angle adjustment, the patient's chin were tilted upward in an attempt to shift the upper incisors superiorly, the posterior occiput would simultaneously be shifted inferiorly.

- This inferior shift of the occiput would obscure the dens and possibly the atlantoaxial joint. The dens and atlantoaxial joint space may also be obscured if a 5-degree cephalad central ray angle was used but the occlusal plane and base of the skull were not superimposed. When the base of the skull is positioned inferior to the upper occlusal plane, the image demonstrates the dens and, depending on the degree of mispositioning, the atlantoaxial joint space superimposed onto the posterior occiput (see Image 11). When the occlusal plane is positioned inferior to the base of the skull, the posterior occiput is demonstrated superior to the dens, and the upper incisors are superimposed over a portion of the superior dens (see Image 12).
- *Positioning for trauma.* For the dens and atlantoaxial joint to be demonstrated without incisor or occiput superimposition in a trauma patient, the direction of the central ray must be changed from the standard position. A trauma patient's head and neck cannot be adjusted, so you must angle the central ray until it is aligned parallel with the infraorbitomeatal line (IOML) (imaginary line connecting the inferior orbital rim and the external ear opening). This line is easily accessible in a patient wearing a cervical collar. The exact degree of angulation needed depends on the amount of chin elevation. Most patients in a cervical collar require approximately a 10-degree caudal angle. Once the angle is set, attempt to get the patient to drop the lower jaw. Do not adjust head rotation or tilting. If the cervical collar allows the lower jaw to move without elevating the upper jaw, instruct the patient to drop the lower jaw. If the cervical collar prevents lower jaw movement without elevating the upper jaw, instruct the patient about the importance of

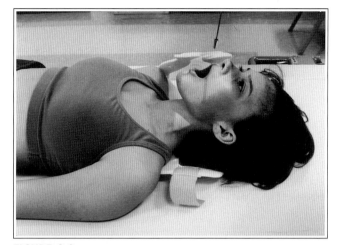

FIGURE 8-9 Proper patient positioning for AP atlas and axis projection taken to evaluate trauma.

holding the head and neck perfectly still; then have the ordering physician remove the front of the cervical collar so that the patient can drop the jaw without adjusting the head or neck position (Figure 8-9). After the patient's jaw is dropped, align the central ray to the midsagittal plane at a level 0.5 inch (1.25 cm) inferior to the occlusal plane. Immediately after the image is taken, the physician should return the front of the cervical collar to its proper position. For trauma positioning, insufficient caudal angulation causes the upper incisors to be demonstrated superior to the dens and the dens to be superimposed over the posterior occiput (see Image 13). If the central ray was angled too caudally, the posterior occiput is demonstrated superior to the dens and the upper incisors are superimposed over the dens (see Image 14).

The atlantoaxial joint is open, and the axis's spinous process is demonstrated in the midline and slightly inferior to the dens.

- AP neck extension and flexion determine the alignment of the atlantoaxial joint with the imaging table and the position of the axis's spinous process to the dens. When the occlusal plane and base of the skull are aligned perpendicular to the imaging table, the atlantoaxial joint should be open.
- *Effect of cervical column flexion and extension.* If the cervical column is flexed, the atlantoaxial joint is closed and the spinous process of the axis is demonstrated closer to the dens (see Image 15). If the cervical column is extended, the atlantoaxial joint is closed and the spinous process of the axis is demonstrated more inferiorly to the dens.

The dens is centered within the exposure field. The atlantoaxial and occipitoatlantal joints, the atlas's lateral masses and transverse processes, and the axis's dens and body are included within the collimated field.

- Center the central ray through the open mouth to the midsagittal plane to center the dens to the center of the exposure field.
- Open the longitudinally collimated field to the patient's external ear opening. Transverse collimation should be to a 5-inch (12.5-cm) field size.
- An 8- × 10-inch (18- × 24-cm) IR placed lengthwise should be adequate to include all the required anatomic structures.

Anteroposterior Cervical Atlas and Axis Projection Analysis

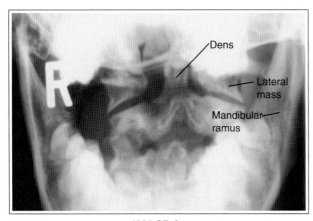

IMAGE 9

Analysis. The distances from the atlas's lateral masses to the dens and from the mandibular rami to the dens are narrower on the left side than on the right side, and the axis's spinous process is shifted from the midline toward the left. The face was rotated toward the right side.

Correction. Rotate the face toward the left side until the mandibular angles and mastoid tips are positioned at equal distances from the imaging table or upright grid holder.

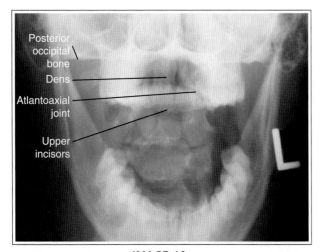

IMAGE 10

Analysis. The upper incisors are demonstrated approximately 1 inch (2.5 cm) inferior to the base of the skull, obscuring the dens and atlantoaxial articulation. The base of the skull is demonstrated directly superior to the dens.

Correction. If the upper occlusal plane and the base of the skull were aligned perpendicular to the imaging table and a perpendicular central ray was used for this image, do not adjust patient positioning; simply direct the central ray 5 degrees cephalad. If a 5-degree cephalad angulation was used for this image, do not adjust patient positioning; simply increase the cephalad angulation by 5 degrees. The incisors will shift approximately 1 inch (2.5 cm) for every 5 degrees of central ray angulation. (This angle adjustment is based on a 40-inch [102-cm] SID; if a longer SID is used, less angle adjustment is required; if a shorter SID is used, more angle adjustment is required.)

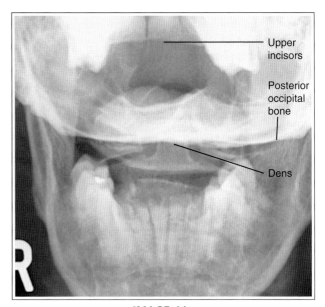

IMAGE 11

Analysis. The dens is superimposed over the posterior occiput. The upper incisors are demonstrated approximately 1.5 inches (3.75 cm) superior to the base of the skull. The patient's head was not accurately positioned.

Correction. Tuck the chin toward the chest until an imaginary line connecting the upper occlusal plane with the base of the skull is aligned perpendicular to the IR. The needed movement is equal to half the distance demonstrated between the upper incisors and base of the skull. For this patient, the chin should be tucked approximately 0.75 inch (2 cm).

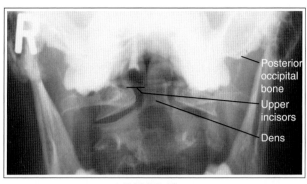

IMAGE 12

Analysis. The upper incisors are superimposed over the dens. The base of the skull is demonstrated approximately 0.5 inch (1.25 cm) superior to the upper incisors and 0.25 inch (0.6 cm) superior to the dens. The upper occlusal plane was positioned inferior to the base of the skull.

Correction. Elevate the upper jaw until an imaginary line connecting the upper occlusal plane with the base of the skull is aligned perpendicular to the IR. The needed movement is equal to half the distance demonstrated between the upper incisors and the base of the skull. For this patient, the upper occlusal plane should be elevated approximately 0.25 inch (0.6 cm).

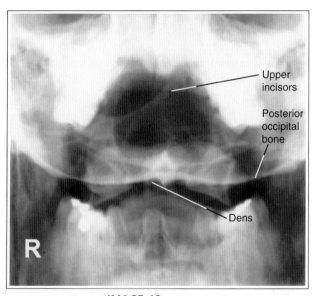

IMAGE 13 Trauma.

Analysis. The upper incisors are demonstrated superior to the dens and the base of the skull, and the dens is superimposed over the posterior occiput. The central ray angulation was not directed enough caudally.

Correction. Angle the central ray approximately 5 degrees caudad for every 1 inch (2.5 cm) demonstrated between the upper incisors and the base of the skull. (This angle adjustment is based on a 40-inch [102-cm] SID.) Because approximately 1 inch (2.5 cm) is demonstrated between the upper incisors and base of the skull on this image, the central ray angulation should be adjusted approximately 5 degrees caudally.

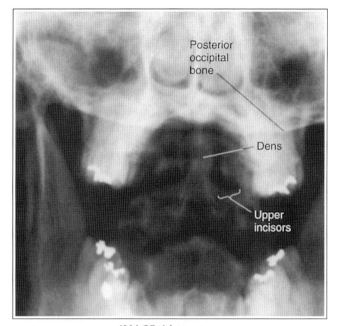

IMAGE 14 Trauma.

Analysis. The upper incisors are superimposed over the dens, and the base of the skull is situated superior to the dens and upper incisors. The central ray was angled too caudally.

Correction. Angle the central ray approximately 5 degrees cephalically for every 1 inch (2.5 cm) demonstrated between the upper incisors and base of the skull.

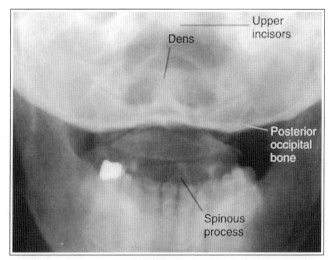

IMAGE 15

Analysis. The atlantoaxial joint is closed, the posterior occipital bone is superimposed over the dens, the upper incisors appear superior to the posterior occipital bone, and the axis's spinous process is demonstrated too inferior to the dens. The patient's head was not accurately positioned, and the cervical column was extended.

Correction. Tuck the chin toward the chest until an imaginary line connecting the upper occlusal plane with the base of the skull is aligned perpendicular to the IR.

CERVICAL VERTEBRAE: LATERAL PROJECTION

See Figure 8-10 and Box 8-4.

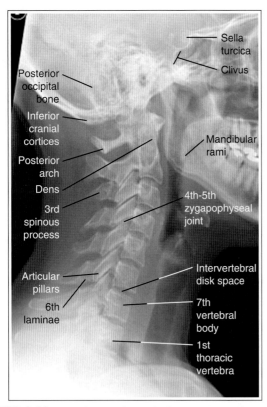

FIGURE 8-10 Lateral cervical vertebral projection with accurate positioning.

Contrast and density are adequate to demonstrate the prevertebral fat stripe.

- *Prevertebral fat stripe.* The soft tissue structure of interest on a lateral cervical projection is the prevertebral fat stripe. It is located anterior to the cervical vertebrae and is visible on correctly exposed lateral cervical projections with accurate positioning (Figure 8-11). The reviewer evaluates the distance between the anterior surface of the cervical vertebrae and the prevertebral fat stripe. Abnormal widening of this space is used for the detection and localization of fractures, masses, and inflammation.

The cervical vertebrae demonstrate a lateral projection. The anterior and posterior aspects of the right and left articular pillars and the right and left zygapophyseal joints of each cervical vertebra are superimposed, and the spinous processes are in profile.

- A lateral cervical vertebral projection is obtained by placing the patient in an upright position with the midcoronal plane positioned perpendicular to the IR (Figure 8-12). In this position the right and left sides of each cervical vertebra are superimposed, demonstrating the spinous processes and vertebral bodies in profile. To prevent rotation, superimpose the patient's shoulders, mastoid tips, and mandibular rami.
- *Effect of rotation.* The upper and lower cervical vertebrae can demonstrate rotation simultaneously or separately, depending on which part of the body

BOX 8-4 | **Lateral Cervical Vertebrae Projection Analysis Criteria**

- Contrast and density are adequate to visualize the prevertebral fat stripe.
- The anterior and posterior aspects of the right and left articular pillars and the right and left zygapophyseal joints of each cervical vertebra are superimposed, and the spinous processes are in profile.
- The posterior arch of C1 and spinous process of C2 are in profile without posterior occiput superimposition. Their bodies are seen without mandibular superimposition, cranial cortices and the mandibular rami are superimposed, the superior and inferior aspects of the right and left articular pillars and zygapophyseal joints of each cervical vertebra are superimposed, and the intervertebral disk spaces are open.
- The long axis of the cervical vertebral column is aligned with the long axis of the exposure field.
- The fourth cervical vertebra is at the center of the exposure field.
- The sella turcica, clivus, first through seventh cervical vertebrae, and superior half of the first thoracic vertebra and the surrounding soft tissue are included within the collimated field.

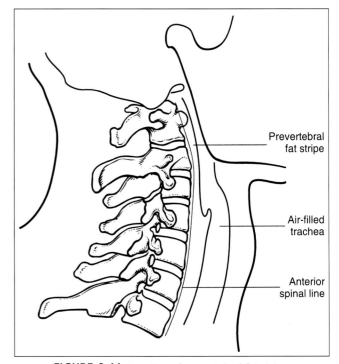

FIGURE 8-11 Location of prevertebral fat stripe.

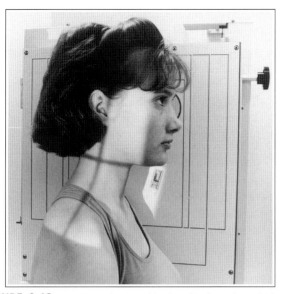

FIGURE 8-12 Proper patient positioning for lateral cervical vertebrae projection.

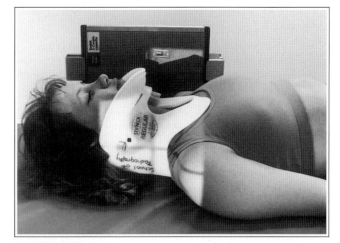

FIGURE 8-13 Proper patient positioning for lateral cervical vertebrae projection taken to evaluate trauma.

is rotated. If the head was rotated and the thorax remained in a lateral projection, the upper cervical vertebrae demonstrate rotation. If the thorax was rotated and the head remained in a lateral projection, the lower cervical vertebrae demonstrate rotation. If the patient's head and thorax were rotated simultaneously, the entire cervical column demonstrates rotation.

- *Detecting rotation.* Rotation can be detected on a lateral cervical projection by evaluating each vertebra for anterior and posterior pillar superimposition and for zygapophyseal joint superimposition. When the patient is rotated, the pillars and zygapophyseal joints on one side of the vertebra move anterior to those on the other side (see Images 16 and 17). Because the two sides of the vertebra are mirror images, it is very difficult to determine from a rotated lateral cervical projection which side of the patient is rotated anteriorly and which is rotated posteriorly. The magnification of the side situated farther from the IR may provide a moderately reliable clue at the articular pillar regions.
- *Positioning for trauma.* When cervical vertebral projections are taken of a trauma patient with suspected subluxation or fracture, take the lateral projection with the patient's position left as is. Do not attempt to remove the cervical collar or adjust head or body rotation, mandible position, or vertebral tilting. This might result in increased injury to the vertebrae or spinal cord. A trauma lateral cervical vertebral projection is obtained by placing a lengthwise IR against the patient's shoulder and directing a horizontal beam to the cervical vertebrae (Figure 8-13). Such an image should meet as many of the analysis requirements listed

for a nontrauma lateral projection as possible without moving the patient. A 10- × 12-inch (24- × 30-cm) IR may be needed to include all the required structures.

The posterior arch of C1 and the spinous process of C2 are in profile without posterior occiput superimposition, and their bodies are demonstrated without mandibular superimposition. The cranial cortices and the mandibular rami are superimposed, the superior and inferior aspects of the right and left articular pillars and the zygapophyseal joints of each cervical vertebra are superimposed, and the intervertebral disk spaces are open.

- When the patient is positioned for a lateral cervical projection, place the head in a lateral projection with the midsagittal plane aligned parallel with the IR and the chin is elevated until the acanthiomeatal line is aligned parallel with the floor and the interpupillary line is aligned perpendicular to the IR. This positioning accomplishes five goals: alignment of the cervical vertebral column parallel with the IR; demonstration of C1 and C2 without occiput or mandibular superimposition; superimposition of the anterior and posterior and superior and inferior aspects of the cranial and mandibular cortices, and of the superior and inferior aspects of the right and left articular pillars and zygapophyseal joints.
- *Effect of mandibular rotation and elevation on C1 and C2 visualization.* The position of the mandible and demonstration of C1 and C2 on a lateral cervical vertebrae projection are affected by head positioning. The posterior cortices of the mandibular rami are superimposed when the head's midsagittal plane was aligned parallel with the IR. If the posterior cortices of the mandibular rami are not superimposed on a lateral cervical vertebrae projection, one mandibular ramus is superimposed

over the bodies of C1 and/or C2 and the other is situated anteriorly (see Image 18).

If the chin was elevated adequately to place the acanthiomeatal line parallel with the floor, the mandibular rami are demonstrated anterior to the vertebral column. If the patient's chin was not adequately elevated, the mandibular rami are superimposed over the bodies of C1 and/or C2 (see Image 19).

- *Detecting head and shoulder tilting that causes lateral cervical flexion.* If the patient's head is tilted toward or away from the IR enough to flex the upper cervical column laterally, or if the shoulders are not placed on the same plane but are tilted enough to flex the lower cervical column laterally, the lateral cervical projection will demonstrate a superoinferior separation between the right and left articular pillars and zygapophyseal joints of the flexed vertebrae (see Images 18 and 20). Head tilting will also result in a superoinferior separation between the cranial cortices and between the mandibular rami; this can be avoided by positioning the interpupillary line (imaginary line connecting the outer corners of the eyelids) parallel with the floor. If the head was tilted toward the IR, neither the superior or the inferior cortices of the cranium nor the mandibular rami are superimposed, and the vertebral foramen of C1 is demonstrated (see Image 20). If the head and upper cervical vertebral column were tilted away from the IR, neither the inferior cortices of the cranium nor the mandibular rami are superimposed, and the posterior arch of C1 remains in profile (see Image 18).

The long axis of the cervical vertebral column is aligned with the long axis of the exposure field.

- Aligning the long axis of the cervical vertebral column with the long axis of the exposure field ensures against flexion or extension of the cervical column and allows for tight collimation. This alignment is obtained by positioning the patient's neck vertically and aligning the midline of the patient's neck with the collimator's longitudinal light line; it places the cervical column in a neutral position.

- *Hyperflexion and hyperextension positioning to evaluate AP mobility of cervical vertebrae.* Hyperflexion and hyperextension lateral cervical vertebrae projections are obtained to evaluate AP vertebral mobility. For hyperflexion, instruct the patient to tuck the chin into the chest as far as possible (Figure 8-14). For patients who demonstrate extreme degrees of flexion, it may be necessary to place the IR crosswise to include the entire cervical column on the same image. Such an image should meet all the analysis requirements listed for a neutral lateral projection, except that the long axis demonstrates forward bending (see Image 21). For hyperextension, instruct the patient to extend the chin up and backward as far as possible (Figure 8-15). Such an image should meet all the analysis requirements listed for a neutral lateral projection, except that the long axis demonstrates backward bending (see Image 22). If the lateral projection is used with the patient in hyperflexion or hyperextension, an arrow pointing in the direction the neck is moving or a flexion or extension marker should be included to indicate the direction of neck movement.

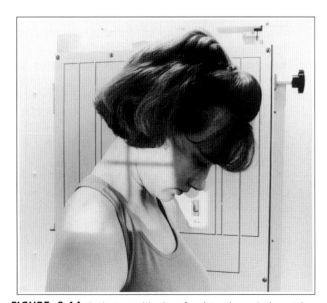

FIGURE 8-14 Patient positioning for lateral cervical vertebrae projection with hyperflexion.

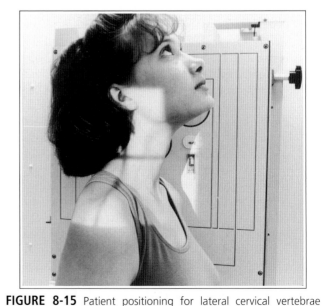

FIGURE 8-15 Patient positioning for lateral cervical vertebrae projection with hyperextension.

The fourth cervical vertebra is centered within the exposure field. The sella turcica, clivus, first through seventh cervical vertebrae, and superior half of the first thoracic vertebra and the surrounding soft tissue are included within the collimated field.

- Center a perpendicular central ray to the midcoronal plane at a level halfway between the EAM and the jugular notch to center C4 to the exposure field.
- Open the longitudinally and transversely collimated field enough to include the clivus and sella turcica, which is at a level 0.75 inch (2 cm) anterosuperior to the EAM. (The clivus, a slanted structure that extends posteriorly off the sella turcica, and the dens are used to determine cervical injury. A line drawn along the clivus should point to the tip of the dens on the normal upper lateral cervical vertebrae projection.)
- An 8- × 10-inch (18- × 24-cm) IR placed lengthwise should be adequate to include all the required anatomic structures.
- ***Demonstration of C7 and T1 vertebrae.*** The seventh cervical vertebra and first thoracic vertebra are located between the patient's shoulders. This location makes it difficult to demonstrate them because of the great difference in lateral thickness between the neck and the shoulders. The best method to demonstrate C7 is to have the patient hold 5- or 10-lb weights on each arm to depress the shoulders and attempt to move them inferior to C7. Weights are best placed on each arm rather than in each hand, because sometimes the patient's shoulders will elevate when weights are placed in the hands. Without weights, it is often difficult to demonstrate more than six cervical vertebrae (see Image 23). Taking the image on expiration also aids in lowering the shoulders.
- ***Visualization of C7 and T1 in trauma or recumbency.*** For trauma or recumbent patients who do not have upper extremity or shoulder injuries, depress the shoulders by having a qualified assistant, with the consent of a physician, pull down on the patient's arms while the image is taken. To accomplish this, instruct an assistant to wear a protection apron and stand at the end of the imaging table or stretcher, with the patient's feet resting against the assistant's abdomen and the assistant's hands wrapped around the patient's wrists. The assistant should slowly pull on the patient's arms until the shoulders are moved inferiorly as much as possible.
- ***Demonstration C7.*** If even after using weights to depress the patient's shoulders C7 cannot be demonstrated in its entirety, a special image known as the lateral cervicothoracic projection (Twining method, Swimmer's technique) should be taken. Refer to page 449 for specifics.

Lateral Cervical Vertebrae Projection Analysis

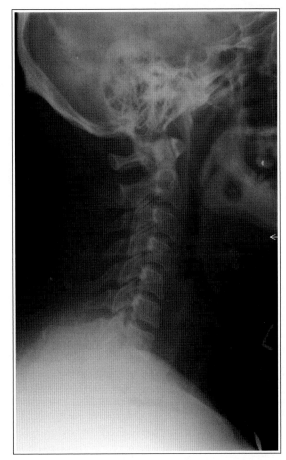

IMAGE 16

Analysis. The articular pillars and zygapophyseal joints on one side of the patient are situated anterior to those on the other side. The patient was rotated.

Correction. Rotate the patient until the midcoronal plane is aligned perpendicular to the IR.

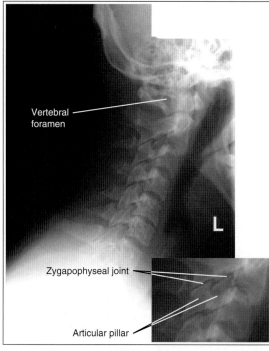

IMAGE 17

Analysis. The articular pillars and zygapophyseal joints on one side of the patient are situated anterior to those on the other side. The patient was rotated. The inferior cortices of the cranium and mandible are demonstrated without superimposition, and the vertebral foramen of C1 is visualized. The patient's head and upper cervical vertebral column were tilted toward the IR.

Correction. Rotate the patient until the midcoronal plane is aligned perpendicular to the IR, and tilt the head away from the IR until the interpupillary line is perpendicular to the IR.

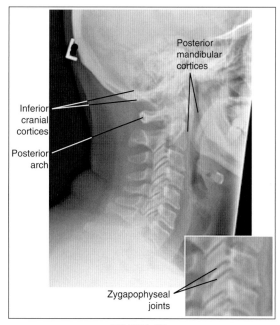

IMAGE 18

Analysis. The inferior and posterior cortices of the cranium and the mandible are not superimposed; the posterior arch of C1 is in profile, and the right and left articular pillars and zygapophyseal joints demonstrate a superoinferior separation. The patient's head was rotated and the patient's head and upper cervical vertebrae were tilted away from the IR.

Correction. Rotate the patient until the midsagittal plane is aligned parallel with the IR, and then tilt the head toward the IR until the interpupillary line is perpendicular to the IR.

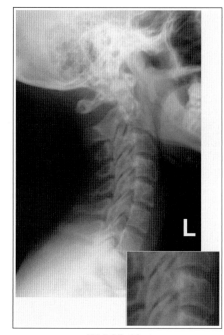

IMAGE 19

Analysis. The articular pillars and zygapophyseal joints on one side of the patient are situated anterior to those on the other side. The patient was rotated. The cranial and mandibular cortices are accurately aligned, and the mandibular rami are superimposed over the body of C2. The patient's chin was not adequately elevated.

Correction. Rotate the patient until the midcoronal plane is aligned perpendicular to the IR. Elevate the chin until the acanthiomeatal line is aligned parallel with the floor.

Analysis. The long axis of the cervical vertebral column is not aligned with the long axis of the collimated field. The cervical vertebral column is tilted forward. The patient was in hyperflexion.

Correction. Extend the patient's chin until the eyes are facing forward and the long axis of the neck is aligned with the long axis of the collimated field. If this examination is being performed to evaluate AP mobility, no corrective movement is required.

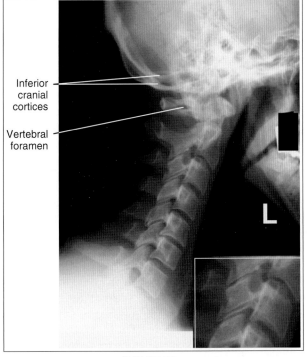

Inferior cranial cortices

Vertebral foramen

IMAGE 20

Analysis. The inferior cortices of the cranium and mandible are demonstrated without superimposition, the vertebral foramen of C1 is visualized, and the right and left articular pillars and zygapophyseal joints demonstrate a superoinferior separation. The patient's head and upper cervical vertebrae were tilted toward the IR.

Correction. Tilt the head away from the IR until the interpupillary line is aligned perpendicular to the IR.

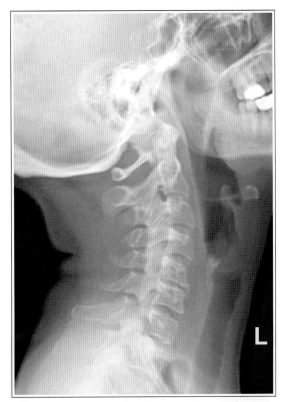

IMAGE 22

Analysis. The long axis of the cervical vertebral column is not aligned with the long axis of the collimated field. The cervical vertebral column is tilted backward. The patient was in hyperextension.

Correction. Tuck the patient's chin until the eyes are facing forward and the long axis of the neck is aligned with the long axis of the collimated field. If this examination is being performed to evaluate AP mobility, no corrective movement is required.

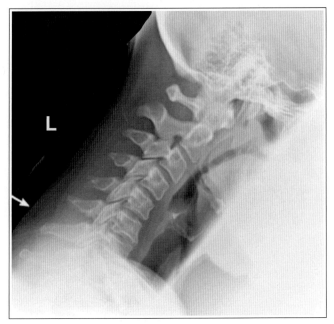

IMAGE 21

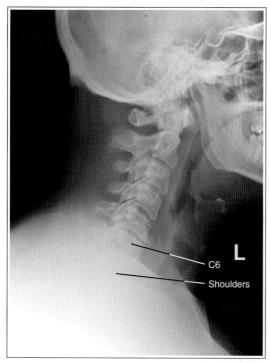

IMAGE 23

Analysis. The vertebral body of C7 is not demonstrated in its entirety and the superior body of T1 is not demonstrated. The shoulders were not adequately depressed.

Correction. If possible, have the patient hold 5- to 10-lb weights on each arm to depress the shoulders. If the patient cannot hold weights or if the weights do not sufficiently drop the shoulders, a special image known as the cervicothoracic lateral projection (Twining method) should be taken to demonstrate this area (refer to page 449 for details).

CERVICAL VERTEBRAE: POSTEROANTERIOR OR ANTEROPOSTERIOR AXIAL OBLIQUE PROJECTION (ANTERIOR AND POSTERIOR OBLIQUE POSITIONS)

See Figures 8-16 and 8-17 and Box 8-5.

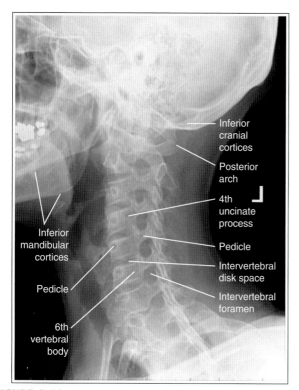

FIGURE 8-16 PA axial oblique cervical vertebrae projection with cranium in lateral projection and accurate positioning.

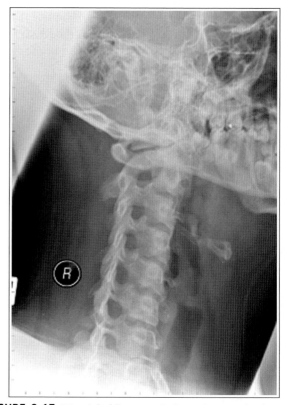

FIGURE 8-17 PA axial oblique cervical vertebrae projection with cranium in PA oblique projection and accurate positioning.

BOX 8-5 | **Posteroanterior-Anteroposterior Axial Oblique Cervical Vertebrae Image Analysis Criteria**

- The second through seventh intervertebral foramina are open, demonstrating uniform size and shape, the pedicles of interest are shown in profile, and the opposite pedicles are aligned with the anterior vertebral bodies.
- The intervertebral disk spaces are open, the cervical bodies are seen as individual structures and are uniform in shape, and the posterior arch of the atlas is seen without foreshortening, demonstrating the vertebral foramen.
- The inferior outline of the outer cranial cortices and the mandibular rami are seen without superimposition.
- Oblique cranium: The upper cervical vertebrae are seen with posterior occipital and mandibular superimposition.
- Lateral cranium: The upper cervical vertebrae are seen without occipital or mandibular superimposition, and the right and left posterior cortices of the cranium and the mandible are aligned.
- The fourth cervical vertebra is at the center of the exposure field.
- The first through seventh cervical vertebrae, the first thoracic vertebra, and the surrounding soft tissue are included within the collimated field.

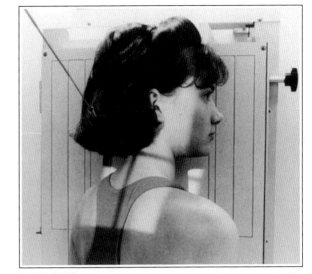

FIGURE 8-18 Proper patient positioning for PA axial oblique cervical vertebrae projection.

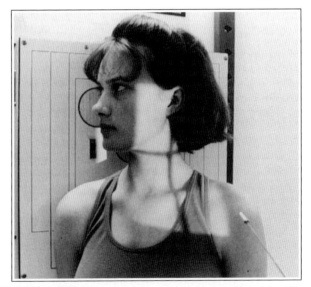

FIGURE 8-19 Proper patient positioning for AP axial oblique cervical vertebrae projection.

The cervical vertebrae have been rotated 45 degrees. The second through seventh intervertebral foramina are open, demonstrating uniformity in size and shape, the pedicles of interest are in profile, and the opposite pedicles are aligned with the anterior vertebral bodies. The sternum and sternoclavicular joints, when visible, are demonstrated without vertebral column superimposition.

- To position the intervertebral foramina and pedicles of interest in profile, begin by placing the patient in a recumbent or upright PA-AP axial oblique projection. Rotate the patient from this position until the midcoronal plane is at a 45-degree angle to the imaging table or upright IR. To demonstrate the foramina and pedicles on both sides of the cervical vertebrae, right and left oblique projections must be taken. When PA axial oblique projections (Figure 8-18) are obtained, the foramina and pedicles situated closer to the IR are demonstrated, whereas AP axial oblique projections (Figure 8-19) demonstrate the foramina and pedicles situated farther from the IR.
- *Effect of incorrect rotation.* If the cervical vertebral rotation is insufficient, the intervertebral foramina are narrowed or obscured, the pedicles are foreshortened, and a portion of the sternum, one sternoclavicular joint, and the vertebral column are superimposed (see Image 24). If the cervical vertebrae are rotated more than 45 degrees, one side of the pedicles is partially foreshortened but the other side is aligned with the midline of the vertebral bodies, and the zygapophyseal joints—demonstrated without vertebral body superimposition—are open (see Image 25). Because it is possible for the upper

and lower cervical vertebrae to be rotated to different degrees on the same image, one needs to evaluate the entire cervical vertebrae for proper rotation (see Image 26).

- *Positioning for trauma.* When imaging the cervical vertebrae of a trauma patient with suspected subluxation or fracture, obtain the trauma AP axial and lateral projections and have them evaluated before the patient is moved for the AP axial oblique projection. The trauma AP axial oblique projection of the cervical vertebrae is accomplished by elevating the supine patient's head, neck, and thorax enough to place a lengthwise IR beneath the neck. If the right vertebral foramina and pedicles are of interest, the IR should be shifted to the left enough to align the right mastoid tip with the longitudinal

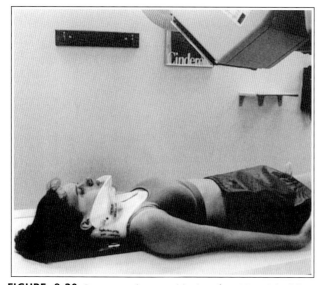

FIGURE 8-20 Proper patient positioning for AP axial oblique cervical vertebrae projection taken to evaluate trauma.

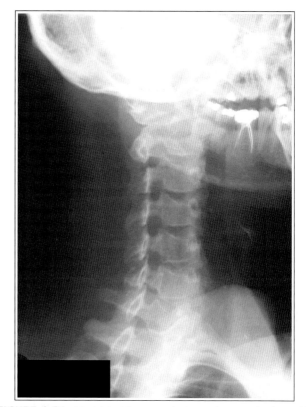

FIGURE 8-21 AP axial oblique cervical vertebrae projection with accurate positioning taken to evaluate trauma.

axis of the IR and inferior enough to position the right gonion (C3) with the transverse axis of the IR. Direct the central ray 45 degrees medially to the right side of the patient's neck and 15 degrees cephalically, and then center it halfway between the AP surfaces of the neck at the level of the thyroid cartilage (C4) (Figure 8-20). If the left vertebral foramina and pedicles are of interest, shift the IR to the right enough to align the right mastoid tip with the longitudinal axis of the IR and inferior enough to position the left gonion with the transverse axis of the IR. The central ray should be angled and centered as described earlier, except that it should be directed to the left side of the patient's neck. A trauma AP axial oblique cervical projection should meet all the analysis requirements listed for a regular AP axial oblique cervical projection; the cranium will be in an AP oblique projection (Figure 8-21).

The intervertebral disk spaces are open, the cervical bodies are demonstrated as individual structures and are uniform in shape, and the posterior arch of the atlas is demonstrated without self-superimposition, demonstrating the vertebral foramen. The inferior outline of the outer cranial cortices and the mandibular rami are demonstrated without superimposition.

- The cervical vertebral column demonstrates a lordotic curvature. This curvature, along with the shape of the cervical bodies, causes the disk-articulating surfaces of the vertebral bodies to slant downward posteriorly to anteriorly.
- *Importance of central ray angulation.* To obtain open intervertebral disk spaces and undistorted, uniformly shaped vertebral bodies, the central ray must be angled in the same direction as the slope of the vertebral bodies. This is accomplished by

angling the central ray 15 to 20 degrees caudally for PA axial oblique projections and 15 to 20 degrees cephalically for AP axial oblique projections. This angle will also result in demonstration of the atlas's vertebral foramen on the projections.

- *Effect of inaccurate central ray angulation.* If the central ray is not accurately angled with the intervertebral disk spaces, they are closed and the cervical bodies are not demonstrated as individual structures (see Images 27 and 28). Because this examination can be performed using AP or PA axial oblique projections that require differing central ray angulations, and the typical cervical vertebral series requires the radiographer to change angle directions several times, radiographers should be able to identify an image that was taken with an incorrect angle. Image 27 was taken using a perpendicular central ray, and Image 28 was taken with the central ray angled in the wrong direction. Note the closed intervertebral disk spaces, distorted cervical bodies, and demonstration of the posterior tubercles within the intervertebral foramina.
- *Positioning for kyphosis.* In patients with severe kyphosis, the lower cervical vertebrae are angled toward the IR because of the greater lordotic curvature of this area. To demonstrate the lower cervical vertebrae with open intervertebral disk spaces and undistorted cervical bodies, the central ray will need to be angled more than the suggested 15 to 20

degrees for the AP-PA oblique projection. The patient in Image 29 had kyphosis. Note the decrease in intervertebral disk space openness and vertebral body distortion and the demonstration of the zyga-pophyseal joints through the cervical bodies between the upper and lower cervical regions.

- *Mandibular rami and cranial demonstration.* The distances demonstrated between the inferior cortical outlines of the cranium and the mandibular rami are a result of the angulation placed on the central ray. On PA axial oblique cervical projections, the caudal angle projects the cranial cortex situated farther from the IR approximately 0.25 inch (0.6 cm) inferiorly and the mandibular ramus situated farther from the IR approximately 0.5 inch (1.25 cm) inferiorly. The ramus is projected farther inferiorly because it is located at a larger OID than the cranial cortex. On AP axial oblique projections, the cephalic angle projects the cranial cortex and mandibular rami situated farther from the IR superiorly.

  The distance between these two cortical out-lines will be increased or decreased if the patient's head is allowed to tilt toward or away from the IR. Such tilting also causes the upper cervical verteb-rae to lean toward or away from the IR. To avoid head and cervical column tilting, position the interpupillary line parallel with the floor.

- *Detecting head tilting.* On PA axial oblique projec-tions, if the head and upper cervical column are allowed to tilt, the atlas and its posterior arch are distorted. From such an image, one can determine whether the head and upper cervical vertebrae were tilted toward or away from the IR by evaluating the distance demonstrated between the inferior cranial cortices and the inferior mandibular rami. If these distances are increased, the head and upper cervical vertebrae were tilted away from the IR (see Image 30). If these distances are decreased, the head and upper cervical vertebrae were tilted toward the IR.

The cranium is in an oblique or lateral projection as defined by the facility.

Oblique cranium: The upper cervical vertebrae are demonstrated with posterior occipital and mandibular superimposition (see Figure 8-16).

- The desired position of the patient's head for an AP axial oblique cervical projection varies among facil-ities. If an AP oblique cranium projection is desired, rotate the patient's head 45 degrees with the body. If a lateral cranium projection is desired, turn the patient's face away from the side of interest until the head's midsagittal plane is aligned parallel with the IR.

Lateral cranium: The upper cervical vertebrae are demonstrated without occipital or mandibular superimpo-sition, and the right and left posterior cortices of the cra-nium and mandible are aligned (see Figure 8-17).

- To demonstrate the upper cervical vertebrae with-out mandibular superimposition and aligned right and left cranial and mandibular cortices on an AP axial oblique cervical projection, place the patient's cranium in a lateral projection and adjust chin elevation until the acanthiomeatal line is aligned parallel with the floor. If the patient's chin is not properly elevated and/or the patient's head is rotated, the mandibular rami are superimposed over C1 and C2 (see Image 31).

The fourth cervical vertebra is centered within the expo-sure field. The first through seventh cervical vertebrae, the first thoracic vertebra, and the surrounding soft tis-sue are included within the collimated field.

- Center a 15- to 20-degree cephalically angled cen-tral ray for the AP axial oblique or a 15- to 20-degree caudally angled central ray for the PA axial oblique to the patient's midsagittal plane at a level halfway between the EAM and the jugular notch to center C4 to the exposure field.
- Open the longitudinal collimation to the EAM and the jugular notch. Transverse collimation should be to within 0.5 inch (1.25 cm) of the neck skin line.
- An 8- × 10-inch (18- × 24-cm) IR placed length-wise should be adequate to include all the required anatomic structures.

Posteroanterior Axial Oblique Cervical Vertebrae Projection Analysis

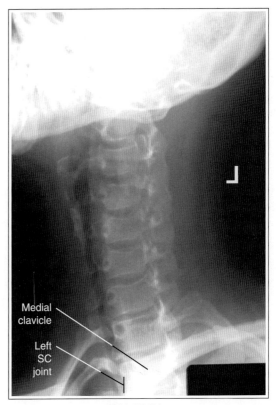

IMAGE 24

Analysis. This patient was in a left PA axial oblique projection (anterior oblique [LAO] position), with the head in a PA projection. The pedicles and intervertebral foramina are obscured, and portions of the left sterno-clavicular joint and medial clavicular end are superimposed by the vertebral column. The patient was not rotated the required 45 degrees.

Correction. Increase the patient obliquity until the midcoronal plane is placed at a 45-degree angle with the IR.

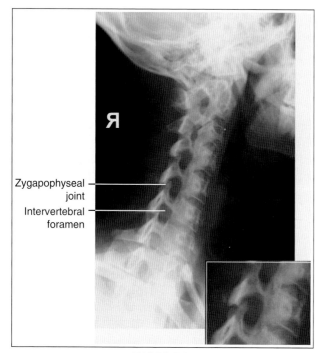

Zygapophyseal joint

Intervertebral foramen

IMAGE 25

Analysis. This patient was in a right PA axial oblique projection (anterior oblique [RAO] position), with the patient's head in a lateral projection. The intervertebral foramina are demonstrated, the right pedicles are shown, although they are not in true profile, the left pedicles are demonstrated in the midline of the vertebral bodies, and the right zygapophyseal joints are demonstrated. The patient was rotated more than 45 degrees.

Correction. Decrease the patient rotation until the midcoronal plane is placed at a 45-degree angle with the IR.

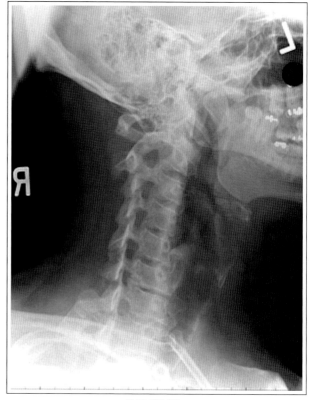

IMAGE 26

Analysis. This patient was in a right PA axial oblique projection (RAO position) with the patient's head in a lateral projection. The upper cervical vertebrae demonstrate open and uniformly shaped intervertebral foramina, and the left pedicles are aligned with the anterior vertebral body, indicating that the patient's upper vertebrae were adequately rotated. The lower cervical vertebrae demonstrate the right zygapophyseal joints, narrowed and distorted intervertebral foramina, and the left pedicles aligned closer toward the midline of the vertebral bodies, indicating that the patient's torso was overrotated.

Correction. While maintaining the degree of upper cervical rotation, decrease patient torso rotation until the midcoronal plane is placed at a 45-degree angle with the IR.

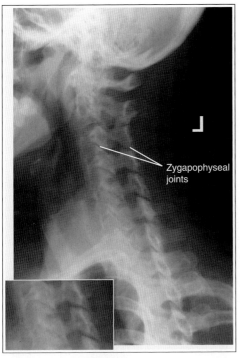

IMAGE 27

Analysis. This patient was in a left PA axial oblique projection (LAO position), with the head in a lateral projection. The intervertebral disk spaces are closed, the cervical bodies are distorted, the posterior tubercles are demonstrated within the intervertebral foramina, the C1 vertebral foramen is not demonstrated, and the inferior mandibular rami and cranial cortices are demonstrated with superimposition. The central ray was directed perpendicular to the IR.

Correction. Angle the central ray 15 to 20 degrees caudally for PA axial oblique projections.

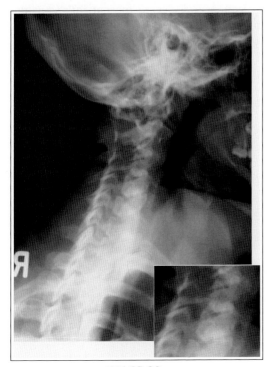

IMAGE 28

Analysis. This patient was in a right PA axial oblique projection (RAO position), with the head in a lateral projection. The intervertebral disk spaces are closed, the cervical bodies are distorted, the posterior tubercles are demonstrated within the intervertebral foramina, the C1 intervertebral foramen is demonstrated, and the inferior mandibular rami and cranial cortices are shown without superimposition. The central ray was angled 15 to 20 degrees cephalically.

Correction. Angle the central ray 15 to 20 degrees caudally for PA axial oblique projections.

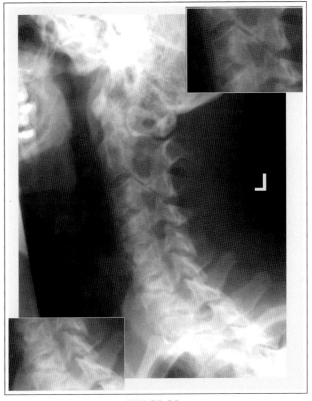

IMAGE 29

Analysis. This patient is in a left PA axial oblique projection (LAO position), with the head in a lateral projection. A decrease in intervertebral disk space openness and vertebral body distortion are present, and demonstration of the zygapophyseal joints through the cervical bodies in the lower cervical vertebrae (C5 through C7) is increased. The patient is kyphotic, and the entire cervical spine was not aligned parallel with the IR.

Correction. Align the entire cervical spine parallel with the IR or increase the central ray angulation over the 15 to 20 degrees required for a routine PA axial oblique projection to demonstrate the fifth through seventh cervical vertebrae better.

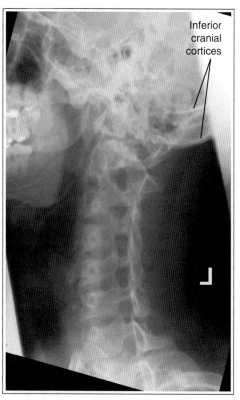

IMAGE 30

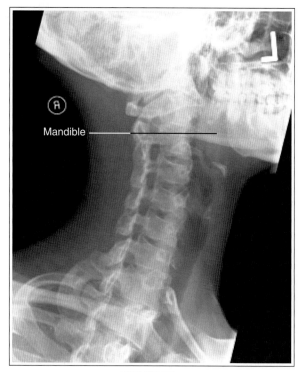

IMAGE 31

Analysis. This patient was in a left PA axial oblique projection (LAO position), with the head in a lateral projection. The atlas and its posterior arch are obscured. The inferior cranial cortices demonstrate more than 0.25 inch (0.6 cm) between them, and the inferior cortices of the mandibular rami demonstrate more than 0.5 inch (1.25 cm) between them. The first thoracic vertebra is not included in its entirety. The head and the upper cervical vertebrae were tilted away from the IR, and the central ray and IR were positioned too superiorly.

Correction. Tilt the patient's head toward the IR until the interpupillary line is aligned perpendicular to the IR, and move the central ray and IR inferiorly.

Analysis. This patient was in a right PA axial oblique projection (RAO position), with the head in a PA oblique projection. The mandibular ramus is superimposed over the body of C2.

Correction. To demonstrate C2 without mandibular ramus superimposition, place the patient's head in a lateral projection and elevate the patient's chin until the acanthiomeatal line is aligned parallel with the floor.

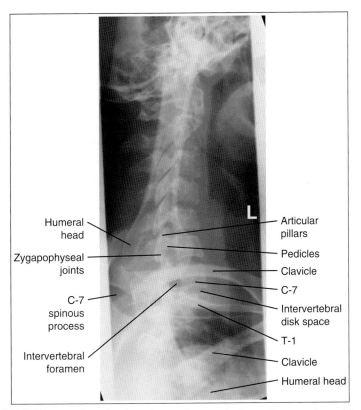

Humeral head — Zygapophyseal joints — C-7 spinous process — Intervertebral foramen

L — Articular pillars — Pedicles — Clavicle — C-7 — Intervertebral disk space — T-1 — Clavicle — Humeral head

FIGURE 8-22 Lateral cervicothoracic vertebrae projection with accurate positioning.

CERVICOTHORACIC VERTEBRAE

CERVICOTHORACIC VERTEBRAE: LATERAL PROJECTION (TWINING METHOD; SWIMMER'S TECHNIQUE)

This examination is performed when the routine lateral cervical projection does not adequately demonstrate the seventh cervical vertebra or when the routine lateral thoracic projection does not demonstrate the first through third thoracic vertebrae. See Figure 8-22 and Box 8-6.

The cervicothoracic vertebrae are demonstrated in a lateral projection. The humerus elevated above the patient's head is aligned with the vertebral column, the right and left cervical zygapophyseal joints and articular

pillars are superimposed, and the posterior ribs are superimposed.

• Position the patient in an upright or a recumbent lateral projection. Whether the right or left side of the patient is positioned against the imaging table or upright IR is not significant, although left-side positioning is easier for the technologist. For the recumbent position, flex the patient's knees and hips for support. For the upright position, instruct the patient to evenly distribute weight on both feet. Elevate the arm positioned closer to the IR above the patient's head as high as the patient allows. The forearm and hand may be rested on the head for support in the erect position. Place the other arm against the patient's side, and instruct the patient to depress this shoulder (Figure 8-23) and move it slightly anteriorly. This supplementary lateral cervicothoracic projection moves the shoulders in opposite directions, overlapping one onto the upper cervical region and the other onto the lower thoracic region, allowing visualization of the cervicothoracic area without shoulder superimposition. To demonstrate the fifth through seventh cervical vertebrae and the first through third thoracic vertebrae without shoulder superimposition, the shoulder positioned away from the IR is depressed. Taking the image on expiration will also aid in lowering the shoulder. A 5-degree caudal central ray angulation may be

> BOX 8-6 | **Lateral Cervicothoracic Vertebrae Projection Analysis Criteria**
>
> • The humerus elevated above the patient's head is aligned with the vertebral column, right and left cervical zygapophyseal joints, and articular pillars, and the posterior ribs are superimposed.
> • The intervertebral disk spaces are open, and the vertebral bodies are demonstrated without distortion.
> • The first thoracic vertebra is at the center of the exposure field.
> • The fifth through seventh cervical vertebrae are included within the collimated field.

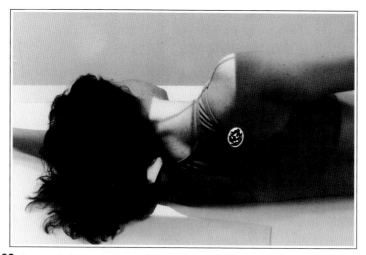

FIGURE 8-23 Proper patient positioning for recumbent lateral cervicothoracic vertebrae projection.

used for a patient who is unable to depress the shoulder positioned farther from the IR adequately. This angle projects the shoulder inferiorly.

Once the shoulders are positioned, adjust patient head and body rotation to obtain a lateral projection. You can avoid cervical rotation by placing the head in a lateral projection and thoracic rotation by resting your extended flat palm against the patient's shoulders and the inferior posterior ribs, and then adjusting patient rotation until your hand is positioned perpendicular to the imaging table or upright grid holder.

- *Detecting rotation.* If the patient is rotated, the articular pillars, posterior ribs, zygapophyseal joints, and humeri move away from each other, obscuring the pedicles and distorting the vertebral bodies. When rotation is demonstrated on a lateral cervicothoracic projection, determine which side was rotated anteriorly or posteriorly by evaluating the position of the humeral head positioned closer to the IR. If the patient was rotated anteriorly, the humeral head farther from the IR is positioned anteriorly (see Image 32). If the patient was

rotated posteriorly, the humeral head closer to the IR is positioned anteriorly and the humeral head farther from the IR is positioned posteriorly (see Image 33).

- *Positioning for trauma.* When routine cervical projections are obtained in a trauma patient with suspected subluxation or fracture and the seventh lateral cervical vertebra is not demonstrated, obtain the lateral cervicothoracic projection with the patient's head, neck, and body trunk left as is. Instruct the patient to elevate the arm farther from the x-ray tube and to depress the arm closer to the tube. Then place a grid cassette against the patient's lateral body surface, centering its transverse axis at a level 1 inch (2.5 cm) superior to the jugular notch (Figure 8-24). Position the central ray horizontal to the posterior neck surface and the center of the grid cassette. If the shoulder closer to the central ray is not well depressed, a 5-degree caudal angulation is recommended.

The intervertebral disk spaces are open, and the vertebral bodies are demonstrated without distortion.

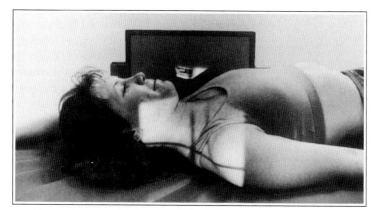

FIGURE 8-24 Proper patient positioning for lateral cervicothoracic vertebrae projection taken to evaluate trauma.

- To obtain open disk spaces and undistorted vertebral bodies, position the head in a lateral projection, with the interpupillary line perpendicular to and the midsagittal plane parallel with the upright grid holder or imaging table.
- If the patient is in a recumbent lateral projection, it may be necessary to elevate the head on a sponge to place it in a lateral projection, preventing cervical column tilting (see Image 34).

The first thoracic vertebra is centered within the exposure field. The fifth through seventh cervical vertebrae and the first through fourth thoracic vertebrae are included within the collimated field.

- Center a perpendicular central ray to the midcoronal plane at a level 1 inch (2.5 cm) superior to the jugular notch or at the level of the vertebral prominens. The seventh cervical vertebra can be identified on a lateral cervicothoracic projection by locating the elevated clavicle, which is normally shown traversing the seventh cervical vertebra.
- Open the longitudinal collimated field to the patient's mandibular angle. Transverse collimation should be to within 0.5 inch (1.25 cm) of the cervical skin line.
- A 10- × 12-inch (24- × 30-cm) IR placed lengthwise should be adequate to include all the required anatomic structures.

Lateral Cervicothoracic Vertebrae Projection Analysis

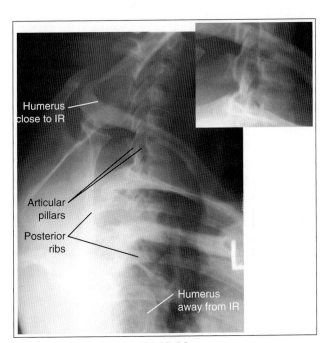

IMAGE 32

Analysis. The right and left articular pillars, zygapophyseal joints, and posterior ribs are demonstrated without superimposition. The patient's thorax was rotated. The humerus that was raised and situated closer to the IR is demonstrated posterior to the vertebral column. The shoulder that was depressed and positioned farther from the IR was rotated anteriorly.

Correction. Rotate the shoulder positioned farther from the IR posteriorly, until your flat palms placed against the shoulders or posterior ribs, respectively, are aligned perpendicular to the imaging table and upright grid holder.

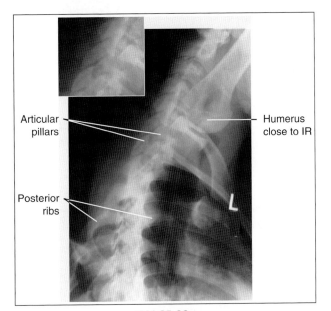

IMAGE 33

Analysis. The right and left articular pillars, zygapophyseal joints, and posterior ribs are demonstrated without superimposition. The patient's thorax was rotated. The humerus that was raised and situated closer to the IR is demonstrated anterior to the vertebral column. The shoulder that was depressed and positioned farther from the IR was rotated posteriorly.

Correction. Rotate the shoulder positioned farther from the IR anteriorly until your flat palms placed against the shoulders and posterior ribs, respectively, are aligned perpendicular to the imaging table and upright IR.

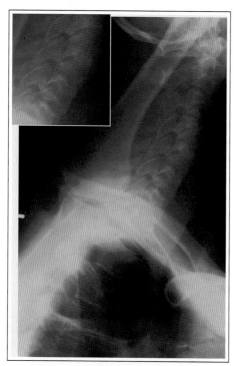

IMAGE 34

Analysis. The intervertebral disk spaces are closed, and the vertebral bodies are distorted. The patient's cervical vertebral column was not positioned parallel with the IR.

Correction. Position the midsagittal plane of the head and cervical vertebral column parallel with the IR. It may be necessary to prop the head on a sponge to help the patient maintain the position.

THORACIC VERTEBRAE

THORACIC VERTEBRAE: ANTEROPOSTERIOR PROJECTION

See Figure 8-25 and Box 8-7.

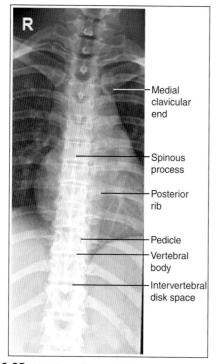

FIGURE 8-25 AP thoracic vertebral projection with accurate positioning.

BOX 8-7	**Anteroposterior Thoracic Vertebrae Projection Analysis Criteria**

- There is uniform density across the thoracic vertebrae.
- The spinous processes are aligned with the midline of the vertebral bodies; the distances from the vertebral column to the sternal clavicular ends and from the pedicles to the spinous processes are equal on the two sides.
- The intervertebral disk spaces are open, and the vertebral bodies are seen without foreshortening.
- The seventh thoracic vertebra is at the center of the exposure field.
- The seventh cervical vertebra, first through twelfth thoracic vertebrae, first lumbar vertebra, and 2.5 inches (6.25 cm) of the posterior ribs and mediastinum on each side of the vertebral column are included within the collimated field.

There should be uniform density across the thoracic vertebrae.

- When an exposure (mAs) is set that adequately demonstrates the lower thoracic vertebrae (T6 to T12), the upper thoracic vertebrae (T1 to T5) are often overexposed because of the difference in AP body thickness between these two regions. Two methods may be used to achieve uniform density in spite of this difference in thickness. The first method uses a wedge compensating filter and the second method uses the anode heel effect.

• *Wedge filter.* The wedge filter absorbs x-ray photons before they reach the patient, thereby decreasing the number of photons exposing the IR where the filter is located (see discussion in Chapter 1). The number of the upper thoracic vertebrae that should be covered by the filter's shadow depends on the slope of the patient's sternum and upper thorax. Position the thin edge of the wedge filter's shadow at the inferior sternum and thorax, at the level at which they begin to decline (Figures 8-26 and 8-27). If the wedge filter has been accurately positioned, there will be uniform image density throughout the thoracic column. If the wedge filter was inaccurately positioned, a definite density difference will define

where the wedge filter was and was not placed. Positioning the filter too inferiorly on the patient results in an underexposed area where the filter was misplaced (see Image 35). Positioning the filter too superiorly results in an overexposed area where the filter should have been placed.

• *Anode heel effect.* The anode heel effect works similarly to a filter; it decreases the number of photons reaching the upper thoracic vertebrae and results in decreased density in this area. This method works sufficiently in patients who have very little difference in AP body thickness between their upper and lower thoracic vertebrae but does not provide an adequate density decrease in patients with larger thickness differences. For the latter patients, use the anode heel effect in combination with a wedge filter. To use the anode heel effect, position the patient's head and upper thoracic vertebrae at the anode end of the tube and the feet and lower thoracic vertebrae at the cathode end. Then set an exposure (mAs) that adequately demonstrates the middle thoracic vertebrae. Because the anode will absorb some of the photons aimed at the anode end of the IR, the upper thoracic vertebrae will receive less exposure than the lower vertebrae.

• *Expiration versus inspiration.* Patient respiration determines the amount of contrast and density difference demonstrated between the mediastinum and vertebral column. These differences are a result of the variation in atomic density that exists between the thoracic cavity and the vertebrae. The thoracic cavity is largely composed of air, which contains very few atoms in a given area; the same area of bone, as in the vertebrae, contains many compacted atoms. As radiation goes through the patient's body, fewer photons are absorbed in the thoracic cavity than in the vertebral column, because fewer atoms with which the photons can interact are present in the thoracic cavity. Consequently, more photons will penetrate the thoracic cavity to expose the IR than will penetrate the vertebral column. Taking the exposure on full suspended expiration can help decrease the thoracic cavity's image density by reducing the air volume and compressing the tissue in this area (see Figure 8-25). This decreased image density allows better visualization of the posterior ribs and mediastinum region. If the AP thoracic vertebrae projection is exposed while the patient is in full suspended inspiration, the thoracic cavity demonstrates increased image density compared with the vertebral column (see Image 36). It should be noted, however, that the contrast created on an AP thoracic vertebrae projection taken on inspiration can be valuable in detecting thoracic tumors or disease.

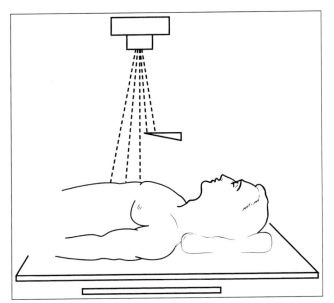

FIGURE 8-26 Proper patient positioning for AP thoracic vertebrae projection with compensating filter.

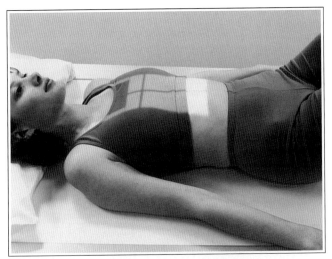

FIGURE 8-27 Proper placement of compensating filter.

The thoracic vertebral column demonstrates an AP projection. The spinous processes are aligned with the midline of the vertebral bodies, the distances from the vertebral column to the medial (sternal) ends of the clavicles are equal, and the distances from the pedicles to the spinous processes are equal on the two sides.

- An AP thoracic vertebrae projection is obtained by placing the patient supine on the imaging table. Position the shoulders and ASISs at equal distances from the imaging table to prevent rotation, and draw the patient's arms away from the thoracic area to keep them from being tucked beneath the patient (Figure 8-28).
- *Effect of rotation.* The upper and lower thoracic vertebrae can demonstrate rotation independently or simultaneously, depending on which section of the body is rotated. If the patient's shoulders and upper thorax were rotated and the pelvis and lower thorax remained supine, the upper thoracic vertebrae demonstrate rotation. If the patient's pelvis and lower thorax were rotated and the thorax and shoulders remained supine, the lower thoracic vertebrae demonstrate rotation. If the patient's thorax and pelvis were rotated simultaneously, the entire thoracic column demonstrates rotation.
- *Detecting rotation.* Rotation is effectively detected on an AP thoracic projection by comparing the distances between pedicles and spinous processes on the same vertebra and the distances between the vertebral column and medial ends of the clavicles. When no rotation is present, the comparable distances are equal. If one side demonstrates a larger distance, vertebral rotation is present. The side demonstrating a larger distance is the side of the patient positioned closer to the imaging table and the IR (see Image 37).

- *Distinguishing rotation from scoliosis.* In patients with spinal scoliosis, the thoracic bodies may appear rotated because of the lateral twisting of the vertebrae. Scoliosis of the vertebral column can be very severe, demonstrating a large amount of lateral deviation, or it can be subtle, demonstrating only a small amount of deviation (Figure 8-29). Severe scoliosis is very obvious and is seldom mistaken for patient rotation, whereas subtle scoliotic changes may be easily mistaken for rotation. Although both conditions demonstrate unequal distances between the pedicles and spinous processes, certain clues can be used to distinguish subtle scoliosis from rotation. The long axis of a rotated vertebral column remains straight, whereas the scoliotic vertebral column demonstrates lateral deviation. When the thoracic vertebrae demonstrate rotation, it has been caused by the rotation of the upper or lower torso. Rotation of the middle thoracolumbar vertebrae does not occur unless the upper and lower thoracic vertebrae also demonstrate rotation. On an image from a patient with scoliosis, the thoracolumbar vertebrae may demonstrate rotation without corresponding upper or lower vertebral rotation. Familiarity with the difference between a rotated thoracic vertebral column and a scoliotic one prevents unnecessarily repeated procedures in patients with spinal scoliosis.

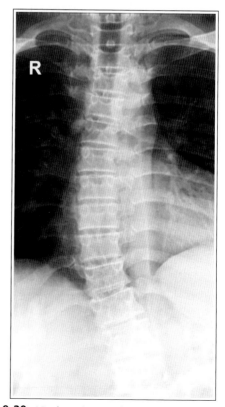

FIGURE 8-29 AP thoracic vertebrae projection demonstrating spinal scoliosis.

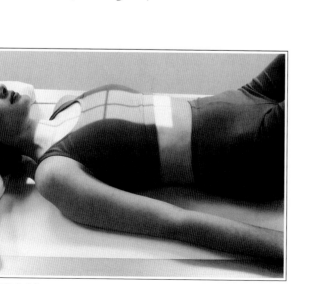

FIGURE 8-28 Proper patient positioning for AP thoracic vertebrae projection without compensating filter.

The intervertebral disk spaces are open, and the vertebral bodies are demonstrated without distortion.

- The thoracic vertebral column demonstrates a kyphotic curvature. Because the thoracic vertebrae have very limited flexion and extension movements, it is difficult to achieve a significant reduction of this curvature. A small reduction can be obtained by placing the patient's head on a thin pillow or sponge and flexing the hips and knees until the lower back rests firmly against the imaging table; both procedures improve the relationship of the upper and lower vertebral disk spaces and bodies with the x-ray beam. The head position reduces the upper vertebral curvature, and the hip and knee position reduces the lower vertebral curvature. If the disk spaces are not aligned parallel with the x-ray beam and the vertebral bodies are not aligned perpendicular to the x-ray beam, it is difficult for the reviewer to evaluate the height of the disk spaces and vertebral bodies (see Image 38).
- *Positioning for kyphosis.* To demonstrate open disk spaces and undistorted vertebral bodies in a patient with excessive spinal kyphosis, it may be necessary to angle the central ray until it is perpendicular to the vertebral area of interest. Because it is painful for such a patient to lie supine on the imaging table, it is best to perform the examination with the patient upright or recumbent in a lateral projection with use of a horizontal beam.

The seventh thoracic vertebra is centered within the exposure field. The seventh cervical vertebra, first through twelfth thoracic vertebrae, first lumbar vertebra, and 2.5 inches (6.25 cm) of the posterior ribs and mediastinum on each side of the vertebral column are included within the collimated field.

- Center a perpendicular central ray to the patient's midsagittal plane at a level halfway between the jugular notch and the xiphoid to position the seventh thoracic vertebra in the center of the exposure field.
- Open the longitudinal collimation the full 17-inch (43-cm) IR length for adult patients. Transverse collimation should be to approximately an 8-inch (20-cm) field.
- A 14- × 17-inch (35- × 43-cm) IR placed lengthwise should be adequate to include all the required anatomic structures.

Anteroposterior Thoracic Vertebrae Projection Analysis

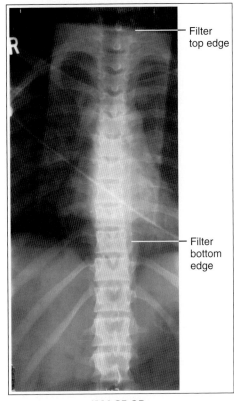

Filter top edge

Filter bottom edge

IMAGE 35

Analysis. The sixth through ninth thoracic vertebrae are underexposed. The wedge compensating filter was positioned too inferiorly.

Correction. Position the shadow of the wedge filter's thin edge at the beginning of the downward slope of the patient's sternum and upper thorax, as shown in Figure 8-26.

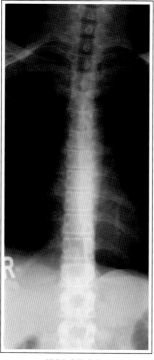

IMAGE 36

Analysis. The thoracic cavity is overexposed. The image was taken on inspiration.

Correction. Expose the image with the patient in full expiration. If a mediastinal tumor or disease is in question, however, no correction is needed.

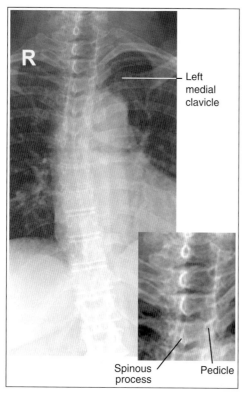

Left medial clavicle

Spinous process — Pedicle

IMAGE 37

Analysis. The upper cervical vertebrae demonstrate more distance from the left pedicle to the spinous process than from the right pedicle to the spinous process, and the left medial clavicle is demonstrated away from the vertebral column. The patient was rotated toward the left side.

Correction. Rotate the patient toward the right side until the shoulders and ASISs are at equal distances from the imaging table.

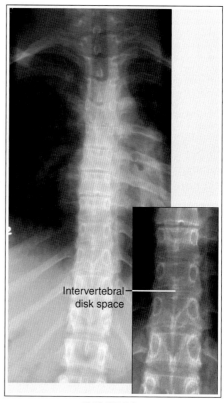

Intervertebral disk space

IMAGE 38

Analysis. The eighth through twelfth intervertebral disk spaces are obscured, and the vertebral bodies distorted. The patient's legs were extended.

Correction. Flex the patient's hips and knees, placing the feet and back firmly against the imaging table.

THORACIC VERTEBRAE: LATERAL PROJECTION

See Figure 8-30 and Box 8-8.

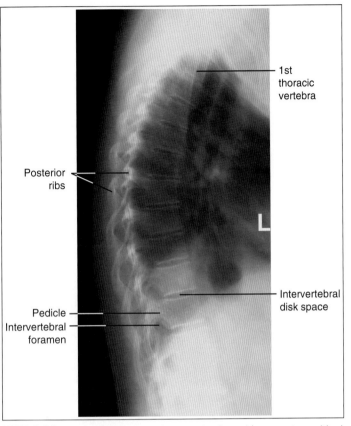

1st thoracic vertebra

Posterior ribs

Intervertebral disk space

Pedicle

Intervertebral foramen

FIGURE 8-30 Lateral thoracic vertebrae projection with accurate positioning.

BOX 8-8 | **Anteroposterior Thoracic Vertebrae Projection Analysis Criteria**

- The thoracic vertebrae are seen through overlying lung and rib structures.
- The intervertebral foramina are clearly demonstrated, pedicles are in profile, posterior surfaces of each vertebral body are superimposed, and no more than ½ inch (1.25 cm) of space is demonstrated between the posterior ribs.
- The intervertebral disk spaces are open, and the vertebral bodies are demonstrated without distortion.
- The seventh thoracic vertebra is at the center of the exposure field.
- The seventh cervical vertebra, first through twelfth thoracic vertebrae, and first lumbar vertebra are included within the collimated field.

The thoracic vertebrae are demonstrated through overlying lung and rib structures.

- *Breathing technique.* The thoracic vertebrae have many overlying structures, including the axillary ribs and lungs. Using a long exposure time (3 to 4 seconds) and requiring the patient to breathe shallowly (costal breathing) during the exposure forces a slow and steady, upward and outward

movement of the ribs and lungs. This technique is often referred to as breathing technique. This movement causes blurring of the ribs and lung markings on the image, providing greater thoracic vertebral demonstration. Deep breathing, which requires movement (elevation) of the sternum and a faster and expanded upward and outward movement of the ribs and lungs, should be avoided during the breathing technique, because deep breathing results in motion of the thoracic cavity and vertebrae (see Image 39).

- NOTE: If patient motion cannot be avoided when using the extended 3 to 4 seconds for breathing technique, take the image on suspended expiration to reduce the air volume within the thoracic cavity.

The thoracic vertebrae demonstrate a lateral projection. The intervertebral foramina are clearly demonstrated, the pedicles are in profile, the posterior surfaces of each vertebral body are superimposed, and no more than 0.5 inch (1.25 cm) of space is demonstrated between the posterior ribs.

- To obtain a lateral thoracic vertebrae projection, place the patient on the imaging table in a lateral recumbent projection. Whether the patient is lying

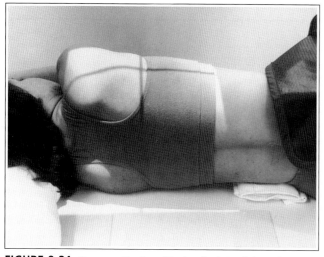

FIGURE 8-31 Proper patient positioning for lateral thoracic vertebrae projection.

the superimposition of the right and left posterior surfaces of the vertebral bodies and the amount of posterior rib superimposition. On a nonrotated lateral thoracic projection, the posterior surfaces are superimposed and the posterior ribs are almost superimposed. Because the posterior ribs positioned farther from the IR were placed at a greater OID than the other side, they demonstrate more magnification. This magnification prevents the posterior ribs from being directly superimposed but positions them approximately 0.5 inch (1.25 cm) apart. This distance is based on a 40-inch (102-cm) SID. If a longer SID is used, the distance between the posterior ribs is decreased and, if a shorter SID is used, the distance is increased. On rotation, the right and left posterior surfaces of the vertebral bodies are demonstrated one anterior to the other on a lateral projection.

Because the two sides of the thorax and vertebrae are mirror images, it is very difficult to determine from a rotated lateral thoracic projection which side of the patient was rotated anteriorly and which posteriorly. If the patient was only slightly rotated, one way of determining which way the patient was rotated is to evaluate the amount of posterior rib superimposition. If the patient's elevated side was rotated posteriorly, the posterior ribs demonstrate more than 0.5 inch (1.25 cm) of space between them (see Image 40). If the patient's elevated side was rotated anteriorly, the posterior ribs are superimposed on slight rotation (see Image 41) and demonstrate greater separation as rotation of the patient increases. Another method is to view the scapulae and humeral heads when visible. The scapula and humeral head demonstrating the greatest magnification will be the ones situated farthest from the IR (see Image 42).

- **Distinguishing rotation from scoliosis:** On the image of a patient with spinal scoliosis, the lung field may appear rotated because of the lateral deviation of the vertebral column (see Image 12, Chapter 3). On such an image, the posterior ribs demonstrate differing degrees of separation depending on the severity of the scoliosis. View the accompanying AP thoracic projection (see Image 3, Chapter 3) to confirm this patient condition.

The intervertebral disk spaces are open, and the vertebral bodies are demonstrated without distortion.

- The thoracic vertebral column is capable of lateral flexion. When the patient is placed in a recumbent lateral projection, the vertebral column may not be aligned parallel with the imaging table and IR but may sag at the level of the lower thoracic vertebrae, especially in a patient who has wide hips and a narrow waist (Figure 8-32). If the patient's

on the right or left side is not significant, although left-side positioning is easier for the technologist (Figure 8-31). One exception to this guideline is the scoliotic patient, who should be placed on the imaging table so the central ray is directed into the spinal curve. Abduct the patient's arms to a 90-degree angle with the body to prevent the humeri or their soft tissue from obscuring the thoracic vertebrae. Flex the patient's knees and hips for support, and position a pillow or sponge between the knees. The thickness of the pillow or sponge should be enough to prevent the side of the pelvis situated farther from the IR from rotating anteriorly but not so thick as to cause posterior rotation. To avoid vertebral rotation, align the shoulders, the posterior ribs, and the posterior pelvic wings perpendicular to the imaging table and IR by resting an extended flat palm against each, respectively, and then adjusting patient rotation until the hand is positioned perpendicular to the IR.

- **Effect of rotation.** The upper and lower thoracic vertebrae can demonstrate rotation independently or simultaneously, depending on which section of the torso was rotated. If the shoulders and the superoposterior ribs were not placed on top of each other but the posterior pelvic wings and inferoposterior ribs were aligned, the upper thoracic vertebrae demonstrate rotation and the lower thoracic vertebrae demonstrate a true lateral projection. If the posterior pelvic wings and inferoposterior ribs were rotated but the shoulders and superoposterior ribs were placed on top of each other, the lower thoracic vertebrae demonstrate rotation and the upper vertebrae demonstrate a lateral projection.

- **Detecting rotation.** Rotation can be detected on a lateral thoracic vertebrae projection by evaluating

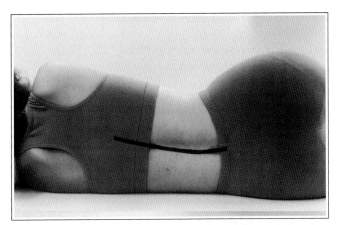

FIGURE 8-32 Poor alignment of vertebral column with imaging table.

thoracic column is allowed to sag, the diverging x-ray beams are not aligned parallel with the intervertebral disk spaces and perpendicular with the vertebral bodies. Lateral flexion on a lateral thoracic vertebrae projection is most evident at the lower thoracic vertebral bodies, where closed disk spaces and distorted vertebral bodies are present (see Image 43). For a patient who has a sagging thoracic column, it may be necessary to tuck an immobilization device between the lateral body surface and imaging table just superior to the iliac crest, elevating the sagging area. The radiolucent sponge should be thick enough to bring the thoracic vertebral column parallel with the imaging table and IR (see Figure 8-31)

- An alternative method of obtaining open disk spaces and undistorted vertebral bodies in a patient whose thoracic column is sagging is to angle the central ray 10 degrees cephalically for female patients and 15 degrees for male patients. The degree of cephalic angulation used should align the central ray perpendicular to the thoracic vertebral column.

The seventh thoracic vertebra is centered within the exposure field. The seventh cervical vertebra, the first through 12th thoracic vertebrae, and the first lumbar vertebra are included within the collimated field.

- Center a perpendicular central ray to the inferior scapular angle. With the patient's arm positioned at a 90-degree angle with the body, the inferior scapular angle is placed over the seventh thoracic vertebra.
- Open the longitudinal collimation the full 17-inch (43-cm) IR length for adult patients. Transverse collimation should be to an 8-inch (20-cm) field.
- A 14- × 17-inch (35- × 43-cm) IR placed lengthwise should be adequate to include all the required anatomic structures.
- *Verifying inclusion of all thoracic vertebrae.* When viewing a lateral thoracic projection, you can be sure that the twelfth thoracic vertebra has been

included by locating the vertebra that has the last rib attached to it; this is the twelfth vertebra. To confirm this finding, follow the posterior vertebral bodies of the lower thoracic and upper lumbar vertebrae, watching for the subtle change in curvature from kyphotic to lordotic. The twelfth thoracic vertebra is located just above it. The first thoracic vertebra can be identified on a lateral thoracic projection by counting up from the twelfth thoracic vertebra or by locating the seventh cervical vertebral prominens. The first thoracic vertebra is at the same level as this prominens.

- *Lateral cervicothoracic projection (Twining method).* Because of shoulder thickness and the superimposition of the shoulders over the first through third thoracic vertebrae, it may be necessary to take a supplementary image of this area to demonstrate the thoracic vertebrae. Refer to page 449 for details.

Lateral Thoracic Vertebrae Projection Analysis

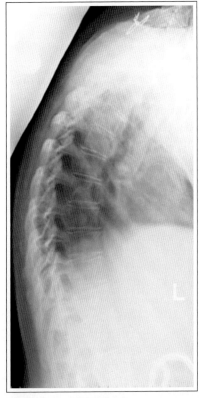

IMAGE 39

Analysis. The thoracic vertebrae, ribs, and lung markings demonstrate a blurring of the recorded details. The image was exposed using deep breathing technique during the exposure, causing patient motion.

Correction. Instruct the patient to breath shallowly. If the patient is unable to perform costal breathing, take the exposure on suspended expiration.

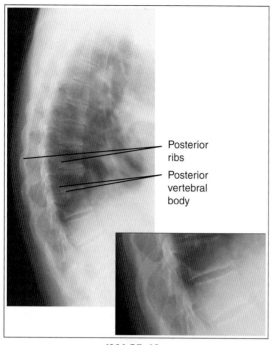

Posterior ribs

Posterior vertebral body

IMAGE 40

Analysis. The posterior surfaces of the vertebral bodies are demonstrated without superimposition, and more than 0.5 inch (1.25 cm) of space is demonstrated between the posterior ribs. The elevated side of the thorax was rotated posteriorly.

Correction. Rotate the elevated thorax anteriorly until a flat palm placed against the shoulders, posterior ribs, and posterior pelvic wings is aligned perpendicular to the imaging table. All three areas need to be checked to prevent rotation across the entire spine. The amount of rotation required is half the distance demonstrated between the posterior surfaces of the vertebral bodies.

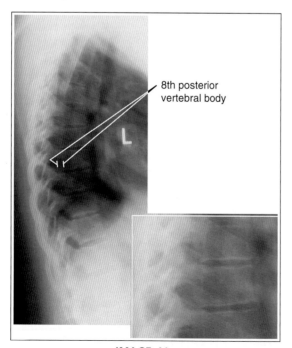

8th posterior vertebral body

IMAGE 41

Analysis. The posterior surfaces of the vertebral bodies are demonstrated without superimposition, and the posterior ribs are superimposed. The elevated side of the thorax was rotated anteriorly.

Correction. Rotate the elevated thorax posteriorly until a flat palm placed against the shoulder, posterior ribs, and posterior pelvic wings is aligned perpendicular to the imaging table. The amount of rotation required is half the distance demonstrated between the posterior surfaces of the vertebral bodies.

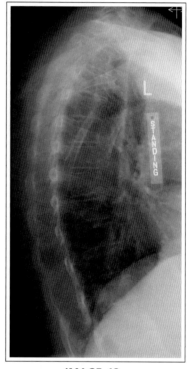

IMAGE 42

Analysis. The posterior surfaces of the vertebral bodies are demonstrated without superimposition, more than 0.5 inch (1.25 cm) of space is demonstrated between the posterior ribs, and the more magnified (right side) scapula and humeral head is positioned posterior to the less magnified (left side) scapula and humeral head. The elevated side of the thorax was rotated posteriorly.

Correction. Rotate the elevated thorax anteriorly until a flat palm placed against the shoulder, posterior ribs, and posterior pelvic wings is aligned perpendicular to the imaging table.

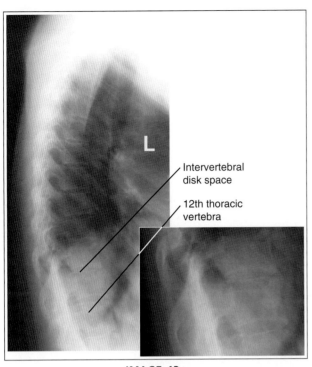

Intervertebral disk space

12th thoracic vertebra

IMAGE 43

Analysis. The T8 through T12 intervertebral disk spaces are obscured, and the vertebral bodies are distorted. The thoracic vertebral column was not aligned parallel with the imaging table.

Correction. Position a radiolucent sponge between the lateral body surface and imaging table just superior to the iliac crest. The radiolucent sponge should be thick enough to align the thoracic vertebral column parallel with the imaging table. If a sponge cannot be used, the central ray can be angled cephalically until it is perpendicular to the thoracic vertebral column.

9

Lumbar Vertebrae, Sacrum, and Coccyx

OUTLINE

OBJECTIVES

After completion of this chapter, you should be able to do the following:

- Identify the required anatomy on lumbar, sacral, and coccygeal projections.
- Describe how to properly position the patient, image receptor (IR), and central ray for lumbar, sacral, and coccygeal projections.
- State how to properly mark and display lumbar, sacral, and coccygeal projections.
- List the image analysis requirements for lumbar, sacral, and coccygeal projections with accurate positioning and state how to reposition the patient when less than optimal images are produced.
- Describe how the upper and lower lumbar vertebrae can move simultaneously and independently.
- Describe how spinal scoliosis is distinguished from rotation on an AP lumbar projection.
- State which zygapophyseal joints are demonstrated when AP and PA oblique lumbar projections are produced.

- List the anatomic structures that make up the parts of the "Scottie dogs" demonstrated on an AP oblique lumbar projection with accurate positioning.
- Explain which procedures are used to produce lateral lumbar, L5-S1 spot, sacral, and coccygeal projections with the least amount of scatter radiation reaching the IR.
- State two methods of positioning the long axis of the lumbar column parallel with the long axis of the imaging table for a lateral lumbar projection.
- Describe how the patient is positioned to demonstrate AP mobility of the lumbar vertebral column.
- State why the patient is instructed to empty the bladder and colon before an AP sacral or coccygeal projection is taken.

KEY TERM

interiliac line

IMAGE ANALYSIS CRITERIA

The following image analysis criteria are used for all adult and pediatric lumbar vertebral, sacral, and coccygeal projections and should be considered when completing the analysis for each projection presented in this chapter (Box 9-1).

- *Visibility of lumbar, sacral, and coccygeal details.* An optimal kVp technique, as shown in Table 9-1, sufficiently penetrates lumbar vertebrae and sacral or coccygeal structures and provides the contrast scale necessary to visualize the vertebral details. A grid is used to absorb the scatter radiation produced by the lumbar vertebrae, sacrum, and coccyx, increasing detail visibility. To obtain optimal density, set milliampere seconds (mAs) manually based on the patient's structure thickness, or choose the appropriate automatic exposure control (AEC) chamber (see Box 9-1 for specifics).

BOX 9-1	Lumbar Vertebrae, Sacrum, and Coccyx Imaging Analysis Criteria

- The facility's identification requirements are visible.
- A right or left marker identifying the correct side of the patient is present on the image and is not superimposed over the anatomy of interest.
- Good radiation protection practices are evident.
- Bony trabecular patterns and cortical outlines of the anatomic structures are sharply defined.
- Contrast and density are uniform and adequate to demonstrate the soft tissue and bony structures.
- Penetration is sufficient to visualize the bony trabecular patterns and cortical outlines of the vertebral bodies, pedicles, and spinous and transverse processes.
- No evidence of removal artifacts is present.

LUMBAR VERTEBRAE: ANTEROPOSTERIOR PROJECTION

See Figure 9-1 and Box 9-2.

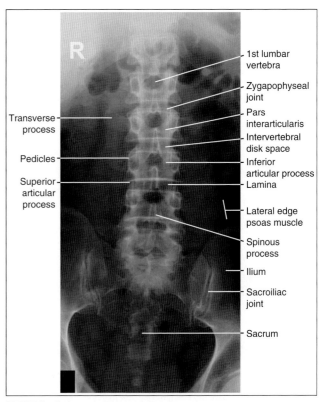

FIGURE 9-1 AP lumbar vertebrae projection with accurate positioning.

The psoas muscles are demonstrated.

- *Soft tissue structures of lumbar vertebrae.* The soft tissue structures that should be visualized on AP lumbar vertebral projections are the psoas muscles. They are located laterally to the lumbar vertebrae, originating at the first lumbar vertebra on each side and extending to the corresponding side's lesser trochanter. They are used in lateral flexion and rotation of the thigh and in flexion of the vertebral column. On an AP lumbar projection, they are visible on each side of the vertebral bodies as long triangular soft tissue shadows.

TABLE 9-1	Lumbar Vertebrae, Sacrum, and Coccyx Technical Data			
Projection	**kVp**	**Grid**	**AEC Chamber(s)**	**SID**
AP, lumber vertebrae	75–80	Grid	Center	40–48 inches (100–120 cm)
AP oblique, lumbar vertebrae	75–85	Grid		40–48 inches (100–120 cm)
Lateral, lumbar vertebrae	85–95	Grid	Center	40–48 inches (100–120 cm)
Lateral, L5-S1 lumbosacral junction	95–100	Grid	Center	40–48 inches (100–120 cm)
AP axial, sacrum	75–80	Grid	Center	40–48 inches (100–120 cm)
Lateral, sacrum	85–95	Grid	Center	40–48 inches (100–120 cm)
AP axial, coccyx	75–80	Grid	Center	40–48 inches (100–120 cm)
Lateral, coccyx	80–85	Grid		40–48 inches (100–120 cm)

AEC, Automatic exposure control; *kVp,* kilovoltage peak; *SID,* source–image receptor distance.

BOX 9-2	Anteroposterior Lumbar Vertebrae Projection Analysis Criteria

- The psoas muscles are demonstrated and the distances from the pedicles to the spinous processes are equal on both sides. The sacrum and coccyx should be centered within the inlet pelvis and aligned with the symphysis pubis.
- The intervertebral disk spaces are open and the vertebral bodies are seen without distortion.
- The spinous processes are aligned with the midline of the vertebral bodies.
- The long axis of the lumbar column is aligned with the long axis of the exposure field.
- 14- × 17-inch (35- × 43-cm) IR: The L4 vertebra and iliac crest are at the center of the exposure field.
- 14- × 17-inch (35- × 43-cm) IR: The twelfth thoracic vertebra, first through fifth lumbar vertebrae, sacroiliac joints, sacrum, coccyx and psoas muscles are included within the collimated field.
- 11- × 14-inch (28- × 35-cm) IR: The L3 vertebra is at the center of the exposure field.
- 11- × 14-inch (28- × 35-cm) IR: The twelfth thoracic vertebra, first through fifth lumbar vertebrae, sacroiliac joints, and psoas muscles are included in the collimated field.

The lumbar vertebrae demonstrate an AP projection. The spinous processes are aligned with the midline of the vertebral bodies, and the distances from the pedicles to the spinous processes are equal. When demonstrated, the sacrum and coccyx should be centered within the inlet pelvis and aligned with the symphysis pubis.

- An AP lumbar vertebral projection is obtained by placing the patient supine on the imaging table. Position the shoulders and anterior superior iliac spines (ASISs) at equal distances from the imaging table to prevent rotation, and draw the arms away from the abdominal area to prevent them from being tucked beneath the body (Figure 9-2).

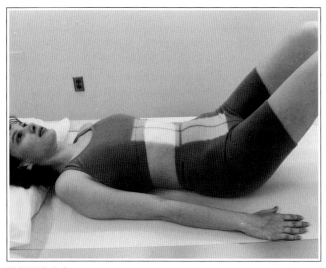

FIGURE 9-2 Proper patient positioning for AP lumbar vertebrae projection.

- *Effect of rotation.* The upper and lower lumbar vertebrae can demonstrate rotation independently or simultaneously, depending on which section of the body is rotated. If the patient's thorax were rotated and the pelvis remained supine, the upper lumbar vertebrae demonstrate rotation. If the patient's pelvis were rotated and the thorax remained supine, the lower lumbar vertebrae demonstrate rotation. If the patient's thorax and pelvis were rotated simultaneously, the entire lumbar column demonstrates rotation.
- *Detecting rotation.* Rotation is effectively detected on an AP lumbar projection by evaluating the alignment of the spinous processes in the vertebral body. If no rotation is present, the spinous processes are aligned with the midline of the vertebral bodies, positioning them at equal distances from the pedicles. On rotation the affected spinous processes move away from the midline and closer to the pedicles, resulting in different distances between the spinous processes and corresponding pedicles (see Image 1). The side toward which the spinous processes rotate and that demonstrates the least distance from the spinous processes to the pedicles is the side of the patient positioned farther from the imaging table and IR.

  Lower lumbar rotation can also be detected by evaluating the position of the sacrum and coccyx within the pelvic inlet. If no rotation was present, they are centered within the pelvic inlet. On rotation, the sacrum and coccyx rotate toward the side of the pelvic inlet positioned farther from the IR.
- *Distinguishing rotation from scoliosis.* In patients with spinal scoliosis, the lumbar bodies may appear rotated because of the lateral twisting of the vertebrae. Scoliosis of the vertebral column can be very severe, demonstrating a large amount of lateral deviation, or it can be subtle, demonstrating only a small amount of deviation. Severe scoliosis is very obvious and is seldom mistaken for patient rotation (see Image 2), whereas subtle scoliotic changes can be easily mistaken for rotation (see Image 3).

  Although both conditions demonstrate unequal distances between the pedicles and spinous processes, certain clues can be used to distinguish subtle scoliosis from rotation. The long axis of a rotated vertebral column remains straight, whereas the scoliotic vertebral column demonstrates lateral deviation. If the lumbar vertebrae demonstrate rotation, it has been caused by the rotation of the upper or lower torso. Rotation of the middle lumbar vertebrae (L3 and L4) does not occur unless the lower thoracic or upper or lower lumbar vertebrae also demonstrate rotation.

On a scoliotic image, the middle lumbar vertebrae may demonstrate rotation without corresponding upper or lower vertebral rotation. Familiarity with the differences between a rotated lumbar vertebral column and a scoliotic one prevents unnecessary repeated procedures in patients with spinal scoliosis.

The intervertebral disk spaces are open, and the vertebral bodies are demonstrated without distortion.

- When the patient is in a supine position with the legs extended, the lumbar vertebrae have an exaggerated lordotic curvature. Obtaining an AP lumbar projection with the patient in this position results in closed intervertebral disk spaces and distorted vertebral bodies because of how the x-ray beams are directed at the disk spaces and vertebral bodies (Figure 9-3). To straighten the lumbar vertebral column—thereby aligning the intervertebral disk spaces parallel with and the vertebral bodies perpendicular to the x-ray beam—flex the patient's knees and hips until the lower back rests firmly against the imaging table (Figure 9-4).
- *Effect of lordotic curvature.* On an AP lumbar projection, determine how well the central ray parallels the intervertebral disk spaces by evaluating the openness of the T12 through L3 intervertebral disk spaces and the visibility of the ischial spines without pelvic brim superimposition. If the lordotic curvature was adequately reduced, the disk spaces are open and the ischial spines are only

partially demonstrated without pelvic brim superimposition. If the lordotic curvature was not adequately reduced, the intervertebral disk spaces are closed and the ischial spines are demonstrated without pelvic brim superimposition (see Image 4).

If a 14-× 17-inch (35- × 43-cm) IR placed lengthwise was used, the L4 vertebra and the iliac crest are centered within the exposure field. The twelfth thoracic vertebra, first through fifth lumbar vertebrae, sacroiliac joints, sacrum, coccyx, and psoas muscles are included within the collimated field.

If an 11- × 14-inch (28- × 35-cm) IR placed lengthwise was used, the L3 vertebra is centered within the exposure field. The twelfth thoracic vertebra, first through fifth lumbar vertebrae, sacroiliac joints, and psoas muscles are included within the collimated field.

- Center a perpendicular central ray to the patient's midsagittal plane at the level of the iliac crest for a 14- × 17-inch (35- × 43-cm) IR and at a level 1.5 inches (4 cm) superior to the iliac crest for a 11- × 14-inch (28- × 35-cm) IR. Center the IR to the central ray.
- Open the longitudinal collimation the full 17-inch (43-cm) or 14-inch (35-cm) IR length for adult patients. Transverse collimation should be to approximately an 8-inch (20-cm) field.

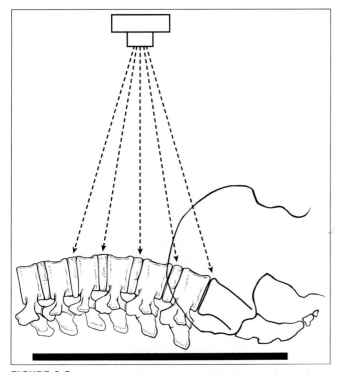

FIGURE 9-3 Alignment of central ray and lumbar vertebrae when legs are not flexed.

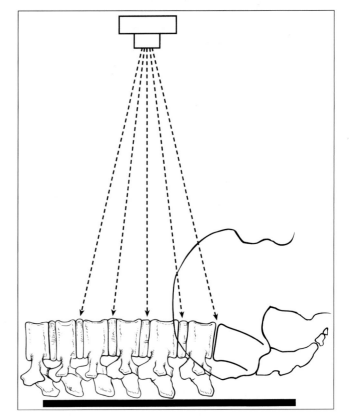

FIGURE 9-4 Alignment of central ray and lumbar vertebrae when legs are flexed.

Anteroposterior Lumbar Projection Analysis

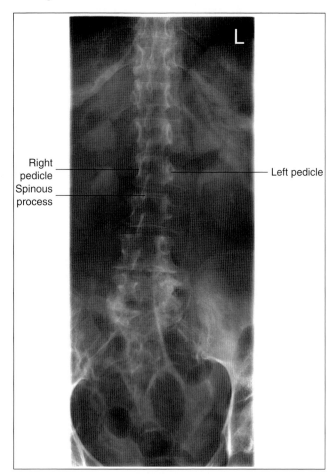

Right pedicle

Spinous process

Left pedicle

IMAGE 1

Analysis. The spinous processes are not aligned with the vertebral midline. The distances from the left pedicles to the spinous processes are greater than the distances from the right pedicles to the spinous processes, and the sacrum and coccyx are rotated toward the right lateral inlet pelvis. The patient was rotated toward the left side.

Correction. Rotate the patient toward the right side until the shoulders and the ASISs are positioned at equal distances from the IR.

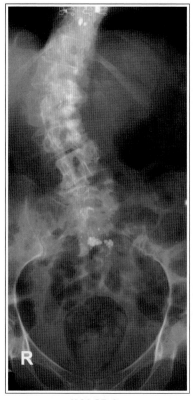

IMAGE 2

Analysis. The vertebral column demonstrates severe spinal scoliosis.

Correction. No corrective movement is required. An AP lumbar projection of a patient with scoliosis appears rotated.

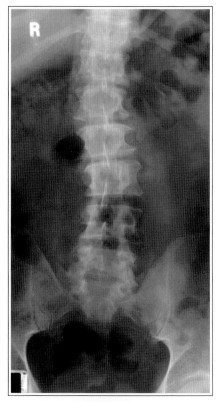

IMAGE 3

Analysis. The vertebral column deviates laterally at the level of the second through fourth lumbar vertebrae, the sacrum is centered within the pelvic inlet, and the distances from the pedicles to the spinous processes of the eleventh thoracic vertebra and fifth lumbar vertebra are almost equal. The vertebral column demonstrates subtle spinal scoliosis.

Correction. No corrective movement is required. An AP lumbar projection of a patient with scoliosis appears rotated.

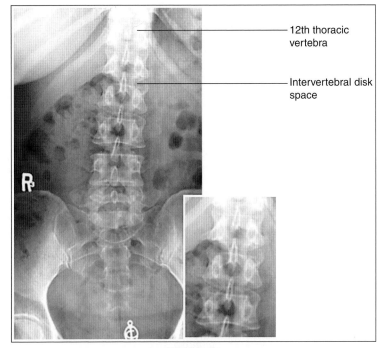

12th thoracic vertebra

Intervertebral disk space

IMAGE 4

Analysis. The T12 to L3 intervertebral disk spaces are closed, and the lumbar bodies are distorted. The ischial spines are demonstrated without pelvic brim superimposition. The lordotic curvature of the spine was not reduced, as shown in Figure 9-3.

Correction. Flex the hips and knees until the lower back rests firmly against the imaging table, restraightening the lumbar vertebrae as shown in Figure 9-4.

LUMBAR VERTEBRAE: ANTEROPOSTERIOR OBLIQUE PROJECTION (RIGHT AND LEFT POSTERIOR OBLIQUE POSITIONS)

See Figure 9-5 and Box 9-3.

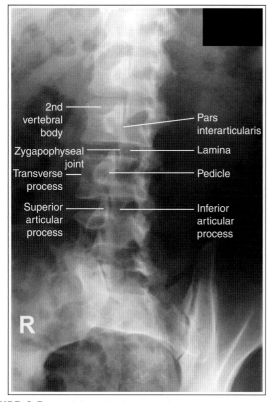

FIGURE 9-5 AP oblique lumbar vertebrae projection with accurate positioning.

BOX 9-3	**Anteroposterior Oblique Lumbar Vertebrae Projection Analysis Criteria**

- The superior and inferior articular processes are in profile, the zygapophyseal joints are demonstrated, and the pedicles are seen halfway between the midpoint of the vertebral bodies and the lateral border of the vertebral bodies.
- The third lumbar vertebra is at the center of the exposure field.
- The twelfth thoracic vertebra, first through fifth lumbar vertebrae, first and second sacral segments, and sacroiliac joints are included within the collimated field.

Zygapophyseal joints are demonstrated with the least amount of magnification.

- This examination can be performed using an AP or PA oblique projection. In the AP oblique projection (right posterior oblique [RPO] and left posterior oblique [LPO] positions; Figure 9-6) the zygapophyseal joints of interest are placed closer to the IR. In the PA oblique projection (right anterior oblique [RAO] and left anterior oblique [LAO]

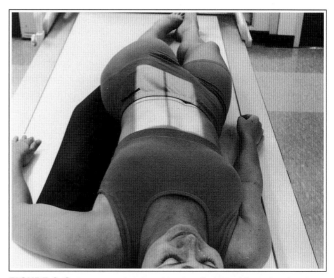

FIGURE 9-6 Proper patient positioning for AP oblique lumbar vertebrae projection.

positions), the zygapophyseal joints of interest are positioned farther from the IR, resulting in greater magnification.

The lumbar vertebrae have been adequately rotated. The superior and inferior articular processes are in profile, the zygapophyseal joints are visualized, and the pedicles are seen halfway between the midpoint of the vertebral bodies and the lateral border of the vertebral bodies. The ears, necks, eyes, feet, and bodies of the "Scottie dogs" are well defined.

- An AP oblique lumbar vertebral projection is obtained by placing the patient supine on the imaging table, and then rotating the patient toward the side until the superior and inferior articular processes are positioned in profile. The knee positioned closer to the imaging table may be flexed as needed for support. The articular processes are placed in profile by rotating the thorax until the midcoronal plane is at a 45-degree angle with the IR (Figure 9-6). To demonstrate the right and left articular processes and zygapophyseal joints of each vertebra, both right and left PA oblique projections must be taken.
- *Scottie dogs and accurate lumbar obliquity.* The accuracy of an AP oblique lumbar projection is often judged by the demonstration of five Scottie dogs stacked on top of one another. Figure 9-7 is a close-up of an accurately positioned oblique lumbar vertebra with the Scottie dog parts outlined and labeled. It should be noted that the Scottie dogs can be identified even on AP oblique lumbar projections with poor positioning. Judge the openness of each zygapophyseal joint to determine whether the lumbar vertebrae have been adequately rotated.
- *Identifying poor obliquity.* If a lumbar vertebra was not rotated enough to position the superior

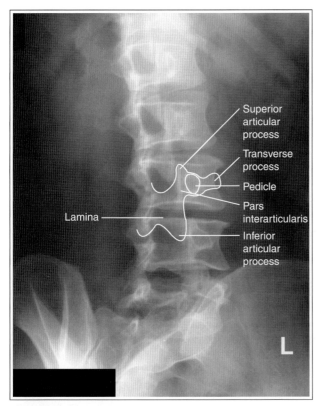

FIGURE 9-7 Identifying "Scottie dogs" and lumbar anatomy.

and inferior articular processes (ear and front leg of Scottie dog) in profile, the corresponding zygapophyseal joint is closed, the pedicle (eye of Scottie dog) is situated closer to the lateral vertebral body border, and more of the lamina (body of Scottie dog) is demonstrated (see Image 5). If a lumbar vertebra was rotated more than needed to position the superior and inferior articular processes in profile, the corresponding zygapophyseal joint is closed, the pedicles are demonstrated closer to the vertebral body midline, and less of the lamina is demonstrated (see Image 6).

The third lumbar vertebra is centered within the exposure field. The twelfth thoracic vertebra, first through fifth lumbar vertebrae, first and second sacral segments, and sacroiliac joints are included within the collimated field.

- To place the third lumbar vertebra in the center of the exposure field, center a perpendicular central ray 2 inches (5 cm) medial to the elevated ASIS at a level 1.5 inches (4 cm) superior to the iliac crest. Center the IR to the central ray.
- Open the longitudinally collimated field the full 14-inch (35-cm) IR length for adult patients. Transverse collimation should be to an 8-inch (20-cm) field.
- An 11- × 14-inch (28- × 35-cm) IR placed lengthwise should be adequate to include all the required anatomic structures.

Anteroposterior Oblique Lumbar Projection Analysis

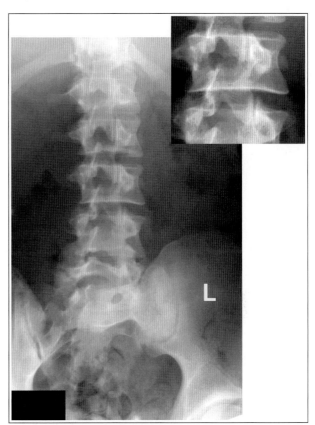

IMAGE 5

Analysis. The first and second lumbar vertebrae are accurately positioned on this image, indicating that the patient's upper torso was adequately rotated. The third, fourth, and fifth lumbar vertebrae's superior and inferior articular processes are not demonstrated in profile, their corresponding zygapophyseal joint spaces are closed, and their pedicles (eyes of Scottie dog) are demonstrated closer to the vertebrae's lateral vertebral body borders than to their midlines. The patient's inferior lumbar vertebrae and pelvis were in insufficient obliquity.

Correction. While maintaining the degree of thoracic and upper lumbar vertebral obliquity, increase the lower lumbar vertebral and pelvic rotation.

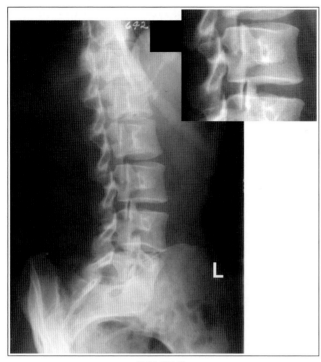

IMAGE 6

Analysis. The lumbar vertebrae's superior and inferior articular processes are not demonstrated in profile, their corresponding zygapophyseal joint spaces are closed, their laminae are obscured, and the pedicles are aligned with the midline of the vertebral bodies. The patient's upper lumbar vertebrae and thorax were in excessive obliquity.

Correction. Decrease the lumbar vertebral and thoracic rotation to 45 degrees.

LUMBAR VERTEBRAE: LATERAL PROJECTION

See Figure 9-8 and Box 9-4.

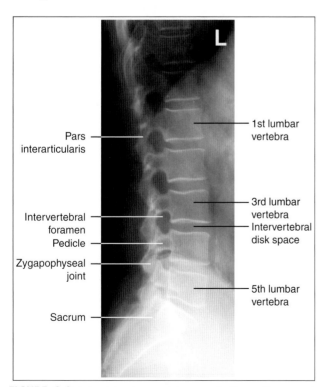

FIGURE 9-8 Lateral lumbar vertebrae projection with accurate positioning.

BOX 9-4	**Lateral Lumbar Vertebrae Projection Analysis Criteria**

- The intervertebral foramina are demonstrated and the spinous processes are in profile. The right and left pedicles and the posterior surfaces of each vertebral body are superimposed.
- The intervertebral disk spaces are open and the vertebral bodies are seen without distortion.
- The lumbar vertebral column is in a neutral position, without anteroposterior flexion or extension.
- The long axis of the lumbar vertebral column is aligned with the long axis of the exposure field.
- 14- × 17-inch (35- × 43-cm) IR: The L4 vertebra and iliac crest are at the center of the exposure field.
- 14- × 17-inch (35- × 43-cm) IR: The eleventh and twelfth thoracic vertebra, first through fifth lumbar vertebrae, and sacrum are included within the collimated field.
- 11- × 14-inch (28- × 35-cm) IR: The L3 vertebra is at the center of the exposure field.
- 11- × 14-inch (28- × 35-cm) IR: The twelfth thoracic vertebra, first through fifth vertebrae, and L5-S1 intervertebral disk space are included in the collimated field.

The lumbar vertebrae demonstrate a lateral projection. The intervertebral foramina are demonstrated, and the spinous processes are in profile. The right and left pedicles and the posterior surfaces of each vertebral body are superimposed.

- To obtain a lateral lumbar projection, place the patient on the imaging table in a lateral recumbent position. Whether the patient is lying on the right or left side is insignificant, although left side positioning is often easier for the technologist. One exception to this guideline is the scoliotic patient, who should be placed on the imaging table so that the central ray is directed into the spinal curve (Figure 9-9) to better demonstrate the intervertebral joint spaces. Determine how the patient's curve is directed by viewing the patient's back and following the curve of the vertebral column and evaluating the AP projection. Figure 9-10 demonstrates AP and lateral lumbar projections taken on a patient with a scoliotic lumbar vertebral column that curves toward the right side of the patient. The lateral projection was taken with the patient lying on the left side. Note how all the intervertebral disk spaces are closed. Once the patient has been placed on the table, flex the patient's knees and hips for support, and position a pillow or sponge between the knees. The pillow or sponge should be thick enough to prevent the side of the pelvis situated farther from the IR from rotating anteriorly, without being so thick as to cause this side to rotate posteriorly (Figure 9-11). To avoid vertebral rotation, align the shoulders, posterior ribs, and posterior pelvic wings perpendicular to the imaging table and IR. This is accomplished by resting your extended flat hand against each structure, individually, and then adjusting the patient's rotation until your hand is perpendicular to the IR.

- **Effect of rotation.** The upper and lower lumbar vertebrae can demonstrate rotation independently or simultaneously, depending on which section of the torso is rotated. If the thorax was rotated but the pelvis remained in a lateral position, the upper lumbar vertebrae demonstrate rotation. If the pelvis was rotated but the thorax remained in a lateral position, the lower lumbar vertebrae demonstrate rotation.

- **Detecting rotation.** Rotation can be detected on a lateral lumbar projection by evaluating the superimposition of the right and left posterior surfaces of the vertebral bodies. On a nonrotated lateral lumbar projection, these posterior surfaces are superimposed, appearing as one. On rotation, these posterior surfaces are not superimposed, but one is demonstrated anterior to the other (see Image 7). Because the two sides of the vertebrae, thorax, and pelvis are mirror projection, it is very difficult to determine from a rotated lateral lumbar projection which side of the patient was rotated anteriorly and which posteriorly, unless the twelfth posterior ribs are demonstrated. The twelfth posterior rib that demonstrates the greatest magnification and is situated inferiorly is adjacent to the side of the patient positioned farther from the IR.

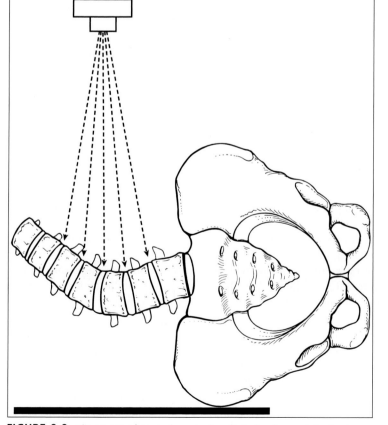

FIGURE 9-9 Alignment of central ray and scoliotic lumbar vertebral column.

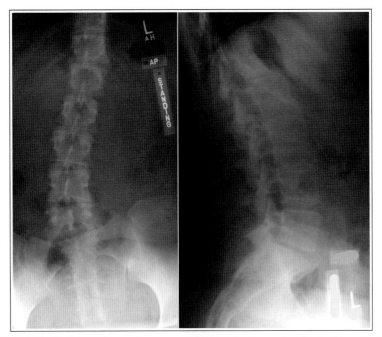

FIGURE 9-10 AP and lateral lumbar vertebrae projections of patient with scoliosis.

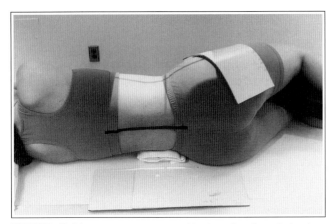

FIGURE 9-11 Proper patient positioning for lateral lumbar vertebrae projection.

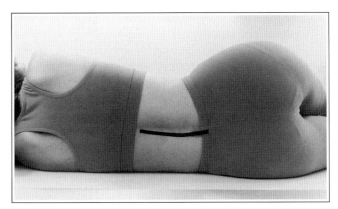

FIGURE 9-12 Poor alignment of vertebral column and imaging table.

The intervertebral disk spaces are open, and the vertebral bodies are demonstrated without distortion.

- The lumbar vertebral column is capable of lateral flexion. Therefore when the patient is placed in a lateral recumbent position, the vertebral column may not be aligned parallel with the imaging table and IR but may sag or curve upwardly at the level of the iliac crest (Figure 9-12). If the patient's lumbar column is allowed to sag, the diverging x-ray beams are not aligned parallel with the intervertebral disk spaces and perpendicular to the vertebral bodies. Lateral lumbar flexion on a lateral vertebrae projection is most evident at the lower lumbar region, where closed disk spaces and distorted vertebral bodies are present (see Image 8). For a patient who has a sagging lumbar column, it may be necessary to tuck a radiolucent sponge between

the lateral body surface and imaging table just superior to the iliac crest, elevating the sagging area. The sponge should be thick enough to bring the lumbar vertebral column parallel with the imaging table and IR (see Figure 9-11).

- An alternative method of obtaining open disk spaces and undistorted vertebral bodies for a patient whose lumbar column is sagging is to angle the central ray 5 to 8 degrees caudally. This caudal angulation should align the central ray perpendicular to the vertebral column and parallel with the interiliac line (imaginary line connecting the iliac crests).

The lumbar vertebral column is in a neutral position, without AP flexion or extension. A lordotic curvature is present.

- A neutral position of the lumbar vertebrae is obtained when the long axis of the patient's body is aligned with the long axis of the imaging table. The thoracic and pelvic regions are aligned.

- *Positioning to evaluate AP mobility of lumbar vertebrae.* If the lumbar vertebrae are being imaged in the lateral projection to demonstrate AP vertebral mobility, two lateral images should be taken, one with the patient in maximum flexion and one in maximum extension. For maximum flexion, instruct the patient to flex the shoulders, upper thorax, and knees anteriorly, rolling into a tight ball (Figure 9-13). The resulting image should meet all the requirements listed for a lateral projection with accurate positioning, except that the lumbar vertebral column demonstrates a very straight longitudinal axis without lordotic curvature (see Image 9). For maximum extension, instruct the patient to arch the back by extending the shoulders, upper thorax, and legs as far posteriorly as possible (Figure 9-14). The resulting image should meet all the requirements listed for a lateral projection with accurate positioning, except that the lumbar vertebral column demonstrates an increased lordotic curvature (see Image 10).

The long axis of the lumbar vertebral column is aligned with the long axis of the exposure field.

- Aligning the long axis of the lumbar vertebral column with the collimator's longitudinal light line allows tight collimation, which is necessary to reduce the production of scatter radiation.
- The lumbar vertebrae are located in the posterior half of the torso. Their exact posterior location can be determined by palpating the ASIS and posterior iliac wing (at the level of the sacroiliac joint) of the side of the patient situated farther from the IR. The long axis of the lumbar vertebral column is aligned with the coronal plane that is situated halfway between these two structures (Figure 9-15).

If a 14- × 17-inch (35- × 43-cm) IR placed lengthwise was used, the iliac crest and fourth lumbar vertebra are centered within the exposure field. The eleventh and twelfth thoracic vertebrae, first through fifth lumbar vertebrae, and sacrum are included within the collimated field.

If an 11- × 14-inch (28- × 35-cm) IR placed lengthwise was used, the third lumbar vertebra is centered within the exposure field. The twelfth thoracic vertebra, first through fifth lumbar vertebrae, and L5-S1 intervertebral disk space are included within the collimated field.

- Center a perpendicular central ray to the coronal plane located halfway between the elevated ASIS and posterior wing at the level of the iliac crest for a 14- × 17-inch (35- × 43-cm) IR, and at a level 1.5 inches (4 cm) superior to the iliac crest for an 11- × 14-inch (28- × 35-cm) IR.

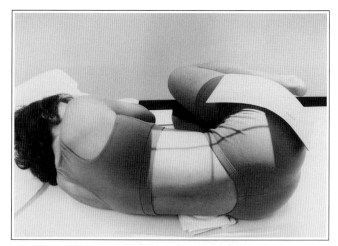

FIGURE 9-13 Proper patient positioning for lateral (flexion) lumbar vertebrae projection.

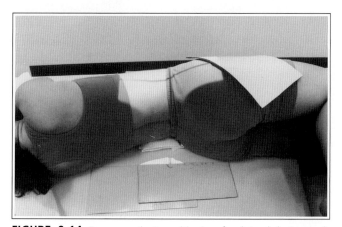

FIGURE 9-14 Proper patient positioning for lateral (extension) lumbar vertebrae projection.

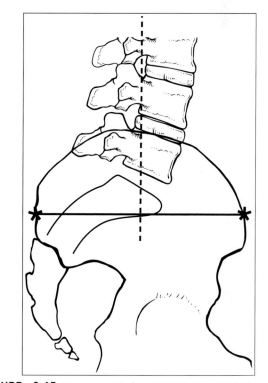

FIGURE 9-15 Proper central ray centering and long axis placement. Asterisks identify the posterior iliac wing and anterior superior iliac spines.

- Open the longitudinal collimation the full 17- or 14-inch (43- or 35-cm) IR length for adult patients. Transverse collimation should be to an 8-inch (20-cm) field.

- *Supplementary projection of the L5-S1 lumbar region.* A coned-down image of the L5-S1 lumbar region is required when a lateral lumbar projection is obtained that demonstrates insufficient image density in this area or the L5-S1 joint space is closed. In patients with wide hips, it is often difficult to set exposure factors that adequately demonstrate the upper and lower lumbar regions concurrently. For these patients, set exposure factors that adequately demonstrate the upper lumbar region. Then obtain a tightly collimated lateral projection of the L5-S1 lumbar region to demonstrate the lower lumbar area.

- *Gonadal shielding.* Use gonadal protection shielding on all patients for this procedure. Begin by palpating the patient's coccyx and elevated ASIS. Next, draw an imaginary line connecting the coccyx with a point 1 inch posterior to the ASIS, and position the longitudinal edge of a large flat contact shield or lead half-apron anteriorly against this imaginary line (Figure 9-16). This shielding method can be safely used for patients being imaged for lateral vertebral, sacral, or coccygeal projections without fear of obscuring areas of interest (Figure 9-17).

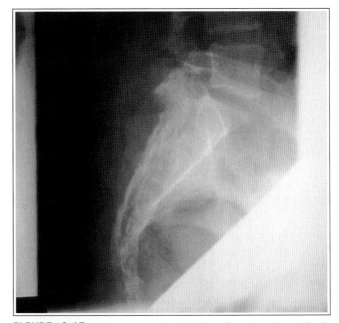

FIGURE 9-17 Proper gonadal shielding for lateral vertebral, sacral, and coccygeal projections.

Lateral Lumbar Vertebrae Projection Analysis

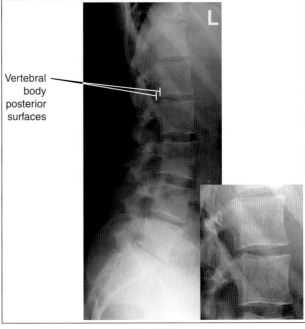

IMAGE 7

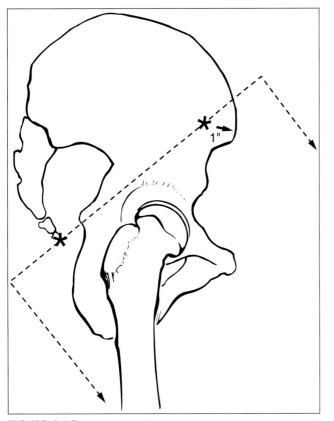

FIGURE 9-16 Gonadal shielding for lateral vertebral, sacral, and coccygeal projections.

Analysis. The posterior surfaces of the first through fourth vertebral bodies and the posterior ribs are demonstrated one anterior to the other. The posterior ribs demonstrating the greater magnification were positioned posteriorly.

Correction. Rotate the side positioned farther from the IR anteriorly until the posterior ribs are superimposed while maintaining posterior pelvic wing superimposition.

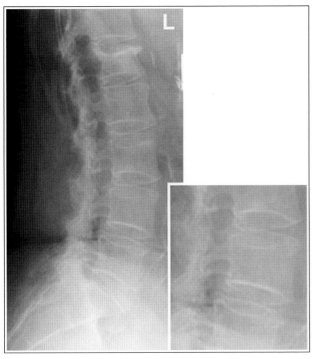

IMAGE 8

Analysis. The L4-L5 and L5-S1 intervertebral disk spaces are closed, and the third through fifth vertebral bodies are distorted. The lumbar vertebral column was not aligned parallel with the imaging table or IR.

Correction. Position a radiolucent sponge between the patient's lateral body surface and the imaging table just superior to the iliac crest. The sponge should be thick enough only to align the lumbar column parallel with the imaging table and IR.

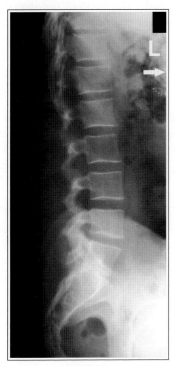

IMAGE 9

Analysis. The lumbar column demonstrates no lordotic curvature. The patient was in a flexed position, as shown in Figure 9-13.

Correction. If a neutral lateral projection is desired, extend the shoulders, upper thorax, and legs posteriorly until the posterior thorax and pelvic wings are aligned with the long axis of the imaging table. If a flexion lateral lumbar projection is being performed to evaluate AP mobility, no corrective movement is required.

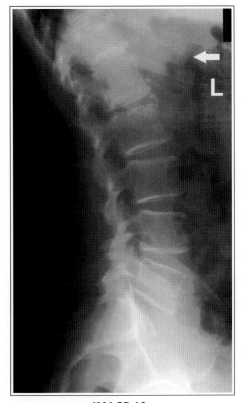

IMAGE 10

Analysis. The lumbar vertebral column demonstrates excess lordotic curvature. The patient was in an extended position, as shown in Figure 9-14.

Correction. If a neutral lateral projection is desired, flex the shoulders, upper thorax, and legs anteriorly until the posterior thorax and pelvic wings are aligned with the long axis of the imaging table. If an extended position is desired to evaluate AP mobility, no corrective movement is required.

L5-S1 LUMBOSACRAL JUNCTION: LATERAL PROJECTION

See Figure 9-18 and Box 9-5.

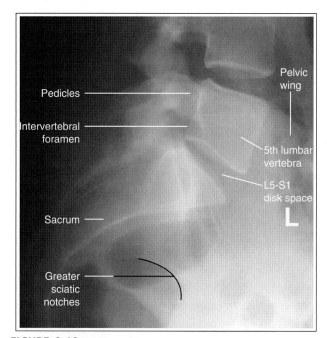

FIGURE 9-18 Lateral L5-S1 lumbosacral junction projection with accurate positioning.

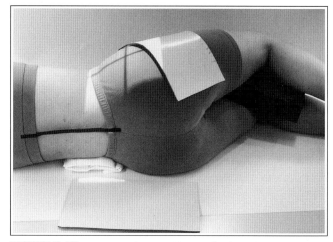

FIGURE 9-19 Proper patient positioning for lateral L5-S1 lumbosacral junction projection.

BOX 9-5	Lateral L5-S1 Lumbosacral Junction Projection Analysis Criteria

- The intervertebral foramina are demonstrated, the right and left pedicles are superimposed and in profile, and the greater sciatic notches and pelvic wings are nearly superimposed.
- The L5-S1 intervertebral disk space is open, the pelvic alae are superimposed, and the sacrum is seen without foreshortening.
- The L5-S1 is at the center of the exposure field.
- The fifth lumbar vertebra and first and second sacral segments are included within the collimated field.

The fifth lumbar vertebra and sacrum demonstrate a lateral projection. The intervertebral foramina are clearly demonstrated, the right and left pedicles are superimposed and demonstrated in profile, and the greater sciatic notches and pelvic wings are nearly superimposed.

- To obtain a lateral L5-S1 lumbosacral junction projection, place the patient on the imaging table in a lateral recumbent position. Whether the patient is lying on the right or left side is not significant, although the left side positioning is easier for the technologist. One exception to this guideline is the scoliotic patient, who should be placed on the imaging table so that the central ray is directed into the spinal curve to better obtain open intervertebral joint spaces. Determine how the patient's curve is directed by viewing the patient's back and following the curve of the vertebral column and evaluating the AP projection.

- Flex the patient's knees and hips for support, and position a pillow or sponge between the knees. The pillow or sponge should be thick enough to prevent the side of the pelvis situated farther from the IR from rotating anteriorly, without being so thick as to cause this side to rotate posteriorly (Figure 9-19).
- To avoid vertebral rotation, align the shoulders, posterior ribs, and posterior pelvic wings perpendicular to the imaging table and IR. This is accomplished by resting your extended flat palm against each structure, individually, and then adjusting the patient's rotation until your hand is perpendicular to the imaging table.
- *Detecting rotation.* Rotation can be detected on a lateral L5-S1 lumbosacral junction projection by evaluating the openness of the intervertebral foramen and the superimposition of the greater sciatic notches and the femoral heads, when seen. On a nonrotated lateral L5-S1 projection, the intervertebral foramen is open, and the greater sciatic notches and femoral heads are superimposed. On rotation, neither the greater sciatic notches nor the femoral heads are superimposed, but are demonstrated one anterior to the other (see Image 11). Because the two sides of the pelvis are mirror images, it is difficult to determine which side of the patient was rotated anteriorly and which posteriorly on a lateral L5-S1 lumbosacral junction poor projection with poor positioning. When rotation has occurred, it is most common for the side of the patient situated farther from the IR to be rotated anteriorly, because of the gravitational forward and downward pull on this side's arm and leg, if a sponge is not placed between the patient's knees. If the patient's femoral heads are visible on the image, they may be used to determine rotation. The femoral head that is projected more inferiorly and demonstrates the greatest magnification is the one situated farther from the IR.

The L5-S1 intervertebral disk space is open, the pelvic alae are superimposed, and the sacrum is demonstrated without foreshortening.

- To obtain an open L5-S1 intervertebral disk space to demonstrate superimposed pelvic alae and to demonstrate the sacrum without foreshortening, the vertebral column is aligned parallel with the imaging table, the interiliac line is aligned perpendicular to the imaging table, and a perpendicular central ray is used.
- *Detecting lateral lumbar flexion.* The lumbar vertebral column is capable of lateral flexion. If this flexion is not considered during positioning, the diverging x-ray beams will not be aligned parallel with the L5-S1 disk space and perpendicular to the long axis of the sacrum. Lateral lumbar flexion can be detected on a lateral L5-S1 projection by evaluating the superimposition of the pelvic alae and the openness of the L5-S1 disk space. A laterally flexed projection demonstrates the pelvic alae without superoinferior alignment and a closed L5-S1 disk space (see Image 12).
- *Adjusting for the sagging vertebral column.* The vertebral column of a patient with wide hips and a narrow waist may sag toward the imaging table at the level of the iliac crest (see Figure 9-12). Two methods may be used to achieve accurate positioning in such a patient:
  1. Place a radiolucent sponge between the patient's lateral body surface and imaging table just superior to the iliac crest to elevate the vertebral column, aligning it parallel with the imaging table (see Figure 9-19); use a perpendicular central ray.
  2. Leave the patient positioned as is and angle the central ray caudally until it parallels the interiliac line.
- *Adjusting for the upwardly curved vertebral column.* The vertebral column of a patient with a large waist may curve upwardly (Figure 9-20). For such a patient, angle the central ray cephalically until it parallels the interiliac line.

The L5-S1 intervertebral disk space is at the center of the exposure field. The fifth lumbar vertebra and the first and second sacral segments are included within the collimated field.

- To place the L5-S1 intervertebral disk space in the center of the exposure field, center a perpendicular central ray to a point 2 inches (5 cm) posterior to the elevated ASIS and 1.5 inches (4 cm) inferior to the iliac crest. Center the IR to the central ray.
- Longitudinally collimate 1 inch (2.5 cm) superior to the iliac crest. Transverse collimation should be to an 8-inch (20-cm) field.
- An 8- × 10-inch (18- × 24-cm) IR placed lengthwise should be adequate to include all the required anatomic structures.

- *Gonadal shielding.* Use gonadal protection shielding on all patients for this procedure (see Figures 9-16 and 9-17).

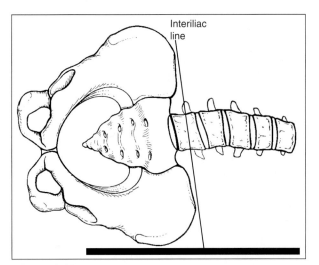

FIGURE 9-20 Adjusting for upwardly curved vertebral column.

Lateral L5-S1 Projection Analysis

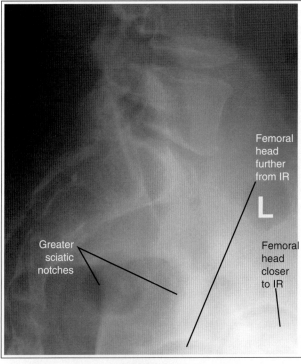

IMAGE 11

Analysis. The L5-S1 intervertebral foramen is obscured and the greater sciatic notches and the femoral heads are demonstrated without superimposition. The femoral head positioned closer to the IR was rotated anteriorly.

Correction. Rotate the patient's hip that was positioned farther from the IR toward the opposite hip until the posterior ribs and the posterior pelvic wings are superimposed. From the original position, the amount of rotation should be approximately 1 inch (2.5 cm).

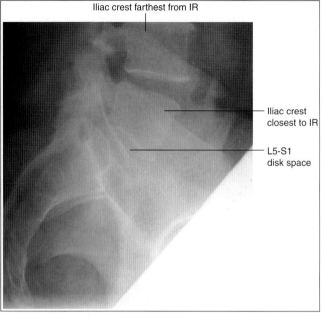

Iliac crest farthest from IR

Iliac crest closest to IR

L5-S1 disk space

IMAGE 12

Analysis. The L5-S1 intervertebral disk space is closed, and the pelvic alae are not superimposed. The long axis of the lumbar vertebral column and the sacrum were not aligned parallel with the imaging table, and the iliac crests were positioned at different transverse levels.

Correction. Position a radiolucent sponge between the patient's lateral body surface and the imaging table just superior to the patient's iliac crest. The sponge should be just thick enough to align the long axis of the vertebral column and sacrum parallel with the imaging table and to place the iliac crests at the same transverse level.

SACRUM

SACRUM: ANTEROPOSTERIOR AXIAL PROJECTION

See Figure 9-21 and Box 9-6.

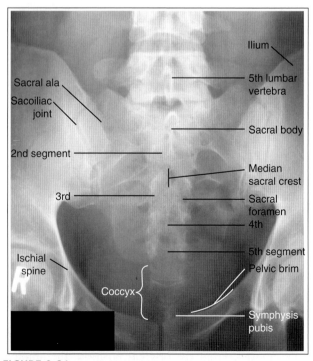

Sacral ala

Sacoiliac joint

2nd segment

3rd

Ischial spine

Coccyx

Ilium

5th lumbar vertebra

Sacral body

Median sacral crest

Sacral foramen

4th

5th segment

Pelvic brim

Symphysis pubis

FIGURE 9-21 AP axial sacral projection with accurate positioning.

BOX 9-6 | **Anteroposterior Axial Sacral Projection Analysis Criteria**

- No evidence of urine, gas, or fecal material superimposing the sacrum.
- The ischial spines are equally demonstrated and are aligned with the pelvic brim, and the median sacral crest and coccyx are aligned with the symphysis pubis.
- The first through fifth sacral segments are seen without foreshortening, the sacral foramina demonstrate equal spacing, and the symphysis pubis is not superimposed over any portion of the sacrum.
- The third sacral segment is at the center of the exposure field.
- The fifth lumbar vertebra, first through fifth sacral segments, first coccygeal vertebra, symphysis pubis, and sacroiliac joints are included within the collimated field.

No evidence suggests that urine, gas, or fecal material is superimposed over the sacrum.

- The patient's urinary bladder should be emptied before the procedure. It is also recommended that the colon be free of gas and fecal material. Elimination of urine, gas, and fecal material from the area superimposed over the sacrum improves its demonstration (see Image 13).

The sacrum demonstrates an AP projection. The ischial spines are equally demonstrated and are aligned with the pelvic brim, and the median sacral crest and coccyx are aligned with the symphysis pubis.

- An AP sacrum projection is obtained by positioning the patient supine on the imaging table with

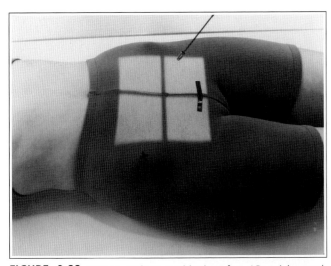

FIGURE 9-22 Proper patient positioning for AP axial sacral projection.

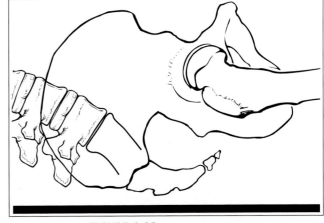

FIGURE 9-23 Sacral curvature.

the legs extended. Position the shoulders and ASISs at equal distances from the imaging table to prevent rotation (Figure 9-22).

- *Detecting rotation.* Rotation is effectively detected on an AP axial sacral projection by comparing the amount of iliac spine demonstrated without pelvic brim superimposition and by evaluating the alignment of the median sacral crest and coccyx with the symphysis pubis. If the patient was rotated away from the AP projection, the sacrum shifts toward the side positioned farther from the imaging table and IR, and the pelvic brim and symphysis shift toward the side positioned closer to the imaging table and IR. If the patient was rotated into an LPO position, the left ischial spine is demonstrated without pelvic brim superimposition, and the median sacral crest and coccyx are not aligned with the symphysis pubis but are rotated toward the patient's right side (see Image 14). If the patient is rotated into an RPO position, the opposite is true—the right ischial spine is demonstrated without pelvic brim superimposition, and the median sacral crest and coccyx are rotated toward the patient's left side (see Image 15).

The first through fifth sacral segments are shown without foreshortening, the sacral foramina demonstrate equal spacing, and the symphysis pubis is not superimposed over any portion of the sacrum.

- When the patient is in a supine position with the legs extended, the lumbar vertebral column demonstrates a lordotic curvature and the sacrum demonstrates a kyphotic curvature (Figure 9-23). To demonstrate the sacrum without foreshortening, a 15-degree

cephalad central ray angulation is used. This angle will align the central ray perpendicular to the long axis of the sacrum and parallel with the L5-S1 intervertebral disk space.

- *Effect of misalignment or mispositioning.* If an AP axial sacral projection was taken with a perpendicular central ray, the first, second, and third sacral segments are foreshortened (see Image 15). If the image was taken with the patient's legs flexed, the lordotic curvature of the lumbar vertebral column is reduced, and the long axis of the sacrum is positioned closer to parallel with the imaging table and IR. For this positioning a 15-degree cephalad angulation causes elongation of the sacrum and superimposition of the symphysis pubis onto the inferior sacral segments (see Image 16). The same elongation results if the patient's legs remain extended and the central ray is angled more than 15 degrees cephalad.

The third sacral segment is at the center of the exposure field. The fifth lumbar vertebra, first through fifth sacral segments, first coccygeal vertebra, symphysis pubis, and sacroiliac joints are included within the collimated field.

- To place the third sacral segment in the center of the exposure field, center the central ray to the patient's midsagittal plane at a level halfway between an imaginary line connecting the ASISs and the superior symphysis pubis (2 inches superior to the superior symphysis pubis). Center the IR to the central ray, and open the longitudinally collimated field to the symphysis pubis. Transverse collimation should be to approximately an 8-inch (20-cm) field size.
- A 10- × 12-inch (24- × 30-cm) IR placed lengthwise should be adequate to include all the required anatomic structures.

Anteroposterior Axial Sacrum Projection Analysis

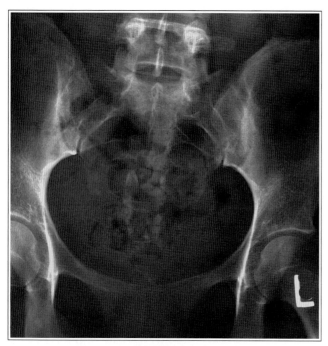

IMAGE 13

Analysis. Fecal material is superimposed over the sacrum, preventing its visualization.

Correction. Have the patient empty the colon of gas and fecal material before the sacrum is imaged.

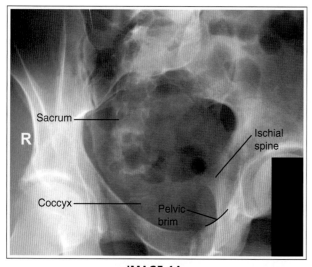

IMAGE 14

Analysis. The left ischial spine is demonstrated without pelvic brim superimposition, and the median sacral crest and coccyx are rotated toward the right hip. The patient was rotated onto the left side (LPO).

Correction. Rotate the patient toward the right hip until the ASISs are positioned at equal distances from the imaging table.

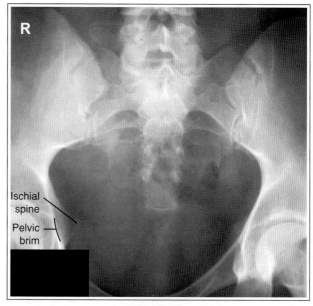

IMAGE 15

Analysis. The right ischial spine is demonstrated without pelvic brim superimposition, and the first, second, and third sacral segments are foreshortened. The patient was rotated onto the right side (RPO), and the central ray was not angled cephalically enough to align it perpendicular to the long axis of the sacrum.

Correction. Rotate the patient toward the left hip until the ASISs are positioned at equal distances from the imaging table and the patient's legs are fully extended and then angle the central ray 15 degrees cephalad.

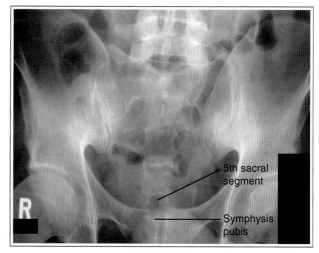

IMAGE 16

Analysis. The sacrum is elongated and the symphysis pubis is superimposed over the fifth sacral segment. Either the central ray was angled too cephalically or the patient's legs were not fully extended and a 15-degree central ray angle was used.

Correction. If the patient's legs were extended, decrease the central ray angulation approximately 5 degrees for every 1 inch (2.5 cm) you wish to move the symphysis pubis. This angulation adjustment is based on a 40-inch (102-cm) source–image receptor distance (SID); if a shorter SID is used, the angle adjustment needs to be increased, and if a longer SID is used, the angle adjustment needs to be decreased. For this patient the angulation should be decreased 5 degrees. If the patient's legs were flexed and a 15-degree central ray angle was used, fully extend the patient's legs and use the same angulation.

SACRUM: LATERAL PROJECTION

See Figure 9-24 and Box 9-7.

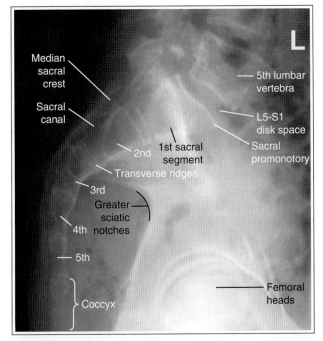

FIGURE 9-24 Lateral sacral projection with accurate positioning.

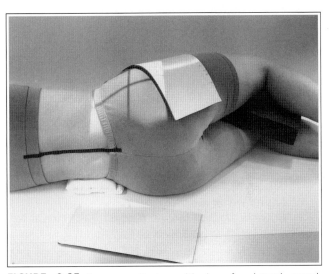

FIGURE 9-25 Proper patient positioning for lateral sacral projection.

BOX 9-7	Lateral Sacral Projection Analysis Criteria

- The median sacral crest is in profile, and the greater sciatic notches and pelvic wings are almost superimposed.
- The L5-S1 disk space is open, the greater sciatic notches are superimposed, and the sacrum is seen without foreshortening.
- The third sacral segment is at the center of the exposure field.
- The fifth lumbar vertebra, first through fifth sacral segments, promontory, and first coccygeal vertebra are included within the collimated field.

The sacrum demonstrates a lateral projection. The median sacral crest is in profile, and the greater sciatic notches and pelvic wings are almost superimposed.

- To obtain a lateral sacral projection, place the patient on the imaging table in a lateral recumbent position. Whether the patient is lying on the right or left side is not significant, although the left side

positioning is easier for the technologist. Flex the patient's knees and hips for support, and position a pillow or sponge between the knees. The thickness of the pillow or sponge should be sufficient to prevent the side of the pelvis situated farther from the IR from rotating anteriorly, without being so thick as to cause this side to rotate posteriorly (Figure 9-25). To avoid vertebral rotation, align the shoulders, posterior ribs, and posterior pelvic wings perpendicular to the imaging table and IR. This is accomplished by resting your extended flat palm against each structure, individually, and then adjusting the patient's rotation until your hand is positioned perpendicular to the imaging table.

- ***Detecting rotation.*** Rotation can be detected on a lateral sacral projection by evaluating the openness of the intervertebral foramen and the superimposition of the greater sciatic notches and femoral heads, when seen. On a nonrotated lateral sacral projection, the intervertebral foramen is open and the greater sciatic notches and femoral heads are superimposed. On rotation, neither the greater sciatic notches nor femoral heads are superimposed but are demonstrated one anterior to the other (see Image 17). Because the two sides of the pelvis are mirror images, it is difficult to determine which side of the patient was rotated anteriorly and which posteriorly on a lateral sacral projection with poor positioning. When rotation has occurred, it is most common for the side of the patient situated farther from the IR to be rotated anteriorly because of the gravitational forward and downward pull on this side's arm and leg, if a sponge is not placed between the patient's knees. When visible, the patient's femoral heads may be used to determine rotation. The femoral head that is projected more inferiorly and demonstrates the greater magnification is the one situated farther from the IR.

The L5-S1 intervertebral disk space is open, the greater sciatic notches are superimposed, and the sacrum is demonstrated without foreshortening.

- To obtain an open L5-S1 intervertebral disk space and superimposed greater sciatic notches and to demonstrate the sacrum without foreshortening, the vertebral column is aligned parallel with the imaging table, the interiliac line is aligned perpendicular to the imaging table, and a perpendicular central ray is used.
- *Detecting lateral lumbar flexion.* If the lateral vertebral column is allowed to flex laterally, causing it to sag or curve upwardly, for a lateral sacral projection, the image will demonstrate the greater sciatic notches without superoinferior alignment and a closed L5-S1 disk space (see Image 18).
- *Adjusting for the sagging vertebral column.* The vertebral column of a patient with wide hips and a narrow waist may sag toward the imaging table at the level of the iliac crest (see Figure 9-12). Two methods may be used to achieve accurate positioning for such a patient:

1. Place a radiolucent sponge between the patient's lateral body surface and the imaging table just superior to the iliac crest to elevate the vertebral column, aligning it parallel with the imaging table (see Figure 9-25), and use a perpendicular central ray.
2. Leave the patient positioned as they are and angle the central ray caudally until it parallels the interiliac line.

- *Adjusting for the upwardly curved vertebral column.* The vertebral column of a patient with a large waist may curve upwardly (see Figure 9-20). For such a patient, angle the central ray cephalically until it parallels the interiliac line.

The third sacral segment is at the center of the exposure field. The fifth lumbar vertebra, first through fifth sacral segments, promontory, and first coccygeal vertebra are included within the collimated field.

- To place the third sacral segment in the center of the exposure field, center a perpendicular central ray to the coronal plane located 3 to 4 inches (7.5 to 10 cm) posterior to the elevated ASIS. Center the IR to the central ray, and open the longitudinal collimation to include the iliac crest and coccyx. Transverse collimation should be to an 8-inch (20-cm) field.
- A 10- × 12-inch (24- × 30-cm) IR placed lengthwise should be adequate to include all the required anatomic structures.
- *Gonadal shielding.* Use gonadal protection shielding on all patients for this procedure (see Figures 9-16 and 9-17).

Lateral Sacrum Projection Analysis

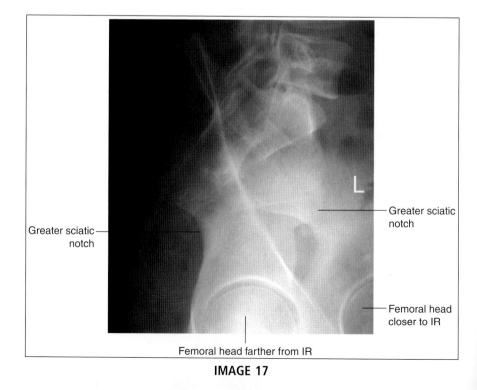

Greater sciatic notch

Greater sciatic notch

Femoral head closer to IR

Femoral head farther from IR

IMAGE 17

Analysis. The L5-S1 intervertebral foramen is obscured, and the greater sciatic notches and the femoral heads are demonstrated without superimposition. The femoral head positioned closer to the IR was rotated anteriorly.

Correction. Rotate the patient's hip that was positioned farther from the IR toward the opposite hip until the posterior ribs and posterior pelvic wings are superimposed. From the original position, the amount of rotation should be approximately 1 inch (2.5 cm).

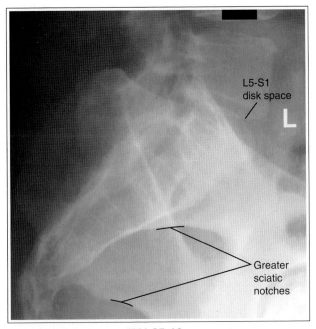

IMAGE 18

COCCYX

COCCYX: ANTEROPOSTERIOR AXIAL PROJECTION

See Figure 9-26 and Box 9-8.

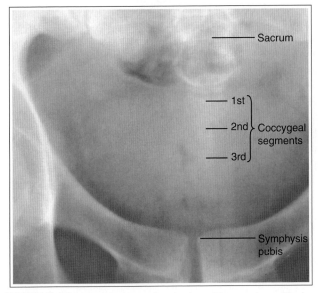

FIGURE 9-26 AP axial coccygeal projection with accurate positioning.

Analysis. The L5-S1 intervertebral disk space is closed, the sacrum is foreshortened, and the greater sciatic notches are demonstrated without superoinferior superimposition. The patient's long axis was not aligned parallel with the imaging table.

Correction. Position the long axis of the lumbar vertebral column and sacrum parallel with the IR. It may be necessary to place a radiolucent sponge between the patient's lateral body surface and imaging table just superior to the iliac crest. The sponge should be just thick enough to align the lumbar column parallel with the imaging table.

BOX 9-8	Anteroposterior Axial Coccygeal Projection Analysis Criteria

- No evidence of urine, gas, or fecal material is superimposed over the coccyx.
- The coccyx is aligned with the symphysis pubis and is at equal distances from the lateral walls of the inlet pelvis.
- The first through third coccygeal vertebrae are seen without foreshortening and without symphysis pubis superimposition.
- The coccyx is at the center of the exposure field.
- The fifth sacral segment, three coccygeal vertebrae, symphysis pubis, and pelvic brim are included within the collimated field.

No evidence suggests that urine, gas, or fecal material is superimposed over the coccyx.

- The patient's urinary bladder should be emptied before the procedure. It is also suggested that the colon be free of gas and fecal material. Both procedures will prevent overlap of these materials onto the coccyx, thereby improving its visualization (see Images 19 and 20).

The coccyx demonstrates an AP projection. The coccyx is aligned with the symphysis pubis and is at equal distances from the lateral walls of the inlet pelvis.

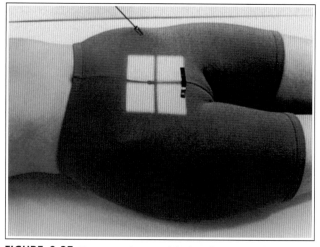

FIGURE 9-27 Proper patient positioning for AP axial coccygeal projection.

The coccyx is at the center of the exposure field. The fifth sacral segment, the three coccygeal vertebrae, the symphysis pubis, and the pelvic brim are included within the collimated field.

- To place the coccyx in the center of the exposure field, center the central ray to the patient's midsagittal plane at a level 2 inches (5 cm) superior to the symphysis pubis. Center the IR to the central ray.
- Open the longitudinal collimation to the symphysis pubis. Transverse collimation should be to approximately a 6-inch (15-cm) field size.
- An 8- × 10-inch (18- × 24-cm) IR placed lengthwise should be adequate to include all the required anatomic structures.

Anteroposterior Axial Coccyx Projection Analysis

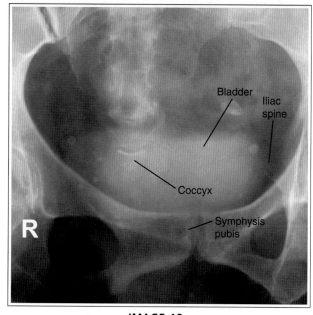

IMAGE 19

Analysis. The urinary bladder is dense and creating a shadow over the coccyx. The coccyx is not aligned with the symphysis pubis but is situated closer to the right lateral wall of the inlet pelvis. The patient did not empty the urinary bladder and was rotated onto the left side (LPO).

Correction. Have the patient empty the urinary bladder, and rotate the patient toward the right side until the ASISs are positioned at equal distances from the imaging table and IR.

- An AP coccygeal projection is obtained by positioning the patient supine on the imaging table with the legs extended. Position the patient's shoulders and ASISs at equal distances from the imaging table to prevent rotation (Figure 9-27).
- *Detecting rotation.* Rotation is detected on an AP coccyx projection by evaluating the alignment of the long axis of the coccyx with the symphysis pubis and by comparing the distances from the coccyx to the lateral walls of the inlet pelvis. If the patient was rotated away from the supine position, the coccyx moves in a direction opposite the direction of the symphysis pubis and is positioned closer to the lateral pelvic wall situated farther from the imaging table and IR. If the patient was rotated into an LPO position, the coccyx is rotated toward the patient's right side (see Image 19). If the patient was rotated into an RPO position, the coccyx is rotated toward the patient's left side.

The first through third coccygeal vertebrae are demonstrated without foreshortening and without symphysis pubis superimposition.

- When the patient is in a supine position with the legs extended, the coccyx curves anteriorly and is located beneath the symphysis pubis. To demonstrate the coccyx without foreshortening and without overlap by the symphysis pubis, a 10-degree caudal central ray angulation is used. This angle aligns the central ray perpendicular to the coccyx and projects the symphysis pubis inferiorly. If the AP projection of the coccyx is taken with a perpendicular central ray, the second and third coccygeal vertebrae are foreshortened and are superimposed by the symphysis pubis (see Image 21).

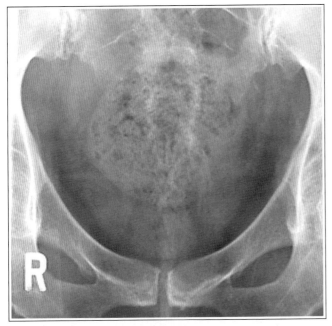

IMAGE 20

Analysis. Fecal material is superimposed over the coccyx, preventing its visualization.

Correction. Have the patient empty the colon of gas and fecal material before the coccyx is imaged.

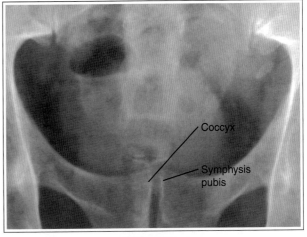

IMAGE 21

Analysis. The symphysis pubis is superimposed over the coccyx, and the second and third coccygeal vertebrae are foreshortened. The central ray was not angled caudally.

Correction. Angle the central ray approximately 5 degrees for every 1 inch (2.5 cm) you wish to move the symphysis pubis. This angulation adjustment is based on a 40-inch (102-cm) SID; if a shorter SID is used, the angle adjustment needs to be increased and, if a longer SID is used, the angle adjustment needs to be decreased. For this patient, the angulation should be angled 10 degrees caudally.

COCCYX: LATERAL PROJECTION

See Figure 9-28 and Box 9-9.

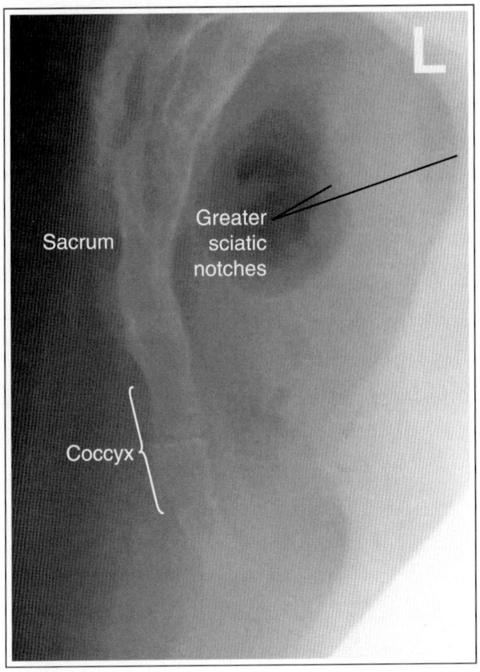

FIGURE 9-28 Lateral coccygeal projection with accurate positioning.

<table>
<tr><td>**BOX 9-9**</td><td>**Lateral Coccygeal Projection Analysis Criteria**</td></tr>
</table>

- The median sacral crest is in profile and greater sciatic notches are superimposed.
- The coccyx is seen without foreshortening
- The coccyx is at the center of the exposure field.
- The fifth sacral segment, first through third coccygeal vertebrae, and inferior median sacral crest are included within the collimated field.

The coccyx demonstrates a lateral projection. The median sacral crest is demonstrated in profile, and the greater sciatic notches are superimposed.

- To obtain a lateral coccyx projection, place the patient on the imaging table in a lateral recumbent position. Whether the patient is lying on the right or left side is not significant, although the left side positioning is easier for the technologist. Flex the patient's knees and hips for support, and position a pillow or sponge between the knees. The thickness of the pillow or sponge should be sufficient to prevent the side of the pelvis situated farther from the IR from rotating anteriorly, without being so thick as to cause this side to rotate posteriorly (Figure 9-29).

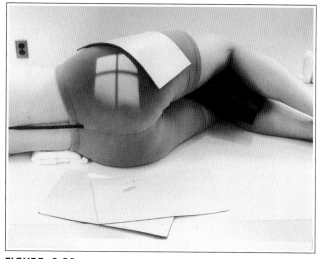

FIGURE 9-29 Proper patient positioning for lateral coccygeal projection.

- To avoid vertebral rotation, align the shoulders, posterior ribs, and posterior pelvic wings perpendicular to the IR. This is accomplished by resting your extended flat palm against each structure, individually, and then adjusting the patient's rotation until your hand is perpendicular to the imaging table and IR.
- *Detecting rotation.* Rotation can be detected on a lateral coccyx projection by evaluating the superimposition of the greater sciatic notches. On a nonrotated lateral coccygeal projection, the greater sciatic notches are superimposed. On rotation the greater sciatic notches are not superimposed but are demonstrated one anterior to the other, and the coccyx and posteriorly situated ischium are almost superimposed on slight rotation and truly superimposed on severe rotation (see Image 22). Because the two sides of the pelvis are mirror images, it is difficult to determine which side of the patient was rotated anteriorly and which posteriorly on a lateral coccygeal projection with poor positioning. When rotation has occurred, it is most common for the side of the patient situated farther from the IR to have been rotated anteriorly, if a sponge was not placed between the patient's knees, because of the gravitational forward and downward pull on this side's arm and leg.

The coccyx is demonstrated without foreshortening.

- To demonstrate the coccyx without foreshortening, the vertebral column is aligned parallel with

the imaging table, the interiliac line is aligned perpendicular to the imaging table, and a perpendicular central ray is used.

- *Adjusting for the sagging vertebral column.* The vertebral column of a patient with wide hips and a narrow waist may sag toward the imaging table at the level of the iliac crest (see Figure 9-12). Two methods may be used to achieve accurate positioning in such a patient:
  1. Place a radiolucent sponge between the patient's lateral body surface and the imaging table just superior to the iliac crest to elevate the vertebral column, aligning it parallel with the imaging table (see Figure 9-25), and use a perpendicular central ray.
  2. Leave the patient positioned as is, and angle the central ray caudally until it parallels the interiliac line.
- *Adjusting for the upwardly curved vertebral column.* The vertebral column of a patient with a large waist may curve upwardly (see Figure 9-20). For such a patient, angle the central ray cephalically until it parallels the interiliac line.

The coccyx is at the center of the exposure field. The fifth sacral segment, first through third coccygeal vertebrae, and inferior median sacral crest are included within the collimated field.

- To place the coccyx in the center of the exposure field, center a perpendicular central ray approximately 3.5 inches (9 cm) posterior and 2 inches (5 cm) inferior to the elevated ASIS to place the coccyx in the center of the collimated field.
- Because tight collimation is essential to obtain optimal recorded detail visibility, collimate longitudinally and transversely to a 4-inch (10-cm) field. The third coccygeal vertebra is situated slightly more anteriorly than the first coccygeal vertebra. With injury, this anterior position may be increased, causing the coccyx to align transversely (see Image 23). When this condition is suspected, transverse collimation should not be too tight.
- An 8- × 10-inch (18- × 24-cm) IR placed lengthwise should be adequate to include all the required anatomic structures.
- *Gonadal shielding.* Use gonadal protection shielding on all patients for this procedure (see Figures 9-15 and 9-16).

Lateral Coccyx Projection Analysis

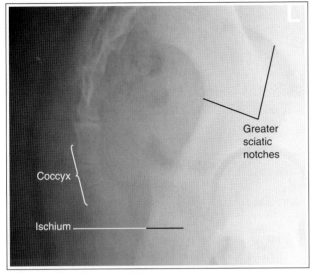

IMAGE 22

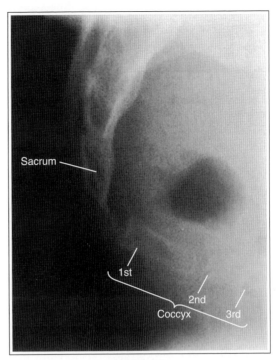

IMAGE 23

Analysis. The greater sciatic notches are demonstrated one anterior to the other, and the ischium is almost superimposed over the third coccygeal segment. The pelvis, sacrum, and coccyx were rotated.

Correction. When rotation has occurred, it is most common for the elevated side of the patient to have been rotated anteriorly. Rotate the elevated pelvic wing posteriorly until the posterior pelvic wings are aligned perpendicular to the IR. It may be necessary to position a sponge or pillow between the patient's knees to help maintain this positioning.

Analysis. The coccyx is aligned transversely and the third coccygeal vertebra is not included within the collimated field. The transversely collimated field was collimated too tightly.

Correction. Open the transversely collimated field enough to include the third coccygeal vertebra.

10

Sternum and Ribs

OBJECTIVES

After completion of this chapter, you should be able to do the following:

- Identify the required anatomy on sternal and rib projections.
- Describe how to properly position the patient, image receptor (IR), and central ray on sternal and rib projections.
- State how to properly mark and display sternal and rib projections.
- List the image analysis requirements for sternal and rib projections with accurate positioning and state how to reposition the patient when less than optimal projections are produced.
- Describe how the patient is positioned to achieve homogeneous density on PA oblique sternal projections.

- Explain why a 30-inch (76 cm) source–image receptor distance (SID) is used on PA oblique sternal projections.
- Define costal breathing, and discuss the advantages of using it for PA oblique sternal projections.
- Describe how thoracic thickness affects how far the sternum is positioned from the vertebral column when the patient is rotated.
- List ways of reducing the amount of scatter radiation that reaches the IR when the sternum is imaged in the lateral projection.
- Discuss when it is appropriate to take an AP projection of the ribs rather than a PA projection and why the AP oblique projection is preferred over the PA oblique projection when the axillary ribs are imaged.

KEY TERMS

breathing technique   costal breathing   homogeneous

STERNUM

The following image analysis criteria are used for all adult and pediatric sternum and rib projections and should be considered when completing the analysis for each projection presented in this chapter (Box 10-1).

- *Visibility of sternum and rib details.* An optimal kVp technique, as shown in Table 10-1, sufficiently penetrates the sternal and rib structures and provides the contrast scale necessary to demonstrate the recorded details. To obtain optimal density, a milliampere seconds (mAs) level is set manually based on the patient's thoracic thickness.

BOX 10-1	Sternum and Ribs Imaging Analysis Criteria

- The facility's identification requirements are visible.
- A right or left marker identifying the correct side of the patient is present on the image and is not superimposed over the anatomy of interest.
- Good radiation protection practices are evident.
- The bony trabecular patterns and cortical outlines of the anatomic structures are sharply defined.
- Sternum: Contrast and density are adequate to demonstrate the bony structures of the sternum.
- Ribs: Contrast and density are adequate to demonstrate the surrounding chest and intra-abdominal soft tissue, cortical outlines of the anterior, posterior, and axillary ribs, and vertebral column.
- Penetration is sufficient to visualize the bony trabecular patterns and cortical outlines of the sternum or ribs.
- No evidence of removal artifacts is present.

STERNUM: POSTEROANTERIOR OBLIQUE PROJECTION (RIGHT ANTERIOR OBLIQUE POSITION)

See Figure 10-1 and Box 10-2.

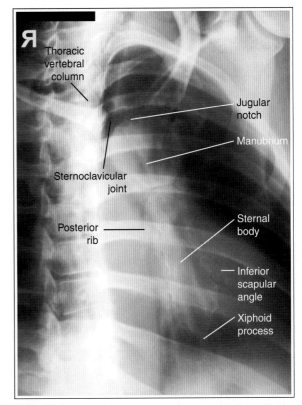

FIGURE 10-1 PA oblique sternum projection (RAO position) with accurate positioning.

BOX 10-2	Posteroanterior Oblique Sternum Projection Analysis Criteria

- The sternum demonstrates homogeneous density.
- The sternum is demonstrated without motion or distortion. Ribs and lung markings are blurred, and the posterior ribs and left scapulae are magnified.
- The manubrium, SC joints, sternal body, and xiphoid process are demonstrated within the heart shadow without vertebral superimposition.
- The midsternum is at the center of the exposure field.
- The jugular notch, SC joints, sternal body, and xiphoid process are included within the collimated field.

SC, Sternoclavicular.

TABLE 10-1	Sternum and Rib Technical Data		
Projection	**kVp**	**Grid**	**SID**
PA oblique, sternum	60–70	Grid	30–40 inches (75–100 cm)
Lateral, sternum	70–75	Grid	72 inches (180 cm)
AP or PA, upper ribs	65–70	Grid	40–48 inches (100–120 cm)
AP or PA, lower ribs	70–75	Grid	40–48 inches (100–120 cm)
PA oblique, upper ribs	70–80	Grid	40–48 inches (100–120 cm)
PA oblique, lower ribs	75–85	Grid	40–48 inches (100–120 cm)

AEC, Automatic exposure control; *kVp,* kilovoltage peak; *SID,* source–image receptor distance.

The sternum demonstrates homogeneous density.

- *Importance of choosing the right AP oblique projection (RAO position).* The right AP oblique projection (RAO position) is used to rotate the sternum from beneath the thoracic vertebrae. It is chosen over the left anterior oblique (LAO) position because the RAO position superimposes the heart shadow over the sternum (see Image 1). Because the air-filled lungs and heart shadow have different densities, they demonstrate distinctly different degrees of density on an image produced using the same exposure factors. The air-filled lungs demonstrate greater image density than the heart shadow. Positioning the sternum in the heart shadow ensures homogeneous density across the entire sternum. Any portion of the sternum positioned outside the heart shadow demonstrates a darker density than the portion positioned within the heart shadow.

The sternum is demonstrated without motion or distortion. The ribs and lung markings are blurred, and the posterior ribs and left scapulae are magnified.

- In the PA oblique projection, the sternum has many overlying structures—the posterior ribs, lung markings, heart shadow, and left inferior scapula. Specific positioning techniques should be followed to show a sharply defined sternum while magnifying and blurring these overlying structures.
- *Blurring overlying sternal structures.* The SID recommended for the PA oblique sternum varies among positioning textbooks. It ranges from 30 inches (76 cm) to 40 inches (100 cm). A short (30-inch) SID provides increased magnification and blurring of the posterior ribs and left scapula but also results in a higher patient entrance skin dosage. Facility protocol dictates the SID. Using a breathing technique, which requires a long exposure time (3 to 4 seconds) and requires the patient to breathe shallowly (costal breathing) during the exposure, forces upward and outward and downward and inward movements of the ribs and lungs, thus blurring the posterior ribs and lung markings on the image. Deep breathing requires movement (elevation) of the sternum to provide deep lung expansion and should be avoided during breathing technique because this sternal motion would blur the sternum on the image (see Image 2).

  If breathing technique is not used, the details and cortical outlines of the posterior ribs, left scapula and lung markings are sharply defined, and the increased recorded detail obscures the details of the sternum (see Image 3).

The manubrium, sternoclavicular (SC) joints, sternal body, and xiphoid process are demonstrated within the heart shadow without vertebral superimposition.

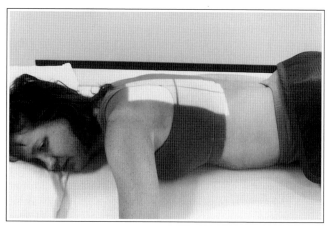

FIGURE 10-2 Proper patient positioning for PA oblique sternum projection (RAO position).

- Rotating the patient until the midcoronal plane is angled 15 to 20 degrees to the IR draws the sternum from beneath the thoracic vertebrae (Figure 10-2). This degree of obliquity provides you with a PA oblique projection of the sternum with only a small amount of rotation. To evaluate an anatomic structure sufficiently, two images of the area of interest, taken 90 degrees from each other, are obtained. The PA oblique (RAO) and lateral projections are obtained to fulfill this requirement for the sternum. Although these are not exactly 90 degrees from each other, it is necessary to rotate the patient slightly for the PA oblique projection to demonstrate the sternum without vertebral superimposition.
- *Determining the required obliquity.* To determine the exact obliquity needed to rotate the sternum away from the thoracic vertebral column on a prone patient, place the fingertips of one hand on the right SC joint and the fingertips of the other hand on the spinous processes of the upper thoracic vertebrae. Rotate the patient until your fingers on the SC joint are positioned just to the left of the fingers on the spinous processes.
- *Evaluating accuracy of obliquity.* When evaluating a PA oblique sternal projection, note that patient obliquity was sufficient when the sternum is located within the heart shadow and the manubrium and right SC joint are shown without vertebral superimposition. If the patient was not adequately rotated, the right SC joint and manubrium are positioned beneath the vertebral column (see Image 4). If patient obliquity was excessive, the sternum is rotated to the left of the heart shadow and the sternum demonstrates excessive transverse foreshortening (see Image 3).

The midsternum is at the center of the exposure field. The jugular notch, SC joints, sternal body, and xiphoid process are included within the collimated field.

- To position the midsternum in the center of the exposure field, align the midsternum to the central ray and midline of the IR (approximately 3 inches to the left of the thoracic spinous processes), and then position the top of the IR approximately 1.5 inches (3.75 cm) superior to the jugular notch and center a perpendicular central ray to the IR.

- *Determining IR size and collimation.* The size of the IR and amount of collimation used for a PA oblique sternum projection depends on the age and gender of the patient. The adult male sternum is approximately 7 inches (18 cm) long, but the female sternum is considerably shorter. A 10- × 12-inch (24- × 30-cm) IR should sufficiently accommodate male and female adult patients. Because chest depth from the thoracic vertebrae to the manubrium is less than from the thoracic vertebrae to the xiphoid process, the manubrium remains closer to the thoracic vertebrae than the xiphoid process when the patient is rotated. The sternum, then, is not aligned with the longitudinal plane but is slightly tilted. Because of this sternal tilt, the transverse collimation should be confined to the thoracic spinous processes and the left inferior angle of the scapula.

Posteroanterior Oblique Sternum Projection Analysis

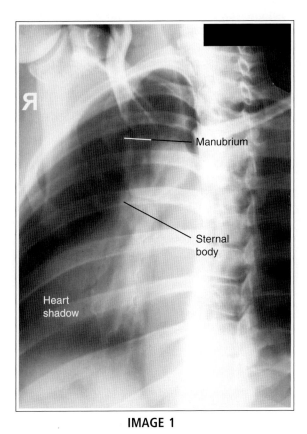

IMAGE 1

Analysis. The patient was positioned in an LAO position. The thoracic vertebrae are superimposed over the heart shadow, and the sternum is demonstrated to the right of the heart shadow.

Correction. Place the patient in an RAO position.

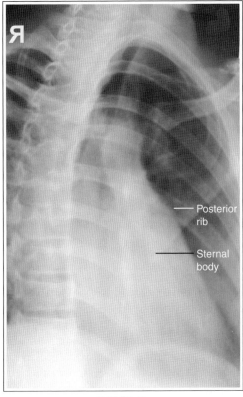

IMAGE 2

Analysis. The right SC joint is sharply defined, but the sternal body, posterior ribs, and lung markings are blurry. Breathing technique was used for this image, but the patient was breathing deeply instead of shallowly, causing the sternum to move and blur.

Correction. Instruct the patient to breathe shallowly.

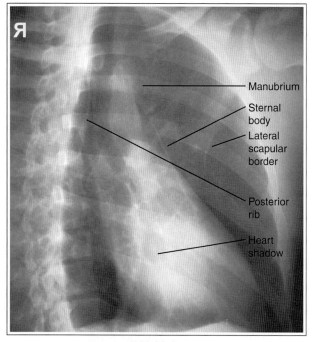

IMAGE 3

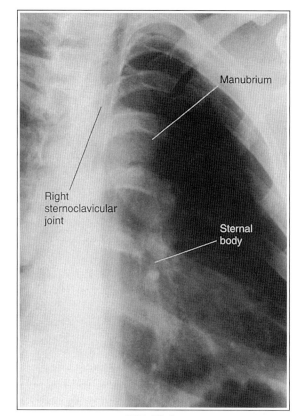

IMAGE 4

Analysis. The lung markings, posterior ribs, and left scapula are demonstrated without magnification or blurring, making it difficult to distinguish the sternum through these overlying structures. The SID was not shortened, and the patient's breathing was halted for this image. Also, patient obliquity was excessive, as indicated by the position of the sternum to the left of the heart shadow and by the amount of sternum rotation.

Correction. Shorten the SID to 30 inches (76 cm) if it is your facility's protocol, take the exposure while the patient is breathing shallowly, and decrease the degree of patient obliquity.

Analysis. The right SC joint and right side of the manubrium are superimposed by the thoracic vertebrae. The patient was not rotated enough to move the entire manubrium from beneath the thoracic vertebrae.

Correction. Increase the patient obliquity. Rotate the patient until the palpable right SC joint is positioned to the left of the thoracic vertebrae.

STERNUM: LATERAL PROJECTION

See Figure 10-3 and Box 10-3.

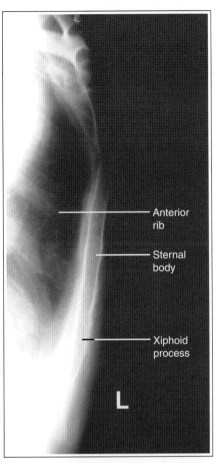

FIGURE 10-3 Lateral sternum projection with accurate positioning.

BOX 10-3	Lateral Sternum Projection Analysis Criteria

- The sternum demonstrates homogeneous density.
- The manubrium, sternal body, and xiphoid process are in profile, and the anterior ribs are not superimposed over the sternum.
- No superimposition of humeral soft tissue over the sternum is present.
- The midsternum is at the center of the exposure field.
- The jugular notch, sternal body, and xiphoid process are included within the collimated field.

Sternum demonstrates homogeneous density.

- Homogeneous density over the entire sternum region is difficult to obtain because the lower sternum is superimposed by the pectoral (chest) muscles or by the female breast tissue, whereas the upper sternum is free of this superimposition. The amount of density difference between the two halves of the sternum depends on the development of the patient's pectoral muscles and the amount of female breast tissue. Enlargement of either tissue

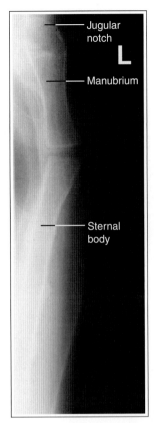

FIGURE 10-4 Superior lateral sternum projection with accurate positioning.

requires an increase in exposure to obtain sufficient density to demonstrate the sternum through them. This increase may overexpose the upper sternum region on the image, requiring an additional image to be taken with a lower exposure so the entire sternum can be demonstrated (Figure 10-4).

- *Reduce scatter radiation.* A remarkable amount of scatter radiation is evident on a lateral sternal projection anterior to the sternum. One can be certain that if scatter is demonstrated here, it is also overlying the image of the sternum, decreasing the overall image contrast. To eliminate some of this scatter radiation and produce a higher contrast image, tightly collimate, use a grid, and place a lead sheet anterior to the sternum close to the patient's skin line (Figure 10-5). For the upright patient the lead sheet may be taped to the upright IR holder.

The sternum and chest demonstrate no rotation, the manubrium, sternal body, and xiphoid process are in profile, and the anterior ribs are not superimposed over the sternum.

- To obtain a lateral sternum projection, place the patient in an upright position with the right or left lateral aspect of the body against the upright IR holder (see Figure 10-5). Avoid chest rotation by aligning the shoulders, posterior ribs, and posterior pelvic wings perpendicular to the IR. This

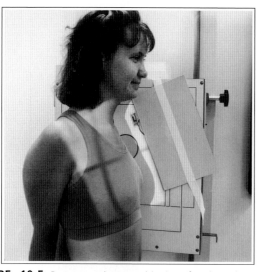

FIGURE 10-5 Proper patient positioning for lateral sternum projection.

alignment, which superimposes each of these posterior body parts on the image, is accomplished by resting your extended flat hand against each structure, individually, and then adjusting the patient's rotation until your hand is perpendicular to the IR. When the thorax is demonstrated without rotation, the sternum is in profile and the anterior ribs are superimposed over each other instead of over or under the sternum.

- *Lateral sternal projection in supine position.* If the patient is unable to be positioned upright, a lateral sternum projection can be obtained with the patient supine. In this position, rest the patient's arms against the sides, position a grid cassette vertically against the patient's arm, and use a horizontal beam. All other positioning and analysis requirements are the same as for an upright image.

- *Detecting rotation and determining how to reposition the rotated patient.* Rotation is effectively detected on a lateral sternum projection by evaluating the degree of anterior rib and sternal superimposition. If a lateral sternum projection demonstrates rotation, the right and left anterior ribs are not superimposed; one side is positioned anterior to the sternum and the other side is positioned posterior to the sternum.

Determine how to reposition after obtaining a rotated lateral sternal projection by using the heart shadow to identify the right and left anterior ribs. Because the heart shadow is located in the left chest cavity and extends anteroinferiorly, outlining the superior border of the heart shadow enables recognition of the left side of the chest. If the left lung and ribs were positioned anterior to the sternum, as shown in Figure 10-6, the outline of the superior heart shadow continues beyond the sternum and into the anteriorly located lung (see Image 5). If the right lung and ribs were positioned

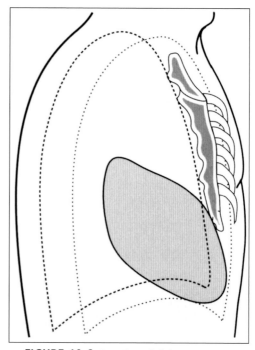

FIGURE 10-6 Rotation—left lung anterior.

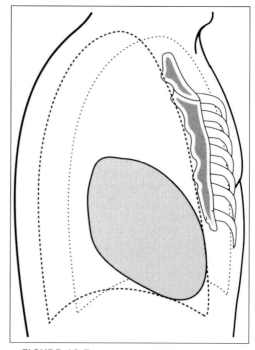

FIGURE 10-7 Rotation—right lung anterior.

anterior to the sternum, as shown in Figure 10-7, the superior heart shadow does not continue into the anteriorly situated lung, but ends at the sternum (see Image 6). Once the right and left sides of the chest have been identified, reposition the patient by rotating the thorax. If the left lung and ribs were anteriorly positioned, rotate the left thorax posteriorly. If the right lung and ribs were anteriorly positioned, rotate the right thorax posteriorly.

- *Respiration.* Elevation of the sternum, resulting from deep suspended inspiration, aids in better sternal demonstration by drawing the sternum away from the anterior ribs.

No superimposition of humeral soft tissue over the sternum is present.

- Extending the patient's arms behind the back with the hands clasped positions the humeral soft tissue away from the sternum.

The midsternum is at the center of the exposure field. The jugular notch, sternal body, and xiphoid process are included within the collimated field.

- To position the midsternum in the center of the exposure field, place the top edge of the IR 1.5 inches (4 cm) above the jugular notch, and then align the image receptor's long axis and a perpendicular central ray to the midsternum. Use the sternal skin surface when determining the location of the midsternum. Do not be thrown off by the vastness of the patient's pectoral muscles or breast tissue; these structures are situated anterior to the sternum and its skin surface.
- A 72-inch (180-cm) SID is used to minimize the sternal magnification that would result because of the long sternum to IR distance.

Lateral Sternum Projection Analysis

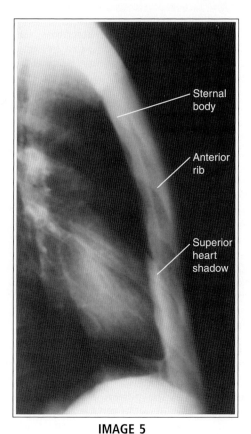

IMAGE 5

Analysis. The anterior ribs are not superimposed, and the sternum is not in profile, indicating that the chest was rotated. The superior heart shadow extends anterior to the sternum and into the anteriorly situated lung, verifying it as the left lung. The patient was positioned with the left thorax rotated anteriorly and the right thorax rotated posteriorly.

Correction. Position the right thorax slightly anteriorly.

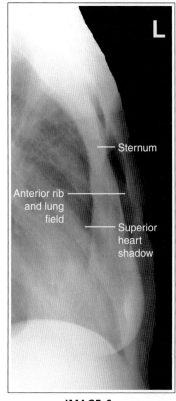

IMAGE 6

Analysis. The anterior ribs are not superimposed and the sternum is not in profile, indicating that the chest was rotated. The superior heart shadow does not extend beyond the sternum, verifying that the right lung is situated anterior to the sternum and the left lung is situated posterior. The patient was positioned with the right thorax rotated anteriorly and the left thorax rotated posteriorly.

Correction. Position the left thorax anteriorly.

RIBS

- *Soft tissue structures of interest.* The demonstration of the soft tissue structures that surround the ribs is very important. When an upper rib fracture is suspected, the surrounding upper thorax, axillary, and neck soft tissues and vascular lung markings are carefully studied for signs (e.g., hematoma, presence of air) that indicate associated lung pathology (e.g., pneumothorax, interstitial emphysema) or rupture of the trachea, bronchus, or aorta. When a lower rib fracture is suspected, the upper abdominal tissue is examined for signs of associated injury to the kidney, liver, spleen, or diaphragm.

- *A rib marker is present when requested by facility.* Many facilities require that the technologist tape a rib marker (lead "BB") on the patient's skin near the area where the ribs are tender. This aids the reviewer in pinpointing the exact location of potential injury.

RIBS: ANTEROPOSTERIOR OR POSTEROANTERIOR PROJECTION (ABOVE OR BELOW DIAPHRAGM)

See Figures 10-8 and 10-9 and Box 10-4.

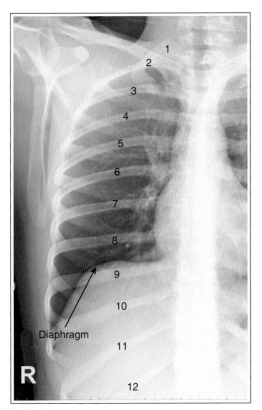

FIGURE 10-8 AP above-diaphragm rib projection with accurate positioning.

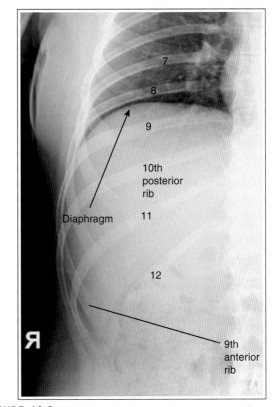

FIGURE 10-9 PA below-diaphragm rib projection with accurate positioning.

BOX 10-4	**Anteroposterior or Posteroanterior Ribs Projection Analysis Criteria**

- Rib magnification is kept to a minimum.
- The thoracic vertebrae–rib head articulations are demonstrated, the sternum and vertebral column are superimposed, and the distances from the vertebral column to the sternal ends of the clavicles, when seen, are equal.

Above diaphragm:
- The scapulae are outside the lung field, and the chin does not obscure the superior ribs.
- Nine posterior ribs are seen above the diaphragm.
- The seventh posterior rib is at the center of the exposure field.
- The affected side's first through ninth ribs and vertebral column are included within the collimated field.

Below diaphragm:
- The eighth through twelfth posterior ribs are demonstrated below the diaphragm.
- The tenth posterior rib is at the center of the exposure field.
- Part of the thoracic and lumbar vertebral column and the eighth through twelfth ribs of the affected side of the patient are included within the collimated field.

Rib magnification is kept to a minimum.

- *AP versus PA projection.* When the patient complains of anterior rib pain, obtain the image in a PA projection to place the anterior ribs closer to the IR. When the posterior ribs are the affected ribs, take the image in an AP projection to place the posterior ribs closer to the IR. Compare the difference in posterior rib detail sharpness in Figures 10-8 and 10-9. Figure 10-8 was obtained in an AP projection and Figure 10-9 in a PA projection. Note how the posterior ribs in Figure 10-9 are magnified, demonstrating less detail sharpness than the posterior ribs in Figure 10-8, which were positioned closer to the IR for the image.

The thorax demonstrates no rotation. The thoracic vertebrae–rib head articulations are demonstrated and the sternum and vertebral column are superimposed. The distances from the vertebral column to the sternal ends of the clavicles, when shown, are equal.

- Thoracic and rib rotation are avoided on the AP projection by flexing the patient's knees and placing the feet flat against the table. The shoulders should also be positioned at equal distances from the imaging table (Figure 10-10).

    For the kyphotic patient, it may be necessary to place a sponge under each shoulder or obtain the image with the patient in an upright position to avoid rotation of the upper thorax. Preventing rotation in the PA projection is slightly more difficult. It is best accomplished by placing the patient's chin on a radiolucent sponge so that he or she can look straight ahead and still be able to breathe, as well as by positioning shoulders and anterosuperior iliac spines (ASISs) at equal distances from the table (Figure 10-11).

    For the patient who has excessive abdominal tissue and has a tendency to roll to one side in the PA projection, it may be necessary to place a radiolucent sponge under the side of the lower abdomen toward which the patient is leaning or to obtain the image with the patient in an upright position to avoid thoracic rotation.

- *Detecting rotation.* Rotation is effectively detected on an AP or PA rib projection by evaluating the sternum and vertebral column superimposition and by comparing the distances between the

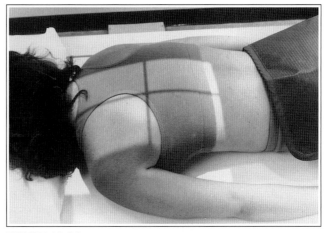

FIGURE 10-11 Proper patient positioning for PA above-diaphragm rib projection.

vertebral column and the sternal ends of the clavicles. When an image of the ribs demonstrates rotation and the patient was in an AP projection, the side of the patient positioned closer to the IR demonstrates the sternum and SC joint without vertebral column superimposition (see Image 7). The opposite is true for a PA projection—the side of the chest positioned farther from the IR demonstrates the sternum and the SC joint without vertebral column superimposition (see Image 8).

- *Rotation versus scoliosis.* In images of patients with spinal scoliosis, the ribs and vertebral column will appear rotated because of the lateral deviation of the vertebrae (see Image 9). Become familiar with this condition to prevent unnecessarily repeated procedures on these patients.

RIBS: ANTEROPOSTERIOR AND POSTEROANTERIOR PROJECTIONS ABOVE DIAPHRAGM

The scapulae are located outside the lung field, and the chin does not obscure the superior ribs.

- For the AP projection, position the scapulae outside the lung field by placing the back of the patient's hands on the hips or under the patient's head and rotating the elbows and shoulders anteriorly.
- For the PA projection, position the scapulae outside the lung field by abducting and internally rotating the patient's arms, forcing the shoulders to rotate anteriorly.
- To avoid rotation, it is best to position the two arms in the same manner, even when only one side of the thorax is being imaged. If the scapula is not drawn away from the lung field, it is demonstrated in the upper ribs (see Image 10).
- Elevate the chin to position it superior to the upper ribs.

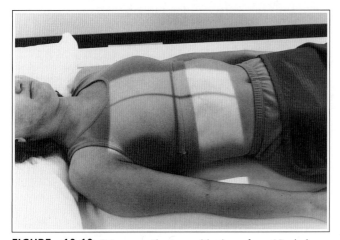

FIGURE 10-10 Proper patient positioning for AP below-diaphragm rib projection.

Nine posterior ribs are demonstrated above the diaphragm, indicating full lung aeration.

- The number of ribs demonstrated above the diaphragm is determined by the depth of patient inspiration. In full inspiration, when the patient is recumbent, approximately nine posterior ribs are demonstrated above the diaphragm. When the patient is in an upright position, 10 or 11 posterior ribs will be demonstrated. If the patient does not fully inhale, the inferior ribs are demonstrated below the diaphragm. Any ribs situated below the diaphragm are not well demonstrated because an increase in exposure would be needed to penetrate the abdominal tissue they surround. To maximize the number of ribs located above the diaphragm, the exposure should be taken with the patient in full inspiration.

The seventh posterior rib is at the center of the exposure field. The affected side's first through ninth ribs and the vertebral column are included within the collimated field.

- In the AP projection, to place the seventh posterior rib at the center of the exposure field, center a perpendicular central ray halfway between the midsagittal plane and the affected lateral rib surface at a level halfway between the jugular notch and the xiphoid process.
- In the PA projection, center a perpendicular central ray halfway between the midsagittal plane and the affected lateral rib surface at the level of the inferior scapular angle. Palpate the scapular angle with the arm next to the patient's body. After accurate centering has been accomplished, abduct the arm to position it out of the collimated field. Abducting the arm shifts the inferior scapular angle laterally and inferiorly, so centering should be accomplished before arm abduction.
- Once the central ray is centered, collimate transversely to the thoracic vertebral column and the patient's lateral skin line. Because above-diaphragm ribs are imaged on inspiration, causing the thorax to expand transversely, perform the transverse collimation with the patient in deep inspiration. Open the longitudinal collimation the full 17-inch (43-cm) IR length.
- A 14- × 17-inch (35- × 43-cm) IR placed lengthwise should be adequate to include all the required anatomic structures.
- *Alternative IR size and centering method when both sides of the ribs are on the same image.* It should be noted that some positioning textbooks suggest that PA or AP above- and below-diaphragm rib images be taken to include both sides of the ribs on the same image. For this positioning, the IR is positioned crosswise and centering is to the midsagittal plane instead of halfway between the midsagittal plane and lateral rib surface.

RIBS: ANTEROPOSTERIOR AND POSTEROANTERIOR PROJECTIONS BELOW DIAPHRAGM

The eighth through twelfth posterior ribs are demonstrated below the diaphragm.

- The number of ribs demonstrated below the diaphragm is determined by the depth of patient inspiration. In full inspiration, up to 10 posterior ribs may be demonstrated above the diaphragm (see Image 11). To maximize demonstration of the lower ribs the exposure should be obtained on expiration. In expiration, only seven or eight posterior ribs are clearly visible above the diaphragm, and four or five ribs are demonstrated below the diaphragm. When below-diaphragm ribs are imaged, it is necessary to use a higher kVp and exposure than needed for above-diaphragm ribs to penetrate the denser abdominal tissue. Any ribs situated above the diaphragm for this image may be too dark to evaluate.

The tenth posterior rib is at the center of the exposure field. A portion of the thoracic and lumbar vertebral column and the eighth through twelfth ribs of the affected side of the patient are included within the collimated field.

- To center the tenth posterior rib in the center of the field and include the eighth through twelfth ribs on the AP and PA below-diaphragm rib projections, place the lower edge of the IR at the level of the iliac crest and center the image receptor's long axis halfway between the midsagittal plane and the affected lateral rib surface. Center a perpendicular central ray to the IR.
- For a hypersthenic patient with a short wide thorax, the centering needs to be positioned slightly higher. Place the lower border of the IR approximately 2 inches (5 cm) above the iliac crest.
- Transversely collimate to the vertebral column and the patient's lateral skin line. Open the longitudinal collimation the full 17-inch (43-cm) field size.
- A 14- × 17-inch (35- × 43-cm) IR placed lengthwise should be adequate to include all the anatomic structures.

Anteroposterior or Posteroanterior Rib Projection Analysis

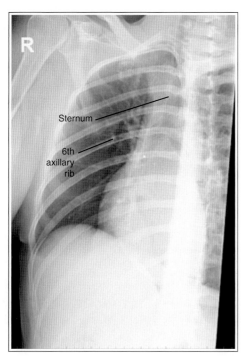

IMAGE 7 AP projection.

Analysis. The sternum is demonstrated to the right of the patient's vertebral column. The patient was rotated. In an AP projection, the sternum is rotated toward the side that was positioned closer to the IR. For this image, the patient was rotated toward the right side.

Correction. Position the patient in an AP projection by flexing his or her knees and placing his or her shoulders at equal distances from the imaging table.

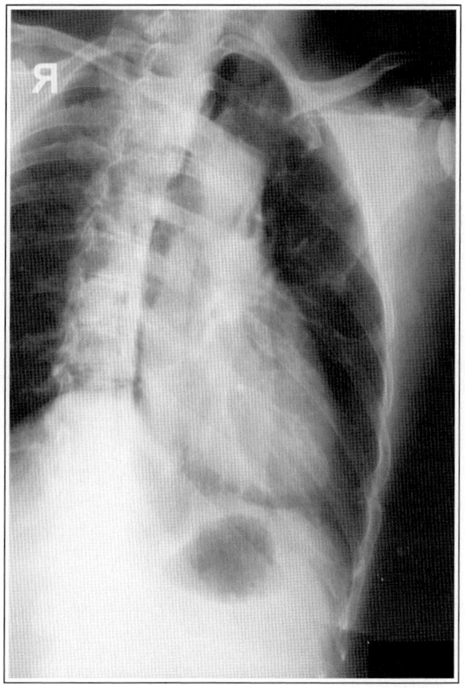

Analysis. The sternum and the SC joints are demonstrated to the left of the patient's vertebral column. The patient was rotated. In a PA projection the sternum and SC joints are rotated toward the side that was positioned farther from the IR. For this image, the patient was rolled toward the right side, away from the left side.

Correction. Position the patient in a PA projection by having the patient look straight ahead, with the chin elevated on a sponge. The shoulders and ASISs should be positioned at equal distances from the imaging table.

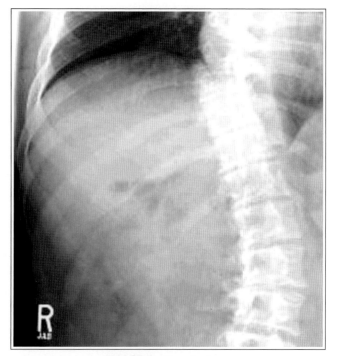

IMAGE 9 AP projection.

Analysis. The distances from the vertebral column to the lateral rib edges down the length of the thoracic region vary, indicating that the patient has spinal scoliosis.

Correction. No corrective movement is required.

IMAGE 8 PA projection.

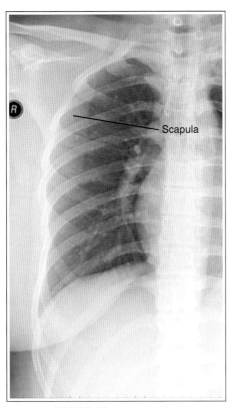

IMAGE 10 AP projection.

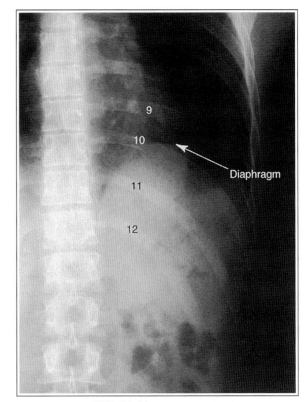

IMAGE 11 PA projection.

Analysis. The left scapula is superimposed over the upper lateral rib field. The left elbow and shoulder were not rotated anteriorly.

Correction. If the patient's condition allows, place the back of the patient's hands on the hips, and rotate the elbows and shoulders anteriorly.

Analysis. For this below-diaphragm rib image, only three posterior ribs are demonstrated below the diaphragm. The image was exposed after the patient had taken a deep breath.

Correction. To demonstrate more posterior ribs below the diaphragm, the image should be exposed after the patient exhales.

RIBS: ANTEROPOSTERIOR OBLIQUE PROJECTION (RIGHT AND LEFT POSTERIOR OBLIQUE POSITIONS)

See Figure 10-12 and Box 10-5.

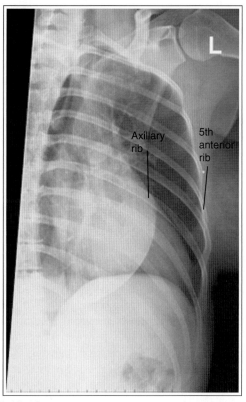

FIGURE 10-12 AP oblique above-diaphragm rib projection (RPO position) with accurate positioning.

BOX 10-5	Anteroposterior Oblique Ribs Projection Analysis Criteria

- Rib magnification is kept to a minimum.
- The inferior sternal body is located halfway between the lateral rib surface and the vertebral column, and the axillary ribs are demonstrated without foreshortening.
- The axillary ribs are demonstrated without superimposition and are located in the center of the collimated field; the anterior ribs are located at the lateral edge.

Above diaphragm:
- Ten axillary ribs are demonstrated above the diaphragm.
- The seventh axillary rib is at the center of the exposure field.
- The first through tenth axillary ribs of the affected side and thoracic vertebral column are included within the collimated field.

Below diaphragm:
- The ninth through twelfth axillary ribs are demonstrated below the diaphragm.
- The tenth axillary rib is at the center of the exposure field.
- Part of the thoracic and lumbar vertebral column and the eighth through twelfth axillary ribs of the affected side of the patient are included within the collimated field.

Rib magnification is kept to a minimum.

- *AP oblique versus PA oblique projections.* Oblique ribs may be performed using AP and PA oblique projections but, to provide maximum axillary rib detail, the AP oblique projection (right posterior oblique [RPO] and left posterior oblique [LPO] positions) should be routinely performed. In the AP oblique projection (Figure 10-13), the axillary ribs are placed closer to the IR than in the PA oblique projection (see Image 12), resulting in less rib magnification and greater recorded detail.

The thorax has been rotated 45 degrees. The inferior sternal body is located halfway between the lateral rib surface and the vertebral column, and the axillary ribs are seen without foreshortening. The axillary ribs are demonstrated without superimposition and are located in the center of the collimated field, and the anterior ribs are located at the lateral edge.

- To open up the curvature of the axillary ribs, rotate the patient toward the affected side until the midcoronal plane is angled 45 degrees with the IR, placing the axillary ribs parallel with the IR (Figures 10-14 and 10-15). If the patient is rotated in the opposite direction, the axillary ribs demonstrate increased foreshortening (see Image 13).
- *Determining accuracy of rotation.* Because the sternum rotates toward the affected axillary ribs

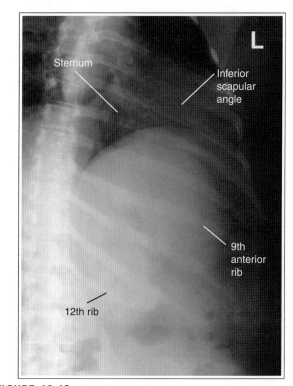

FIGURE 10-13 AP oblique below-diaphragm rib projection (RPO position) with accurate positioning.

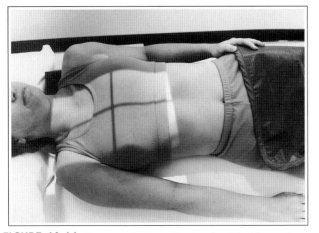

FIGURE 10-14 Proper patient positioning for AP oblique above-diaphragm rib projection (RPO position).

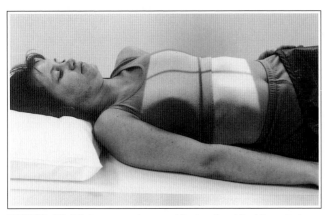

FIGURE 10-15 Proper patient positioning for AP oblique below-diaphragm rib projection (RPO position).

on thoracic rotation, the position of the sternum can be used to identify the accuracy of patient rotation. If the inferior sternum is positioned halfway between the vertebral column and the anterior ribs, the patient was rotated 45 degrees and the axillary ribs are "opened." When the desired 45-degree obliquity has not been obtained, view the position of the inferior sternum to determine how to reposition the patient. If the sternal body is demonstrated next to the vertebral column, the patient was insufficiently rotated (see Image 14). If the inferior sternal body is demonstrated laterally, the patient was rotated more than 45 degrees.

RIBS: ABOVE DIAPHRAGM

Ten axillary ribs are demonstrated above the diaphragm, indicating full lung aeration.

- The number of ribs demonstrated above the diaphragm is determined by the depth of patient

inspiration. In full inspiration, when the patient is recumbent, 10 axillary ribs are usually demonstrated above the diaphragm. When the patient is in an upright position, 10 or 11 axillary ribs are demonstrated. If the patient does not fully inhale, the inferior axillary ribs are positioned below the diaphragm. Any ribs situated below the diaphragm are not well demonstrated because an increase in exposure would be needed to penetrate the abdominal tissue they surround. To maximize the number of ribs located above the diaphragm, take the exposure with the patient in full inspiration.

The seventh axillary rib is at the center of the exposure field. The first through tenth axillary ribs of the affected side and thoracic vertebral column are included within the collimated field.

- For the above-diaphragm AP oblique axillary rib projections (RPO or LPO positions), the seventh posterior rib is placed at the center of the image by centering a perpendicular central ray halfway between the midsagittal plane and the affected lateral rib surface at a level halfway between the jugular notch and the xiphoid process.
- Once the central ray is centered, collimate transversely to the thoracic vertebral column and the patient's lateral skin line. Because above-diaphragm ribs are imaged on inspiration, causing the thorax to expand transversely, perform the transverse collimation with the patient in deep inspiration. Open the longitudinal collimation the full 17-inch (43-cm) IR length.
- A 14- × 17-inch (35- × 43-cm) IR placed lengthwise should be adequate to include all the required anatomic structures.

RIBS: BELOW DIAPHRAGM

The ninth through twelfth axillary ribs are demonstrated below the diaphragm.

- The number of ribs located below the diaphragm is determined by the depth of patient inspiration. In full suspended inspiration, up to 10 axillary ribs may be demonstrated above the diaphragm. In expiration, only seven or eight axillary ribs are clearly visible above the diaphragm, and four or five ribs are demonstrated below the diaphragm. When below-diaphragm ribs are imaged, it is necessary to use a higher kVp and exposure than needed for the above-diaphragm ribs to penetrate the denser abdominal tissue. Any ribs situated above the diaphragm for this image may be too dark to evaluate. To maximize the number of ribs located below the diaphragm, take the exposure on full suspended expiration.

The tenth axillary rib is at the center of the exposure field. A portion of the thoracic and lumbar vertebral column and the eighth through twelfth axillary ribs of the affected side of the patient are included within the collimated field.

- To place the tenth axillary rib in the center of the exposure field for below-diaphragm AP oblique axillary rib projections, place the lower edge of the IR at the level of the iliac crest and center the image receptor's long axis halfway between the midsagittal plane and the affected lateral rib surface. Center a perpendicular central ray to the IR.

    For a hypersthenic patient with a short wide thorax, the centering needs to be positioned slightly higher. Place the lower border of the IR approximately 2 inches (5 cm) above the iliac crest.
- Transversely collimate to the vertebral column and the patient's lateral skin line. Open the longitudinal collimation the full 17-inch (43-cm) field size.
- A 14- × 17-inch (35- × 43-cm) IR placed lengthwise should be adequate to include all the anatomic structures.

Anteroposterior Oblique Rib Projection Analysis

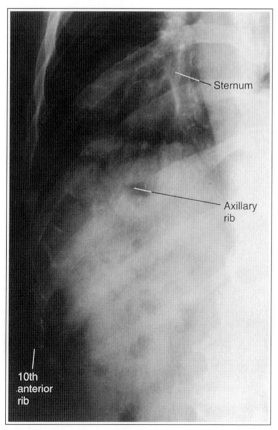

IMAGE 12

Analysis. This is a PA oblique projection of the lower ribs. The sternum demonstrates sharply defined cortical outlines, but the axillary ribs are magnified and demonstrate little definition.

Correction. The axillary ribs would demonstrate greater definition if an AP oblique projection had been taken instead. Replace an RAO position with an LPO position to demonstrate the left axillary ribs. Replace an LAO position with an RPO position to demonstrate the right axillary ribs.

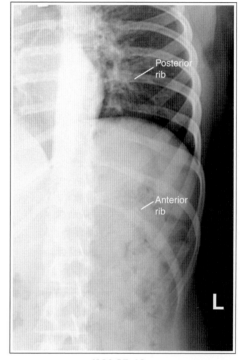

IMAGE 13

Analysis. The axillary ribs demonstrate increased foreshortening and the sternum is rotated away from the affected ribs. The patient was rotated in the wrong direction.

Correction. For AP oblique projections, rotate the patient toward the affected side. For PA oblique projections, rotate the patient away from the affected side.

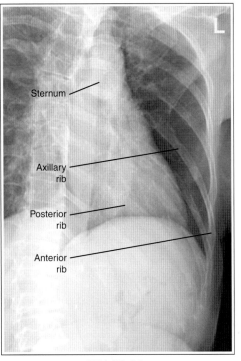

Sternum

Axillary
rib

Posterior
rib

Anterior
rib

IMAGE 14

Analysis. The sternal body is not positioned halfway between the vertebral column and the affected lateral rib surface. The sternum is situated next to the vertebral column. The patient was rotated less than 45 degrees.

Correction. Increase the degree of patient obliquity until the midcoronal plane is angled 45 degrees with the IR.

Cranium

OUTLINE

OBJECTIVES

After completion of this chapter, you should be able to do the following:

- Identify the required anatomy on cranial, facial bone, mandible, and sinus projections.
- Describe how to properly position the patient, image receptor (IR), and central ray on cranial, facial bone, mandible, and sinus projections.
- State how to properly mark and display cranial, facial bone, mandible, and sinus projections.
- List the image analysis requirements for cranial, facial bone, mandible, and sinus projections with accurate positioning and state how to reposition the patient when less than optimal projections are produced.

- State how the central ray is adjusted to obtain accurate cranial positioning when the patient has a suspected cervical injury or is unable to adequately align the head with the IR.
- Define and state the common abbreviations used for the cranial positioning lines.
- Discuss why the parietoacanthial projection (Waters method) is taken with the patient's mouth open.
- Explain how the patient and central ray are positioned to demonstrate accurate air-fluid levels in the sinus cavities.

KEY TERMS

glabelloalveolar line
infraorbital
infraorbitomeatal line

interpupillary line
mentomeatal line
orbitomeatal line

supraorbital

IMAGE ANALYSIS CRITERIA

The following image analysis criteria are used for all adult and pediatric cranium, facial bones, sinuses, and mandible projections and should be considered when completing the analysis for each projection presented in this chapter (Box 11-1).

- *Visibility of details.* An optimal kilovoltage peak (kVp) technique, as shown in Table 11-1, sufficiently penetrates the structures as indicated and provides a contrast scale necessary to visualize the needed details. Use a grid to absorb the scatter radiation, providing a higher-contrast image. To obtain optimal density, set the milliampere-seconds (mAs) level manually based on the patient's part thickness, or choose the appropriate automatic exposure control (AEC) chamber when recommended.

BOX 11-1	**Cranium, Facial Bones, Sinuses, and Mandible Imaging Analysis Criteria**

- The facility's identification requirements are visible.
- A right or left marker identifying the correct side of the patient is present on the image and is not superimposed over the anatomy of interest.
- Good radiation protection practices are evident.
- The bony trabecular patterns and cortical outlines of the cranium, facial bones, sinuses, and petromastoid portion are sharply defined.
- Contrast and density are adequate to demonstrate the air-filled cavities, sinuses, and mastoids, when present, and bony structures of the cranium, facial bones, and mandible, when present.
- Penetration is sufficient to visualize the bony trabecular patterns and cortical outlines.
- No evidence of removal artifacts is present.

CRANIUM AND MANDIBLE: POSTEROANTERIOR OR ANTEROPOSTERIOR PROJECTION

See Figures 11-1, 11-2, and 11-3 and Box 11-2.

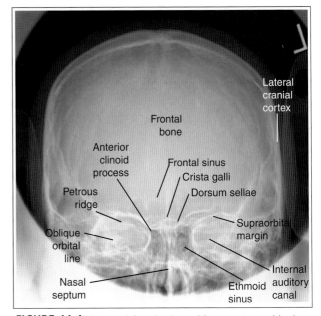

FIGURE 11-1 PA cranial projection with accurate positioning.

The cranium and mandible demonstrate a PA projection. The distances from the lateral margin of orbits to the lateral cranial cortex, from the crista galli to the lateral cranial cortices, and from the mandibular rami to the lateral cervical vertebrae on both sides are equal.

TABLE 11-1	**Cranium, Facial Bones, Sinuses, Mandible, and Petromastoid Portion Technical Data**				
Projection	**Structure**	**kVp**	**Grid**	**AEC Chamber(s)**	**SID**
AP or PA	Cranium	70-80	Grid	Center	40-48 inches (100-120 cm)
	Mandible	70-80	Grid		
PA axial (Caldwell method)	Cranium	70-80	Grid	Center	40-48 inches (100-120 cm)
	Facial bones	70-80	Grid	Center	
	Sinuses	70-80	Grid	Center	
AP axial (Towne method)	Cranium	70-80	Grid	Center	40-48 inches (100-120 cm)
	Mandible	70-80	Grid		
Lateral	Cranium	70-80	Grid	Center	40-48 inches (100-120 cm)
	Facial bones	70-80	Grid	Center	
	Sinuses	50-60	Grid		
	Nasal bones	70-80	Grid		
Submentovertex (Schueller method)	Cranium	70-80	Grid	Center	40-48 inches (100-120 cm)
	Mandible	70-80	Grid	Center	
	Sinuses	70-80	Grid	Center	
	Zygomatic arches	60-70	Nongrid		
Parietoacanthial (Waters method)	Facial bones	70-80	Grid	Center	40-48 inches (100-120 cm)
	Sinuses	70-80	Grid	Center	
Tangential	Nasal bones	50-60	Nongrid		40-48 inches (100-120 cm)

AEC, Automatic exposure control; *kVp,* kilovoltage peak; *SID,* source–image receptor distance.

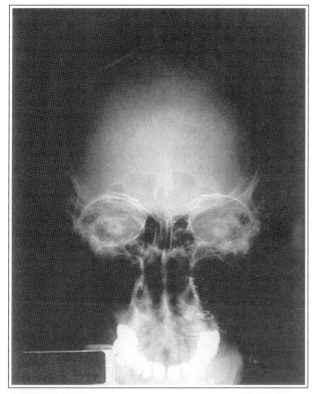

FIGURE 11-2 Trauma AP cranial projection with accurate positioning.

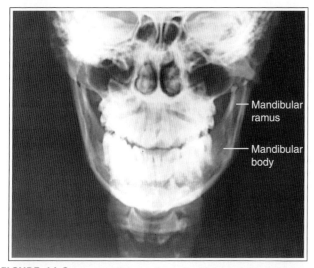

Mandibular ramus

Mandibular body

FIGURE 11-3 PA mandible projection with accurate positioning. *(From Frank ED, Long BW, Smith BJ. Merrill's atlas of radiographic positions and radiologic procedures, vol 2, ed 10, St. Louis, 2005, Elsevier, p. 368).*

BOX 11-2 | **Posteroanterior Cranium and Mandible Projection Analysis Criteria**

- The distances from the lateral margin of orbits to the lateral cranial cortices, from the crista galli to the lateral cranial cortices, and from the mandibular rami to the lateral cervical vertebrae on both sides are equal.
- The anterior clinoids and dorsum sellae are seen superior to the ethmoid sinuses.
- The petrous ridges are superimposed over the supraorbital margins and the internal acoustic meatus and visualized horizontally through the center of the orbits.
- Mandible: The mouth is closed with the teeth together.
- The crista galli and nasal septum are aligned with the long axis of the exposure field, and the supraorbital margins and TMJs are demonstrated on the same horizontal plane.
- Cranium: The dorsum sellae is at the center of the exposure field.
- Cranium: The outer cranial cortex and the maxillary sinuses are included within the collimated field.
- Mandible: A point midway between the mandibular rami is at the center of the exposure field.
- The entire mandibular rami is included within the collimated field.

TMJ, Temporomandibular joint.

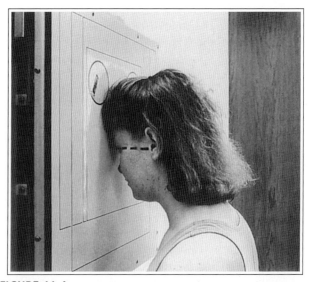

FIGURE 11-4 Proper patient positioning for PA cranial projection.

- A PA projection of the cranium is obtained by positioning the patient in an upright or recumbent prone position with the nose and forehead resting against the upright IR holder or imaging table (Figure 11-4). Positioning the midsagittal plane perpendicular to the IR prevents cranium rotation. The best method of accomplishing this goal is to place an extended flat palm next to each lateral parietal bone. Then adjust the head rotation until your hands are perpendicular to the IR and parallel with each other.

- **Detecting head rotation.** Head rotation is present on a PA projection if the distance from the lateral margins of orbit to the lateral cranial cortices on one side is greater than on the other side, the distance from the crista galli to the lateral cranial margin on one side is greater than on the other side, and the distance from the mandibular rami on one side is greater than on the other side (see Images 1 and 2). The patient's face was rotated away from the side demonstrating the greater distance.

- *AP projection of cranium.* For the AP projection of the cranium, the patient is placed supine on the imaging table. If injury to the cervical vertebrae is suspected, do not adjust the patient's head rotation. Take the image with the head positioned as is. If a cervical vertebral injury is not in question, adjust the patient's head until the midsagittal plane is perpendicular to the IR to prevent rotation. An AP cranium projection, should meet all the requirements listed for the PA cranial projection, although some features of the cranium appear different. The AP projection demonstrates increased orbital magnification and less distance from the oblique orbital line to the lateral cranial cortices than the PA projection. These differences result from greater magnification of the anatomy situated farther from the IR. In the AP projection, the orbits are positioned farther from the IR than the lateral parietal bones, whereas in the PA projection the lateral parietal bones are farther from the IR.

The anterior clinoids and dorsum sellae are demonstrated superior to the ethmoid sinuses. The petrous ridges are superimposed over the supraorbital margins, and the internal acoustic meatus is demonstrated horizontally through the center of the orbits.

- To position the anterior clinoids and dorsum sellae superior to the ethmoid sinuses, lower or tuck the patient's chin toward the chest until the orbitomeatal line (OML) is perpendicular to the IR. This positioning moves the frontal bone inferiorly, until it is parallel with the IR, and the orbits inferiorly, until the supraorbital margins are situated beneath the petrous ridges, and places the petrous pyramids and internal acoustic meatus within the orbits.
- *Adjusting central ray for poor OML alignment.* If the patient is unable to tuck the chin adequately to position the OML perpendicular to the IR, the central ray angle may be adjusted to compensate. Instruct the patient to tuck the chin to place the OML as close as possible to perpendicular to the IR. Then angle the central ray parallel with the patient's OML; this is easily accomplished by aligning the collimator's transverse light line with the patient's OML.
- *Detecting poor OML alignment.* Poor OML alignment can be detected on a PA cranial or mandibular projection by evaluating the relationship of the petrous ridges and supraorbital margin. If the patient's chin was not adequately tucked to bring the OML perpendicular to the IR, the petrous ridges are demonstrated inferior to the supraorbital margins, the internal acoustic meatus are obscured by the infraorbital margins, and the dorsum sellae and anterior clinoids are demonstrated within the ethmoid sinuses (see Images 2 and 3). If the patient's chin was tucked more than needed to

bring the OML perpendicular to the IR, the petrous ridges are demonstrated superior to the supraorbital margins, the internal acoustic meatus are distorted, and the dorsum sellae and anterior clinoids are visualized more clearly superior to the ethmoid sinuses (see Images 4 and 5). When adjusting for poor OML alignment, adjust the patient's head the full distance demonstrated between the petrous ridges and supraorbital margins.

- *Trauma AP projection.* For a trauma AP projection of the cranium or mandible when a cervical vertebrae injury is not in question, adjust the patient's head as described for the PA projection. If a cervical vertebral injury is suspected, do not adjust the patient's head position or greater cervical injury may result. Instead, angle the central ray through the OML, as shown in Figure 11-5. The angulation required varies according to the chin elevation provided by the cervical collar but is most often between 10 and 15 degrees caudad.
- *Correcting the central ray angulation for a trauma AP projection.* For the trauma AP projection, the central ray angulation determines the relationship of the petrous ridges and the supraorbital margins. For a trauma AP skull projection that demonstrates poor supraorbital margin and petrous ridge superimposition, adjust the angulation in the direction in which the orbits are to move. If the petrous ridges are demonstrated inferior to the supraorbital margins, the central ray was angled too cephalically and should be decreased (adjusted caudally; see Images 6 and 7). If the petrous ridges are

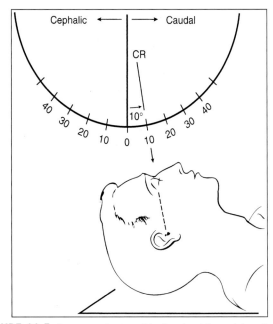

FIGURE 11-5 Proper patient positioning for AP cranial projection. *CR,* Central ray. *(Reproduced with permission from Martensen K. Trauma Skulls [In-Service Reviews in Radiologic Technology, vol 15, no 5], Birmingham, Ala, 1991, Educational Reviews.)*

demonstrated superior to the supraorbital margins, the central ray was not angled cephalically enough and should be increased (see Image 8).

Mandible: **The mouth is closed with the teeth and lips together.**

- The patient's jaw is closed, with teeth and lips placed together to place the mandible in a PA instead of a PA axial projection.
- *Patients who are unable to close jaw.* For patients who are unable to close the jaw for the PA projection, the mandible will be tilted (see Image 7). For a PA projection of the mandible, the central ray should be angled cephalically until it is aligned with the palpable posterior mandibular rami.

The crista galli and nasal septum are aligned with the long axis of the exposure field, and the supraorbital margins and temporomandibular joints (TMJs) are demonstrated on the same horizontal plane.

- Aligning the head's midsagittal plane with the long axis of the IR ensures that the crista galli and nasal septum are aligned with the long axis of the exposure field and the canium and mandible are demonstrated without tilting. Head tilting does not change any anatomic relationships for this position, although severe tilting prevents tight collimation and makes viewing the image slightly more awkward.

Cranium: **The dorsum sellae is centered within the exposure field. The outer cranial cortex and the maxillary sinuses are included within the collimated field.**

- Center a perpendicular central ray to the glabella (area located on the midsagittal plane at the level of the eyebrows) to place the dorsum sellae in the center of the collimated field and include the top of the cranium. Center the IR to the central ray.
- Open the longitudinal and transverse collimation to within 0.5 inch (1.25 cm) of the head skin line, or use a circle diaphragm.
- A 10- × 12-inch (24- × 30-cm) IR placed lengthwise should be adequate to include all the required anatomic structures.

Mandible: **A point midway between the mandibular rami is centered within the exposure field. The entire mandible is included within the collimated field.**

- Center a perpendicular central ray to exit the acanthion (junction of nose and upper lip). Center the IR to the central ray.
- Open the longitudinal collimation to include the patient's orbits and chin, and transversely collimate to within 0.5 inch (1.25 cm) of the lateral skin line or use a circle diaphragm.
- An 8- × 10-inch (18- × 24-cm) IR placed lengthwise should be adequate to include all the required anatomic structures.

Posteroanterior or Anteroposterior Cranium and Mandible Projection Analysis

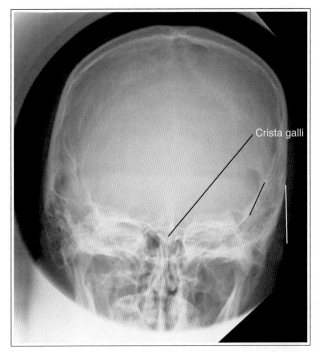

Crista galli

IMAGE 1 PA projection skull.

Analysis. The distances from the lateral orbital margins to the lateral cranial cortices and from the crista galli to the lateral cranial cortex on the right side are greater than the same distances on the left side. The patient's face was rotated toward the left side.

Correction. Rotate the patient's face toward the right side until the midsagittal plane is aligned perpendicular to the IR.

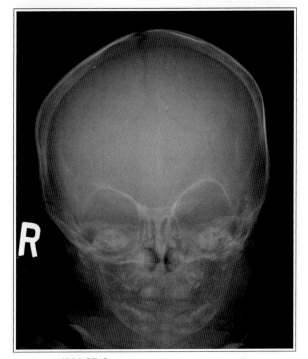

IMAGE 2 Pediatric AP projection skull.

Analysis. The distances from the lateral orbital margins to the lateral cranial cortices on the right side are greater than the same distances on the left side. The patient's face was rotated toward the left side. The petrous ridges are demonstrated inferior to the supraorbital margins. The patient's chin was not tucked enough to position the OML perpendicular to the IR.

Correction. Rotate the patient's face toward the right side until the midsagittal plane is aligned perpendicular to the IR. Tuck the chin until the OML is aligned perpendicular to the IR or adjust the central ray angulation caudally.

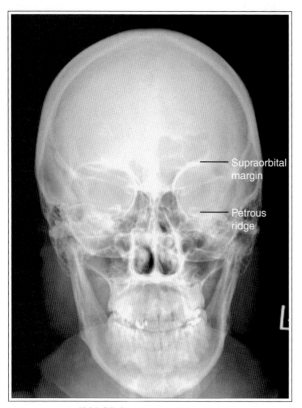

IMAGE 3 PA projection skull.

Analysis. The petrous ridges are demonstrated inferior to the supraorbital margins and the dorsum sellae and anterior clinoids are demonstrated within the ethmoid sinuses. The patient's chin was not tucked enough to position the OML perpendicular to the IR.

Correction. Tuck the chin until the OML is aligned perpendicular to the IR or move it the full distance demonstrated between the petrous ridges and supraorbital margins.

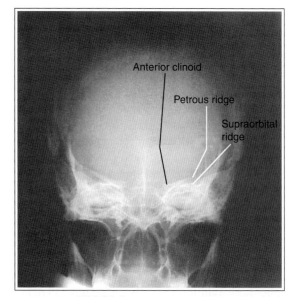

IMAGE 4 PA projection skull.

Analysis. The petrous ridges are demonstrated superior to the supraorbital margins and the internal acoustic meatus are obscured. The patient's chin was tucked more than needed to position the OML perpendicular to the IR.

Correction. Extend the chin, moving it away from the thorax until the OML is aligned perpendicular to the IR or move it the full distance demonstrated between the petrous ridges and supraorbital margins.

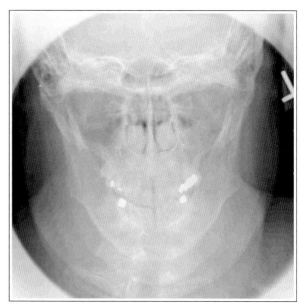

IMAGE 5 PA projection mandible.

Analysis. The petrous ridges are demonstrated superior to the supraorbital margins and the internal acoustic meatus are obscured. The patient's chin was tucked more than needed to position the OML perpendicular to the IR.

Correction. Extend the chin, moving it away from the thorax until the OML is aligned perpendicular to the IR or move it the full distance demonstrated between the petrous ridges and supraorbital margins.

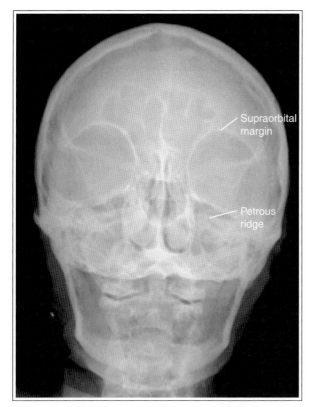

IMAGE 6 Trauma AP projection skull.

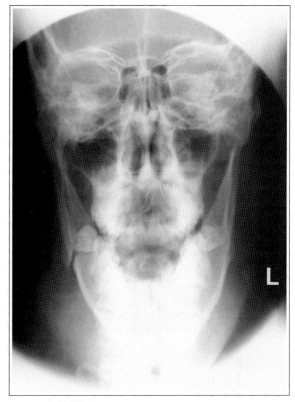

IMAGE 7 Trauma AP projection mandible.

Analysis. The petrous ridges are demonstrated inferior to the supraorbital margins and the dorsum sellae and anterior clinoids are demonstrated within the ethmoid sinuses. The chin was not tucked enough to position the OML perpendicular to the IR or the central ray was angled too cephalically.

Correction. The supraorbital margins need to be moved toward the petrous ridges. To accomplish this, tuck the chin until the OML is aligned perpendicular to the IR or adjust the central ray angulation caudally. The amount of adjustment needed is approximately 5 degrees for every 0.5 inch (1.25 cm) of distance demonstrated between the petrous ridges and the supraorbital margins.

Analysis. The petrous ridges are demonstrated inferior to the supraorbital margins, the dorsum sellae and anterior clinoids are demonstrated within the ethmoid sinuses, and the mandible is elongated. The patient's chin was not tucked enough to position the OML perpendicular to the IR or the central ray was not aligned parallel with the OML. The patient's jaw was not closed because of a fracture.

Correction. If the patient is able, tuck the chin until the OML is perpendicular to the IR and close the patient's mouth. If the patient is unable to move, adjust the central ray angulation caudally until it is aligned parallel with the OML to demonstrate the TMJ area best. To demonstrate the mandible best when the jaw is open in an AP projection, angle the central ray cephalically until it is aligned with the posterior mandibular rami.

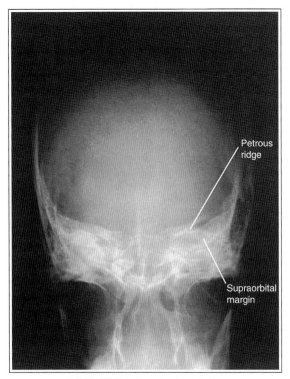

IMAGE 8 AP projection skull.

Analysis. The petrous ridges are demonstrated superior to the supraorbital margins. The chin was tucked more than needed to position the OML perpendicular to the IR or the central ray was not angled cephalically enough to align it parallel with the OML.

Correction. The supraorbital margins need be moved toward the petrous ridges. To accomplish this, elevate the chin until the OML is aligned perpendicular to the IR or adjust the central ray angulation cephalically until it is parallel with the OML.

CRANIUM, FACIAL BONES, AND SINUSES: POSTEROANTERIOR AXIAL PROJECTION (CALDWELL METHOD)

See Figures 11-6 and 11-7 and Box 11-3.

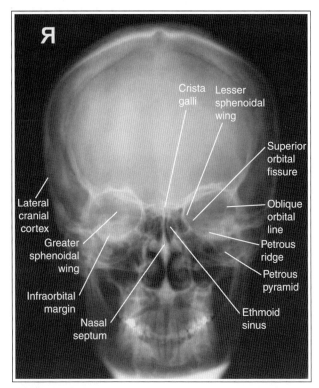

FIGURE 11-6 PA axial cranial projection (Caldwell method) with accurate positioning.

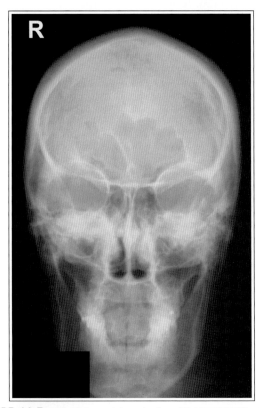

FIGURE 11-7 AP axial cranial projection (Caldwell method) with accurate positioning.

BOX 11-3 | **Posteroanterior Axial Cranium, Facial Bones, and Sinuses Projection Analysis Criteria**

- The distances from the lateral orbital margins to the lateral cranial cortices on both sides and from the crista galli to the lateral cranial cortices on both sides are equal.
- The petrous ridges are demonstrated horizontally through the lower third of the orbits, the petrous pyramids are superimposed over the infraorbital margins, and the superior orbital fissures are seen within the orbits.
- The crista galli and nasal septum are aligned with the long axis of the exposure field, and the supraorbital margins are demonstrated on the same horizontal plane.
- The ethmoid sinuses are at the center of the exposure field.
- Cranium: The outer cranial cortex and ethmoid sinuses are included within the collimated field.
- Facial bones and sinuses: The frontal and ethmoid sinuses and lateral cranial cortices are included within the collimated field.

The cranium is demonstrated without rotation. The distances from the lateral orbital margins to the lateral cranial cortices on both sides and from the crista galli to the lateral cranial cortices on both sides are equal.

- A PA axial projection (Caldwell method) of the cranium is obtained by positioning the patient in an upright or recumbent prone position, with the nose and forehead resting against the upright IR holder or imaging table (Figure 11-8). Position the midsagittal plane perpendicular to the IR to prevent rotation.
- *Detecting rotation.* Head rotation is present on PA axial projection if the distance from the lateral orbital margin to the lateral cranial cortex on

one side is greater than that on the other side and if the distance from the crista galli to the lateral cranial cortex is greater on one side than on the other side (see Image 9). The patient's face was rotated away from the side demonstrating the greater distance.

- *Positioning for AP axial projection.* For the AP axial cranium projection, the patient is placed supine on the imaging table. If a cervical vertebral injury is suspected, do not adjust the patient's head rotation. Take the image with the head positioned as is. If a cervical vertebral injury is not in question, adjust the patient's head until the midsagittal plane is perpendicular to the IR to prevent rotation.
- An AP axial projection should meet all the requirements listed for a PA axial projection, although some features of the cranium appear different. The AP axial projection demonstrates greater orbital magnification and less distance from the oblique orbital lines to the lateral cranial cortices than the PA axial projection. (Compare Figures 11-6 and 11-7.)

The petrous ridges are demonstrated horizontally through the lower third of the orbits, the petrous pyramids are superimposed over the infraorbital margins, and the superior orbital fissures are demonstrated within the orbits.

- Accurate petrous ridge and pyramid placement within the lowest third of the orbits is accomplished when the patient's chin is lowered or tucked toward the chest until the OML is aligned perpendicular to the IR. This positioning moves the frontal bone inferiorly until it is parallel with the IR, it moves the orbits inferiorly until the supraorbital margins are situated beneath the petrous ridges, and it places the pyramids and internal acoustic meatus within the orbits just as they are positioned for a PA cranium projection.

    For the PA axial projection, a 15-degree caudal central ray angulation is then used to align the central ray perpendicular to the frontal and ethmoid sinuses, orbital margins, superior orbital fissures, nasal septum, and anterior nasal spine. This angulation also projects the petrous ridges and pyramids inferiorly onto the lowest third of the orbits.
- *Adjusting the central ray for poor OML alignment.* For a patient who is unable to tuck the chin adequately to position the OML perpendicular to the IR, the central ray angulation may be adjusted to compensate. Instruct the patient to tuck the chin to position the OML as close as possible to perpendicular to the IR. Angle the central ray parallel with the patient's OML; this is easily accomplished by aligning the collimator's transverse light line

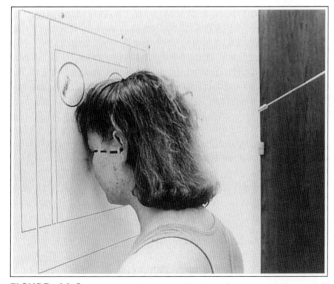

FIGURE 11-8 Proper patient positioning for PA axial cranial projection (Caldwell method).

with the patient's OML. Then adjust the central ray 15 degrees caudally from the angle that resulted when the central ray was parallel with the OML.

- *Detecting poor OML–central ray alignment* Poor OML–central ray alignment can be detected on the image by evaluating the relationship of the petrous ridges and the orbits. If the patient's chin was not adequately tucked to bring the OML perpendicular to the IR, or if the OML was adequately positioned but the central ray was angled more than 15 degrees caudally, the petrous ridges are demonstrated inferior to the infraorbital margins (see Image 10). If the patient's chin was tucked more than needed to bring the OML perpendicular to the IR, or if the OML was adequately positioned but the central ray was angled less than 15 degrees caudally, the petrous ridges and pyramids are demonstrated in the upper half of the orbits (see Image 11).

- *Central ray angulation for a trauma AP axial projection.* For a trauma AP axial projection of the cranium if no possibility of a cervical vertebrae injury exists, adjust the patient's head as described for the PA axial projection. If a cervical vertebrae injury is suspected, do not adjust the patient's head position or increased cervical injury may result. Instead, begin by angling the central ray parallel with the OML, as shown in Figure 11-9. The angulation required to do this varies according to

the chin elevation provided by the cervical collar, but is most often between 10 and 15 degrees caudad. From this angulation, adjust the central ray 15 degrees cephalad (a cephalic angulation is used instead of a caudal angle because the patient is now in an AP projection) to align the angle 15 degrees from the OML, as shown in Figure 11-9. For example, if a 10-degree caudal angle were needed to position the central ray parallel with the OML, a 5-degree cephalic angulation would be required for the AP axial projection, 15 degrees cephalad from the OML.

- *Correcting the central ray angulation for a trauma AP axial projection.* For the trauma AP axial projection, the central ray angulation determines the relationship of the petrous ridges and the orbits. For an AP axial cranial projection that demonstrates a poor petrous ridge and orbital relationship, adjust the central ray angulation in the direction in which you want the orbits to move. If the petrous ridges are demonstrated inferior to the infraorbital margins, the central ray was angled too cephalically and should be decreased. (The petrous ridge and orbital relationship obtained would be similar to that shown in Image 10.) If the petrous ridges are demonstrated in the superior half of the orbits, the central ray was not angled cephalically enough and should be increased. (The petrous ridge and orbital relationship obtained would be similar to that shown in Image 11.)

The crista galli and nasal septum are aligned with the long axis of the exposure field, and the supraorbital margins are demonstrated on the same horizontal plane.

- Aligning the head's midsagittal plane with the long axis of the IR ensures that the patient's cranium is aligned with the long axis of the exposure field and is demonstrated without tilting. Slight tilting does not change any anatomic relationships for this position, although it does prevent tight collimation and makes viewing the image slightly more awkward.

Cranium: **The ethmoid sinuses are centered within the exposure field. The outer cranial cortex and the ethmoid sinuses are included within the collimated field.**

- Centering a 15-degree caudally angled central ray to exit at the nasion (depression at the bridge of the nose) places the ethmoid sinuses in the center of the collimated field. A slightly higher centering may be needed if the entire cranial cortex is required on the image. Center the IR to the central ray.

- Open the longitudinal and transverse collimation to within 0.5 inch (1.25 cm) of the head skin line, or use a circle diaphragm, for an image of the cranium.

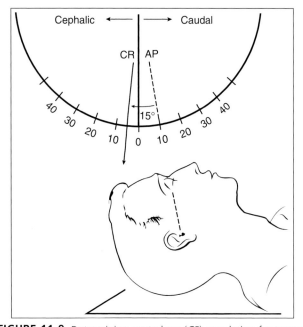

FIGURE 11-9 Determining central ray (*CR*) angulation for trauma AP axial cranial projection (Caldwell method). *(Reproduced with permission from Martensen K: Trauma Skulls [In-Service Reviews in Radiologic Technology, vol 15, no 5], Birmingham, Ala, 1991, Educational Reviews.)*

- An 8- × 10-inch (18- × 24-cm) IR placed lengthwise is sufficient when facial bones and sinuses are imaged.

Facial bones and sinuses: The ethmoid sinuses are centered within the exposure field. The frontal and ethmoid sinuses and the lateral cranial cortices are included within the collimated field.

- Centering a 15-degree caudally angled central ray to exit at the nasion places the ethmoid sinuses in the center of the exposure field. A slightly higher centering may be needed if the entire cranial cortex is required on the image. Center the IR to the central ray.
- Open the longitudinal and transverse collimation to within 1 inch (2.5 cm) of the sinus cavities, or use a circle diaphragm, for an image of the facial bones or sinuses.
- A 10- × 12-inch (24- × 30-cm) IR placed lengthwise should be adequate to include all required anatomic structures when the cranium is imaged.

Posteroanterior Axial Cranium, Facial Bone, and Sinus Projection Analysis

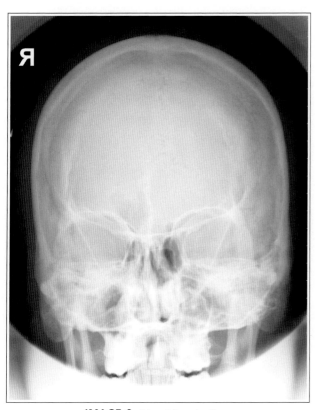

IMAGE 9 PA axial projection.

Analysis. The distances from the lateral orbital margins to the lateral cranial cortices and from the crista galli to the lateral cranial cortex are greater on the left side than on the right side. The patient's face was rotated toward the right side. The petrous ridges are demonstrated inferior to the infraorbital margins. The patient's chin was not tucked enough to position the OML perpendicular to the IR.

Correction. Rotate the patient's face toward the left side and tuck the chin to bring the OML perpendicular to the IR.

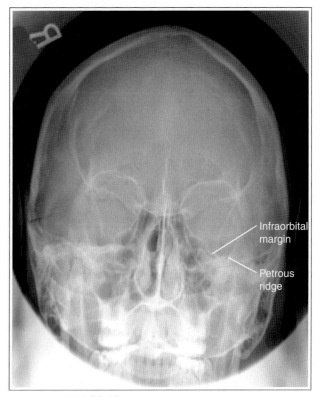

IMAGE 10 Trauma AP axial projection.

Analysis. The petrous ridges are demonstrated inferior to the infraorbital margins. The patient's chin was not tucked enough to position the OML perpendicular to the IR or the central ray was angled too cephalically.

Correction. The infraorbital margins need to be moved toward the petrous ridges. To accomplish this, tuck the chin until the OML is aligned perpendicular to the IR or adjust the central ray angulation caudally. The amount of adjustment needed is approximately 5 degrees for every 0.5 inch (1.25 cm) of distance demonstrated between where the petrous ridges are and where they should be on a PA axial projection with accurate positioning.

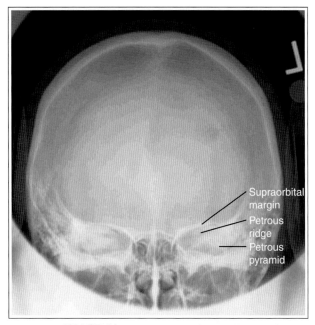

IMAGE 11 Trauma AP axial projection.

Analysis. The petrous ridges and pyramids are demonstrated in the superior half of the orbits. The patient's chin was tucked more than needed to position the OML perpendicular to the IR or the central ray was angled more caudally.

Correction. Elevate the chin until the OML is perpendicular to the IR or adjust the central ray angulation

CRANIUM AND MANDIBLE: ANTEROPOSTERIOR AXIAL PROJECTION (TOWNE METHOD)

See Figures 11-10 and 11-11 and Box 11-4.

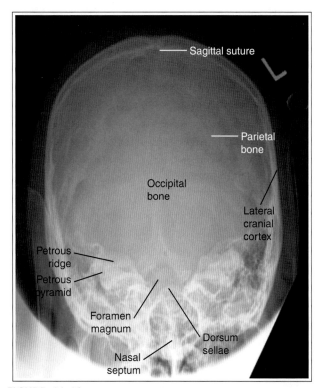

FIGURE 11-10 AP axial cranial and mastoid projection (Towne method) with accurate positioning.

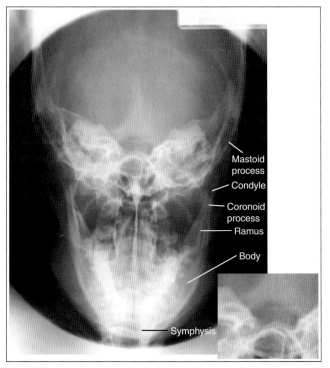

FIGURE 11-11 AP axial mandible projection (Towne method) with accurate positioning.

The cranium is demonstrated without rotation. The distances from the posterior clinoid process to the lateral borders of the foramen magnum on both sides and the mandibular necks to the lateral cervical vertebrae on both sides are equal, the petrous ridges are symmetrical, and the dorsum sellae is centered within the foramen magnum.

BOX 11-4 | **Anteroposterior Axial Cranium and Mandible Projection Analysis Criteria**

- The distances from the posterior clinoid process to the lateral borders of the foramen magnum on both sides and the mandibular necks to the lateral cervical vertebrae on both sides are equal, the petrous ridges are symmetrical, and the dorsum sellae is centered within the foramen magnum.
- Cranium: The dorsum sellae and posterior clinoids are seen within the foramen magnum without foreshortening or superimposition of the atlas's posterior arch.
- Mandible: The dorsum sellae and posterior clinoids are at the level of the superior foramen magnum and the mandibular condyles and fossae are clearly demonstrated, with minimal mastoid superimposition.
- The sagittal suture and nasal septum are aligned with the long axis of the exposure field.
- Cranium: The inferior occipital bone is at the center of the exposure field.
- Cranium: The outer cranial cortex, petrous ridges, dorsum sellae, and foramen magnum are included within the collimated field.
- Mandible: A point midway between the mandibular rami is at the center of the exposure field.
- Mandible: The entire mandible and temporomandibular fossae are included within the collimated field.

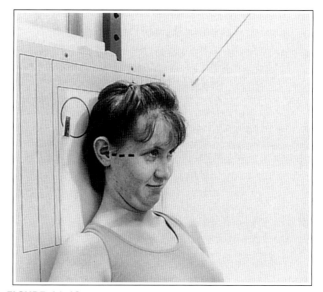

FIGURE 11-12 Proper patient positioning for AP axial cranial projection (Towne method).

Cranium and petromastoid portion: The dorsum sellae and posterior clinoids are demonstrated within the foramen magnum without foreshortening or superimposition of the atlas's posterior arch.

Mandible: The dorsum sellae and posterior clinoids are at the level of the superior foramen magnum. The mandibular condyles and fossae are clearly demonstrated, with minimal mastoid superimposition.

- An AP axial projection (Towne method) of the cranium, petromastoid portion, or mandible is obtained by positioning the patient in an upright AP or supine projection with the posterior head resting against the upright IR holder or imaging table (Figure 11-12). Position the midsagittal plane perpendicular to the IR to prevent cranial rotation. The best method of accomplishing this goal is to place an extended flat palm next to each lateral parietal bone and then to adjust patient head rotation until your hands are perpendicular to the IR and parallel with each other.
- *Detecting head rotation.* Head rotation was present on an AP axial projection if the distance from the posterior clinoid process and dorsum sellae to the lateral border of the foramen magnum is greater on one side and the distance from the mandibular neck to the cervical vertebrae is greater on one side than on the other side. The patient's face was rotated toward the side demonstrating the least distance from the posterior clinoid process and dorsum sellae to the lateral foramen magnum (see Image 12) and from the mandibular neck to the cervical vertebrae.
- *Positioning for trauma.* For a trauma AP axial projection of the cranium and mandible, the patient is positioned supine on the imaging table. If a cervical vertebral injury is suspected, do not adjust the patient's head rotation. Take the image with the head positioned as is. If no possibility of a cervical vertebral injury exists, adjust the patient's head until the midsagittal plane is positioned perpendicular to the IR, to prevent rotation.

- A combination of patient positioning and central ray angulation accurately demonstrates the dorsum sellae and posterior clinoids within the foramen magnum. To accomplish proper patient positioning, tuck the chin until the OML is aligned perpendicular to the IR. This positioning aligns an imaginary line connecting the dorsum sellae and foramen magnum at a 30-degree angle with the IR and the OML.
- *Mandible.* To position the dorsum sellae at the level of the superior foramen magnum and align the central ray with the TMJs, a 35- to 40-degree caudal angulation is used for the AP axial projection of the mandible.
- *Poor OML alignment.* If a patient tucked the chin less than needed to position the OML perpendicular to the IR, the dorsum sellae will be demonstrated superior to the foramen magnum (see Images 13 and 14). If the patient tucked the chin more than needed to align the OML perpendicular to the IR, the dorsum sellae will be foreshortened and will be superimposed over the atlas's posterior arch (see Image 15).
- *Adjusting for poor OML alignment and determining central ray angulation for trauma patients.* In a patient who is unable to tuck the chin adequately to position the OML perpendicular to the IR because of cervical trauma or stiffness, the central ray angulation may be adjusted to compensate. If the patient is able to place the infraorbitomeatal line (IOML)

perpendicular to the IR, use a 37-degree caudal angle. If the patient is unable to tuck until the IOML or OML is perpendicular, instruct the patient to tuck the chin to position the OML as close as possible to perpendicular to the IR. Angle the central ray parallel with the OML (easily accomplished by aligning the collimator's transverse light line with the patient's OML), and then adjust the central ray 30 degrees caudally from the angle obtained when the central ray was parallel with the OML to obtain an AP axial cranium and mastoid projection (Figure 11-13) and 35 to 40 degrees caudally from the angle obtained to obtain an AP axial mandible projection. The angle used for this projection should not exceed 45 degrees or excessive distortion will result.

The sagittal suture and nasal septum are aligned with the long axis of the exposure field.

- Aligning the head's midsagittal plane with the long axis of the collimator's longitudinal light line ensures that the patient's cranium is demonstrated without tilting. Head tilting changes the alignment of the central ray, dorsum sellae, and foramen magnum by positioning the dorsum sellae laterally to the central ray and foramen magnum.

Cranium portion: **The inferior occipital bone is centered within the exposure field. The outer cranial cortex, petrous ridges, dorsum sellae, and foramen magnum are included within the collimated field.**

- Center the central ray to the midsagittal plane at a level 2.5 inches (6 cm) above the glabella. Center the IR to the central ray.

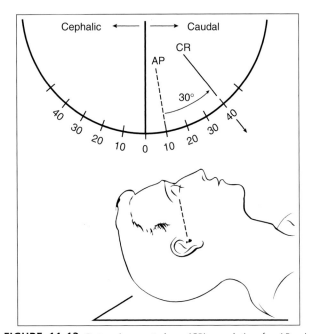

FIGURE 11-13 Determine central ray (CR) angulation for AP axial cranial projection in a trauma patient. *(Reproduced with permission from Martensen K: Trauma Skulls. [In-Service Reviews in Radiologic Technology, vol 15, no 5.] Birmingham, AL: Educational Reviews, 1991.)*

- Open the longitudinally and transversely collimated field to within 0.5 inch (1.25 cm) of the head skin line, or use a circle diaphragm.
- A 10- × 12-inch (24- × 30-cm) IR placed lengthwise should be adequate to include all the required anatomic structures.

Mandible: **A point midway between the mandibular rami is centered within the exposure field. The entire mandible and temporomandibular fossae are included within the collimated field.**

- Center the central ray to the midsagittal plane at the level of the glabella. Center the IR to the central ray.
- Open the longitudinally and transversely collimated field to within 0.5 inch (1.25 cm) of the head skin line, or use a circle diaphragm.
- An 8- × 10-inch (18- × 24-cm) IR placed lengthwise should be adequate to include all the required anatomic structures.

Anteroposterior Axial Cranium, Mandible, and Petromastoid Portion Projection Analysis

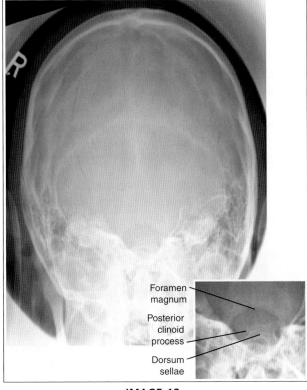

IMAGE 12

Analysis. The distance from the posterior clinoid process to the lateral foramen magnum is less on the patient's left side than on the right side. The patient's face was rotated toward the left side.

Correction. Rotate the patient's face toward the right side until the midsagittal plane is perpendicular to the IR.

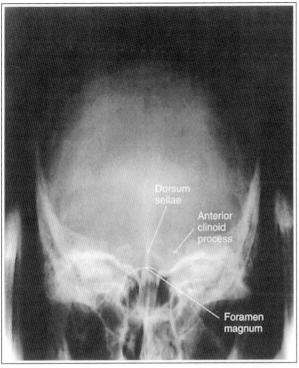

IMAGE 13

Analysis. The dorsum sellae and anterior clinoids are demonstrated superior to the foramen magnum. Either the patient's chin was not tucked enough or the central ray was not angled caudally enough to form a 30-degree angle with the OML.

Correction. Tuck the patient's chin until the OML is perpendicular to the IR. The amount of movement needed is the full distance demonstrated between where the foramen magnum is located and where it should be located on an AP axial projection with accurate positioning. If the patient is unable to tuck the chin any further, leave the patient's chin positioned as is. Angle the central ray caudally approximately 5 degrees for every 0.5 inch (1.25 cm) of distance demonstrated between where the foramen magnum is located on this image and where it should be on an AP axial projection with accurate positioning.

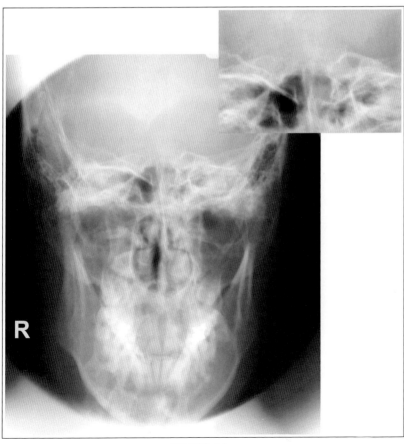

IMAGE 14

Analysis. The dorsum sellae and anterior clinoids are demonstrated superior to the foramen magnum. Either the patient's chin was not tucked enough or the central ray was not angled caudally enough to form a 30-degree angle with the OML.

Correction. Tuck the patient's chin until the OML is perpendicular to the IR. The amount of movement needed is the full distance demonstrated between where the foramen magnum is located and where it should be located on an AP axial projection with accurate positioning. If the patient is unable to tuck the chin any further, leave the patient's chin positioned as is and adjust the central ray angulation caudally.

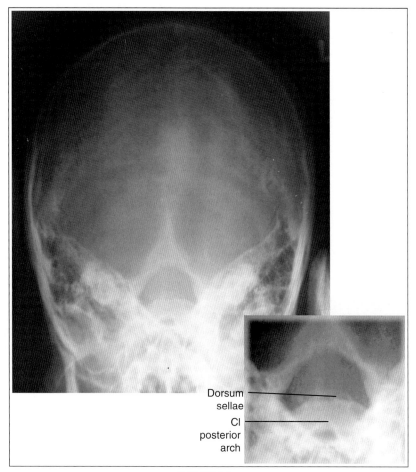

Dorsum
sellae

CI
posterior
arch

IMAGE 15

Analysis. The dorsum sellae is foreshortened and is superimposed over the atlas's posterior arch. Either the patient's chin was tucked more than needed to bring the OML perpendicular to the IR or the central ray was angled more caudally than needed to form a 30-degree angle with the OML.

Correction. Elevate the patient's chin until the OML is perpendicular to the IR. The amount of movement needed is the full distance needed to position the posterior arch inferior to the dorsum sellae. If the patient is unable to tuck the chin any further, angle the central ray cephalically approximately 5 degrees for every 0.5 inch (1.25 cm) of the posterior arch that is demonstrated.

CRANIUM, FACIAL BONES, NASAL BONES, AND SINUSES: LATERAL PROJECTION

See Figures 11-14 through 11-17 and Box 11-5.

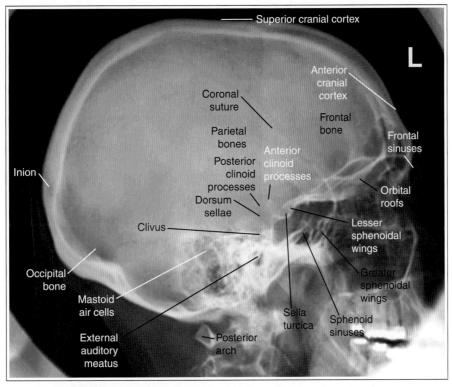

FIGURE 11-14 Lateral cranial projection with accurate positioning.

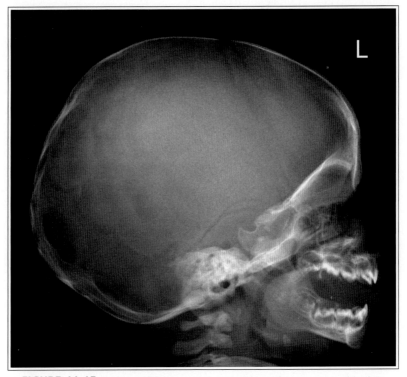

FIGURE 11-15 Pediatric lateral cranial projection with accurate positioning.

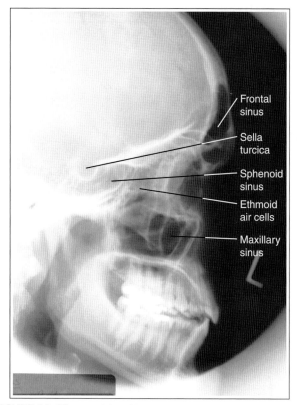

FIGURE 11-16 Lateral facial bone and sinus projection with accurate positioning.

BOX 11-5   **Lateral Cranium, Facial Bones, Nasal Bones, and Sinuses Projection Analysis Criteria**

- When visualized, the sella turcica is seen in profile. The orbital roofs, mandibular rami, greater wings of the sphenoid, external acoustic canals, zygomatic bones, and cranial cortices are superimposed.
- Cranium: The posteroinferior occipital bones and posterior arch of the atlas are free of superimposition.
- Cranium: An area 2 inches (5 cm) superior to the external auditory meatus is at the center of the exposure field.
- Cranium: The outer cranial cortex is included within the collimated field.
- Facial bones and sinuses: The zygoma and greater wings of the sphenoid are at the center of the exposure field.
- Facial bones and sinuses: The frontal, ethmoid, sphenoid, and maxillary sinuses, greater wings of the sphenoid, orbital roofs, sella turcica, zygoma, and mandible are included within the collimated field.
- Nasal bones: The nasal bones are at the center of the exposure field.
- Nasal bones: The nasal bones, with surrounding soft tissue, anterior nasal spine of maxilla, and the most anterior aspects of the cranial cortices, orbital roofs, and zygomatic bones, are included within the collimated field.

The cranium, facial bones, sinuses, and nasal bones are in a lateral projection. When visualized, the sella turcica is demonstrated in profile, and the orbital roofs, mandibular rami, greater wings of the sphenoid, external acoustic canals, zygomatic bones, and cranial cortices are superimposed.

- Achieve a lateral projection of the cranium, facial bones, sinuses, and nasal bones by placing the patient in an upright or recumbent prone PA projection, with the affected side of the head against the upright IR holder or imaging table.
- To demonstrate air-fluid levels within the sinus cavities, this projection should be taken in an upright position. In this position the thick, gelatin-like sinus

fluid settles to the lowest position, creating an air-fluid line that shows the reviewer the amount of fluid present.

- Rotate the patient's head and body as needed to place the head in a lateral position, with the head's midsagittal plane parallel with the IR and the interpupillary line (IPL) perpendicular to the IR (Figure 11-18). It may be necessary to position a sponge beneath the patient's chin or head to help maintain precise positioning.
- *Positioning for trauma.* A trauma lateral cranial projection is accomplished by placing a crosswise IR vertically against the patient's lateral cranium and directing a horizontal beam to a point 2 inches (5 cm) superior to the external acoustic meatus (EAM). For a patient whose head position can be manipulated, elevate the occiput on a radiolucent sponge and adjust the head

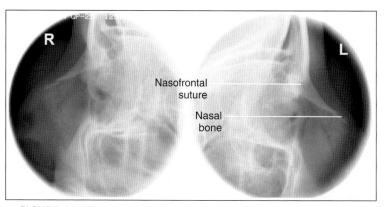

FIGURE 11-17 Lateral nasal bone projection with accurate positioning.

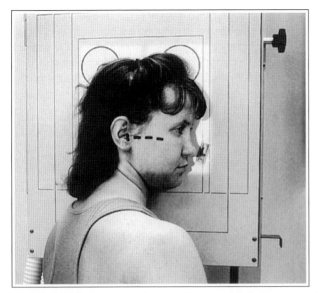

FIGURE 11-18 Proper patient positioning for lateral cranial projection.

until the midsagittal plane is parallel with the IR. If a cervical vertebral injury is suspected, do not adjust the patient's head; take the image with the head positioned as is, and position the IR 1 inch (2.5 cm) below the occipital bone.

- *Detecting head rotation.* Accurate positioning of the head's midsagittal plane is essential to prevent rotation and tilting of the cranium, facial bones, sinuses, and nasal bones. If the patient's head was not adequately turned to position the midsagittal plane parallel with the IR, rotation results. Rotation causes distortion of the sella turcica and situates one of the mandibular rami, greater wings of the sphenoid, external acoustic canals, zygomatic bones, and anterior cranial cortices anterior to the other on a lateral projection (see Image 16). Because the two sides of the cranium are mirror images, it is very difficult to determine which way the face was rotated when studying lateral projections with poor positioning. Paying close attention to initial positioning may give you an idea as to which way the patient has a tendency to lean. Routinely, patients tend to rotate their faces and lean the tops of their heads toward the IR.

- *Detecting head tilting.* If the patient's head was tilted toward or away from the IR, preventing the midsagittal plane from aligning parallel with the IR or the IPL from aligning perpendicular to the IR, tilting of the cranium, facial bones, sinuses, and nasal bones results. Tilting can be distinguished from rotation on lateral projections by studying the superimposition of the orbital roofs, the greater wings of the sphenoid, the external acoustic canals, the zygomatic bones, and the inferior cranial cortices. If the patient's head was tilted, one of each corresponding structure is demonstrated superior

to the other. The direction of the head tilt, toward or away from the IR, can be determined by evaluating the degree of atlas (C1) vertebral foramen visualization. If the top of the head is tilted toward the IR, the foramen will not be visualized and, if the tip of the head is tilted away from the IR, the foramen will be seen (see Image 17).

Cranium: **The posteroinferior occipital bone and posterior arch of the atlas are free of superimposition.**

- Adjusting the chin to bring the IOML perpendicular to the front edge of the IR positions the posteroinferior cranium superior to the posterior arch of the atlas, preventing their superimposition.

Cranium: **An area 2 inches (5 cm) superior to the EAM is centered within the exposure field. The outer cranial cortex is included within the collimated field.**

- Centering a perpendicular central ray to a point 2 inches (5 cm) superior to the EAM positions the cranium in the center of the exposure field.
- Open the longitudinally and transversely collimated field to within 0.5 inch (1.25 cm) of the patient's head skin line, or use a circle diaphragm.
- A 10- × 12-inch (24- × 30-cm) IR placed crosswise should be adequate to include all the required anatomic structures.

Facial bones and sinuses: **The zygoma and greater wings of the sphenoid are centered within the exposure field. Included within the field are the frontal, ethmoid, sphenoid, and maxillary sinuses, greater wings of the sphenoid, orbital roofs, sella turcica, zygoma, and mandible.**

- Centering a perpendicular central ray to the zygoma (midway between the outer canthus and EAM) positions the zygoma and greater wings of the sphenoid in the center of the exposure field. Center the IR to the central ray.
- Open the longitudinally and transversely collimated field to include the mandible and frontal sinuses and transversely collimate to within 0.5 inch (1.25 cm) of the anterior skin line or use a circle diaphragm.
- An 8- × 10-inch (18- × 24-cm) IR placed lengthwise should be adequate to include all the required anatomic structures.

Nasal bones: **The nasal bones are centered within the exposure field. Included within the collimated field are the nasal bones with surrounding soft tissue, anterior nasal spine of maxilla, and the most anterior aspects of the cranial cortices, orbital roofs, and zygomatic bones.**

- Center a perpendicular central ray 0.5 inch (1.25 cm) inferior to the nasion to center the nasal bones to the center of the exposure field. Center the IR to the central ray.

- Open the longitudinal field to include the frontal sinuses and transversely collimated field to within 0.5 inch (1.25 cm) of the nose skin line or use a small circle diaphragm.
- An 8- × 10-inch (18- × 24-cm) IR placed lengthwise should be adequate to include all the required anatomic structures. A small focal spot will increase detail sharpness. Both right and left lateral projections of the nasal bones are routinely requested.

Lateral Cranium, Facial Bone, Sinus, and Nasal Bone Projection Analysis

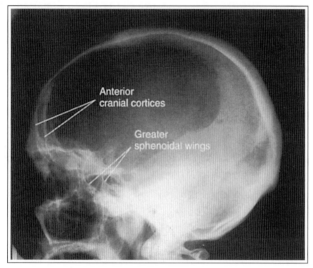

IMAGE 16

Analysis. The greater wings of the sphenoid and the anterior cranial cortices are demonstrated without superimposition. One of each corresponding structure is demonstrated anterior to the other. The patient's head was rotated.

Correction. Position the cranium's midsagittal plane parallel with the IR.

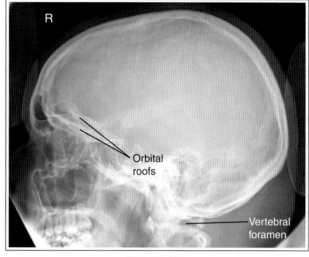

IMAGE 17

Analysis. The orbital roofs, the EAM, and the inferior cranial cortices are demonstrated without superimposition. One of each corresponding structure is demonstrated superior to the other and the atlas vertebral foramen is visualized. The patient's head was tilted away from the IR.

Correction. Tilt the top of the head toward the IR until the cranium's midsagittal plane is parallel with the IR and the IPL is perpendicular to the IR.

CRANIUM, MANDIBLE, AND SINUSES: SUBMENTOVERTEX PROJECTION (SCHUELLER METHOD)

See Figures 11-19 and 11-20 and Box 11-6.

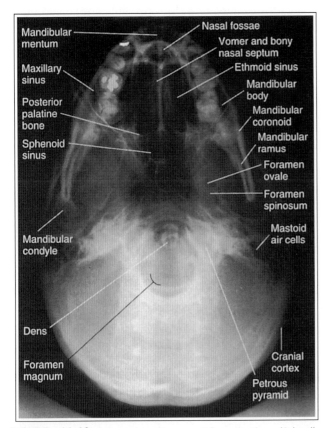

FIGURE **11-19** Submentovertex cranial projection (Schueller method) with accurate positioning.

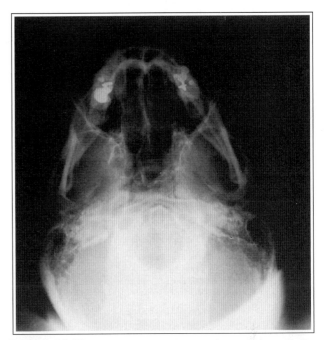

FIGURE **11-20** Submentovertex sinus and mandible projection (Schueller method) with accurate positioning.

BOX 11-6	Submentovertex Cranium, Mandible, and Sinuses Projection Analysis Criteria

- The mandibular mentum and nasal fossae are demonstrated just anterior to the ethmoid sinuses.
- The distances from the mandibular ramus and body to the lateral cranial cortex on both sides are equal.
- The vomer, bony nasal septum, and dens are aligned with the long axis of the exposure field.
- Cranium: The dens is at the center of the exposure field.
- Cranium: The mandible and the outer cranial cortices are included within the collimated field.
- Sinuses and mandible: The sphenoid sinuses are at the center of the exposure field.
- The mandible, lateral cranial cortices, and mastoid air cells are included within the collimated field.

The mandibular mentum and nasal fossae are demonstrated just anterior to the ethmoid sinuses.

- The submentovertex (SMV) projection (Schueller method) is accomplished by placing the patient in an upright AP projection, with the cranial vertex resting against the upright IR holder or imaging table. Continue to elevate the chin and hyperextend the patient's neck until the IOML is parallel to the upright IR holder or imaging table (Figure 11-21). For a patient with a retracted jaw, it may be necessary to raise the chin and extend the patient's neck beyond the IOML to position the mandibular mentum anterior to the frontal bone.
- If the patient is unable to align the IOML parallel with the imaging table, extend the patient's neck as far as possible and angle the central ray cephalad until it is aligned perpendicular to the IOML.
- *Effect of mispositioning IOML.* Mispositioning of the mandibular mentum and ethmoid sinuses on an SMV projection obscures the nasal fossae and

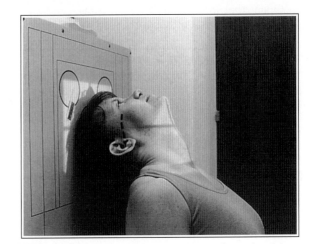

FIGURE **11-21** Proper patient positioning for submentovertex cranial projection (Schueller method).

ethmoid sinuses. If the patient's neck was overextended, the mandibular mentum is demonstrated too far anterior to the ethmoid sinuses (see Image 18). If the patient's neck was underextended, the mandibular mentum is demonstrated posterior to the ethmoid sinuses (see Image 19).

The distances from the mandibular ramus and body to the lateral cranial cortex on both sides are equal.

- Positioning the cranium's midsagittal plane perpendicular to the IR prevents cranial tilting.
- *Detecting head tilting.* Cranial tilting can be identified on an SMV projection of the head by comparing the distances from the mandibular ramus and body with the distance to the corresponding lateral cranial cortex on either side. If the head was not tilted, the distances are equal. If the head was tilted, the distance is greater on the side toward which the cranial vertex was tilted (see Image 20).

The vomer, bony nasal septum, and dens are aligned with the long axis of the exposure field.

- Turning the patient's face until the midsagittal plane is aligned with the long axis of the collimator's longitudinal light line ensures that the patient's head is not rotated and that the vomer, bony nasal septum, and dens are aligned with the long axis of the exposure field. Rotation does not change any anatomic relationships for this position, although it does prevent tight collimation and makes viewing of the image slightly more awkward.

Cranium: **The dens is centered within the exposure field. The mandible and the outer cranial cortices are included within the collimated field.**

- Centering a perpendicular central ray to the midsagittal plane (midway between the mandibular angles) 0.75 inch (2 cm) anterior to the level of the EAM places the dens in the center of the exposure field. Center the IR to the central ray.
- Open the longitudinally and transversely collimated field to within 0.5 inch (1.25 cm) of the patient's lateral head skin line and mandibular mentum, or use a circle diaphragm.
- A 10- × 12-inch (24- × 30-cm) IR placed lengthwise should be adequate to include all the required anatomic structures.

Sinuses and mandible: **The sphenoid sinuses are centered within the exposure field. The mandible, lateral cranial cortices, and mastoid air cells are included within the collimated field.**

- Centering a perpendicular central ray to the midsagittal plane at a level 1.5 to 2 inches (4 to 5 cm) inferior to the mandibular symphysis places the ethmoid sinuses in the center of the exposure field.
- Open the longitudinally and transversely collimated field to within 0.5 inch (1.25 cm) of the patient's lateral head skin line and mandibular symphysis, or use a circle diaphragm.
- An 8- × 10-inch (18- × 24-cm) IR placed lengthwise should be adequate to include all the required anatomic structures.

Submentovertex Cranium, Sinus, and Mandible Projection Analysis

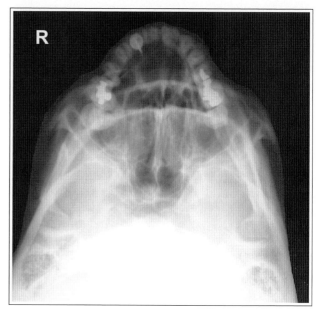

IMAGE 18

Analysis. The mandibular mentum is demonstrated too far anterior to the ethmoid sinuses. The patient's neck was overextended, preventing the IOML from being positioned parallel with the IR. If the central ray was angled to accomplish this image, it was angled too cephalically.

Correction. Depress the patient's chin until the IOML is aligned parallel with the IR. The amount of movement needed is half the distance demonstrated between the mandibular mentum and the ethmoid sinuses. If the central ray was angled, adjust the angulation caudally until it is perpendicular to the IOML.

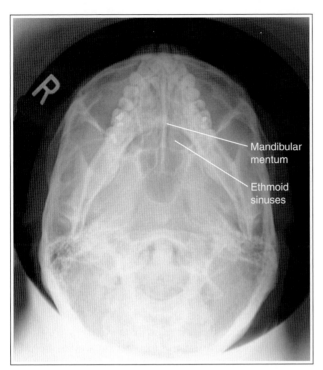

IMAGE 19

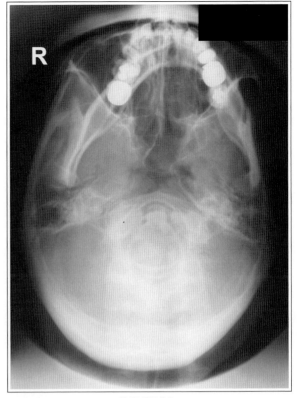

IMAGE 20

Analysis. The mandibular mentum is demonstrated posterior to the ethmoid sinuses. The patient's neck was underextended, preventing the IOML from being positioned parallel with the IR.

Correction. Elevate the patient's chin until the IOML is aligned parallel with the IR. The amount of movement needed is half the distance demonstrated between the mandibular mentum and the ethmoid sinuses. If the patient is unable to elevate the chin or hyperextend the neck any further, leave the position as is and angle the central ray cephalad until it is perpendicular to the IOML.

Analysis. The distance from the right mandibular ramus and body to its corresponding lateral cranial cortex is greater than the distance from the left mandibular ramus and body to its corresponding lateral cranial cortex. The patient's cranial vertex was tilted toward the right side. The mandibular mentum is demonstrated posterior to the ethmoid sinuses. The patient's neck was underextended, preventing the IOML from being positioned parallel with the IR.

Correction. Tilt the patient's cranial vertex toward the left side until the cranium's midsagittal plane is perpendicular to the IR and elevate the patient's chin until the IOML is aligned parallel with the IR.

FACIAL BONES AND SINUSES: PARIETOACANTHIAL AND ACANTHIOPARIETAL PROJECTION (WATERS AND OPEN-MOUTH METHODS)

See Figure 11-22 and Box 11-7.

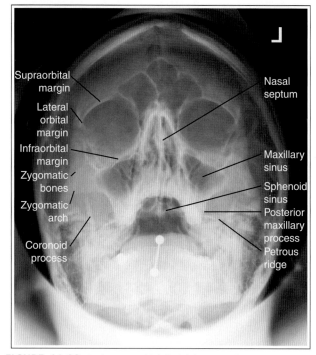

FIGURE 11-22 Parietoacanthial facial bone and sinus projection (Waters method) with accurate positioning.

Labels: Supraorbital margin, Lateral orbital margin, Infraorbital margin, Zygomatic bones, Zygomatic arch, Coronoid process, Nasal septum, Maxillary sinus, Sphenoid sinus, Posterior maxillary process, Petrous ridge

BOX 11-7	**Parietoacanthial and Acanthioparietal Projection Analysis Criteria**

- The distances from the lateral orbital margin to the lateral cranial cortex and the distance from the bony nasal septum to the lateral cranial cortex on both sides are equal.
- The petrous ridges are demonstrated inferior to the maxillary sinuses and extend laterally from the posterior maxillary alveolar process.
- The bony nasal septum is aligned with the long axis of the exposure field, and the infraorbital margins are demonstrated on the same horizontal plane.
- The anterior nasal spine is at the center of the exposure field.
- The frontal and maxillary sinuses and lateral cranial cortices are included within the collimated field.

The cranium is demonstrated without rotation. The distances from the lateral orbital margin to the lateral cranial cortex and the distance from the bony nasal septum to the lateral cranial cortex on both sides are equal.

- The parietoacanthial cranium projection (Waters method) is obtained by positioning the patient in an upright or recumbent prone position, with the

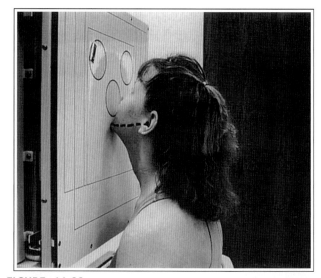

FIGURE 11-23 Proper patient positioning for parietoacanthial facial bone and sinus projection (Waters method).

neck extended and the chin resting against the upright IR holder or imaging table (Figure 11-23).

- To demonstrate air-fluid levels within the maxillary sinus cavities, this projection should be taken with the patient in an upright position. The thick gelatin-like sinus fluid then settles to the lowest level in the sinus cavity, creating an air-fluid line that shows the reviewer the amount of fluid present.
- To prevent cranial rotation, position an extended flat palm next to each lateral parietal bone. Then adjust the head rotation until your hands are perpendicular to the IR and parallel with each other.
- *Detecting head rotation.* Head rotation is present on a parietoacanthial projection if the distance from the lateral orbital margin to the lateral cranial cortex on one side is greater than on the other side and if the distance from the bony nasal septum to the lateral cranial cortex on one side is greater than on the other side (see Image 21). The patient's face was rotated away from the side demonstrating the greater distance.
- *Positioning for trauma acanthioparietal (Waters) projection.* For the trauma acanthioparietal cranium projection, the patient is supine on the imaging table. If a cervical vertebral injury is suspected, do not adjust the patient's head rotation, but take the image with the head positioned as is. If a cervical vertebral injury is not in question, adjust the patient's head to prevent rotation. An acanthioparietal projection should meet all the requirements listed for a parietoacanthial projection, although some features of the cranium appear different. The acanthioparietal projection demonstrates greater orbital magnification and less distance from the lateral orbital margin to the lateral cranial cortices than the parietoacanthial projection

(compare Figure 11-22 and Image 24). These differences result from greater magnification of the anatomy situated farther from the IR. With the acanthioparietal projection the orbits are situated farther from the IR than the parietal bones, whereas in the parietoacanthial projection, the parietal bones are positioned farther from the IR.

The petrous ridges are demonstrated inferior to the maxillary sinuses and extend laterally from the posterior maxillary alveolar process.

- To position the petrous ridges inferior to the maxillary sinuses accurately, elevate the patient's chin until the OML is at a 37-degree angle with IR. Chin elevation moves the maxillary sinuses superior to the petrous ridges. This is best accomplished by positioning the mentomeatal line (MML) perpendicular to the IR. If an open-mouth Waters method is required, do not have patient drop the jaw until after the MML has been positioned perpendicular to the IR (Figure 11-24).
- *Adjusting the central ray for poor MML alignment.* For a patient who is unable to elevate the chin adequately to position the MML perpendicular to the IR, the central ray may be adjusted to compensate. Instruct the patient to elevate the chin to position the MML as close as possible to perpendicular to the IR. Then angle the central ray until it is parallel with the MML. This method should not be used if the maxillary sinuses are being evaluated for air-fluid levels. Unless the central ray remains horizontal, the air-fluid level is obscured or appears higher.
- *Detecting poor MML positioning.* Poor MML positioning can be detected by evaluating the positions of the petrous ridges and posterior maxillary alveolar process. If the patient's chin was not

adequately elevated to bring the MML perpendicular to the IR, the petrous ridges are demonstrated superior to the posterior maxillary alveolar process superimposing the maxillary sinuses (see Images 21 and 22). If the patient's chin was elevated more than needed to position the MML perpendicular to the IR, the petrous ridges are demonstrated inferior to the maxillary sinuses and posterior maxillary alveolar process, and the maxillary sinuses are superimposed over the posterior molars and alveolar process (see Image 23).

- *Central ray angulation for acanthioparietal projection.* For the acanthioparietal cranium projection, if a cervical vertebrae injury is not suspected, adjust the patient's head as described for the parietoacanthial projection. If a cervical vertebrae injury is suspected, do not adjust the patient's head position or increased cervical injury might result. Instead, angle the central ray cephalically until it is aligned parallel with the MML. If the MML is difficult to use or the patient's mouth is open, the central ray may also be adjusted 37 degrees cephalically from the OML to obtain identical anatomic relationships (Figure 11-25).
- *Correcting the central ray angulation for a trauma acanthioparietal projection.* For the trauma acanthioparietal projection, the central ray angulation determines the relationship of the petrous ridges to the maxillary sinuses and posterior maxillary alveolar process. For an acanthioparietal projection that demonstrates poor petrous ridge positioning, adjust the central ray angulation in the direction in which you want the maxillary sinuses and posterior maxillary alveolar process to

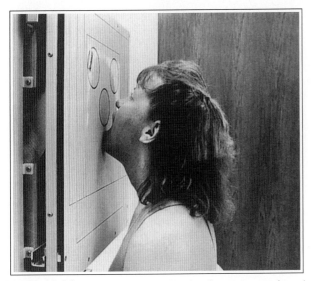

FIGURE 11-24 Proper patient positioning for open-mouth parietoacanthial sinus projection (Waters method).

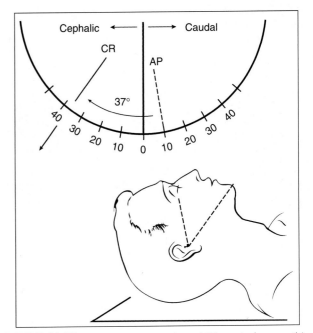

FIGURE 11-25 Determining central ray (*CR*) angle for acanthioparietal facial bone and sinus projection in a trauma patient.

move. Because they are situated farther from the IR than the petrous ridges, their position is most affected by an angulation change. If the petrous ridges are demonstrated within the maxillary sinuses and superior to the posterior maxillary alveolar process, the central ray was angled too caudally (see Image 24). If the petrous ridges are demonstrated inferior to the maxillary sinuses and posterior maxillary alveolar process, and the posterior molars and maxillary alveolar process are superimposed over the maxillary sinuses, the central ray was angled too cephalically. (The petrous ridge and posterior maxillary alveolar relationship would be similar to that shown in Image 23.)

- *Modified Waters method.* A modified Waters method is used to position the orbital floors perpendicular to the IR and parallel to the central ray for increased demonstration of the orbital floors, a modified Waters method. This examination is commonly done to rule out fractures of the orbits and demonstrate foreign bodies in the eyes. The modified Waters method is accomplished by positioning the patient as described for the Waters method, with one exception—the patient's chin is elevated only until the OML is at a 55-degree angle with the IR. In this position, the petrous ridges will be demonstrated within the maxillary sinuses rather than inferior to them (Figure 11-26).

The bony nasal septum is aligned with the long axis of the exposure field, and the infraorbital margins are demonstrated on the same horizontal plane.

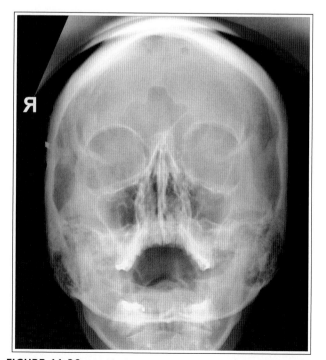

FIGURE 11-26 Modified Waters facial bone and sinus projection with accurate positioning.

- Aligning the cranium's midsagittal plane with the collimator's longitudinal light line controls tilting of the patient's head. Tilting does not change any anatomic relationships for this projection, but it does prevent tight collimation and makes viewing the image slightly more awkward.

The anterior nasal spine is at the center of the exposure field. The frontal and maxillary (and sphenoid on the open-mouth position) sinuses and the lateral cranial cortices are included within the collimated field.

- Centering a perpendicular central ray to the acanthion (area located at the midsagittal plane where the nose and upper lip meet) places the anterior nasal spine in the center of the exposure field. Center the IR to the central ray.
- Open the longitudinally and transversely collimated fields to within 1 inch (2.5 cm) of palpable orbits and zygomatic arches, or use a circle diaphragm.
- An 8- × 10-inch (18- × 24-cm) IR placed lengthwise should be adequate to include all required anatomic structures.

Parietoacanthial and Acanthioparietal Facial Bone and Sinus Projection Analysis

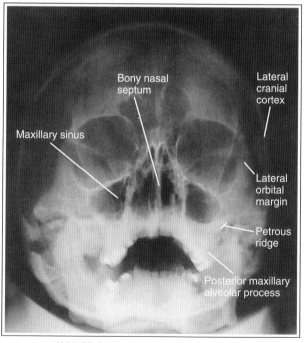

IMAGE 21 Parietoacanthial projection.

Analysis. The distances from the lateral orbital margin to the lateral cranial cortex and from the bony nasal septum to the lateral cranial cortex on the right side of the patient are greater than the same distances on the left side. The petrous ridges are demonstrated within the maxillary sinuses and superior to the posterior maxillary alveolar process. The patient's face was rotated toward the left side, and the chin was not elevated enough to position the MML perpendicular to the IR.

Correction. Rotate the patient's face toward the right side until the midsagittal plane is perpendicular with the IR. Elevate the patient's chin until the MML is perpendicular to the IR. The amount of movement needed is the full distance demonstrated between the petrous ridges and posterior maxillary alveolar process. If the patient is unable to elevate the chin any further, leave the chin positioned as is and angle the central ray caudally approximately 5 degrees for every 0.5 inch (1.25 cm) of distance demonstrated between the petrous ridges and the posterior maxillary alveolar process.

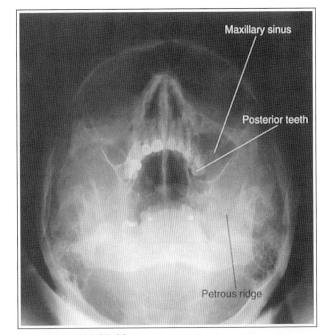

IMAGE 23 Parietoacanthial projection.

Analysis. The petrous ridges are inferior to the maxillary sinuses and the posterior maxillary alveolar process. The patient's chin was elevated more than needed to align the MML perpendicular to the IR.

Correction. Depress the patient's chin until the MML is perpendicular to the IR. The amount of movement needed is the full distance demonstrated between the petrous ridges and posterior maxillary alveolar process.

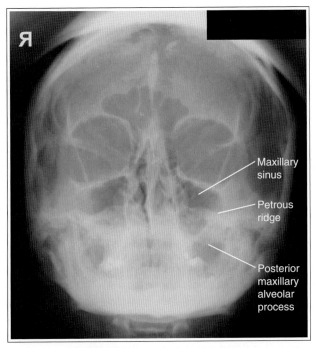

IMAGE 22 Parietoacanthial projection.

Analysis. The petrous ridges are demonstrated within the maxillary sinuses and superior to the posterior maxillary alveolar process. The patient's chin was not elevated enough to position the MML perpendicular to the IR. If this petrous ridge and posterior maxillary alveolar process relationship was obtained on a trauma acanthioparietal projection, the central ray was angled too caudally.

Correction. Elevate the patient's chin until the MML is perpendicular to the IR. The amount of movement needed is the full distance between the petrous ridges and the posterior maxillary alveolar process. If the patient is unable to elevate the chin farther, leave the patient's chin positioned as is and angle the central ray caudally approximately 5 degrees for every 0.5 inch (1.25 cm) of distance demonstrated between the petrous ridges and the posterior maxillary alveolar process. This should align the central ray parallel with the MML when the patient's mouth is closed.

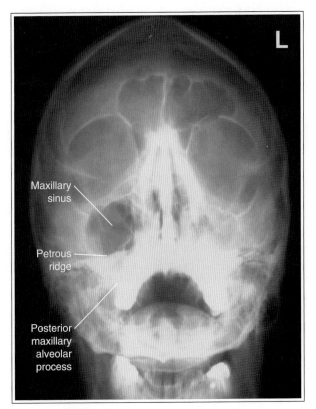

IMAGE 24 Acanthioparietal projection.

Analysis. The petrous ridges are demonstrated within the maxillary sinuses and superior to the posterior maxillary alveolar process. Either the patient's chin was not elevated enough to position the MML perpendicular to the IR or the central ray was angled too caudally.

Correction. Elevate the patient's chin until the MML is perpendicular to the IR. The amount of movement needed is the full distance demonstrated between the petrous ridges and the posterior maxillary alveolar process. If the patient is unable to elevate the chin any further, leave the patient's chin positioned as is and angle the central ray cephalically approximately 5 degrees for every 0.5 inch (1.25 cm) of distance demonstrated between the petrous ridges and the posterior maxillary alveolar process.

NASAL BONES: TANGENTIAL PROJECTION (SUPEROINFERIOR PROJECTION)

See Figure 11-27 and Box 11-8.

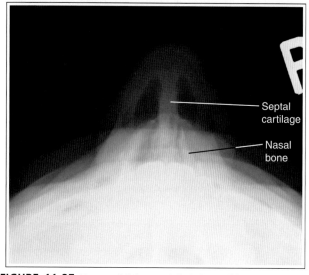

Septal cartilage

Nasal bone

FIGURE 11-27 Tangential (superoinferior) nasal bone projection with accurate positioning.

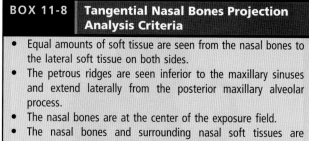

BOX 11-8	**Tangential Nasal Bones Projection Analysis Criteria**

- Equal amounts of soft tissue are seen from the nasal bones to the lateral soft tissue on both sides.
- The petrous ridges are seen inferior to the maxillary sinuses and extend laterally from the posterior maxillary alveolar process.
- The nasal bones are at the center of the exposure field.
- The nasal bones and surrounding nasal soft tissues are included within the collimated field.

Equal amounts of soft tissue are demonstrated from the nasal bones to the lateral soft tissue on both sides.

- The tangential nasal bones projection is obtained by having the patient seated in a chair at the end of the imaging table or in a prone position on the imaging table. The chin is extended and placed on an IR that is resting on a 45-degree angled sponge. Chin elevation and depression are adjusted until the glabelloalveolar line (GAL) is perpendicular to the IR (Figure 11-28). To obtain equal amounts of soft tissue on both sides of the nasal bones, tilt the head as needed to align the cranial midsagittal plane perpendicular to the IR.
- If the cranial midsagittal plane is not aligned perpendicular to the IR, more soft tissue width will be demonstrated from the nasal bone to the lateral soft tissue on the side toward which the patient's chin is rotated and less on the side toward which the patient's cranium is rotated.

The petrous ridges are demonstrated inferior to the maxillary sinuses and extend laterally from the posterior maxillary alveolar process.

- When the GAL is aligned perpendicular to the IR, the posterior nasal bones are demonstrated without glabella and alveolar ridge superimposition. If the GAL is not aligned perpendicular to the IR, the posterior nasal bones will be obscured. If the patient is unable to elevate the chin enough to position the GAL perpendicular to the IR, the central ray may be angled toward the patient until it is aligned parallel with the GAL.

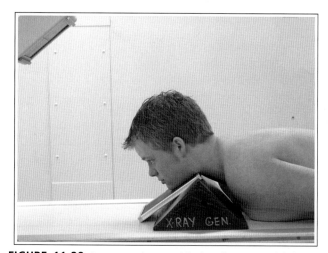

FIGURE 11-28 Proper patient positioning for tangential (superoinferior) nasal bone projection.

The nasal bones are at the center of the exposure field. The nasal bones and surrounding nasal soft tissue are included within the collimated field.

- Centering a perpendicular central ray to the nasion positions the nasal bones in the center of the collimated field.
- An 8- × 10-inch (18-×24-cm) IR placed lengthwise should be adequate to include all the required anatomic structures. A small focal spot will increase detail sharpness.
- Open the longitudinally and transversely collimated fields to within 0.5 inch (1.25 cm) of the nasal skin line or use a circle diaphragm.

OBJECTIVES

After completion of this chapter, you should be able to do the following:

- Identify the required anatomy on upper and lower gastrointestinal projections.
- Describe how to properly position the patient, image receptor (IR), and central ray for upper and lower gastrointestinal projections.
- State how to properly mark and display upper and lower gastrointestinal projections.
- Explain the patient preparation procedure used before upper and lower gastrointestinal examinations to prevent residual debris and fluid from obscuring areas of interest.
- List the image analysis requirements for upper and lower gastrointestinal images with accurate positioning and state how to reposition the patient when less than optimal projections are produced.
- Describe the differences in size, shape, and position of the stomach and abdominal cavity placement of the

small and large intestinal structures among the different types of habitus.
- Define the difference in the barium suspension that is ingested for upper and for lower gastrointestinal projections.
- State how a woman who has had one breast removed may have to be positioned at a greater object–image receptor distance (OID) for PA projections.
- Describe the differences in the appearance of the stomach on projections of patients with different types of body habitus.
- State where the barium and air will be situated for the different upper and lower gastrointestinal double-contrast projections.
- Explain why the small intestine is imaged at set time intervals for a small intestine study.

KEY TERMS

negative contrast

NPO

positive contrast

PREPARATION PROCEDURES

- *Esophagram preparation.* No preparation procedures are required when the esophagus is imaged, but if an esophagus and stomach examination is being performed, the stomach and duodenum preparation is to be followed.
- *Stomach and duodenum preparation.* Adequate preparation of the upper gastrointestinal (GI) system eliminates residual stomach debris, which may obscure abnormalities, and prevents excessive fluid from accumulating in the stomach, which could dilute the barium suspension enough to interfere with optimal mucosal coating (see Image 5). The preparation procedure for the upper GI system includes NPO (nothing orally) after midnight or at least 8 hours before the examination, and avoidance of gum and tobacco products before the procedure.
- *Small intestine preparation.* Optimal preparation of the small intestine for a small bowel study is obtained through a patient preparation procedure that includes a low-residue diet for 1 to 2 days before the examination, NPO after midnight and until the examination, and avoidance of gum and tobacco products before the examination (these are thought to increase salivation and gastric secretions).
- *Large intestine preparation.* Adequate cleansing of the large intestine for a barium enema is obtained through a patient preparation procedure including a low-residue diet for 2 to 3 days before the examination, followed by a clear liquid diet 1 day before the examination, laxatives the afternoon before the examination, and a suppository or cleansing enema the morning of the examination. Remaining fecal material may obscure the mucosal surfaces and, when barium-coated, may mimic polyps and small tumors; remaining residual fluid causes dilution of the barium suspension, resulting in poor mucosal coating and coating artifacts (see Image 11).

    On arrival in the fluoroscopic department, the patient should be queried to determine whether proper preparation instructions were given and followed. Adequate preparation can be assumed if the patient's last bowel movement lacked solid fecal material.

IMAGE ANALYSIS CRITERIA

The following image analysis criteria are used for all adult and pediatric digestive system images and should be considered when completing the analysis for each projection presented in this chapter (Box 12-1).

- *Visibility of Digestive System Details.* An optimal kilovoltage peak (kVp) technique, as shown in Table 12-1, sufficiently penetrates the barium-

BOX 12-1	Digestive System Imaging Analysis Criteria

- The facility's identification requirements are visible.
- A right or left marker identifying the correct side of the patient is present on the image and is not superimposed over the anatomy of interest.
- Good radiation protection practices are evident.
- The GI structures and cortical outlines of the bony structures are sharply defined.
- Contrast, density, and penetration are adequate to demonstrate the barium-coated mucosal surface patterns and intestinal contours while providing uniform grayness within the air-filled stomach or intestine.
- The long axis of the lumbar vertebral column is aligned with the long axis of the exposure field.
- The required upper and lower intestinal structures are included within the collimated field, adjusting to accommodate the patient's habitus.
- The image was taken on full suspended expiration. The diaphragm dome is located superior to the ninth posterior rib.
- No evidence of removal artifacts is present.

coated mucosal surface and provides the contrast needed to distinguish the mucosal patterns. Use a grid to reduce the scatter radiation that reaches the IR, thereby reducing fog, increasing the visibility of the recorded details, and providing a higher contrast image. To obtain optimal density, set a milliampere-seconds (mAs) level manually based on the patient's abdominal thickness or choose the appropriate automatic exposure control (AEC). For double-contrast examinations, using the AEC may be contraindicated because choosing the cell beneath the barium pool may result in overexposure of the area containing the air contrast (see Image 6).

- *Pendulous breasts.* Pendulous breasts may overlap and prevent clear visualization of the colic flexures unless they are shifted superiorly and laterally. Such movement also prevents excessive radiation exposure to the breasts.
- *Exposure times.* Short exposure times are needed when imaging the digestive system to control the image blur that may result from peristaltic activity within the system. Peristalsis is the contraction and relaxation movement of the smooth muscles in the walls of the digestive system that mixes food and secretions and moves the materials through the system. Peristaltic activity of the stomach and large or small intestine can be identified on an image by sharp bony cortices and blurry gastric and intestinal gases or barium (see Image 9).

The required upper and lower intestinal structures are included on the image. Adjustments in patient positioning, central ray centering, and IR size and direction are made to accommodate the patient's habitus.

TABLE 12-1 Digestive System Technical Data				
Projection	**kVp**	**Grid**	**AEC**	**SID**
Upper Gastrointestinal System				
PA oblique (RAO position), esophagus	SC = 100–110	Grid	Center	40–48 inches (100–120 cm)
Lateral, esophagus	SC = 100–110	Grid	Center	40–48 inches (100–120 cm)
AP or PA, esophagus	SC = 100–110	Grid	Center	40–48 inches (100–120 cm)
PA oblique (RAO position), stomach	SC = 100–110 DC = 80–90	Grid	Center	40–48 inches (100–120 cm)
PA, stomach	SC = 100–110 DC = 80–90	Grid	Center	40–48 inches (100–120 cm)
Right lateral, stomach	SC = 100–110 DC = 80–90	Grid	Center	40–48 inches (100–120 cm)
AP oblique (LPO position), stomach	SC = 100–110 DC = 80–90	Grid	Center	40–48 inches (100–120 cm)
AP, stomach	SC = 100–110 DC = 80–90	Grid	Center	40–48 inches (100–120 cm)
Small Intestine				
PA or AP	SC = 100–125	Grid	All three	40–48 inches (100–120 cm)
Large Intestine				
AP or AP	SC = 100–125 DC = 80–90	Grid	All three	40–48 inches (100–120 cm)
Lateral (rectum)	SC = 100–125 DC = 80–90	Grid	Center	40–48 inches (100–120 cm)
AP or PA (lateral decubitus)	SC = 100–125 DC = 80–90	Grid	All three	40–48 inches (100–120 cm)
PA oblique (RAO position)	SC = 100–125 DC = 80–90	Grid	All three	40–48 inches (100–120 cm)
PA oblique (LAO position)	SC = 100–125 DC = 80–90	Grid	All three	40–48 inches (100–120 cm)
PA axial or PA axial oblique (RAO position)	SC = 100–125 DC = 80–90	Grid	All three	40–48 inches (100–120 cm)

AEC, Automatic exposure control; *AP*, anteroposterior; *DC*, double contrast; *kVp*, kilovoltage peak; *LPO*, left posterior oblique; *PA*, posteroanterior; *RAO*, right anterior oblique; *SC*, single contrast; *SID*, source–image receptor distance.

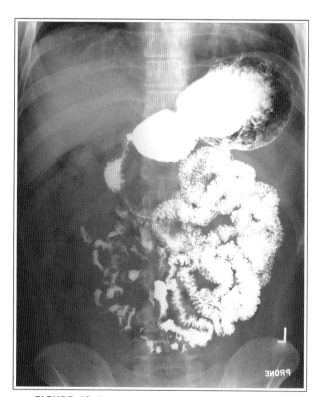

FIGURE 12-1 PA projection of hypersthenic patient.

- *Body habitus.* The body habitus determines the size, shape, and position of the stomach and the abdominal cavity placement of the large intestine. Being familiar with these differences will help the technologist adjust the central ray centering and IR placement for optimal demonstration of the required digestive structures.

  Hypersthenic. The hypersthenic patient's abdomen is broad and deep from anterior to posterior. The stomach is positioned high in the abdomen and lies transversely at the level of the T9 to T12, with the duodenal bulb at the level of T11 to T12. The colic flexures and transverse colon tend to be positioned high in the abdomen (Figure 12-1). Using the sthenic patient as the reference point, this habitus will require a more superior and medial central ray centering and IR placement for AP and PA projections, a more superior and anterior central ray centering and IR placement for the lateral position of the stomach, and two crosswise IRs to include the entire large intestine for barium enema projections.

  Asthenic. The asthenic patient's abdomen is narrow; the stomach is positioned low in the abdomen and runs vertically along the left side of the vertebral column, typically extending from T11 to L5,

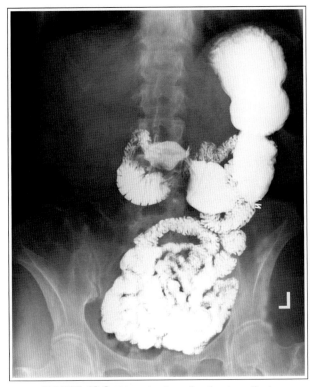

FIGURE 12-2 PA projection of asthenic patient.

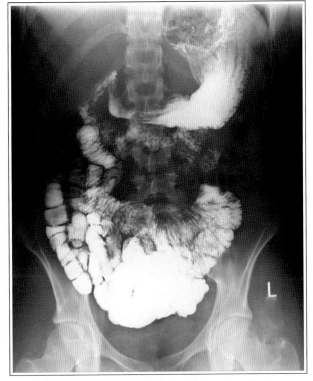

FIGURE 12-3 PA projection of sthenic patient.

with the duodenal bulb at the level of L3 to L4. The small and large intestinal structures tend to be positioned low in the abdomen (Figure 12-2). Using the sthenic patient as the reference point, this habitus will require lower and more lateral centering of the central ray for stomach projections.

Sthenic. The sthenic habitus is the most common. The abdomen is less broad than the hypersthenic habitus, yet not as narrow as the asthenic. The stomach also rests at a position between the hypersthenic and asthenic habitus and typically extends from T10 to L2, with the duodenal bulb at the level of L1 to L2. The small and large intestinal structures tend to be centered in the abdomen (Figure 12-3).

The image was taken on full suspended expiration. The diaphragm dome is located superior to the ninth posterior ribs.

- From full inspiration to expiration the diaphragm position moves from an inferior to a superior position. This movement also changes the pressure placed on the abdominal structures. On full expiration the right side of the diaphragm dome is at the same transverse level as the eighth thoracic vertebrae, whereas on inspiration it may be found at the same transverse level as the ninth or tenth posterior rib. Exposing upper GI and small and large intestine projections on full expiration allows increased abdominal space for the structures to be demonstrated without segment overlapping and foreshortening (see Image 7).

ESOPHAGRAM: UPPER GASTROINTESTINAL SYSTEM

The esophagus is filled with barium, demonstrating its contour.

- *Contrast.* The goal of the esophagram is to demonstrate the workings and appearance of the pharynx and esophagus. This is accomplished through the fluoroscopic procedure and overhead projections that are obtained in an esophagram. Barium is used to demonstrate the pharynx and esophagus during this examination. A 30% to 50% weight or volume barium suspension is ingested continuously during the exposure, or two to three spoonfuls with toothpaste consistency; thick barium is ingested before exposing the esophagus, filling it with barium. The patient may also be asked to swallow cotton balls soaked in thin barium, barium-filled gelatin capsules, barium tablets, or marshmallows when a radiolucent foreign body or stricture is suspected. Adequate filling of the esophagus has occurred when the entire column is filled with barium. Only aspects of the esophagus that are filled with barium will be adequately demonstrated (see Images 1 and 3).

  For the overhead projections, place a cup full of barium in the patient's hand and place the straw in the patient's mouth so that the patient can ingest barium during the exposure, or ask the patient to swallow two spoonfuls of thick barium and then give a third spoonful that is swallowed immediately before the exposure.

ESOPHAGRAM: POSTEROANTERIOR OBLIQUE PROJECTION (RIGHT ANTERIOR OBLIQUE POSITION)

See Figure 12-4 and Box 12-2.

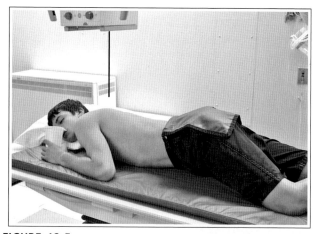

FIGURE 12-5 Proper patient positioning for PA oblique esophagram projection.

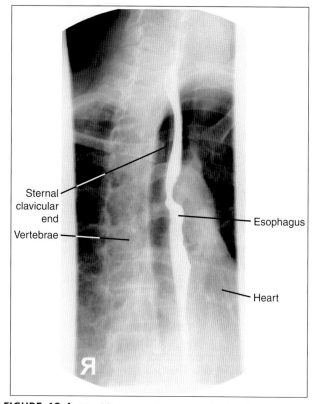

FIGURE 12-4 PA oblique esophagram projection (RAO position) with accurate positioning.

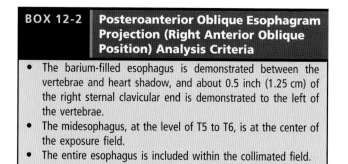

BOX 12-2	Posteroanterior Oblique Esophagram Projection (Right Anterior Oblique Position) Analysis Criteria

- The barium-filled esophagus is demonstrated between the vertebrae and heart shadow, and about 0.5 inch (1.25 cm) of the right sternal clavicular end is demonstrated to the left of the vertebrae.
- The midesophagus, at the level of T5 to T6, is at the center of the exposure field.
- The entire esophagus is included within the collimated field.

The barium-filled esophagus is demonstrated between the vertebrae and heart shadow, and approximately 0.5 inch (1.25 cm) of the right sternal (medial) clavicular end is demonstrated to the left of the vertebrae.

- A PA oblique esophagram projection (right anterior oblique [RAO]) is obtained by placing the patient prone on the imaging table and then

rotating the torso toward the right side until the midcoronal plane is at a 35- to 40-degree angle with the imaging table (Figure 12-5). The patient's left elbow and knee may be flexed and used to support the body rotation.

- **Inaccurate patient rotation.** If less than the desired 35 to 40 degrees of obliquity is obtained on a PA oblique esophagram projection, the vertebrae will be superimposed over the esophagus and the right sternal clavicular end (see Image 2). If the patient is rotated more than 40 degrees, more than 0.5 inch (1.25 cm) of the right sternal clavicular end will be demonstrated to the left of the vertebrae.

The midesophagus, at the level of T5 to T6, is at the center of the exposure field. The entire esophagus is included within the collimated field.

- To place the midesophagus in the center of the exposure field, center a perpendicular central ray approximately 3 inches (7.5 cm) to the left of the spinous processes and 2 to 3 inches (5 to 7.5 cm) inferior to the jugular notch. Center the IR to the central ray.
- Open the longitudinally collimated field the full 17-inch (43-cm) IR length. Transverse collimation should be to a 6-inch (15-cm) field size.
- A 14- × 17-inch (35- × 43-cm) IR placed lengthwise should be adequate to include all the required anatomic structures.

Posteroanterior Oblique Esophagram Projection (RAO Position) Analysis

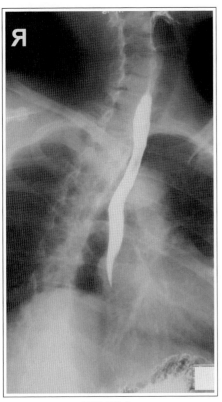

IMAGE 1

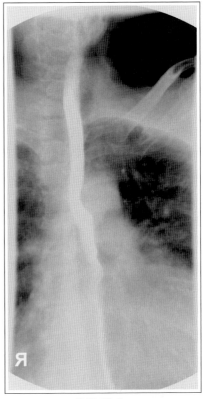

IMAGE 2

Analysis. The superior and inferior ends of the esophagus are not filled with barium.

Correction. The patient should drink barium continuously during the exposure or should swallow two spoonfuls of thick barium and then be given a third spoonful that is swallowed immediately before the exposure.

Analysis. The vertebrae are superimposed over the right sternal clavicular end and a portion of the esophagus. The patient was rotated less than the required 35 to 40 degrees.

Correction. Increase the degree of patient obliquity until the midcoronal plane is at a 35- to 40-degree angle with the imaging table.

ESOPHAGRAM: LATERAL PROJECTION

See Figure 12-6 and Box 12-3.

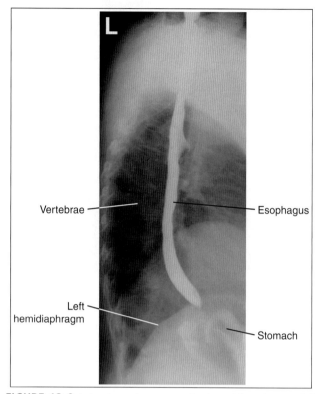

FIGURE 12-6 Lateral esophagram projection with patient on left side.

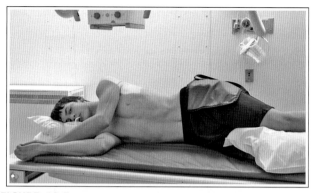

FIGURE 12-7 Proper patient positioning for lateral esophagram projection with arms at 90 degrees.

BOX 12-3	Lateral Esophagram Projection Analysis Criteria

- The esophagus is positioned anterior to the thoracic vertebrae, the posterior surfaces of each vertebral body are superimposed, and no more than 0.5 inch (1.25 cm) of space is demonstrated between the posterior ribs.
- No superimposition of shoulders or humeri over the esophagus is present.
- The midesophagus, at the level of T5 to T6, is at the center of the exposure field.
- The entire esophagus is included within the collimated field.

A barium-filled esophagus in a lateral projection is demonstrated. The esophagus is positioned anterior to the thoracic vertebrae, the posterior surfaces of each vertebral body are superimposed, and no more than 0.5 inch (1.25 cm) of space is demonstrated between the posterior ribs.

- To obtain a lateral esophagram projection, place the patient on the imaging table in a lateral recumbent position. Whether the patient is lying on the right or left side is not significant (Figure 12-7). Flex the patient's knees and hips for support, and position a pillow or sponge between the knees. The pillow or sponge should be thick enough to prevent the side of the pelvis situated farther from the IR from rotating anteriorly but not so thick as to cause posterior rotation. To avoid vertebral rotation, align the shoulders, posterior ribs, and posterior pelvis perpendicular to the imaging table and IR by resting an extended flat palm against each, respectively, and then adjusting patient rotation until the hand is positioned perpendicular to the IR.

- *Detecting thorax rotation.* Rotation can be detected on a lateral esophagram projection by evaluating superimposition of the right and left posterior surfaces of the vertebral bodies and superimposition of the posterior ribs. Because the two sides of the thorax and vertebrae are mirror images, it is very difficult to determine from a rotated lateral esophagram projection which side of the patient was rotated anteriorly and which posteriorly. If the patient was only slightly rotated, one way of determining which way the patient was rotated is to evaluate the amount of posterior rib superimposition. If the patient's elevated side was rotated posteriorly, the posterior ribs demonstrate more than 0.5 inch (1.25 cm) of space between them (see Chapter 8, Image 40). If the patient's elevated side was rotated anteriorly, the posterior ribs are superimposed on slight rotation (see Chapter 8, Image 41) and demonstrate greater separation as rotation of the patient increases.

No superimposition of shoulders or humeri over the esophagus is present.

- *Humeral and shoulder positioning.* Placing the humeri anteriorly at a 90-degree angle with the torso or separating the shoulders by positioning the arm and shoulder closer to the imaging table slightly forward and the arm and shoulder farther

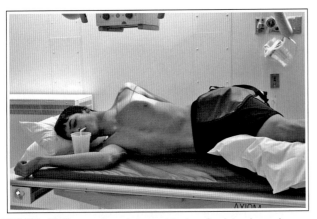

FIGURE 12-8 Proper patient positioning for lateral esophagram projection with shoulders rotated.

away from the imaging table back, while maintaining a lateral thorax (Figure 12-8), prevents the shoulders and humeri from being superimposed over the esophagus.

The midesophagus, at the level of T5 to T6, is at the center of the exposure field. The entire esophagus is included within the collimated field.

- Center a perpendicular central ray to the midcoronal plane at a level 2 to 3 inches (5 to 7.5 cm) inferior to the jugular notch to center the midesophagus at the center of the exposure field. Center the IR to the central ray.
- Open the longitudinally collimated field the full 17-inch (43-cm) IR length. Transverse collimation should be to a 6-inch (15-cm) field size.
- A 14- × 17-inch (35- × 43-cm) IR placed lengthwise should be adequate to include all the required anatomic structures.

Lateral Esophagram Projection Analysis

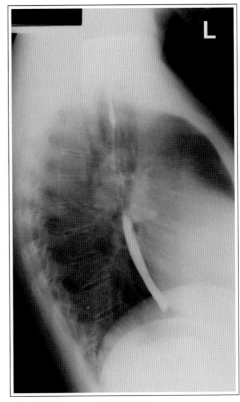

IMAGE 3

Analysis. The superior and middle ends of the esophagus are not filled with barium.

Correction. The patient should drink barium continuously during the exposure or should swallow two spoonfuls of thick barium and then be given a third that is swallowed directly before the exposure.

ESOPHAGRAM: POSTEROANTERIOR PROJECTION

See Figure 12-9 and Box 12-4.

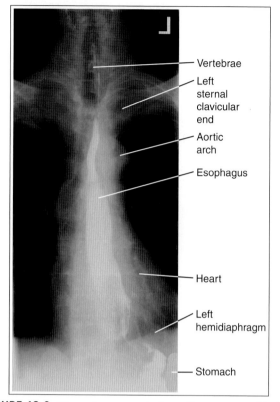

FIGURE 12-9 PA esophagram projection with accurate positioning.

- Vertebrae
- Left sternal clavicular end
- Aortic arch
- Esophagus
- Heart
- Left hemidiaphragm
- Stomach

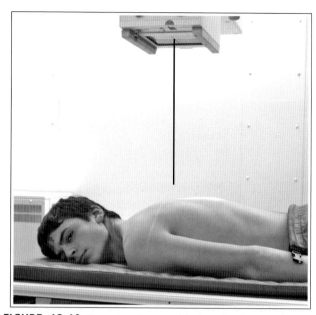

FIGURE 12-10 Proper patient positioning for PA esophagram projection.

BOX 12-4	Posteroanterior Esophagram Projection Analysis Criteria

- The distances from the vertebral column to the sternal ends of the clavicles are equal, and the vertebrae are superimposed over the esophagus.
- The midesophagus, at the level of T5 to T6, is at the center of the exposure field.
- The entire esophagus is included within the collimated field.

- To obtain a PA esophagus projection, place the patient prone on the imaging table. Position the shoulders and anterior superior iliac spines (ASISs) at equal distances from the imaging table to prevent rotation, and draw the patient's arms away from the abdominal area to prevent them from being superimposed over the abdominal region (Figure 12-10). Special attention should be given to female patients who have had one breast removed. The side of the patient on which the breast was removed may need to be placed at a greater OID than the opposite side to prevent rotation.

- *Detecting rotation.* Rotation is readily detected on a PA esophagus projection by evaluating the position of the esophagus with respect to the vertebrae and the distances from the vertebral column to the sternal clavicular ends. On a nonrotated esophagus projection, the vertebrae and esophagus are superimposed and the distances from the vertebrae to the sternal clavicular ends are equal on both sides. On a rotated PA projection, the side of the vertebrae toward which the esophagus is rotated and the sternal clavicular end that demonstrates less vertebral column superimposition represents the side of the chest positioned farther from the IR (see Image 4).

The midesophagus, at the level of T5 to T6, is at the center of the exposure field. The entire esophagus is included within the collimated field.

- Center a perpendicular central ray to the midsagittal plane at a level 2 to 3 inches (5 to 7.5 cm) inferior to the jugular notch for the AP projection and at the level of T5 to T6 (2 to 3 inches superior to the inferior scapular angle) for the PA projection to center the midesophagus at the center of the exposure field. Center the IR to the central ray.
- Open the longitudinally collimated field the full 17-inch (43-cm) IR length. Transverse collimation should be to a 6-inch (15-cm) field size.
- A 14- × 17-inch (35- × 43-cm) IR placed lengthwise should be adequate to include all the required anatomic structures.

Posteroanterior Esophagram Projection Analysis

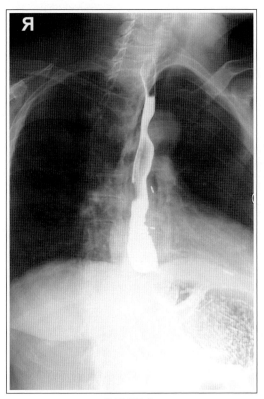

IMAGE 4

Analysis. The esophagus is to the left of the vertebrae and the left sternal clavicular end is demonstrated without vertebral column superimposition. The patient was rotated toward the right side.

Correction. Position the left shoulder closer to the IR until the shoulders are at equal distances from the IR.

STOMACH AND DUODENUM

Single contrast: The stomach and duodenum is barium-filled, demonstrating the contour of the stomach and lumen.

- The single-contrast PA stomach and duodenum projection demonstrates barium-filled organs with normally present gas. The primary goal of a single-contrast upper GI study is to demonstrate abnormalities of the stomach and lumen contour. A 30% to 50% weight or volume barium suspension is typically used for this study.

Double contrast: The stomach and duodenum demonstrate adequate distention and mucosal covering. The rugae (longitudinal gastric folds) are smoothed out, the gastric surface pattern is demonstrated, and a thin, uniform barium line is visible along the contour of the stomach.

- The goal of a double-contrast study is to visualize abnormalities in the mucosal details and contour and lumen of the stomach and duodenum.

  Negative (radiolucent) contrast is most commonly obtained by having the patient swallow effervescent granules, powder, or tablets that rapidly release 300 to 400 mL of carbon dioxide on contact

with the fluid in the stomach. The carbon dioxide causes gastric distention and smoothing of the rugae.

Positive (radiopaque) contrast is obtained by having the patient drink a high-density (up to 250% weight or volume) barium suspension. The barium provides the thin coating that covers the mucosal surface. To obtain adequate mucosal coating of the area, the barium is washed over the gastric surface by having the patient turn 360 degrees and then positioning the patient so that the barium pool will be placed away from the area of interest. Because the barium will slowly flow toward the lowest level after coating, the patient should be rotated between projections or the sequence of projections should be taken to optimize coating of the area of interest to maintain an optimal mucosal covering. Table 12-2 indicates where the barium will pool and which aspect of the upper GI tract is best demonstrated in the most commonly obtained stomach and duodenum projections.

Failure to obtain good mucosal coating may result in missed or simulated lesions. The quality of the mucosal coating depends on the properties of the barium suspension, the volume of barium and gas, the frequency of washing, and the amount of fluid or secretions and viscosity of mucus in the

TABLE 12-2	Double-Contrast Filling of Upper Gastrointestinal System	
Stomach	**Barium-Filled Structures**	**Air-Filled Structures**
PA oblique (RAO position)	Pylorus, duodenum	Fundus
PA projection	Pylorus, duodenum	Fundus
Right lateral projection	Pylorus, duodenum, body	Fundus
AP oblique (LPO position)	Fundus	Pylorus, duodenum
AP projection	Fundus	Pylorus, duodenum, body

stomach. Although proper double-contrast filling is primarily the fluoroscopist's responsibility, the technologist's scope of practice does play a part in some of the causes of poor coating, such as using the wrong type of barium, improperly preparing the barium suspension, or performing poor lower intestine preparation. A thorough mixing of the barium suspension is required before the patient ingests the material.

STOMACH AND DUODENUM: POSTEROANTERIOR OBLIQUE PROJECTION (RIGHT ANTERIOR OBLIQUE POSITION)

See Figures 12-11, 12-12, and 12-13 and Box 12-5.

Contrast distribution: Air contrast is demonstrated in the fundus, and barium is visible in the pylorus, duodenal bulb, and descending duodenum. An optimal PA oblique stomach projection has been obtained when the lumbar vertebrae demonstrate an oblique position, with the degree of obliquity adequate for the body habitus, and when the correct aspect of the stomach, as defined by the body habitus, is in profile.

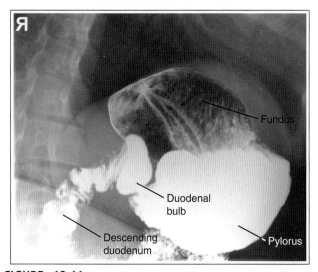

FIGURE 12-11 Hypersthenic PA oblique spot stomach and duodenal projection (RAO position) with accurate positioning.

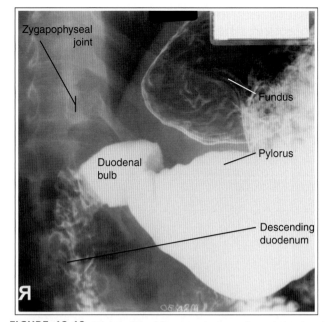

FIGURE 12-12 Sthenic PA oblique spot stomach and duodenal projection (RAO position) with accurate positioning.

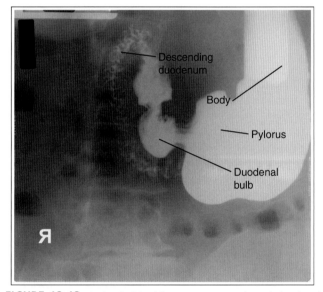

FIGURE 12-13 Asthenic PA oblique spot stomach and duodenal projection (RAO position) with accurate positioning.

- *Hypersthenic habitus.* The patient has been rotated 70 degrees, as identified by the demonstration of the left lumbar zygapophyseal joints in the posterior third of the vertebral bodies. The duodenal bulb and descending duodenum are in profile, and the long axis of the stomach demonstrates foreshortening with a closed lesser curvature (see Figure 12-11).
- *Sthenic habitus.* The patient has been rotated approximately 45 degrees, as identified by the demonstration of the left lumbar zygapophyseal joints at the midline of the vertebral bodies. The duodenal bulb and descending duodenum are in profile, and the long axis of the stomach is partially foreshortened,

BOX 12-5	Posteroanterior Oblique Stomach and Duodenum Projection (Right Anterior Oblique Position) Analysis Criteria

- Air contrast is demonstrated in the fundus and barium is visible in the pylorus, duodenal bulb, and descending duodenum.
- HH: The left lumbar zygapophyseal joints are in the posterior third of the vertebral bodies. The duodenal bulb and descending duodenum are in profile and the long axis of the stomach demonstrates foreshortening, with a closed lesser curvature.
- SH: The left lumbar zygapophyseal joints are at the midline of the vertebral bodies. The duodenal bulb and descending duodenum are in profile, and the long axis of the stomach is partially foreshortened, with a partially closed lesser curvature.
- AH: The left lumbar zygapophyseal joints are in the anterior third of the vertebral bodies. The duodenal bulb and descending duodenum are in profile, the long axis of the stomach is seen without foreshortening, and the lesser curvature is open.
- The pylorus is at the center of the exposure field.
- Stomach and duodenal loop are included within the collimated field.

AH, Asthenic habitus; *HH*, hypersthenic habitus, *SH*, sthenic habitus.

with a partially closed lesser curvature (see Figure 12-12).

- *Asthenic habitus.* The patient has been rotated approximately 40 degrees, as identified by the demonstration of the left lumbar zygapophyseal joints in the anterior third of the vertebral bodies. The duodenal bulb and descending duodenum are in profile, the long axis of the stomach is demonstrated without foreshortening, and the lesser curvature is open (see Figure 12-13).
  - A PA oblique stomach projection (RAO position) is obtained by placing the patient prone on the imaging table and then rotating the torso toward the right side until the midcoronal plane is at a 40- to 70-degree angle with the imaging table (Figure 12-14). The patient's left elbow and knee may be flexed and used to support the body rotation. In general, hypersthenic habitus patients require approximately 70 degrees of obliquity, and the asthenic habitus approximately 40 degrees. The

difference in the degree of obliquity for the body habitus is a result of the difference in the amount of superimposition of the pylorus and duodenal bulb that exists among patients with different habitus.

The pylorus is centered within the exposure field. The stomach and duodenal loop are included within the collimated field.

- To place the pylorus in the center of the exposure field, center a perpendicular central ray halfway between the vertebrae and lateral rib border of the elevated side at a level 1 to 2 inches (2.5 to 5 cm) superior to the inferior rib margin for the sthenic habitus. Center the central ray at a level 2 inches (5 cm) superior to the sthenic patient centering for the hypersthenic habitus, and at a level 2 inches inferior for the asthenic habitus. Center the IR to the central ray.
- Open the longitudinally collimated field the full 14-inch (35-cm) IR length. Transverse collimation should be to the vertebrae and lateral rib border.
- An 11- × 14-inch (28- ×35-cm) IR placed lengthwise should be adequate to include all the required anatomic structures.

STOMACH AND DUODENUM: POSTEROANTERIOR PROJECTION

See Figures 12-15, 12-16, and 12-17 and Box 12-6.
Contrast distribution: Air contrast is demonstrated in the fundus, and barium is visible in the body and pylorus. An optimal PA stomach and duodenum projection has been obtained when the spinous processes are aligned with the midline of the vertebral bodies, the distances from the pedicles to the spinous processes are the

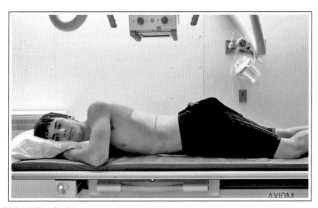

FIGURE 12-14 Proper patient positioning for PA oblique stomach and duodenal projection (RAO position).

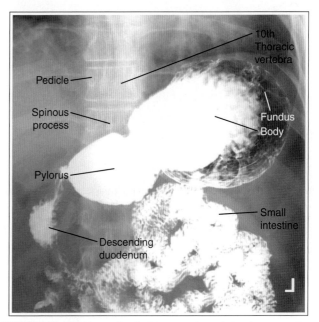

FIGURE 12-15 Hypersthenic PA stomach and duodenum projection with accurate positioning.

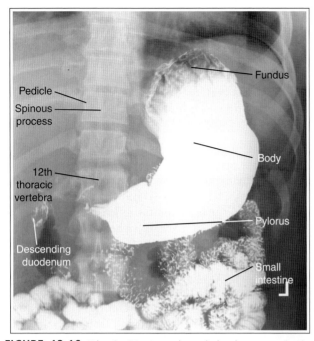

FIGURE 12-16 Sthenic PA stomach and duodenum projection with accurate positioning.

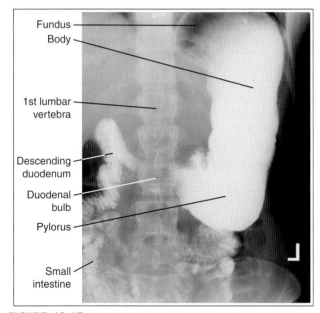

FIGURE 12-17 Asthenic PA stomach and duodenum projection with accurate positioning.

<table>
<tr><td colspan="2">**BOX 12-6**   **Posteroanterior Stomach and Duodenum Projection Analysis Criteria**</td></tr>
</table>

- Air contrast is demonstrated in the fundus and barium is visible in the body and pylorus.
- The spinous processes are aligned with the midline of the vertebral bodies, and the distances from the pedicles to the spinous processes are the same on both sides.
- HH: The stomach is aligned almost horizontally, with the duodenal bulb at the level of T11 to T12. The lesser and greater curvatures are seen almost on end, with the greater curvature being more anteriorly situated and the esophagogastric junction almost on end.
- SH: The stomach is aligned almost vertically, with the duodenal bulb at the level of L1 to L2. The stomach is somewhat J-shaped and its long axis is partially foreshortened. The lesser and greater curvatures, esophagogastric junction, pylorus, and duodenal bulb are in partial profile.
- AH: The stomach is aligned vertically, with the duodenal bulb at the level of L3 to L4. The stomach is J-shaped and its long axis is demonstrated without foreshortening. Lesser and greater curvatures, esophagogastric junction, pylorus, and duodenal bulb are in profile.
- The pylorus is at the center of the exposure field.
- The stomach and descending duodenum are included within the collimated field.

AH, Asthenic habitus; *HH*, hypersthenic habitus, *SH*, sthenic habitus.

The stomach is somewhat J-shaped and its long axis is partially foreshortened. The lesser and greater curvatures, esophagogastric junction, pylorus, and duodenal bulb are in partial profile (see Figure 12-16).

- *Asthenic habitus.* The stomach is aligned vertically, with the duodenal bulb at the level of L3 to L4. The stomach is J-shaped and its long axis is demonstrated without foreshortening. The lesser and greater curvatures, esophagogastric junction, pylorus, and duodenal bulb are in profile (see Figure 12-17).
  - To obtain a PA stomach projection, place the patient prone on the imaging table. Position the shoulders and pelvic ala at equal distances from the imaging table to prevent rotation and draw the patient's arms away from the abdominal area to prevent them from being superimposed over the abdominal region (Figure 12-18).
  - *Detecting abdominal rotation.* Rotation is effectively detected on a PA stomach projection by comparing the distance from the pedicles to the spinous processes on both sides. The side demonstrating the greater distance from the pedicles to the spinous processes is the side positioned farther from the IR.

The pylorus is centered within the exposure field. The stomach and descending duodenum are included within the collimated field.

- To position the pylorus in the center of the collimated field for the sthenic habitus, center a

same on both sides, and the correct aspect of the stomach, as defined by the body habitus, is in profile.

- *Hypersthenic habitus.* The stomach is aligned almost horizontally, with the duodenal bulb at the level of T11 to T12. The lesser and greater curvatures are demonstrated almost on end, with the greater curvature being more anteriorly situated and the esophagogastric junction almost on end (see Figure 12-15).
- *Sthenic habitus.* The stomach is aligned almost vertically, with the duodenal bulb at the level of L1 to L2.

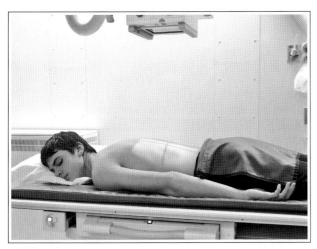

FIGURE 12-18 Proper patient positioning for PA stomach and duodenal projection.

perpendicular central ray halfway between the vertebrae and left lateral rib border at a point approximately 1 to 2 inches (2.5 to 5 cm) superior to the lower rib margin. For the hypersthenic habitus, direct the central ray just to the left of the vertebrae at a level 2 inches (5 cm) superior to the sthenic habitus centering point. For the asthenic habitus, direct the central ray 2 inches inferior to the sthenic habitus centering point. Center the IR to the central ray.

- Open the longitudinally collimated field the full 14-inch (35-cm) IR length. Transverse collimation should be to the vertebrae and lateral rib border.
- An 11- × 14-inch (28- × 35-cm) IR placed lengthwise should be adequate to include all the required anatomic structures.

Posteroanterior Stomach and Duodenum Projection Analysis

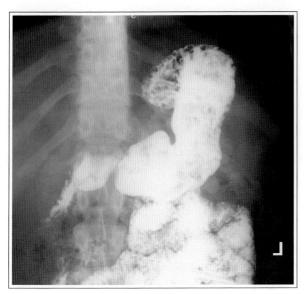

IMAGE 5

Analysis. The stomach demonstrates a blotchy appearance within the barium. The stomach contains residual food particles. The patient did not follow adequate preparation procedure.

Correction. The preparation procedure for the stomach includes NPO after midnight or for at least 8 hours before the examination and avoidance of gum and tobacco products before the procedure.

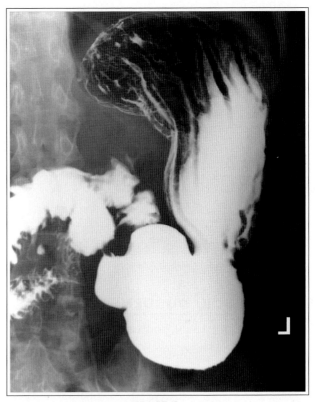

IMAGE 6

Analysis. The air-contrast fundus is overexposed, preventing demonstration of abnormalities. Either the mAs was too high or the AEC was positioned beneath the barium-filled body and pylorus.

Correction. Decrease the mAs enough to demonstrate the fundus or manually set the mAs instead of using the AEC.

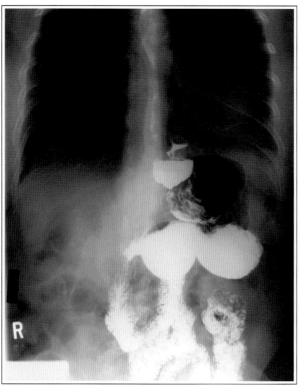

IMAGE 7

Analysis. The examination was obtained after full inspiration, compressing and foreshortening the stomach. Compare this projection with the projections obtained on expiration in Figures 12-3 and 12-16.

Correction. Expose on full suspended expiration.

STOMACH AND DUODENUM: LATERAL PROJECTION (RIGHT LATERAL POSITION)

See Figures 12-19, 12-20, and 12-21 and Box 12-7.

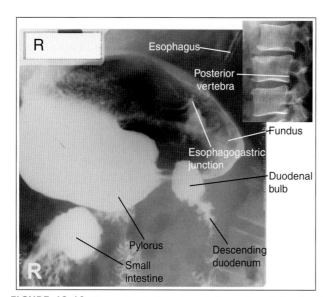

FIGURE 12-19 Hypersthenic lateral spot stomach and duodenal projection (right lateral position) with accurate positioning.

Contrast distribution: Air contrast is demonstrated in the fundus, and barium is visible in the pylorus, duodenum bulb, and descending duodenum.

An optimal right lateral stomach and duodenal projection has been obtained when the thoracic and lumbar

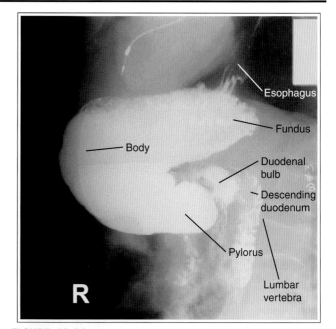

FIGURE 12-20 Sthenic lateral stomach and duodenal projection (right lateral position) with accurate positioning.

vertebrae demonstrate a lateral projection, with the superimposed posterior surfaces of each vertebral body, when the stomach, duodenal bulb, and descending duodenum are anterior to the vertebrae, demonstrating the

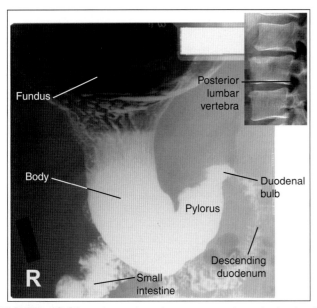

FIGURE 12-21 Asthenic lateral spot stomach and duodenal projection (right lateral position) with accurate positioning.

BOX 12-7	Lateral Stomach and Duodenum Projection Analysis Criteria

- Air contrast is demonstrated in the fundus, and barium is visible in the pylorus, duodenum bulb, and descending duodenum.
- The posterior surfaces of the vertebral bodies are superimposed, the stomach, duodenal bulb, and descending duodenum are anterior to the vertebrae, demonstrating the retrogastric space.
- HH: The duodenal bulb and descending duodenum are in profile and the long axis of the stomach demonstrates foreshortening, with a closed lesser curvature.
- SH: The duodenal bulb and descending duodenum are in profile and the long axis of the stomach is partially foreshortened, with a partially closed lesser curvature.
- AH: The duodenal bulb and descending duodenum are in profile, the long axis of the stomach is demonstrated without foreshortening, and the lesser curvature is open.
- The pylorus is at the center of the exposure field.
- The stomach and duodenal loop are included within the collimated field.

AH, Asthenic habitus; *HH,* hypersthenic habitus, *SH,* sthenic habitus.

retrogastric space, and when the correct aspect of the stomach, as defined by the body habitus, is in profile.

- *Hypersthenic habitus.* The duodenal bulb and descending duodenum are in profile, and the long axis of the stomach demonstrates foreshortening with a closed lesser curvature (see Figure 12-19).
- *Sthenic habitus.* The duodenal bulb and descending duodenum are in profile, and the long axis of the stomach is partially foreshortened with a partially closed lesser curvature (see Figure 12-20).
- *Asthenic habitus.* The duodenal bulb and descending duodenum are in profile, the long axis of the

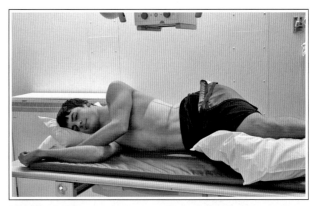

FIGURE 12-22 Proper patient positioning for lateral stomach and duodenal projection (right lateral position).

stomach is demonstrated without foreshortening, and the lesser curvature is open (see Figure 12-21).

- To obtain a lateral stomach projection, place the patient on the imaging table in a right lateral recumbent position. Flex the patient's knees and hips for support (Figure 12-22). To avoid rotation, align the shoulders, posterior ribs, and posterior pelvis perpendicular to the imaging table and IR. This is accomplished by resting your extended flat palm against each structure, individually, and then adjusting the patient's rotation until your hand is positioned perpendicular to the imaging table.
- *Detecting rotation.* Rotation can be detected on a lateral stomach and duodenal projection by evaluating the superimposition of the right and left posterior surfaces of the vertebral bodies. On a nonrotated lateral stomach and duodenal projection, these posterior surfaces are superimposed, appearing as one. On rotation, these posterior surfaces are not superimposed but are demonstrated one anterior to the other (see Image 8).

The pylorus is centered within the exposure field. The stomach and duodenal loop are included within the collimated field.

- To place the pylorus in the center of the exposure field, center a perpendicular central ray halfway between the midcoronal plane and anterior abdomen at the level of the inferior rib margin for the sthenic habitus. For the hypersthenic habitus, direct the central ray at a level 2 inches (5 cm) superior to the sthenic habitus centering point. For the asthenic habitus, direct the central ray 2 inches inferior to the sthenic habitus centering point. Center the IR to the central ray.
- Open the longitudinally collimated field the full 14-inch (35-cm) IR length. Transverse collimation should be to the vertebrae and anterior abdomen border.
- An 11- × 14-inch (28- × 35-cm) IR placed lengthwise should be adequate to include all the required anatomic structures.

Lateral Stomach and Duodenum Projection (Right Lateral Position) Analysis

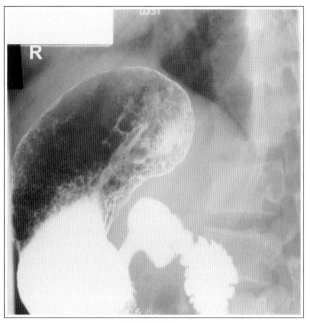

IMAGE 8

Analysis. The descending duodenum is partially superimposed over the duodenal bulb and vertebrae, and the posterior surfaces of the thoracic and lumbar vertebrae are not superimposed. The patient was not in a lateral position.

Correction. Align the shoulders, posterior ribs, and posterior pelvis perpendicular to the imaging table and IR.

STOMACH AND DUODENUM: ANTEROPOSTERIOR OBLIQUE PROJECTION (LEFT POSTERIOR OBLIQUE POSITION)

See Figures 12-23, 12-24, and 12-25 and Box 12-8.

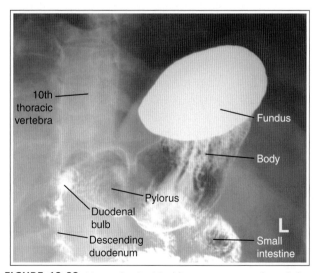

FIGURE 12-23 Hypersthenic AP oblique spot stomach and duodenal projection (LPO position) with accurate positioning.

Contrast distribution: Air contrast is demonstrated in the pylorus, duodenal bulb, and descending duodenum, and barium is visible in the fundus.

An optimal AP oblique stomach and duodenal projection (LPO position) has been obtained when the lumbar vertebrae demonstrate an oblique position with the degree of obliquity adequate for the body habitus and when the correct aspect of the stomach, as defined by the body habitus, is in profile.

- *Hypersthenic habitus.* The patient has been rotated 60 degrees, as identified by the demonstration of the left lumbar zygapophyseal joints in the posterior third of the vertebral bodies. The duodenal bulb and descending duodenum are in profile, and the pylorus is superimposed over the vertebrae (see Figure 12-23).
- *Sthenic habitus.* The patient has been rotated 45 degrees, as identified by the demonstration of the left lumbar zygapophyseal joints at the midline of the vertebral bodies. The duodenal bulb and descending duodenum are in profile, and the vertebrae are demonstrated with little if any pyloric superimposition (see Figure 12-24).
- *Asthenic habitus.* The patient has been rotated 30 degrees, as identified by the demonstration of the left lumbar zygapophyseal joints in the anterior third of the vertebral bodies. The duodenal bulb and descending duodenum are in profile, and the

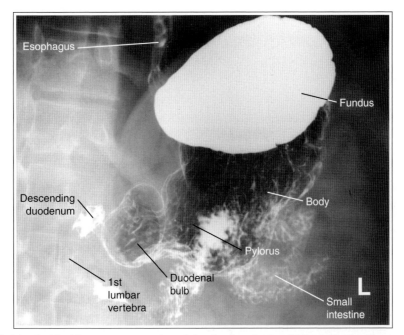

FIGURE 12-24 Sthenic AP oblique spot stomach and duodenal projection (LPO position) with accurate positioning.

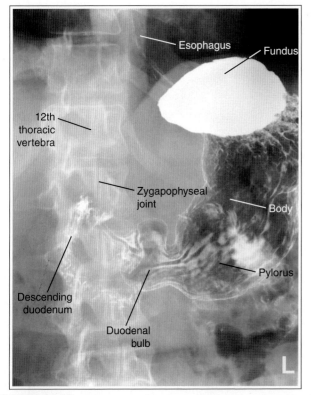

FIGURE 12-25 Asthenic AP oblique spot stomach and duodenal projection (LPO position) with accurate positioning.

BOX 12-8	Anteroposterior Oblique Stomach and Duodenum Projection (Left Posterior Oblique Position) Analysis Criteria

- Air contrast is demonstrated in the pylorus, duodenal bulb, and descending duodenum, and barium is visible in the fundus.
- HH: The left lumbar zygapophyseal joints are seen in the posterior third of the vertebral bodies. The duodenal bulb and descending duodenum are in profile and the pylorus is superimposed over the vertebrae.
- SH: The left lumbar zygapophyseal joints are seen at the midline of the vertebral bodies. The duodenal bulb and descending duodenum are in profile and the vertebrae are demonstrated with little if any pyloric superimposition.
- AH: The left lumbar zygapophyseal joints are seen in the anterior third of the vertebral bodies. The duodenal bulb and descending duodenum are in profile and the vertebrae are demonstrated with little if any pyloric superimposition.
- The pylorus is at the center of the exposure field.
- The stomach and duodenal loop are included within the collimated field.

AH, Asthenic habitus; *HH,* hypersthenic habitus, *SH,* sthenic habitus.

vertebrae are demonstrated with little if any pyloric superimposition (see Figure 12-25).

- An AP oblique stomach and duodenal projection (left posterior oblique [LPO]) is obtained by placing the patient supine on the imaging table and then rotating the patient toward the left side until the midcoronal plane is at a 30- to 60-degree angle with the imaging table (Figure 12-26). The patient's right arm is drawn across the chest, the hand grasps the table edge, and the right knee is flexed for support. A radiolucent sponge positioned beneath the right surface may also help the patient maintain the correct obliquity. Rotate the patient with a hypersthenic habitus approximately 60 degrees and the patient with the asthenic habitus approximately 30 degrees.

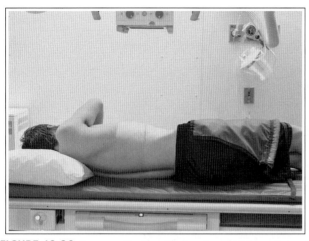

FIGURE 12-26 Proper patient positioning for AP oblique stomach and duodenal projection (LPO position).

The pylorus is centered within the exposure field. The stomach and duodenal loop are included within the collimated field.

- To position the pylorus in the center of the exposure field, center a perpendicular central ray halfway between the vertebrae and left abdominal margin at a level midway between the xiphoid process and inferior rib margin for the sthenic habitus. Center the central ray at a level 2 inches (5 cm) superior to the sthenic habitus central ray centering for the hypersthenic habitus and 2 inches inferior for the asthenic habitus. Center the IR to the central ray.

- Open the longitudinally collimated field the full 14-inch (35-cm) IR length. Transverse collimation should be to the vertebrae and lateral rib border.

- An 11- × 14-inch (28- × 35-cm) IR placed lengthwise should be adequate to include all the required anatomic structures.

Posteroanterior Oblique Stomach and Duodenum Projection (Left Posterior Oblique Position) Analysis

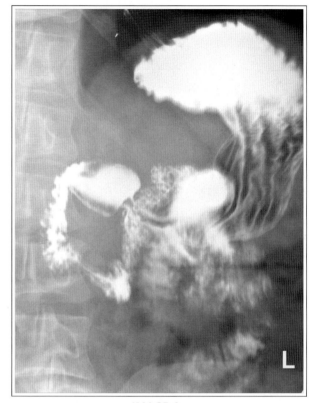

IMAGE 9

Analysis. The bony cortices are sharp and the gastric and intestinal gases and barium are blurry. Peristaltic activity of the stomach and small intestine was occurring during the exposure.

Correction. Use a short exposure time.

STOMACH AND DUODENUM: ANTEROPOSTERIOR PROJECTION

See Figures 12-27, 12-28, and 12-29 and Box 12-9.

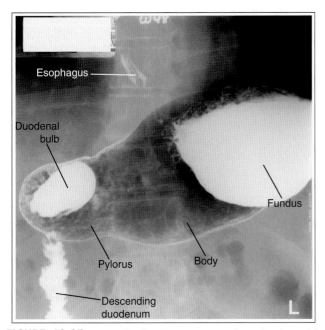

FIGURE 12-27 Hypersthenic AP spot stomach projection with accurate positioning.

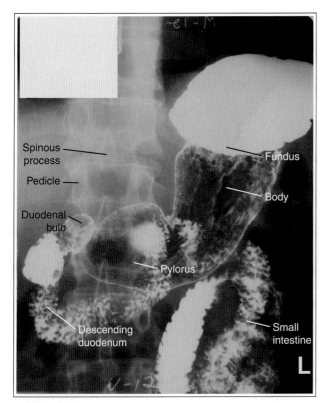

FIGURE 12-28 Sthenic AP spot stomach projection with accurate positioning.

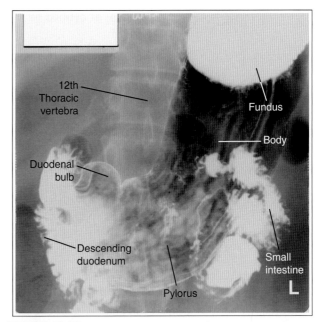

FIGURE 12-29 Asthenic AP spot stomach projection with accurate positioning.

BOX 12-9   Anteroposterior Stomach and Duodenum Projection Analysis Criteria

- Air contrast is demonstrated in the pylorus, duodenal bulb, and descending duodenum, and barium is visible in the fundus.
- The spinous processes are aligned with the midline of the vertebral bodies, and the distances from the pedicles to the spinous processes are the same on both sides.
- HH: The stomach is aligned almost horizontally, with the duodenal bulb at the level of T11 to T12. The lesser and greater curvatures are seen almost on end, with the greater curvature being more anteriorly situated, and the esophagogastric junction is almost on end.
- SH: The stomach is aligned almost vertically, with the duodenal bulb at the level of L1 to L2. The stomach is somewhat J-shaped and its long axis is partially foreshortened. The lesser and greater curvatures, esophagogastric junction, pylorus, and duodenal bulb are in partial profile.
- AH: The stomach is aligned vertically, with the duodenal bulb at the level of L3 to L4. The stomach is J-shaped, its long axis is demonstrated without foreshortening, and the lesser and greater curvatures, esophagogastric junction, pylorus, and duodenal bulb are demonstrated in profile.
- The pylorus is at the center of the exposure field.
- The stomach and duodenal loop are included within the collimated field.

AH, Asthenic habitus; *HH,* hypersthenic habitus, *SH,* sthenic habitus.

Contrast distribution: Air contrast is demonstrated in the pylorus, duodenal bulb, and descending duodenum, and barium is visible in the fundus.

An optimal AP stomach projection has been obtained when the spinous processes are aligned with the midline of the vertebral bodies, the distances from the pedicles to the spinous processes are the same on both sides, and the correct aspect of the stomach, as defined by the body habitus, is in profile.

- *Hypersthenic habitus.* The stomach is aligned almost horizontally, with the duodenal bulb at the level of T11 to T12. The lesser and greater curvatures are demonstrated almost on end, with the greater curvature being more anteriorly situated, and the esophagogastric junction is almost on end (see Figure 12-27).
- *Sthenic habitus.* The stomach is aligned almost vertically, with the duodenal bulb at the level of L1 to L2. The stomach is somewhat J-shaped, and its long axis is partially foreshortened. The lesser and greater curvatures, esophagogastric junction, pylorus, and duodenal bulb are in partial profile (see Figure 12-28).
- *Asthenic habitus.* The stomach is aligned vertically, with the duodenal bulb at the level of L3 to L4. The stomach is J-shaped, its long axis is demonstrated without foreshortening, and the lesser and greater curvatures, esophagogastric junction, pylorus, and duodenal bulb are demonstrated in profile (see Figure 12-29).
  - To obtain an AP stomach and duodenal projection, place the patient supine on the imaging table. Position the shoulders and ASISs at equal distances from the imaging table to prevent rotation, and draw the patient's arms away from the abdominal area to prevent them from being superimposed over the abdominal region (Figure 12-30).
  - *Detecting abdominal rotation.* Rotation is effectively detected on an AP stomach and duodenal projection by comparing the distance from the pedicles to the spinous processes on each side. The side demonstrating the greater distance from the pedicle to the spinous processes is the side positioned closer to the IR.

The pylorus is centered within the exposure field. The stomach and duodenal loop are included within the collimated field.

- To position the pylorus in the center of the exposure field, center a perpendicular central ray halfway between the vertebrae and left abdominal margin at a level midway between the xiphoid process and inferior rib margin sthenic habitus. Center the central ray just medial to the left side of the vertebrae at a level 2 inches (5 cm) superior to the sthenic patient centering for the hypersthenic habitus and at a level 2 inches inferior for the asthenic habitus. Center the IR to the central ray.
- Open the longitudinally collimated field the full 14-inch (35-cm) IR length. Transverse collimation should be to the lateral rib border.
- An 11- × 14-inch (28- × 35-cm) IR placed lengthwise should be adequate to include all the required anatomic structures.

SMALL INTESTINE

SMALL INTESTINE: POSTEROANTERIOR PROJECTION

See Figures 12-31, 12-32, 12-33 and Box 12-10.

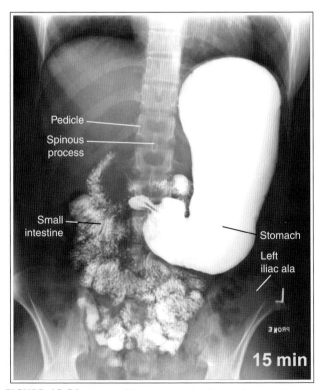

FIGURE 12-31 PA small intestine projection with accurate positioning 15 minutes after ingestion.

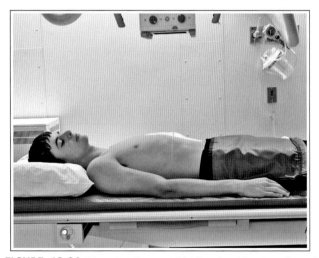

FIGURE 12-30 Proper patient positioning for AP stomach and duodenal projection.

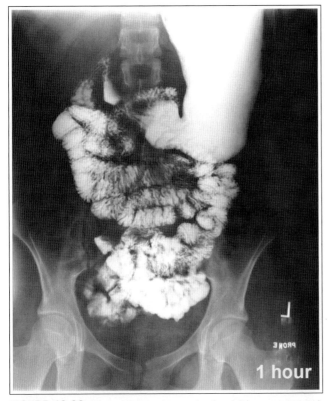

FIGURE 12-32 PA small intestine projection with accurate positioning 1 hour after ingestion.

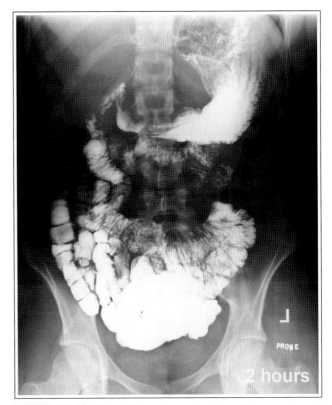

FIGURE 12-33 PA small intestine projection with accurate positioning 2 hours after ingestion.

BOX 12-10	Posteroanterior Small Intestinal Projection Analysis Criteria

- The marker indicates the amount of time that has elapsed since the patient ingested the contrast medium.
- The spinous processes are aligned with the midline of the vertebral bodies, the distances from the pedicles to the spinous processes are the same on both sides, and the iliac alae are symmetrical.
- The small intestine is at the center of the exposure field.
- The stomach and proximal aspects of the small intestine are included within the collimated field on projections taken early in the series, and the small intestine and cecum are included on projections taken later in the series.

AH, Asthenic habitus; *HH,* hypersthenic habitus, *SH,* sthenic habitus.

A marker indicating the amount of time that has elapsed since the patient ingested the contrast medium is included within the collimated field and is not superimposed over anatomic structures of interest.

- For studies of the small intestine, the patient drinks a large amount of barium; then the technologist obtains overhead projections of the stomach and small intestine at timed intervals as peristalsis moves the contrast from the stomach through the small intestine to the cecum. The timing begins when the patient ingests the contrast or as

determined by the radiologist. Typically, the first prone overhead image is obtained at 15 minutes, then at 30 minutes, and then hourly until the barium is demonstrated in the cecum. The barium normally takes 2 to 3 hours to reach the cecum but may vary greatly from patient to patient. Each projection in the timed series must contain a time marker to indicate the amount of time that has passed since the contrast was ingested.

The abdomen demonstrates a PA projection. The spinous processes are aligned with the midline of the vertebral bodies, the distances from the pedicles to the spinous processes are the same on both sides, and the iliac alae are symmetrical.

- To obtain a PA small intestine projection, place the patient prone on the imaging table. Position the shoulders and ASISs at equal distances from the imaging table to prevent rotation, and draw the patient's arms away from the abdominal area to prevent them from being superimposed over the abdominal region (Figure 12-34). The prone position is chosen to demonstrate the small intestine because it will cause compression of the abdominal structures, increasing image quality.
- *Detecting abdominal rotation.* The upper and lower lumbar vertebrae can demonstrate rotation independently or simultaneously, depending on which section of the body is rotated. If the

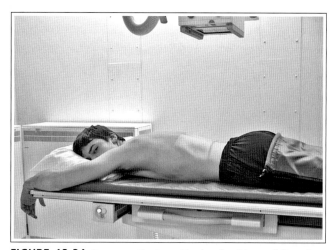

FIGURE 12-34 Proper patient positioning for PA small intestine projection.

Use two 14- × 17-inch (35- × 43-cm) crosswise IRs on *hypersthenic* patients and on other patients who have a transverse abdominal measurement of 14 inches (35 cm) or more to include all the necessary anatomic structures. Take the first projection with the central ray centered to the midsagittal plane at a level halfway between the symphysis pubis and ASIS. Position the bottom of the second IR so it includes 2 to 3 inches (5 to 7.5 cm) of the same transverse section of the peritoneal cavity imaged on the first projection to ensure that no middle peritoneal information has been excluded. It may be necessary to obtain only the superiorly positioned image for the initially obtained image, because the barium may not travel to the inferiorly situated small bowel so soon in the procedure.

patient's thorax was rotated but the pelvis is not, the upper lumbar vertebrae and abdominal cavity demonstrate rotation. If the patient's pelvis was rotated but the thorax was not, the lower vertebrae and abdominal cavity demonstrate rotation. If the patient's thorax and pelvis were rotated simultaneously, the entire abdominal cavity demonstrates rotation. Rotation is effectively detected on a PA small intestine projection by comparing the distances from the pedicles to the spinous processes on both sides and the symmetry of the iliac alae. The side demonstrating the greater distance from the pedicles to the spinous processes and the wider iliac ala is the side positioned farther from the IR.

The small intestine is centered within the exposure field. The stomach and proximal aspects of the small intestine are included within the collimated field on projections taken early in the series, and the small intestine and cecum are included on projections taken later in the series.

- To include the stomach and small intestine on projections obtained earlier in the series, use a perpendicular central ray with the midsagittal plane at a level 2 inches (5 cm) superior to the iliac crest. To include the small intestine and cecum on projections obtained later in the series, direct the central ray to the midsagittal plane at the level of the iliac crest. Center the IR to the central ray (see Image 10).
- The longitudinal collimated field should remain fully open. Transversely collimate to within 0.5 inch (1.25 cm) of the patient's lateral skin line.
- *IR size and direction.* A 14- × 17-inch (35- × 43-cm) lengthwise IR should be adequate to include all the required anatomic structures on sthenic and asthenic patients, as long as the transverse abdominal measurement is less than 14 inches (35 cm).

Posteroanterior Small Intestine Projection Analysis

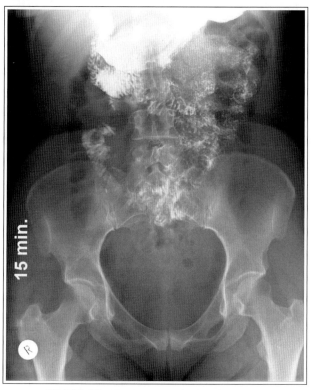

IMAGE 10 15-minute postbarium ingestion.

Analysis. Fifteen minutes after ingestion—the stomach and superior small intestine have not been included on the image. The central ray and IR were positioned too inferiorly.

Correction. Center the central ray 2 inches (5 cm) superior to the iliac crest. Center the IR to the central ray.

LARGE INTESTINE

The large intestine demonstrates adequate distention and mucosal covering. The lumina are distended without mucosal folds, the mucosal surface demonstrates a thin coating of barium, and barium pooling is limited to one third of the intestinal diameter.

- *Good double-contrast lower intestinal filling.* Good gaseous distention is demonstrated when the bowel lumina are distended, eliminating the mucosal folds and allowing all parts of the barium-coated mucosal lining of the colon and any small intraluminal lesions to be visualized. Good lower intestinal barium coating has been obtained when the surface positioned farther from the IR on recumbent projections or superiorly on erect projections, also called the nondependent surface, demonstrates a thin layer of barium coating on the mucosal surface, and when the surface positioned closer to the IR on recumbent projections or inferiorly on erect projections, also called the dependent (decubitus) surface, demonstrates a thin layer of barium coating of the highest structures, with barium pooled in the lower crevices. The barium pools are used to wash away residual fecal material from the dependent surface, coat the mucosal surface, and fill any depressed lesions as the patient is rotated. Ideally, barium should fill one third of the large intestine diameter; overfilling or underfilling may result in obscured lesions or inadequate intestinal washing, respectively. See Table 12-3 to determine where barium pooling will occur on a lower intestine image. Pooling will occur in the anterior surface on prone projections, posterior surface on supine projections and, inferiorly, between the mucosal folds, on erect projections.
- *Poor double contrast.* Poor gaseous distension results in pockets of large barium pools, compacted intestinal segments with tight mucosal folds. Poor mucosal coating is demonstrated by thin, irregular, or interrupted barium coating or excessive barium pooling. Poor coating may cause lesions to be easily missed. Although proper double-contrast filling is primarily the fluoroscopist's responsibility, the technologist's scope of practice may play a part in some of the causes for poor coating, such as using the wrong type of barium, improperly preparing the barium suspension, or performing poor lower intestinal preparation.

LARGE INTESTINE: POSTEROANTERIOR OR ANTEROPOSTERIOR PROJECTION

See Figures 12-35 and 12-36 and Box 12-11.
The abdomen is in a PA or AP projection. The spinous processes are aligned with the midline of the vertebral bodies, the distances from the pedicles to the spinous processes are the same on both sides, and the iliac ala are symmetrical. The ascending and descending limbs of the colic flexures demonstrate some degree of superimposition.

- To obtain a PA large intestine projection, place the patient prone on the imaging table. To obtain an AP large intestine projection, place the patient supine on the imaging table. Position the shoulders and ASISs at equal distances from the imaging table to prevent rotation, and draw the patient's arms away from the abdominal area to prevent them from being superimposed over the abdominal region (Figure 12-37).

TABLE 12-3	Double-Contrast Filling of Large Intestinal Structures	
Large Intestine	**Supine Position**	**Prone Position**
Cecum	Air	Barium
Ascending colon	Barium	Air
Ascending limb right colic (hepatic) flexure	Barium	Air
Descending limb right colic (hepatic) flexure	Barium	Air
Transverse colon	Air	Barium
Ascending limb left colic (splenic) flexure	Air	Barium
Descending limb left colic (splenic) flexure	Barium	Air
Descending colon	Barium	Air
Sigmoid colon	Air	Barium
Rectum	Barium	Air

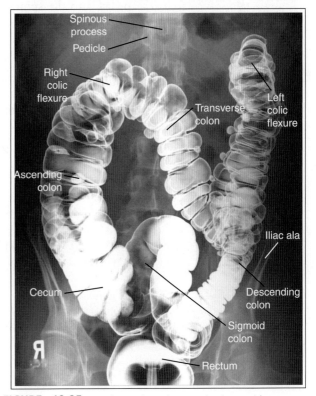

FIGURE 12-35 PA large intestine projection with accurate positioning.

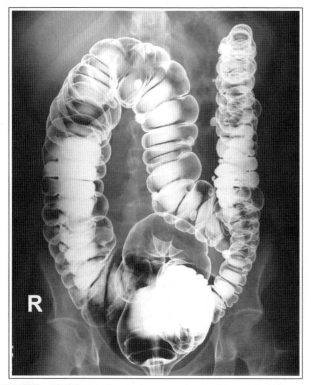

FIGURE 12-36 AP large intestine projection with accurate positioning.

| BOX 12-11 | Posteroanterior-Anteroposterior Large Intestinal Projection Analysis Criteria |

- The spinous processes are aligned with the midline of the vertebral bodies, distances from the pedicles to spinous processes are the same on both sides, and the iliac ala are symmetrical. The ascending and descending limbs of the colic flexure demonstrate some degree of superimposition.
- The fourth lumbar vertebra is at the center of the exposure field.
- The entire large intestine, including the left colic flexure and rectum, is included within the collimated field.

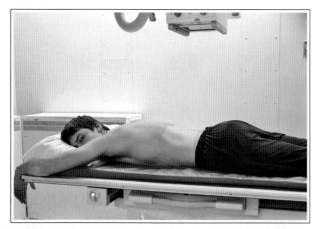

FIGURE 12-37 Proper patient positioning for PA large intestine projection.

- *Detecting abdominal rotation.* Rotation is effectively detected on a PA or AP lower intestine projection by comparing the distances from the pedicles to the spinous processes on both sides, the symmetry of the iliac ala, and the superimposition of the colic flexures.

PA projection. The side demonstrating the greater distance from the pedicles to the spinous processes, wider iliac ala, and colic flexure with greater ascending and descending limb superimposition is the side positioned farther from the IR (see Image 12).

AP projection. The side demonstrating the greater distance from the pedicle to the spinous processes, wider iliac ala, and colic flexure with the greater ascending and descending limb superimposition is the side positioned closer to the IR.

The beam divergence causes very different-appearing iliac alae on an image that is obtained in a supine versus a prone position. Figure 12-38 demonstrates the iliac alae of a supine and prone abdomen; note that the iliac alae in the image obtained with the patient supine are wider than with the patient prone. This information can be used to distinguish whether the image was taken with the patient in a supine or prone position. The narrow iliac ala of a prone projection should not be mistaken for narrowness caused by rotation.

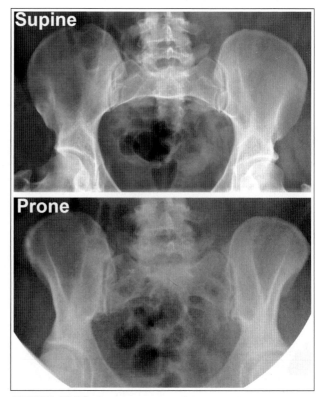

FIGURE 12-38 Iliac alae images of supine and prone patient.

The fourth lumbar vertebra is centered within the exposure field. The entire large intestine, including the left colic (splenic) flexure and rectum, is included within the collimated field.

- To position the fourth lumbar vertebra in the center of the exposure field, center a perpendicular central ray with the patient's midsagittal plane at the level of the iliac crest. Center the IR to the central ray. The longitudinal collimated field should remain fully open. Transversely collimate to within 0.5 inch (0.6 cm) of the patient's lateral skin line.
- *IR size and direction.* A 14- × 17-inch (35- × 43-cm) lengthwise IR should be adequate to include all the required anatomic structures on sthenic and asthenic patients as long as the transverse abdominal measurement is less than 14 inches (35 cm).

   Use two 14- × 17-inch (35- × 43-cm) crosswise IRs on hypersthenic patients and on other patients who have a transverse abdominal measurement of 14 inches (35 cm) or more to include all the necessary anatomic structures (Figure 12-39; see Image 13). Take the first projection with the central ray centered to the midsagittal plane at a level halfway between the symphysis pubis and ASIS. Position the bottom of the second IR so that it includes 2 to 3 inches (5 to 7.5 cm) of the same transverse section of the peritoneal cavity imaged on the first projection to ensure that no middle peritoneal information has been excluded. The top of the IR should extend to the patient's xiphoid (which is at the level of the tenth thoracic vertebra) to make sure that the left colic (splenic) flexure is included.

Posteroanterior or Anteroposterior Large Intestine Projection Analysis

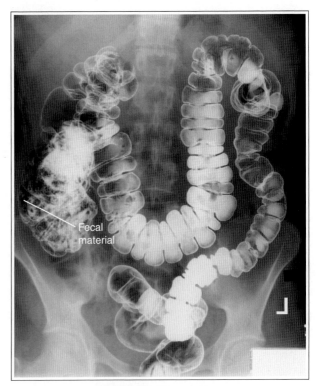

IMAGE 11 PA projection.

Analysis. PA projection—remaining fecal material is visible in the cecum. Fecal material may obscure the mucosal surfaces and, when barium-coated, may mimic polyps and small tumors.

Correction. The patient should follow the large intestinal preparation procedure before examination.

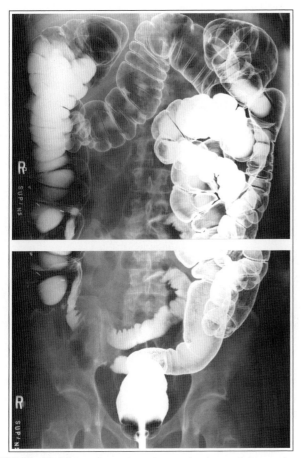

FIGURE 12-39 AP large intestine projections of hypersthenic patient with accurate positioning.

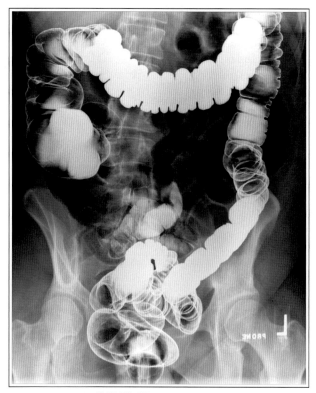

IMAGE 12 PA projection.

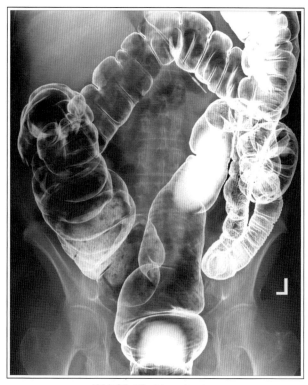

IMAGE 13 PA projection.

Analysis. PA projection—the right iliac ala is narrow, the left iliac ala is wide, the distance from the right pedicles to the spinous processes is narrower than the same distance on the left side, and the left colic (splenic) flexure demonstrates greater ascending and descending limb superimposition. The patient was rotated toward the right side.

Correction. Rotate the patient toward the left side until the shoulders and iliac alae are at equal distances to the imaging table.

Analysis. PA projection—the left colic (splenic) flexure and part of the transverse colon are not included on the image. The IR is not adequate to include the entire large intestine.

Correction. Use two crosswise IRs with 2 to 3 inches of overlap.

LARGE INTESTINE (RECTUM): LATERAL PROJECTION

See Figure 12-40 and Box 12-12.

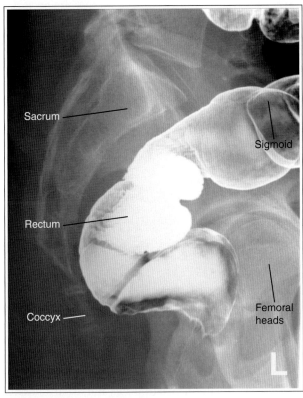

FIGURE 12-40 Lateral large intestine (rectum) projection with accurate positioning.

BOX 12-12	Lateral Large Intestinal (Rectum) Projection Analysis Criteria

- The rectum is in profile. The sacrum demonstrates a lateral projection. The median sacral crest is in profile and the femoral heads are superimposed.
- The rectosigmoid region is at the center of the exposure field.
- The rectum, distal sigmoid, sacrum, and femoral heads are included within the collimated field.

Scatter radiation is controlled.

- A grid and lead sheet are placed on the imaging table at the edge of the posteriorly collimated field to reduce the amount of scatter radiation that reaches the IR, providing higher contrast and better visibility of recorded details.

The rectum is in profile. The sacrum demonstrates a lateral projection. The median sacral crest is in profile, and the femoral heads are superimposed.

- To obtain a lateral sacral projection, place the patient on the imaging table in a lateral recumbent position. Whether the patient is lying on the right or left side is not significant, although the left side positioning is easier for the technologist.

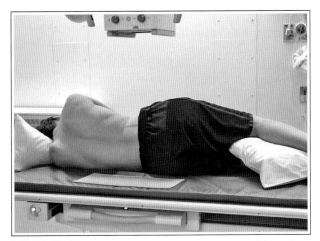

FIGURE 12-41 Proper patient positioning for lateral large intestine projection.

Flex the patient's knees and hips for support, and position a pillow or sponge between the knees. The pillow or sponge should be thick enough to prevent the side of the pelvis situated farther from the IR from rotating anteriorly, without being so thick as to cause this side to rotate posteriorly (Figure 12-41).

To avoid rectal and vertebral rotation, align the shoulders, posterior ribs, and posterior pelvis perpendicular to the imaging table and IR. This is accomplished by resting your extended flat palm against each structure individually and adjusting the patient's rotation until your hand is positioned perpendicular to the imaging table.

- *Detecting rotation.* Rotation can be detected on a lateral rectum projection by evaluating the degree of femoral head superimposition. On a nonrotated lateral rectal projection, the femoral heads are directly superimposed. On rotation, the femoral heads will move away from each other. When rotation has occurred, evaluate the placement of the femoral heads to determine the way in which the patient was rotated. The femoral head that demonstrates the greater magnification is the one situated farther from the IR (see Images 14 and 15).

The rectosigmoid region is at the center of the exposure field. The rectum, distal sigmoid, sacrum, and femoral heads are included within the collimated field.

- To place the rectosigmoid region in the center of the exposure field, center a perpendicular central ray to the midcoronal plane (between the ASIS and posterior sacrum) at the level of the ASIS. Center the IR to the central ray.
- Open the longitudinal and transverse collimation to the full IR field size.
- A 10- × 12-inch (24- × 30-cm) IR placed lengthwise should be adequate to include all the required anatomic structures.

Lateral Large Intestine (Rectum) Projection Analysis

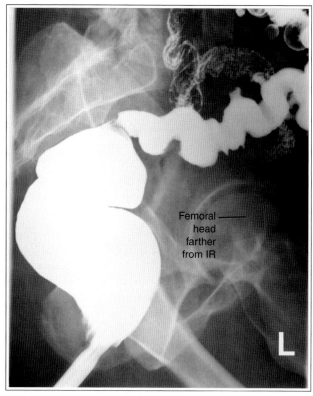

IMAGE 14

Analysis. A lateral position has not been obtained. The femoral heads are not superimposed; the right femoral head is rotated anterior to the left femoral head.

Correction. Rotate the right side of the patient posteriorly until the posterior pelvic wings are superimposed and aligned perpendicular to the imaging table.

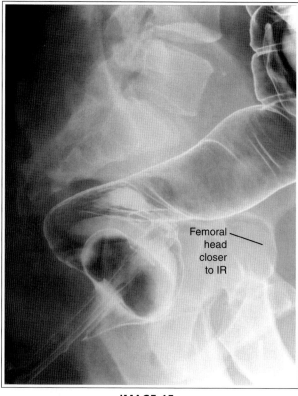

IMAGE 15

Analysis. A lateral position has not been obtained. The femoral heads are not superimposed; the right femoral head is rotated posterior to the left femoral head.

Correction. Rotate the right side of the patient anteriorly until the posterior pelvis wings are superimposed and aligned perpendicular to the imaging table.

LARGE INTESTINE: ANTEROPOSTERIOR OR POSTEROANTERIOR PROJECTION (LATERAL DECUBITUS POSITION)

See Figures 12-42 and 12-43 and Box 12-13.

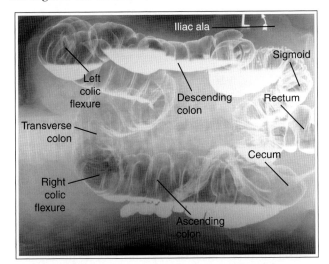

FIGURE 12-42 AP large intestine projection (right lateral decubitus position) with accurate positioning.

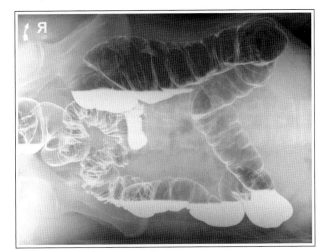

FIGURE 12-43 PA large intestine projection (left lateral decubitus position) with accurate positioning.

An arrow or word marker is present on the image, indicating the side of patient that was positioned up and away from the imaging table or cart.

- Place the marker superiorly, away from anatomic structures of interest, and within the collimated field.

Density is uniform across abdominal structures.

- *Using a wedge-compensating filter.* When an AP-PA (lateral decubitus) large intestine projection is obtained in a patient with excessive abdominal soft tissue, the soft tissue often drops toward the imaging table or cart. This movement results in a smaller AP measurement at the elevated side than at the side closer to the imaging table or cart. To compensate for this thickness difference, a wedge-compensating filter may be used. Attach the wedge-compensating filter to the x-ray collimator head with the thick end positioned toward the patient's "up" side (thinnest part of abdomen) and the thin end toward the patient's "down" side (thickest part of abdomen). Then set a technique that will accurately expose the middle section of the abdomen. When the filter has been accurately positioned, image density is uniform throughout the abdominal structures. Positioning the filter too close to or too far away from the thickest part of the abdomen results in an overexposed or underexposed area on the image, respectively, and a line of density difference. If the compensating filter is inaccurately positioned, a density variation line will appear, defining where the filter was and was not placed over the structures (see Image 16).

BOX 12-13 | **Anteroposterior-Posteroanterior Large Intestinal Projection (Lateral Decubitus Position) Analysis Criteria**

- The arrow or word marker that indicates the side of patient that is positioned up and away from the imaging table or cart is present.
- Density is uniform across abdominal structures.
- The spinous processes are aligned with the midline to the vertebral bodies, the distances from the pedicles to the spinous processes are the same on both sides, and the iliac alae are symmetrical. The ascending and descending limbs of the colic flexures demonstrate some degree of superimposition.
- The abdominal field positioned against the imaging table or cart is seen in its entirety and without artifact lines.
- The fourth lumbar vertebra is at the center of the exposure field.
- The entire large intestine, including the left colic flexure and rectum, is included within the collimated field.

The abdomen demonstrates an AP or PA projection. The spinous processes are aligned with the midline of the vertebral bodies, the distances from the pedicles to the spinous processes are the same on both sides, and the iliac alae are symmetrical. The ascending and descending limbs of the colic flexures demonstrate some degree of superimposition.

- AP or PA large intestine projections (lateral decubitus position) are obtained by placing the patient in left and right lateral recumbent positions on the imaging table or cart with the back or abdomen resting against a grid cassette or the upright IR holder. To avoid rotation, align the shoulders, the posterior ribs, and the posterior pelvis perpendicular to the imaging table or cart (Figure 12-44). Accomplish this alignment by resting an extended flat hand against each, respectively, and then adjusting the patient's rotation until the hand is positioned perpendicular to the imaging table or cart. Flex the patient's knees to support the patient's lateral position, although do not bring them to a 90-degree angle with the torso or they may be superimposed over the lateral aspect of the distal

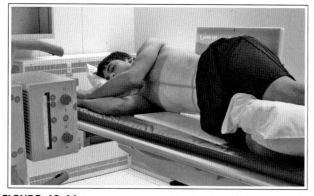

FIGURE 12-44 Proper patient positioning for AP large intestine projection (right lateral decubitus position).

rectum (see Image 17). It is most common for a patient to rotate the elevated thorax and iliac ala anteriorly. A pillow or other support placed between the patient's flexed knees may help eliminate this forward rotation.

- *Detecting abdominal rotation.* Rotation is effectively detected on a PA or AP lower intestine projection (lateral decubitus position) by comparing the distance from the pedicles to the spinous processes on each side, the symmetry of the iliac ala, and the superimposition of the colic flexures.

  PA decubitus projection. The side demonstrating the greater distance from the pedicles to the spinous processes, wider iliac ala, and colic flexure with greater ascending and descending limb superimposition is the side positioned farther from the IR (see Image 18).

  AP decubitus projection. The side demonstrating the greater distance from the pedicle to the spinous processes, wider iliac ala, and colic flexure with greater ascending and descending limb superimposition is the side positioned closer to the IR (see Image 19).

The abdominal field positioned against the imaging table or cart is demonstrated in its entirety and without artifact lines.

- Elevating the patient on a radiolucent sponge or hard surface such as a cardiac board positions the patient's abdomen above the IR's cassette border, preventing part of the abdomen from being clipped and preventing the abdomen from sinking into the table or cart pad. When the patient's body is allowed to sink into the cart pad, artifact lines are superimposed over the lateral abdominal field of the side that is down (see Image 17).

The fourth lumbar vertebra is centered within the exposure field. The entire large intestine, including the left colic (splenic) flexure and rectum, is included within the collimated field.

- To position the fourth lumbar vertebra in the center of the exposure field, center a perpendicular central

ray with the patient's midsagittal plane at the level of the iliac crest. Center the IR to the central ray.

- The longitudinal collimated field should remain fully open. Transversely collimate to within 0.5 inch (1.25 cm) of the patient's lateral skin line.
- *IR size and direction.* A 14- × 17-inch (35- × 43-cm) lengthwise IR should be adequate to include all the required anatomic structures on sthenic and asthenic patients, as long as the transverse abdominal measurement is less than 14 inches (35 cm).
- Use two 14- × 17-inch (35- × 43-cm) crosswise IRs on *hypersthenic* patients and on other patients who have a transverse abdominal measurement of 14 inches (35 cm) or more to include all the necessary anatomic structures. Take the first projection with the central ray centered to the midsagittal plane at a level halfway between the symphysis pubis and ASIS. Position the bottom of the second IR so that it includes 2 to 3 inches (5 to 7.5 cm) of the same transverse section of the peritoneal cavity imaged on the first projection to ensure that no middle peritoneal information has been excluded. The top of the IR should extend to the patient's xiphoid (which is at the level of the tenth thoracic vertebra) to make sure that the left colic (splenic) flexure is included.

Anteroposterior or Posteroanterior Large Intestine Projection (Lateral Decubitus Position) Analysis

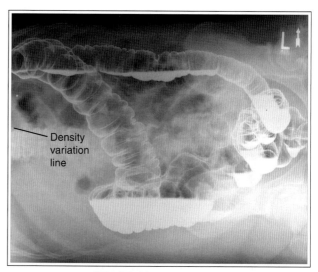

IMAGE 16 AP projection.

Analysis. AP projection—the image density is not uniform across the abdomen. The right side of the abdomen is slightly underexposed, and the left side is slightly overexposed. Too much thickness of the compensating filter was positioned over the right side of the abdomen. A density difference line defines where the filter was and was not placed correctly over the abdomen.

Correction. Move the filter so that less thickness is present over the right side of the abdomen.

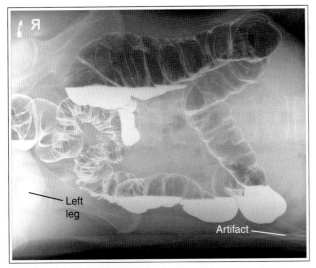

IMAGE 17 PA projection.

Analysis. PA projection—artifact lines are superimposed over the left lateral abdominal region. The patient was not elevated on a radiolucent sponge. An underexposed area is present on the left side of the rectum. The patient's knee was bent to 90 degrees.

Correction. Elevate the patient on a radiolucent sponge or cardiac board to prevent the side of the abdomen from sinking into the table or cart pad. Decrease the amount of knee flexion.

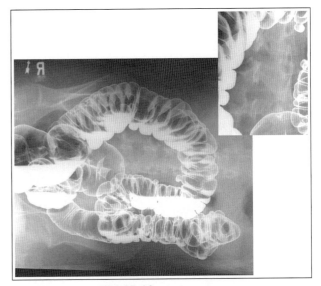

IMAGE 18 PA projection.

Analysis. PA projection—the distance from the right pedicles to the spinous processes is less than the distance from the left pedicles to the spinous processes, the right iliac ala is narrower than the left, and the ascending and descending limbs of the left colic (splenic) flexure demonstrate increased superimposition. The right side of the patient was positioned closer to the IR than the left side.

Correction. Rotate the left side of the patient away from the IR until the shoulders and iliac ala are at equal distances to the IR.

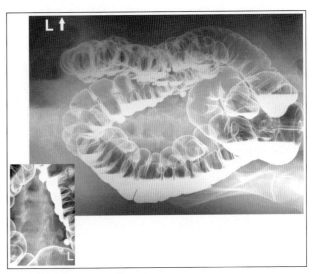

IMAGE 19 AP projection.

Analysis. AP projection—the distance from the right pedicles to the spinous processes is less than the distance from the left pedicles to the spinous processes, the left iliac ala is wider than the right, and the left colic (splenic) flexure demonstrates increased superimposition. The left side of the patient was positioned closer to the IR than the right side.

Correction. Rotate the left side of the patient away from the IR until the shoulders and ASISs are at equal distances from the IR.

LARGE INTESTINE: POSTEROANTERIOR OBLIQUE PROJECTION (RIGHT ANTERIOR OBLIQUE POSITION)

See Figure 12-45 and Box 12-14.

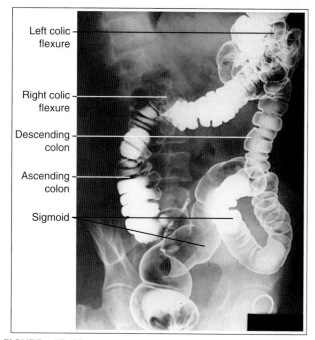

FIGURE 12-45 PA oblique large intestine projection (RAO position) with accurate positioning. *(From Frank ED, Long BW, Smith BJ. Merrill's atlas of radiographic positions and radiologic procedures, vol 2, ed 10, St. Louis, 2007, Mosby, p. 179.)*

BOX 12-14	Posteroanterior Oblique Large Intestinal Projection (Right Anterior Oblique Position) Analysis Criteria

- The ascending and descending limbs of the right colic flexure are seen with decreased superimposition when compared to the PA projection, whereas the limbs of the left colic flexure demonstrate increased superimposition and the rectosigmoid segments are seen without transverse superimposition.
- The right iliac ala is narrower than the left, and the distances from the right pedicles to the spinous processes are narrower than the distances from the left pedicles to the spinous processes.
- The midabdomen is at the center of the exposure field.
- The entire large intestine is included within the collimated field.

The ascending and descending limbs of the right colic (hepatic) flexure are demonstrated with decreased superimposition when compared with the PA projection, whereas the limbs of the left colic (splenic) flexure demonstrate increased superimposition and the rectosigmoid segments are demonstrated without transverse superimposition. The right iliac ala is narrow and the left is

wide, and the distances from the right pedicles to the spinous processes are narrower than the distances from the left pedicles to the spinous processes.

- A PA oblique large intestine projection (RAO position) is obtained by positioning the patient prone on the imaging table and then rotating the torso toward the right side until the midcoronal plane is at a 35- to 45-degree angle with the imaging table. In the PA projection, the descending limb of the right colic (hepatic) flexure is superimposed over the ascending limb and the rectum is superimposed over the distal sigmoid. Rotating the patient toward the right side moves the ascending right colic limb from beneath the descending limb and the distal sigmoid from beneath the rectum (transversely), allowing better visualization of these structures. The left elbow and knee are partially flexed and are used to support the patient and maintain accurate obliquity (Figure 12-46).
- *Detecting inadequate rotation on a PA oblique projection.* Insufficient rotation of the colon is demonstrated on the PA oblique projection when the ascending and descending limbs of the right colic flexure are superimposed and the rectum is superimposed over the distal sigmoid (see Image 20).

The midabdomen is at the center of the exposure field. The entire large intestine is included within the collimated field.

- To place the midabdomen in the center of the exposure field, center a perpendicular central ray approximately 1 to 2 inches (2.5 to 5 cm) to the left of the midsagittal plane at the level of the iliac crest. Center the IR to the central ray.
- The longitudinal collimated field should remain fully open. Transversely collimate to within 0.5 inch (1.25 cm) of the patient's lateral skin line.
- *IR size and direction.* A 14- × 17-inch (35- × 43-cm) IR placed lengthwise should be adequate to include all the required anatomic structures.

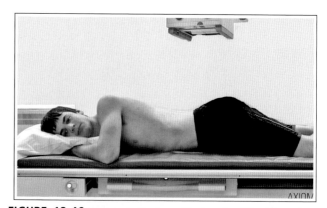

FIGURE 12-46 Proper patient positioning for PA oblique large intestine projection (RAO position).

Posteroanterior Oblique Large Intestine Projection (Right Anterior Oblique Position) Analysis

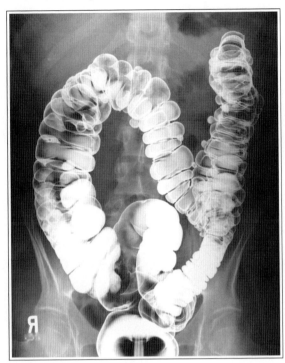

IMAGE 20

Analysis. The ascending and descending limbs of the right colic (hepatic) flexure and the rectum and distal sigmoid, respectively, demonstrate increased superimposition. The iliac ala are uniform in width. The patient was insufficiently rotated.

Correction. Rotate the patient toward the right side until the midsagittal plane is at a 35- to 45-degree angle with the IR.

LARGE INTESTINE: POSTEROANTERIOR OBLIQUE PROJECTION (LEFT ANTERIOR OBLIQUE POSITION)

See Figure 12-47 and Box 12-15.

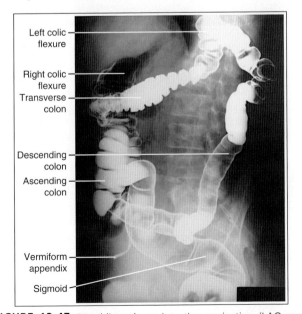

Left colic flexure
Right colic flexure
Transverse colon
Descending colon
Ascending colon
Vermiform appendix
Sigmoid

FIGURE 12-47 PA oblique large intestine projection (LAO position) with accurate positioning. *(Frank ED, Long BW, Smith BJ. Merrill's atlas of radiographic positions and radiologic procedures, vol 2, ed 10, St. Louis, 2007, Mosby, p. 180.)*

BOX 12-15 | **Posteroanterior Oblique Large Intestinal Projection (Left Anterior Oblique Position) Analysis Criteria**

- The ascending and descending limbs of the left colic flexure are seen with decreased superimposition when compared with a PA projection, whereas the limbs of the right colic flexure demonstrate increased superimposition.
- The left iliac ala is narrower than the right and the distances from the left pedicles to the spinous processes are narrower than the distances from the right pedicles to the spinous processes.
- The midabdomen is at the center of the exposure field.
- The entire large intestine is included within the collimated field.

The ascending and descending limbs of the left colic (splenic) flexure are demonstrated with decreased superimposition when compared with the PA projection, whereas the limbs of the right colic (hepatic) flexure demonstrate increased superimposition. The left iliac ala is narrow and the right is wide, and the distances from the left pedicles to the spinous processes are narrower than the distances from the right pedicles to the spinous processes.

- A PA oblique large intestine projection (left anterior oblique [LAO]) is obtained by positioning the

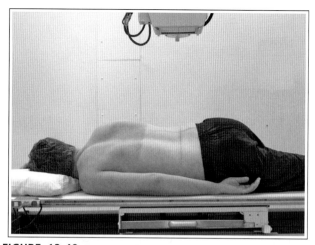

FIGURE 12-48 Proper patient positioning for PA oblique large intestine projection (LAO position).

LARGE INTESTINE: POSTEROANTERIOR AXIAL PROJECTION OR POSTEROANTERIOR AXIAL OBLIQUE PROJECTION (RIGHT ANTERIOR OBLIQUE POSITION)

See Figure 12-49 and Box 12-16.

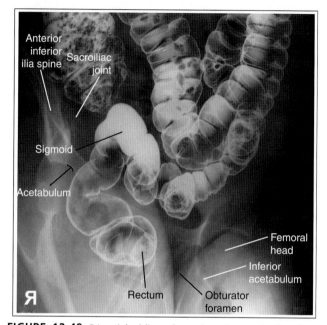

FIGURE 12-49 PA axial oblique large intestine projection (RAO position) with accurate positioning.

BOX 12-16	Posteroanterior Axial Large Intestinal Projection and Posteroanterior Axial Oblique Large Intestinal Projection (Right Anterior Oblique Position) Analysis Criteria

- PA axial: The iliac alae and obturator foramen are symmetrical.
- PA axial oblique: The rectosigmoid segments are seen without transverse superimposition, the right sacroiliac joint is shown just medial to the ASIS, and the left obturator foramen is open.
- The rectosigmoid segment is demonstrated without inferosuperior superimposition, the pelvis is elongated, and the left inferior acetabulum is at the level of the distal rectum.
- The rectosigmoid area is at the center of the exposure field.
- The rectum, sigmoid, and pelvic structures are included within the collimated field.

ASIS, Anterior superior iliac spine.

patient prone on the imaging table and then rotating the torso toward the left side until the midcoronal plane is at a 35- to 45-degree angle with the imaging table. In the PA projection, the descending limb of the left colic (splenic) flexure is superimposed over the ascending limb, and the rectum is superimposed over the distal sigmoid. Rotating the patient toward the left side moves the descending left colic limb from beneath the ascending limb, allowing better visualization of these structures. The right elbow and knee are partially flexed and are used to support the patient and maintain accurate obliquity (Figure 12-48).

- *Detecting inadequate rotation on a PA oblique projection.* Insufficient rotation of the colon is demonstrated on the PA oblique projection when the ascending and descending limbs of the left colic flexure are superimposed.

The midabdomen is at the center of the exposure field. The entire large intestine is included within the collimated field.

- To place the midabdomen in the center of the exposure field, center a perpendicular central ray approximately 1 to 2 inches (2.5 to 5 cm) to the right of the midsagittal plane at the level 1 to 2 inches (2.5 to 5 cm) superior to the iliac crest. Center the IR to the central ray.
- The longitudinal collimated field should remain fully open. Transversely collimate to within 0.5 inch (1.25 cm) of the patient's lateral skin line.
- *IR size and direction.* A 14- × 17-inch (35- × 43-cm) lengthwise IR placed lengthwise should be adequate to include all the required anatomic structures.

PA axial: **The pelvis is demonstrated without rotation. The iliac alae and obturator foramen are symmetrical.**

- A PA axial large intestine projection is obtained by positioning the patient prone on the imaging table with the legs extended. Position the shoulders and ASISs at equal distances from the imaging table to prevent rotation (Figure 12-50).

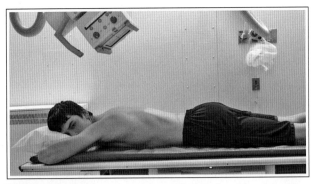

FIGURE 12-50 Proper patient positioning for PA axial oblique large intestine projection (RAO position).

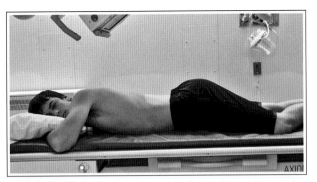

FIGURE 12-51 Proper patient positioning for PA axial large intestine projection.

- *Detecting rotation on a PA axial projection.* Rotation is effectively detected on a PA axial large intestine projection by evaluating the symmetry of the iliac alae and obturator foramen. If the patient was rotated away from the prone position, the iliac ala positioned farther from the IR will increase in width, the iliac ala positioned closer to the IR will narrow, the obturator foramina positioned farther from the IR will narrow, and the obturator foramina positioned closer to the IR will widen.

PA axial oblique projection (RAO position): The pelvis demonstrates adequate rotation when the rectosigmoid segments are demonstrated without transverse superimposition, the right sacroiliac (SI) joint is shown just medial to the ASIS, and the left obturator foramen is open.

- A PA axial oblique large intestine projection (RAO position) is obtained by positioning the patient prone on the imaging table and then rotating the torso toward the right side until the midcoronal plane is at a 35- to 45-degree angle with the imaging table. In the PA projection, the rectum is superimposed over the distal sigmoid, obscuring the rectosigmoid junction. Rotating the patient toward the right side moves the sigmoid from beneath the rectum (transversely), allowing better demonstration of this area. The left elbow and knee are partially flexed and are used to support the patient and maintain accurate obliquity (Figure 12-51).
- *Detecting inadequate rotation on a PA axial oblique projection.* Insufficient pelvic rotation of the rectosigmoid and pelvic area is demonstrated on the PA axial oblique projection when the rectum is superimposed over the sigmoid colon, the right SI joint is too medial to the ASIS, and the left obturator foramen is narrowed. Too much pelvic rotation is demonstrated when the right SI joint is obscured and the left obturator foramen is closed (see Images 21 and 22).

The rectosigmoid segment is demonstrated without inferosuperior superimposition, the pelvis demonstrates elongation, and the left inferior acetabulum is at the level of the distal rectum.

- The PA axial oblique (RAO position) and PA axial projections of the large intestine are obtained to demonstrate the rectosigmoid area with less superimposition. To move the posteriorly situated rectum inferiorly and off the distal sigmoid, a 30- to 40-degree caudal angulation is used, decreasing rectosigmoid superimposition and better demonstrating the area. This angulation also elongates the pelvic structures.
- *Inadequate angulation.* When the rectosigmoid segment demonstrates inferosuperior overlap, the central ray angulation used was inadequate. If the inferior aspect of the left acetabulum is demonstrated superior to the distal rectum, the central ray was insufficient (see Image 21). If the inferior aspect of the left acetabulum is demonstrated inferior to the distal rectum, the central ray angulation was too great (see Image 22).

The rectosigmoid area is at the center of the exposure field. The rectum, sigmoid, and pelvic structures are included within the collimated field.

- *PA axial projection.* To place the rectosigmoid area at the center of the exposure field, center the central ray to exit at the level of the ASIS and to the midsagittal plane.
- *PA axial oblique projection.* To place the rectosigmoid area in the center of the field, center the central ray to the exit at the ASIS and 2 inches (5 cm) to the left of the lumbar spinous processes. Center the IR to the central ray.
- An 11- × 14-inch (28- × 35-cm) or 14- × 17-inch (35- × 43-cm) IR placed lengthwise should be adequate to include all the required anatomic structures.

Posteroanterior Axial Oblique Large Intestine Projection (Right Anterior Oblique Position) Analysis

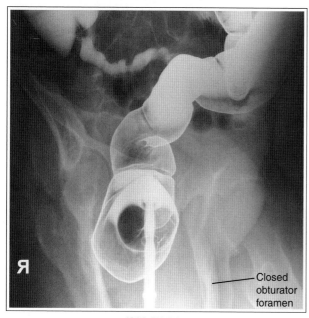

Closed obturator foramen

IMAGE 21

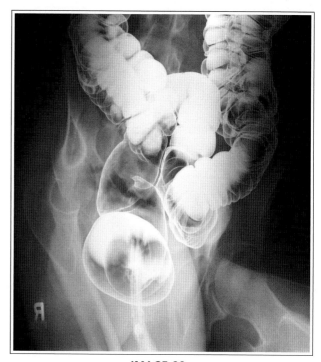

IMAGE 22

Analysis. The right SI joint is obscured. The pelvis was rotated more than 45 degrees. The inferior aspect of the left acetabulum is demonstrated superior to the distal rectum. The central ray was insufficient.

Correction. Decrease pelvic rotation until the mid-coronal plane is at a 30- to 45-degree angle with the imaging table, and increase the degree of central ray angulation.

Analysis. The right SI joint is obscured. The pelvis was rotated more than 45 degrees. The inferior aspect of the left acetabulum is demonstrated inferior to the distal rectum. The central ray angulation was too great.

Correction. Decrease pelvic rotation until the mid-coronal plane is at a 30- to 45-degree angle with the imaging table, and decrease the degree of central ray angulation.

Adler A, Carlton R: *Introduction to radiologic sciences and patient care*, ed 4, St. Louis, 2007, Elsevier.

Bontrager K, Lampignano J: *Textbook of radiographic positioning and related anatomy*, ed 6, St. Louis, 2005, Elsevier.

Bushong SC: *Radiologic science for technologists*, ed 9, St. Louis, 2008, Elsevier.

Carroll QB: *Practical radiographic imaging*, ed 8, Springfield, Ill, 2003, Charles C Thomas.

Ehrlich RA, McCloskey ED, Daly JA: *Patient care in radiography*, ed 6, St. Louis, 2004, Mosby.

Eisenberg RL: *Gastrointestinal radiology: A pattern approach*, ed 4, Philadelphia, 2002, Lippincott Williams & Wilkins.

Fauber TL: *Radiographic imaging and exposure*, ed 3, St. Louis, 2008, Elsevier.

Frank ED, Long BW, Smith BJ: *Merrill's atlas of radiographic positioning and radiologic procedures*, ed 11, St. Louis, Missouri, 2007, Elsevier.

Fraser RG, Colman N, Muller N, Pare P: *Synopsis of diseases of the chest*, ed 3, Philadelphia, 2005, WB Saunders.

Jeffrey RB, Ralls PW, Leung AN, Brant-Zawadzki M: *Emergency imaging*, Philadelphia, 1999, Lippincott Williams & Wilkins.

Levine MS, Rubesin SE, Laufer I: *Double contrast gastro–intestinal radiology*, ed 3, Philadelphia, 2000, WB Saunders.

Rogers LF: *Radiology of skeletal trauma*, ed 3, New York, 2002, Churchill Livingstone.

Shephard CT: *Radiographic image production and manipulation*, New York, 2003, McGraw-Hill.

Standring S: *Gray's anatomy: The anatomical basis of clinical practice*, ed 39, St. Louis, 2004, Churchill Livingstone.

Statkiewicz MA, Visconti PJ, Ritenour ER: *Radiation protection in medical radiography*, ed 5, St. Louis, 2006, Elsevier.

Thornton A, Gyll C: *Children's fracture: A radiological guide to safe practice*, London, 2000, Baillière Tindall.

Tortora GJ, Derrickson BH: *Principles of anatomy and physiology*, ed 12, New York, 2008, John Wiley & Sons.

Ward R, Blickman H: *Pediatric imaging*, St. Louis, 2005, Mosby.

Williamson SL: *Primary pediatric radiology*, Philadelphia, 2002, WB Saunders.

abduct To move an extremity outward, away from the torso. The humerus is abducted when it is elevated laterally.

acanthiomeatal line Imaginary line connecting the point where the upper lip and nose meet with the external ear opening.

additive disease Condition that results in change to the normal bony structures, soft tissues, or air or fluid content of the patient; may require technical changes to compensate for them prior to exposing the patient. Additive diseases cause the tissues to increase density or thickness, resulting in them being more radiopaque.

adduct To move an extremity toward the torso. The humerus is adducted when it is positioned closer to the torso after being abducted.

adductor tubercle Round bony structure located posteriorly on the medial aspect of the femur, just superior to the medial condyle.

air-gap technique Technique of positioning the patient at a distance (10–15 cm) from the image receptor (IR) to reduce the amount of scatter radiation that reaches the IR and increases radiographic contrast.

ALARA Acronym for keeping radiation exposure "*a*s *l*ow as *r*easonably *a*chievable."

algorithm Set of rules or directions for getting a specific outcome from a specific input.

align To bring into line or alignment. *The lower leg and foot are aligned at a 90-degree angle with each other for a lateral foot image.*

anatomic position Refers to positioning the patient with the arms and legs extended and the face, arms, hands, legs, and feet placed in an anteroposterior (AP) projection. This is the starting point from which imaging procedures are referenced.

anode heel effect Absorption of radiation in the heel of the anode that results in less x-ray intensity at the anode side of a long IR when compared to the cathode side.

anterior (antero-) Refers to the front surface of the patient, used to express something situated at or directed toward the front; includes the palms and tops of the feet as in anatomic position. *The sternum is anterior to the vertebral column.*

anterior shoulder dislocation Condition in which the humeral head is demonstrated anteriorly beneath the coracoid.

articulation Joint or place where two bones meet.

artifact Undesirable structure or substance recorded on the image. It may or may not be covering information.

automatic exposure control (AEC) System used in radiography that automatically determines image density by stopping the exposure when adequate intensity has reached the IR.

automatic implantable cardioverter defibrillator (ICD) Used to detect heart arrhythmias and then deliver an electrical shock to the heart to convert it to a normal rhythm.

automatic rescaling Final phase of image processing in digital radiography during which the computer compares the image histogram with the selected lookup table and applies algorithms to the raw data to align the image histogram with the lookup table.

axilla Armpit.

backup timer Maximum time that the AEC x-ray exposure will be allowed to continue before automatically shutting off.

bilateral Both sides.

body habitus Body physique or type. Hypersthenic, sthenic, asthenic, and hyposthenic habitus are discerned in radiography to determine the size of IR to use and locations of the thoracic and peritoneal structures.

bony trabeculae Supporting material in cancellous bone. It is demonstrated on an image as thin white lines throughout a bony structure and is evaluated for changes.

breathing technique Technique in which a long exposure time (3–4 seconds) is used with costal breathing to blur the chest details surrounding the structure of interest.

brightness Describes the degree of luminance seen on the display monitor and refers to the degree of lightness (white) or lack of lightness (black) of the pixels in the image.

Bucky Refers to the Potter-Bucky diaphragm, a device underneath the imaging table that holds the IR and contains a grid to prevent scatter radiation from reaching the IR.

carpal canal Wrist passageway formed anteriorly by the flexor retinaculum, posteriorly by the capitate, laterally by the scaphoid and trapezium, and medially by the pisiform and hamate.

cathode ray tube (CRT) monitor Electronic monitor used for display and/or manipulation of the resulting digital image.

caudal Foot end of the patient. *A caudally angled central ray is directed toward the patient's feet.*

central ray Center of the x-ray beam. It is used to center the anatomic structure and IR.

central venous catheter (CVC) Catheter used to allow infusion of substances that are too toxic for peripheral infusion, such as for chemotherapy, total parenteral nutrition, dialysis, or blood transfusions.

cephalic Head end of the patient. *A cephalically angled central ray is directed toward the patient's head.*

compensating filter Absorbing substance added in the path of the x-ray beam that will remove photons from the beam. The filter is used to even out the density of structures that are imaged at the same time and vary in part thickness, such as the femur or lower leg.

computed radiography Projection radiography that uses photostimulable phosphor plates (imaging plates) as the IR.

concave Curved or rounded inward. *The anterior surface of the metacarpals is concave.*

condyle Rounded projection on a bone that often articulates with another bone.

contrast resolution Ability of an imaging system to resolve low-contrast objects on an image.

contrast Number of shades of gray that represent the different structures on the image.

convex Curved or rounded outward. *The posterior surface of the metacarpals is convex.*

coronal plane Imaginary plane that passes through the body from side to side and divides it into two (not necessarily equal) sections, one anterior and one posterior.

cortical outline Outer layer of a bone demonstrated on an image as the white outline of an anatomic structure.

costal breathing Slow shallow breathing; used with a long exposure time to blur chest details.

decubitus Refers to the patient lying down on a table or cart while a horizontally directed central ray is used; also used with the term *decubitus* is the surface (lateral, dorsal, or ventral) placed adjacent to the table or cart. *The patient is in a left lateral decubitus position.*

density Degree of darkness on an image.

depress To lower or sink down, positioning at a lower level.

destructive disease Condition that results in change to the normal bony structures, soft tissues, or air or fluid content of the patient; may require technical changes to compensate for them prior to exposing the patient. Destructive diseases cause the tissues to decrease mass density or thickness, resulting in them being more radiolucent.

detail Part of the whole structure. *The trabeculae are details in the femoral bone.*

deviate To move away from the normal or routine.

diagnostic specifier In computed radiography, examination indicator chosen by technologist before the plate is processed. It tells you the anatomic structure, position, and projection under which the image plate is to be processed.

differential absorption Radiographic contrast caused by the atomic density, atomic number, and thickness composition differences of the patient's body parts and how differently each tissue composition will absorb x-ray photons.

digital radiography (DR) System that uses detectors to convert x-ray energy to electrical energy that is delivered directly to a computer, where the anatomic image is digitally processed and displayed.

digitization Process of converting an analog image into digital (binary) data for processing by a computer.

distal (disto-) Refers to a structure that is situated away from the source or beginning. *The foot is distal to the ankle.* Or, *The splenic flexure is distal to the hepatic flexure.*

distortion The misrepresentation of the size or shape of the structure being examined.

dorsal (dorso-) See *posterior.*

dorsiflexion Backward bending, as of the hand or foot; brings toes and forefoot upward.

dorsoplantar projection X-ray beam that enters the top of the patient's foot and exits through the bottom of the foot.

dose-area product (DAP) Used in DR systems to monitor the radiation output and dose to the patient per volume of tissue irradiated.

dose equivalent limits Maximum permissible radiation dose limits; used for radiation protection purposes.

dynamic range Range of gray shades that the imaging system can display; measured by the bit capacity for each pixel.

EAM External auditory meatus.

elevate To lift up or raise, positioning at a higher level.

elongation To make one axis of an anatomic structure appear disproportionately longer on the image than the opposite axis. Angling the central ray while the part and IR remain parallel with each other will elongate the axis toward which the central ray is angled.

endotracheal tube (ETT) Stiff thick-walled tube used to inflate the lungs.

entrance skin exposure Absorbed dose to the most superficial layers of skin.

eversion Act of turning the plantar foot surface as far laterally as the ankle will allow.

exposure field recognition Digital radiography process in which the computer distinguishes the raw data representative of information within the exposure field from that which comes from outside the exposure field so that proper automatic rescaling can occur.

exposure indicator Readings obtained in computed radiography that express the amount of light given off by the imaging plate; indicates the amount of radiation exposure to the patient and imaging plate.

extension Movement that results in straightening of a joint. With extension of the elbow, the arm is straightened. Extension of the cervical vertebrae shifts the patient's head posteriorly in an attempt to separate the vertebral bodies.

external (lateral) rotation Act of turning the anterior surface of an extremity outward or away from the patient's torso midline.

fat pad Accumulation of adipose or fatty tissue that by its displacement can indicate joint effusion on radiographic images.

field of view (FOV) Area of the image receptor from where the image data is collected. For computed radiography, the area is the entire imaging plate and for direct or indirect digital radiography it is the detectors that are included in the exposure field, as determined by collimation.

flexion Movement that bends a joint. With flexion of the elbow, the arm is bent. Flexion of the cervical vertebrae shifts the patient's head forward in an attempt to bring the vertebral bodies closer.

foreshorten To make one axis of an anatomic structure appear disproportionately shorter on the image than the opposite axis. Positioning the long axis of the lower leg at a 45-degree angle with the IR while the central ray is perpendicular to the IR foreshortens the image of the lower leg on the image.

frog-leg position Position where the affected leg(s) is flexed and abducted to demonstrate a lateral projection of the hip and proximal femur.

glabelloalveolar line Imaginary line connecting the glabella and alveolar ridge.

gluteal fat plane Fat plane that is superior to the femoral neck.

grid cutoff Reduction in the amount of primary radiation reaching the IR because of poor central ray and grid alignment.

grid Device consisting of lead strips that is placed between the patient and IR to reduce the amount of scatter radiation reaching the receptor.

Hill-Sachs defect Posterolateral humeral head notch defect created by impingement of the articular surface of the humeral head against the anteroinferior rim of the glenoid cavity.

histogram analysis error Image histogram that includes raw data values in the volume of interest that should not be included; this results in a misshapen histogram that will not match the lookup table closely enough for the computer to rescale the data accurately.

histogram Graph that is generated from the raw data that has the pixel brightness value on the x-axis and the number of pixels with that brightness value on the y-axis.

homogeneous Uniformity between structures.

ID plate Area on the resulting image that indicates the patient and facility's identification information, procedure completed, and date and time that the procedure was completed.

iliopsoas fat plane Fat plane that lies within the pelvis medial to the lesser trochanters.

image acquisition Process of collecting x-ray transmission measurements from the patient.

image receptor (IR) Device that receives the radiation leaving the patient. Conventional radiography uses a screen-film system and computed radiography uses an imaging plate.

imaging plate (IP) 1. Plate used in computed radiography that is coated with a photostimulable phosphor material that absorbs the photons exiting the patient, resulting in the formation of a latent image that is released and digitized before being sent to a computer. 2. Thin flexible sheet of plastic with a photostimulable phosphor layer that is placed inside the computed radiography cassette to record the radiographic image; computed radiography's image receptor.

inferior (infero-) Refers to a structure within the patient's torso that is situated closer to the feet; used when comparing the locations of two structures. *The symphysis pubis is inferior to the iliac crest.*

infraorbital Below the orbits.

infraorbitomeatal line (IOML) Imaginary line connecting the inferior orbital margin and external acoustic opening.

interiliac line Imaginary line connecting the iliac crests.

intermalleolar line Imaginary line drawn between the medial and lateral malleoli.

internal (medial) rotation Act of turning the anterior surface of an extremity inward or toward the patient's torso midline.

interpupillary line Imaginary line connecting the outer corners of the eyelids.

intraperitoneal air Presence of free air in the abdominal cavity.

inverse square law Law that states that radiation intensity is inversely proportional to the square of its distance from the x-ray source.

inversion Act of turning the plantar foot surface as far medially as the ankle will allow.

involuntary motion Movement that the patient cannot control.

ionization chamber Chamber in the AEC system that collects radiation. For adequate radiographic density to result, the appropriate chamber must be selected for the part being imaged.

joint effusion Escape of fluid into the joint.

kVp Kilovoltage potential.

kyphosis Excessive posterior convexity of the thoracic vertebrae.

lateral (latero-) Refers to the patient's sides; used to express something that is directed or situated away from the patient's median plane or to express the outer side of an extremity: *The kidneys are lateral to the vertebral column.* Or, *Place the IR against the lateral surface of the knee.*

lateral mortise Talofibular joint.

lateral position Refers to positioning of the patient so that the side of the torso or extremity being imaged is placed adjacent to the IR. When a lateral position of the torso, vertebrae, or cranium is defined, the term *right* or *left* is also included to state which side of the patient is placed closer to the IR. *The patient was in a left lateral position when the chest image was taken.*

Lauenstein method Position in which the affected leg is flexed and abducted and the patient is rotated toward the affected hip as needed to position the femur against the imaging table; this will demonstrate a lateral hip projection with an unforeshortened proximal femur.

law of isometry Used to minimize shape distortion when imaging long bones when the bone and IR cannot be positioned parallel. The law of isometry indicates that the central ray should be set at half the angle formed between the bone and IR.

longitudinal foreshortening Long axis of the structure appears disproportionately shorter on the image than the short axis.

longitudinal or lengthwise (LW) Refers to the long axis of the anatomic structure or object being discussed. A longitudinal axis on a 14- × 17-inch (35- × 43-cm) IR would parallel the IR's longer (17-inch or 43-cm) length. The longitudinal axis of a patient's thorax would parallel the midsagittal plane. To position the IR LW with the patient means to align the IR's longitudinal axis with the patient's longitudinal axis.

lookup table (LUT) Histogram of the brightness values of the ideal image. It is used as a reference to evaluate the raw data of similar images and automatically rescales their values when needed to match those in the LUT.

magnification Proportionately increasing or enlarging both axes of a structure. The gonadal contact shield is magnified on the image if it is placed on top of the patient.

mammary line Imaginary line connecting the nipples.

matrix Columns and rows of pixels (array) that divide the digital image.

medial (medio-) Refers to the patient's median plane; used to express something that is directed or situated toward the patient's median plane or to express the inner side of an extremity. *The sacroiliac joints are medial to the anterior superior iliac spines (ASISs).* Or, *Place the IR against the medial surface of the knee.*

mentomeatal line Imaginary line connecting the chin with the external ear opening.

midcoronal plane Imaginary plane that passes through the body from side to side and divides it into equal anterior and posterior sections or halves.

midsagittal or median plane Imaginary plane that passes through the body anteroposteriorly or posteroanteriorly and divides it into equal right and left sections or halves.

minimum response time Shortest exposure time to which the AEC can respond and still produce an image.

moiré grid artifact Wavy line artifact that occurs when a stationary grid is used in computed radiography and the imaging plate is placed in the plate reader so that the grid's lead strips align parallel with the scanning direction.

negative contrast Contrast medium that is radiolucent, such as effervescent granules that release carbon dioxide on contact with the fluid in the stomach.

nonstochastic effects Biologic response of radiation exposure that can be directly related to the dose received.

normalization (automatic scaling) Process whereby the computed radiography system automatically corrects for a manual setting and automatic exposure errors to produce consistently optimal images.

NPO Nothing orally (by mouth).

object–image receptor distance (OID) Distance from the object being imaged to the IR.

oblique Refers to rotation of a structure away from an AP or PA projection. When obliquity of the torso, vertebrae, or cranium is defined, the terms *right* or *left* and *anterior* or *posterior* are used with the term *oblique* to indicate which side of the patient is placed closer to the IR. In a right anterior oblique (RAO) position the patient is rotated so that the right anterior surface is placed closer to the IR. When obliquity of an extremity is defined, the term *medial* (internal) or *lateral* (external) is used with the term *oblique* to indicate which way the extremity is rotated from anatomic position and which side of the extremity is positioned closer to the IR. For a medial oblique position of the wrist, the medial side of the arm is placed closer to the IR.

obturator internus fat plane Fat plane that lies within the pelvic inlet next to the medial brim.

occlusal plane Chewing surface of maxillary teeth.

optimum kVp kVp that will provide adequate body part penetration and sufficient gray scale.

orbitomeatal line Imaginary line connecting the outer eye canthus and external acoustic opening.

pacemaker Used to regulate the heart rate by supplying electrical stimulation to the heart. This electrical signal will stimulate the heart the amount needed to maintain an effective rate and rhythm.

palmar Anterior surface of the hand.

palpate Act of touching or feeling a structure through the skin.

penetration Ability of x-ray photons to exit the patient's body.

pericapsular fat plane Fat plane.

phantom image Artifact that occurs in computed radiography when the imaging plate is not erased adequately before the next image is exposed on it and two images are recorded onto the plate phosphor.

pixel Single cell within a matrix.

plantar flexion Act of moving the toes and forefoot downward.

plantar Pertaining to the sole of the foot.

plantar-flex Act of moving the toes and forefoot downward (pointing the toes).

pleural drainage tube Thick-walled tube used to remove fluid or air from the pleural space that could result in collapse of the lung.

pleural effusion Fluid in the pleural cavity.

pneumectomy Removal of a lung.

pneumothorax Presence of air in the pleural cavity.

positive contrast Contrast medium that is radiopaque, such as barium.

posterior (postero-) Refers to the back of the patient; used to express something that is situated at or directed toward the back and includes the backs of the hands and bottoms of the feet, as in anatomic position. *The knee joint is posterior to the patella.*

posterior shoulder dislocation Shoulder condition in which the humeral head is demonstrated posteriorly, beneath the acromion process.

prevertebral fat stripe Fat stripe located anterior to the cervical vertebrae.

profile Outline of an anatomic structure: *The glenoid fossa is demonstrated in profile on a Grashey method image.*

project The act of throwing the image of an anatomic structure forward. *An angled central ray projects the anatomic part situated farther away from the IR farther than the anatomic part situated closer to the IR.*

projection Term used to describe the entrance and exit points of the x-ray beam as it passes through the body when an image is taken. In a projection, the path from the first location to the second must be a straight line. These include anteroposterior, inferosuperior, lateromedial, mediolateral, posteroanterior, and superoinferior projections.

pronate To rotate or turn the upper extremity medially until the hand's palmar surface is facing downward or posteriorly.

pronator fat stripe Soft tissue structure demonstrated on lateral wrist images located parallel to the anterior surface of the distal radius.

protract To move a structure forward or anteriorly: *The shoulder is protracted when it is drawn forward.*

proximal (proximo-) Refers to a structure that is closest to the source or beginning. *The shoulder joint is proximal to the elbow joint.* Or, *The hepatic flexure is proximal to the splenic flexure.*

pulmonary arterial catheter (CVC) Catheter used to measure atrial pressures, pulmonary artery pressure, and cardiac output.

quantization Process of converting an analog image into digital (binary) data for processing by a computer.

quantum mottle Mottled or grainy appearance of an image when insufficient milliampere-seconds (mAs) have been used.

quantum noise (mottle) Graininess or random pattern that is superimposed on the image, obscuring information. It is present when photon flux is insufficient.

radial deviation While maintaining PA projection, the distal hand is moved toward the radial side as much as the wrist will allow.

radiolucent Allowing the passage of x-radiation. A radiolucent object appears dark on an image.

radiopaque Preventing the passage of x-radiation. A radiopaque object appears white on an image.

raw data Brightness values that have come from the digital image receptor before rescaling occurs.

recorded detail Sharpness of structures that have been included on the image.

recumbent Lying down.

resolution Differentiation of individual structures or details from one another on an image.

retract To move a structure backward or posteriorly. *The shoulder is retracted when it is drawn backward.*

sagittal plane Imaginary plane that passes through the body anteroposteriorly or posteroanteriorly; divides it into right and left sections that are not necessarily equal.

scaphoid fat stripe Soft tissue structure demonstrated on wrist images located just lateral to the scaphoid.

scatter radiation Radiation that has changed in direction from the primary beam because of an interaction with the patient or other structure. Because it is emitted in a random direction, it carries no useful signal or subject contrast.

scoliosis Spine condition that results in the vertebral column's curving laterally instead of running straight.

shuttering Digital radiography postexposure manipulation that adds a black background around the exposure field, providing a perceived enhancement of image contrast.

situs inversus Total or partial reversal of the body organs.

small detector element (DEL) Element in the DR image receptor that contains the electronic components that store the detected energy.

source–image receptor distance (SID) Distance from the anode's focal spot to the IR.

source–object distance (SOD) Distance from the anode's focal spot to the patient.

source–skin distance (SSD) Distance from the source of radiation (anode) to the patient's skin. Good radiation practices dictate that this distance must be at least 12 inches (30 cm) to prevent unacceptable entrance skin exposure.

spatial frequency Used to define spatial resolution; refers to how often the number of details change in a set amount of space. It is expressed as line pairs per millimeter (lp/mm).

spatial resolution Ability of an imaging system to distinguish small adjacent details from each other in the image.

square law Law that states that a change in the SOD can be compensated for by changing the mAs by the factor SID squared.

stochastic effect Biologic response to radiation in which the chance of occurrence of the effect, rather than the severity of the effect, is proportional to the dose of radiation received.

subject contrast Contrast caused by the x-ray attenuating characteristics (atomic density and number, and thickness) of the subject being imaged.

subluxation Partial dislocation.

superimpose To lie over or above an anatomic structure or object.

superior (supero-) Refers to a structure within the patient's torso that is situated closer to the head; used when comparing the locations of two torso structures. *The thoracic cavity is superior to the peritoneal cavity.*

supination Rotating or turning the upper extremity laterally until the hand's palmar surface is facing upwardly or anteriorly.

supraorbital Above the orbit.

supraspinatus outlet Opening formed between the lateral clavicle, acromion process, and superior scapula when the patient is positioned for a tangential outlet projection of the shoulder.

symmetrical Refers to structures on opposite sides demonstrating the same size, shape, and position.

talar dome Dome shape formed by the most medial and lateral aspects of the talar's trochlear surface when they are in a lateral position.

tarsi sinus Opening between the calcaneus and talus

thin-film transistor (TFT) Component in the DR imaging receptor that receives the remnant radiation.

trabecular pattern Supporting material within cancellous bone. It is demonstrated on an image as thin white lines throughout a bony structure.

transverse foreshortening Short axis of a structure appears disproportionately shorter on the image than the long axis.

transverse, horizontal, or crosswise (CW) Refers to a plane that is at a 90-degree angle from the longitudinal axis of the anatomic structure or object being discussed. The transverse axis of a 14- × 17-inch (35- × 43-cm) IR would parallel the shorter (14-inch or 35-cm) length. The transverse axis on a patient's thorax would be perpendicular to the midsagittal plane.

ulnar deviation While maintaining a PA projection, the distal hand is turned toward the ulnar side as much as the wrist will allow.

umbilical artery catheter (UAC) Found only in neonates because the cord has dried up and fallen off in older infants. Is used to measure oxygen saturation.

umbilical vein catheter (UVC) Catheter used to deliver fluids and medications.

unilateral One side.

valgus deformity Knee deformity in which the lateral side of the knee joint is narrower than the medial side.

varus deformity Knee deformity in which the medial side of the knee joint is narrower than the lateral side.

vascular lung markings White markings in the lung fields that indicate blood vessels on a chest x-ray.

ventral (ventro-) See *anterior.*

volume of interest (VOI) Brightness values (raw data) that represent only the anatomic structures of interest in digital radiography.

voluntary motion Motion that the patient is able to control.

weight-bearing Act of putting weight on the structure, as with a standing lateral foot or AP knee.

windowing 1. In digital radiography, postprocessing manipulation feature whereby the technologist adjusts image contrast and brightness.

Page numbers followed by *b* indicate boxes; *f*, figures; *t*, tables.